Visual Diagnosis and Care of the Patient with Special Needs

Visual Diagnosis and Care of the Patient with Special Needs

EDITORS

Marc B. Taub, OD, MS, FAAO, FCOVD
Chief, Vision Therapy and Rehabilitation
Pediatric and Vision Therapy Residency Supervisor
Southern College of Optometry
Memphis, Tennessee

Mary Bartuccio, OD, FAAO, FCOVD
Assistant Professor
Nova Southeastern University College of Optometry
Fort Lauderdale, Florida

Dominick M. Maino, OD, MEd, FAAO, FCOVD-A
Professor, Pediatrics/Binocular Vision
Illinois College of Optometry
Chicago, Illinois

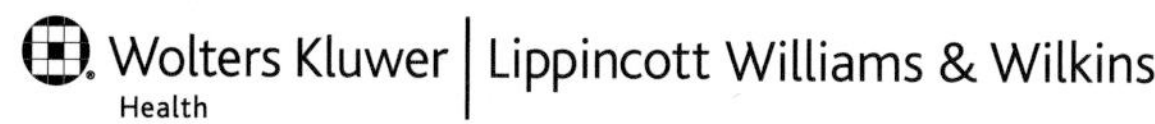

Wolters Kluwer Health | Lippincott Williams & Wilkins

Philadelphia • Baltimore • New York • London
Buenos Aires • Hong Kong • Sydney • Tokyo

Senior Executive Editor: Jonathan W. Pine, Jr.
Senior Product Managers: Marian Bellus, Emilie Moyer
Vendor Manager: Alicia Jackson
Creative Director: Doug Smock
Marketing Manager: Lisa Lawrence
Senior Manufacturing Coordinator: Benjamin Rivera
Prepress Vendor: SPi Global

Printed in China

Library of Congress Cataloging-in-Publication Data

Visual diagnosis and care of the patient with special needs / editors, Marc B. Taub, Dominick M. Maino, Mary Bartuccio.

p. ; cm.

Includes bibliographical references.

ISBN 978-1-4511-1668-7

I. Taub, Marc B. II. Maino, Dominick M. III. Bartuccio, Mary.

[DNLM: 1. Vision Disorders—diagnosis. 2. Disabled Persons. 3. Eye Diseases—diagnosis. 4. Eye Diseases—therapy. 5. Mental Disorders—complications. 6. Optometry. 7. Vision Disorders—therapy.—WW 140]

617.7'5—dc23

2011046046

LWW.com

9 8 7 6 5 4 3 2 1

RRS1202

I dedicate this text to my wife Elissa, sons, Seth and Ari, and parents, Eileen and Joseph; mother- and father-in-law, Marcy and Sam; my rather large extended family; and all of my mentors and teachers who saw something special in me.

Marc B. Taub

I dedicate this text to my husband Francesco and my sons, Nicola and Massimo; my parents, Domenico and Rosa, and my parents-in-law, Maria and Joe; my brother, Antonio and his wife, Ginette, and my niece Victoria Marie and nephew Blake; and my brothers-in-law, Nicola and Joseph.

Mary Bartuccio

I dedicate this text to my wife Sylvia; my son Dominic and his wife Edie; my daughter, Christina; my awesome grandsons, Dominic IV, and Vincenzo; my brother Joseph and his wife Bunny; and the memory of my parents, Lain and Dominic Sr.

Dominick M. Maino

CONTENTS

PREFACE

Who would have known that a simple conversation at an American Academy of Optometry meeting several years ago would have been the spark that started us on such an epic quest? That year, Mary and I gave a lecture on the topic of Special Populations that was very well received. Little did we know that Dominick would also be giving a similar lecture that year. After Mary and I completed our lecture, we began talking about the need for an update to Dr. Dominick Maino's landmark textbook, *Diagnosis and Management of Special Populations* (Mosby, 1995). Since so much had changed in society and medicine with regard to the care of those with special needs, we both agreed that it was time to write another book. Later that day, we happened to "run into" Dominick and decided to pitch him the idea. Even though we did not know this at the time, he had been considering either another edition of his text or writing a new text dealing with the patient with special needs. We decided to join forces and devote our time and talent to not only updating the foundation laid by Dominick's previous book but to increasing the number of topics presented and expanding the breadth of available material in this new work.

As we researched the libraries at our respective institutions, we could not find a single publication, other than Dr. Maino's, that was a comprehensive review of the eye and vision care needs of patients with special needs. Other works had single chapters on certain topics, such as specific conditions or examination techniques, but none brought them all under one cover.

From the title, it may appear that this book is written primarily for eye care practitioners such as optometrists and ophthalmologists. While vision is the overriding topic, this book serves as an excellent resource for a multitude of professions including those engaged in occupational therapy, physical therapy, and speech and language therapy, as well as physiatry, social work, pediatric medicine, and special education, to name but a few. There is literally something of interest for all in this book. Since vision is the dominant sense involved in practically every task we undertake, it is important for all professionals to understand how various anomalies of vision affect their patients' interaction with the environment. These frequently encountered vision dysfunctions often adversely affect the outcome of any therapeutic intervention that our colleagues in rehabilitation may use. All professionals should know how appropriate eye and vision care will enhance the doctor's, therapist's, and special educator's ability to be successful in achieving the goals set forth in the individual's medical and/or educational plan. The publication of this text strongly supports the inclusion of the optometrist as a part of any multidisciplinary care team for individuals with special needs.

This book gives you a better understanding of the most frequently encountered developmental and acquired disabilities seen in the eye care practitioner's office. These disabilities include patients with autism, brain injury, Fragile X syndrome, and Down syndrome, as well as those with psychiatric illness, dual diagnosis, and more. We discuss in great detail the visual issues inherent in these populations and their possible treatment. We have brought together a group of authors with approximately 500 years of experience in the field of eye care and special populations. Our authors often represent the preeminent authorities on the topics about which they write.

While reading this book, please note that many of the treatments used have only been studied in patients *without* special needs. There is a striking lack of randomized, placebo-controlled clinical trials to guide us in many of these areas. Other levels of evidence that include single subject design studies (case reports/series), studies of clinic-based populations, and pilot studies do exist, however. The patients with special needs that we see are often recommended alternative or complementary treatments that are used as an adjunct to or instead of standardized medical intervention. These interventions tend to be highly individualized. Our book, *Visual Diagnosis and Care of the Patient with Special Needs*, gives some insight into how these approaches can fit into the overall recommended treatment regimen as well.

We would like to thank all of the authors who lent their voices to this project. It would not have been possible to see our dream become reality without them. We would like to thank our respective institutions, our administrative leadership, and especially our fellow faculty, for all the assistance they have given along the way. Of particular note (and those due a special thank you) are our librarians and publication specialists who have supported us throughout this project.

We would also like to thank our spouses, children, and extended families for tolerating our unrelenting obsession with this project over these past few years.

We dedicate this book to all patients with special needs and to all those who serve the needs of these individuals. It is our hope that *Visual Diagnosis and Care of the Patient with Special Needs* becomes an essential guide to all disciplines so that our patients receive the best care possible.

Marc B. Taub, OD, MS, FAAO, FCOVD
Mary Bartuccio, OD, FAAO, FCOVD
Dominick M. Maino, OD, M.Ed, FAAO, FCOVD-A

CONTRIBUTORS

Deborah Amster, OD, FAAO, FCOVD
Assistant Professor
Nova Southeastern University College of Optometry
Fort Lauderdale, Florida

Susan R. Barry, PhD
Professor of Biological Sciences
Mount Holyoke College
South Hadley, Massachusetts

Mary Bartuccio, OD, FAAO, FCOVD
Assistant Professor
Nova Southeastern University College of Optometry
Fort Lauderdale, Florida

Curtis Baxstrom, MA, OD, FAAO, FCOVD, FNORA
Vision Northwest
Federal Way, Washington

Elizabeth Berry-Kravis, MD, PhD
Professor of Pediatrics, Neurological Sciences, Biochemistry
Rush University Medical Center
Chicago, Illinois

Elizabeth Bishop, MSSW
Community Education & Dissemination Coordinator
The University of Tennessee Health Science Center
Boling Center for Developmental Disabilities
Memphis, Tennessee

Eric Borsting, OD, M.Ed, FAAO, FCOVD
Professor
Southern California College of Optometry
Fullerton, California

Glenda Brooks, LCSW
The University of Tennessee Health Science Center
Boling Center for Developmental Disabilities
Memphis, Tennessee

R. Terry Browning, PhD
Bartlett, Tennessee

Garth N. Christenson, OD, MS Ed, FAAO, FCOVD
Christenson Vision Care
Hudson, Wisconsin

Kenneth J. Ciuffreda, OD, PhD, FAAO, FCOVD-A
Distinguished Teaching Professor of Vision Sciences
State University of New York College of Optometry
New York, New York

Jason Clopton, OD, FCOVD
Center of Vision Development
Cookeville, Tennessee

Pamela J. Compart, MD
Developmental Pediatrician
HeartLight Healing Arts
Columbia, Maryland

Charles G. Connor, OD, PhD, FAAO
Professor
University of the Incarnate Word Rosenberg School of Optometry
San Antonio, Texas

Jeffrey Cooper, MS, OD, FAAO
Clinical Professor
State University of New York College of Optometry
New York, New York

Rachel A. Coulter, OD, FAAO, FCOVD
Associate Professor
Nova Southeastern University College of Optometry
Fort Lauderdale, Florida

David A. Damari, OD, FCOVD, FAAO
Professor
Chair of the Department of Assessment
Southern College of Optometry
Memphis, Tennessee

Robert Donati, PhD
Associate Professor
Illinois College of Optometry
Chicago, Illinois

Dan Fortenbacher, OD, FCOVD
Wow Vision Therapy
St. Joseph, Michigan

Nadine Girgis, OD
Assistant Professor
Nova Southeastern University College of Optometry
Fort Lauderdale, Florida

Sidney Groffman, OD, MA, FAAO, FCOVD
Professor Emeritus
State University of New York College of Optometry
New York, New York

Bradley Habermehl, OD, FCOVD
Vision Therapy Group
Flint, Michigan

Paul Harris, OD, FCOVD, FACBO, FAAO
Associate Professor
Southern College of Optometry
Memphis, Tennessee

F. Fred Hidaji, MD
Medical Director
Visionary Eye Care
Memphis, Tennessee

Danielle L. Hinton, MD
Medical Director
Baptist Skilled Rehabilitation Unit, Germantown
Baptist Memorial Medical Group-Physiatry
Germantown, Tennessee

Deborah S. Hoffnung, PhD, ABPP-CN
Alegent Health
Omaha, Nebraska

Robert Hohendorf, OD
Vision and Sensory Center of Michigan
Wyoming, Michigan

Angela C. Howell, OD, FAAO
Howell and Wells Eyecare
Paragould, Arkansas

Erin Jenewein, MS, OD, FAAO
Assistant Professor
Nova Southeastern University College of Optometry
Fort Lauderdale, Florida

Robert C. Jespersen, MD
Medical Director
Neumann Family Services
Chicago, Illinois

Neera Kapoor, OD, MS, FAAO, FCOVD-A
Associate Professor
Chief, Vision Rehabilitation Services
State University of New York College of Optometry
New York, New York

Karen A. Kehbein, OD
Assistant Professor
Michigan College of Optometry
Ferris State University
Big Rapids, Michigan

Monika G. Kolwaite, PT, NCS
Brain Injury Coordinator
Baptist Rehabilitation Hospital Germantown
Germantown, Tennessee

Barry S Kran, OD, FAAO
Professor
New England College of Optometry
Boston, Massachusetts

William Kress, OD
Instructor
Southern College of Optometry
Memphis, Tennessee

Patricia S. Lemer, MEd, NCC
Executive Director
Developmental Delay Resources
Pittsburgh, Pennsylvania

Robin D. Lewis, OD, FCOVD
Family Optometry
Chandler, Arizona

Dominick M. Maino, OD, MEd, FAAO, FCOVD-A
Professor
Pediatrics/Binocular Vision
Illinois College of Optometry
Chicago, Illinois

Julie S. Marshall, MA, CCC-SLP
Clinical Associate Professor
Audiology and Speech-Language Pathology
University of Memphis
Memphis, Tennessee

D. Luisa Mayer, PhD, MEd
Associate Professor
New England College of Optometry
Clinical Assistant Professor
Harvard Medical School
Boston, Massachusetts

Kelly Meehan, OD
Clinical Assistant Professor
Midwestern University – Arizona College of Optometry
Glendale, Arizona

John Neal, OD
Instructor
Southern College of Optometry
Memphis, Tennessee

Maryke Nijhuis Neiberg, OD, FAAO
Associate Professor
Western University College of Optometry
Pomona, California

James M. Newman, OD, MS, FAAO
Professor
Southern College of Optometry
Memphis, Tennessee

Yi Pang, OD, PhD, FAAO
Associate Professor
Assistant Dean of Research
Illinois College of Optometry
Chicago, Illinois

Leonard J. Press, OD, FAAO, FCOVD
The Vision and Learning Center
Fairlawn, New Jersey

Ashley S. Reddell, OD
Family EyeCare Center
Vision Development Center
Leavenworth, Kansas

Andrew Rixon, OD, FAAO
Optometry Attending
Memphis Veterans Administration Medical Center
Memphis, Tennessee

Jacqueline Rodena, OD
Assistant Professor
Nova Southeastern University College of Optometry
Fort Lauderdale, Florida

Pamela H. Schnell, OD, FAAO
Assistant Professor
Southern College of Optometry
Memphis, Tennessee

Samantha Slotnick, OD, FAAO, FCOVD
Terri Optics
Dobbs Ferry, New York
Clinical Research Associate
State University of New York College of Optometry
New York, New York

Daniel E. Smith, OD, FAAO
Assistant Professor
Southern College of Optometry
Memphis, Tennessee

Glen T. Steele OD, FCOVD
Professor
Southern College of Optometry
Memphis, Tennessee

Scott B. Steinman, OD, PhD, FAAO, FCOVD-A
Software in Motion
Memphis, Tennessee

Marc B. Taub, OD, MS, FAAO, FCOVD
Chief, Vision Therapy and Rehabilitation
Pediatric and Vision Therapy Residency Supervisor
Southern College of Optometry
Memphis, Tennessee

Yin C. Tea, OD, FAAO
Assistant Professor
Nova Southeastern University College of Optometry
Fort Lauderdale, Florida

Nancy Torgerson, OD, FCOVD
Alderwood Vision Therapy Center
Lynnwood, Washington

Denise A. Valenti, OD, FAAO
Vision Care
Quincy, Massachusetts

Stephen Viola, PhD
Affiliate Assistant Professor
University of Missouri-St. Louis
St. Louis, Missouri

Orli Weisser-Pike, OTR/L, CLVT, SCLV
University of Tennessee Medical Group
Memphis Medical Center
Hamilton Eye Institute
Memphis, Tennessee

J. Margaret Woodhouse, PhD, BSc, FSMC
Senior Lecturer
Cardiff University College of Optometry and Vision Sciences
Cardiff, Wales, United Kingdom

Visual Diagnosis and Care of the Patient with Special Needs

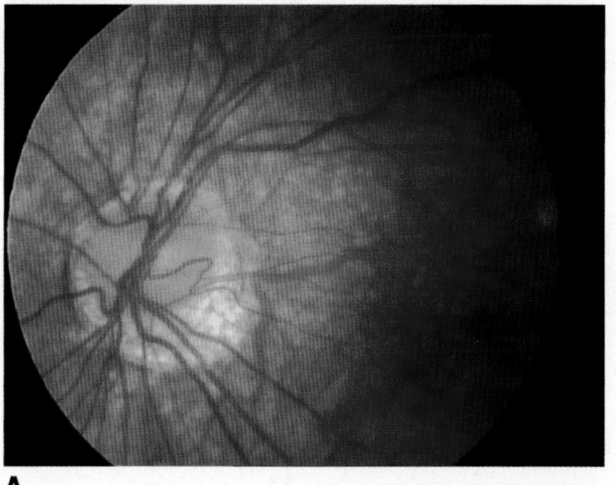

A

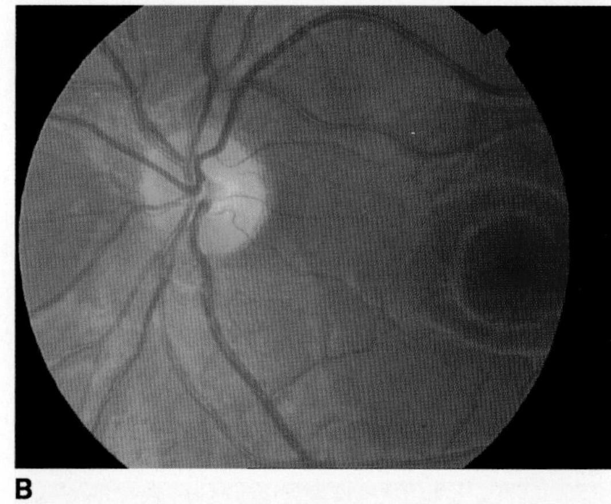

B

FIGURE 4-5. The fundus of **(A)** a young person with DS and **(B)** a control. Both subjects have low hypermetropia.

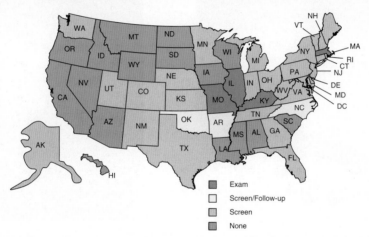

FIGURE 15-1. State preventive vision care requirements for children, United States, 2007. (Reprinted from Abt Associates. Building a comprehensive child vision care system: a Report of the National Commission on Vision and Health. Alexandria, VA, June 2009.)

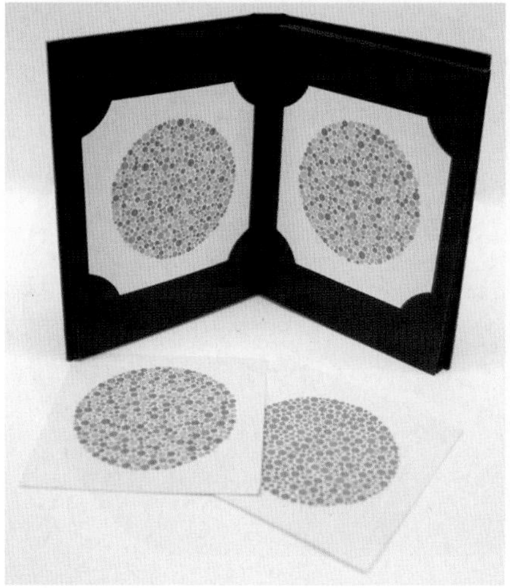

FIGURE 16-11. The Ishihara color vision test.

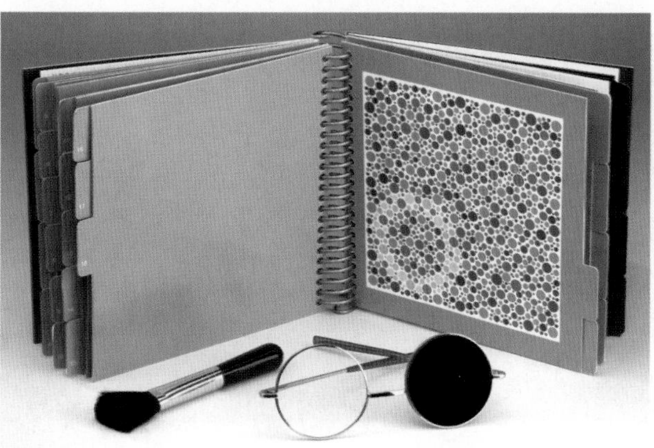

FIGURE 16-12. The Hardy-Rand-Ritter (HRR) test of color vision. (Courtesy of Good-Lite Company.)

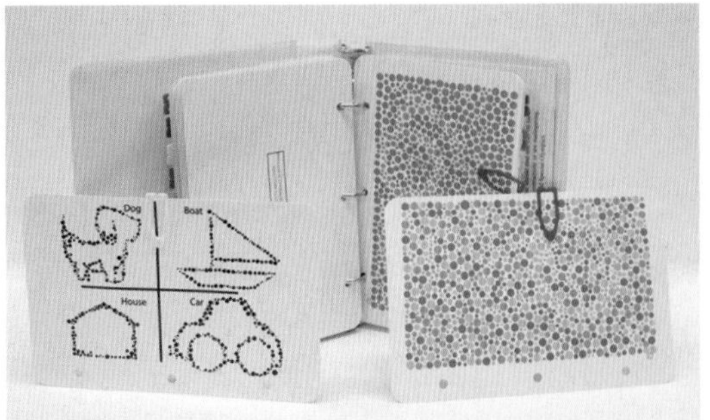

FIGURE 16-13. The color vision made easy color vision test.

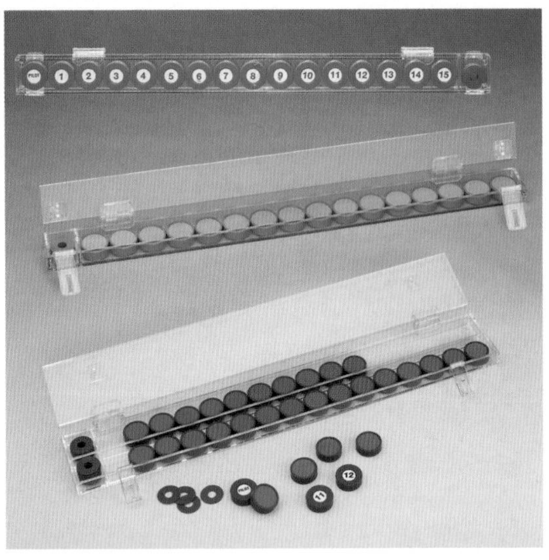

FIGURE 16-14. The Farnsworth D-15 Dichotomous color vision test. (Courtesy of Good-Lite Company.)

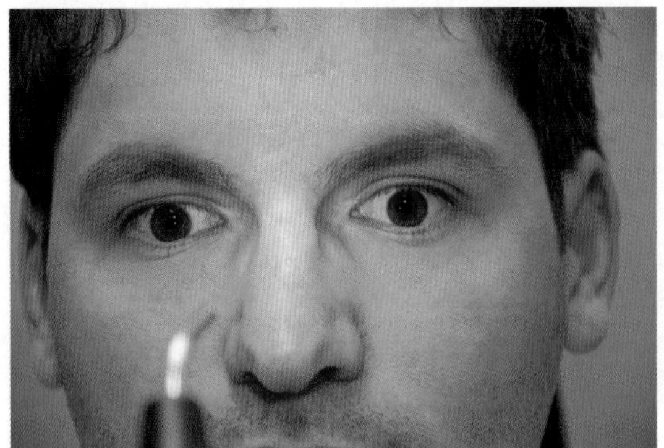

FIGURE 16-27. The Hirschberg test gives a gross estimation of alignment. Notice the white dots on the inner aspects of each iris. This is a normal result.

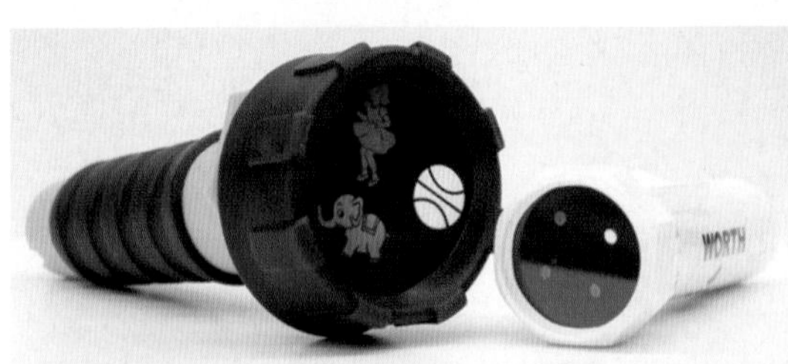

FIGURE 16-29. Adult and pediatric Worth 4 dot tests.

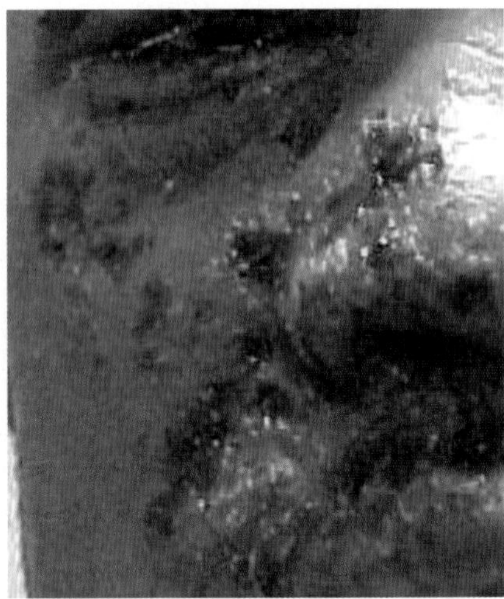

FIGURE 22-1. Herpes zoster (Hutchinson's sign). Photo courtesy of Andrew Gurwood, O.D., F.A.A.O.

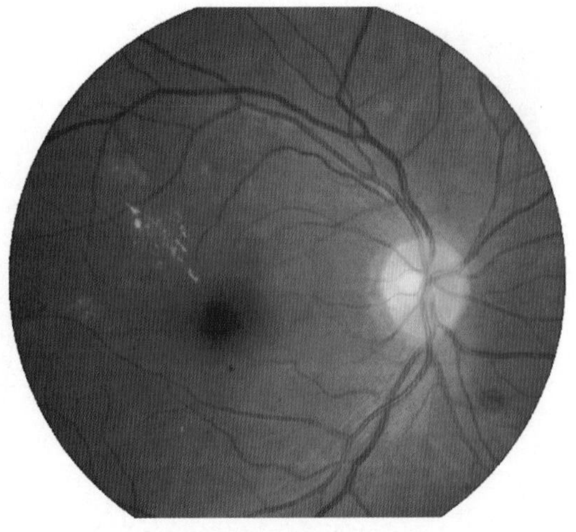

FIGURE 22-2. Diabetic retinopathy. Note the dot hemorrhages and exudates surrounding the macula.

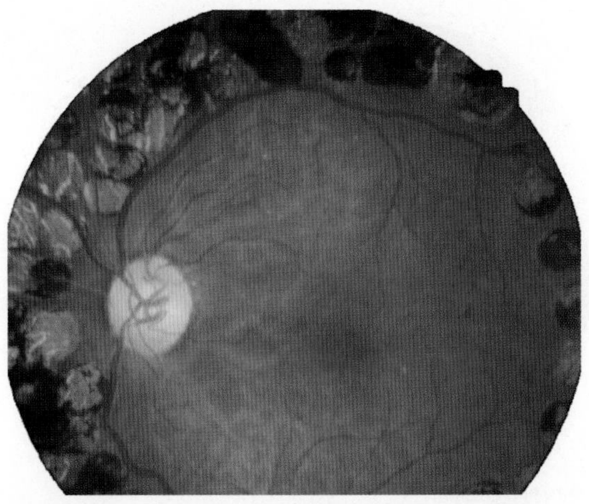

FIGURE 22-3. Pan-retinal photocoagulation for diabetic retinopathy.

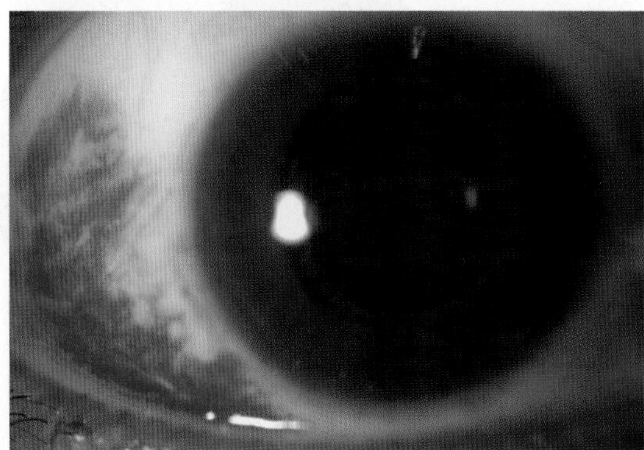

FIGURE 22-6. Subconjunctival hemorrhage.

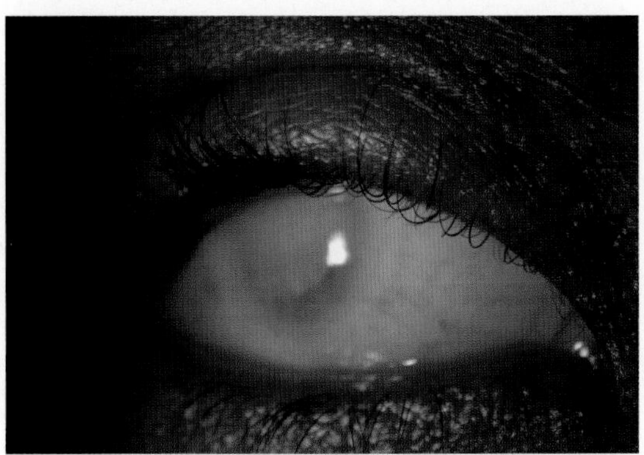

FIGURE 22-4. Simple microphthalmia with corneal opacification.

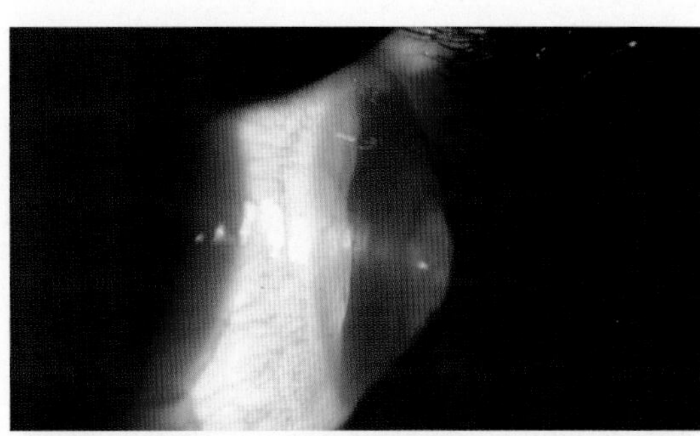

FIGURE 22-7. Advanced keratoconus with central corneal steepening. Photo courtesy of Stephen Byrnes, O.D.

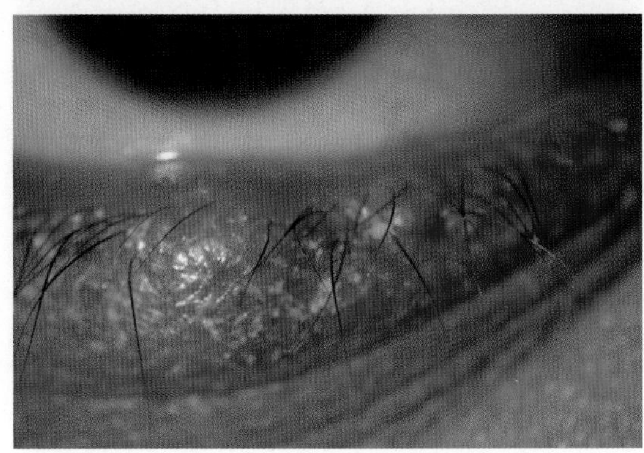

FIGURE 22-5. Anterior blepharitis and small chalazion.

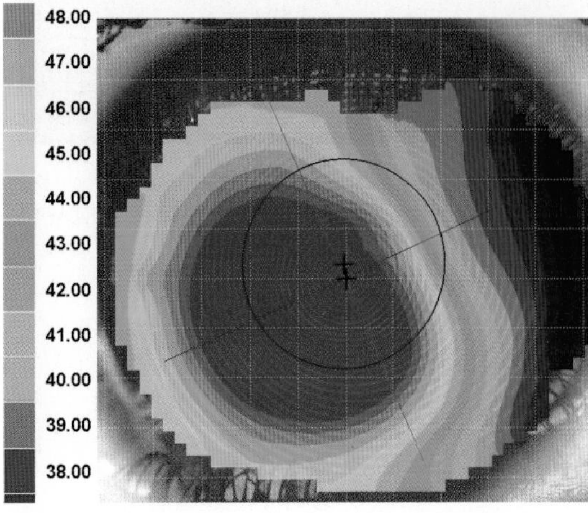

FIGURE 22-8. Keratoconus as viewed on a corneal topography map. Photo courtesy of Daniel Fuller, O.D.

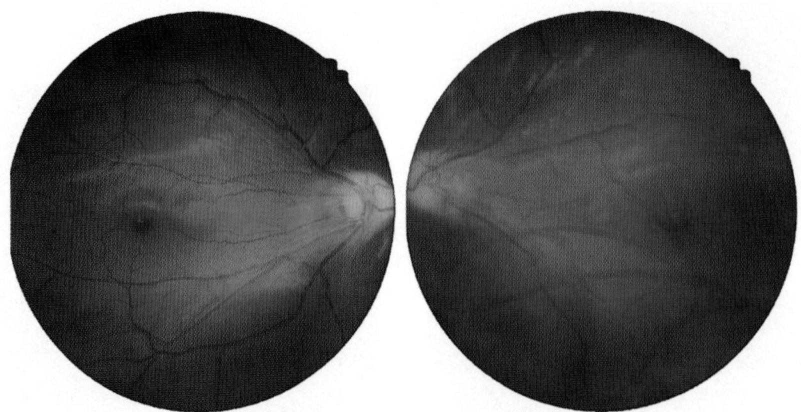

FIGURE 22-9. Retinopathy of prematurity.

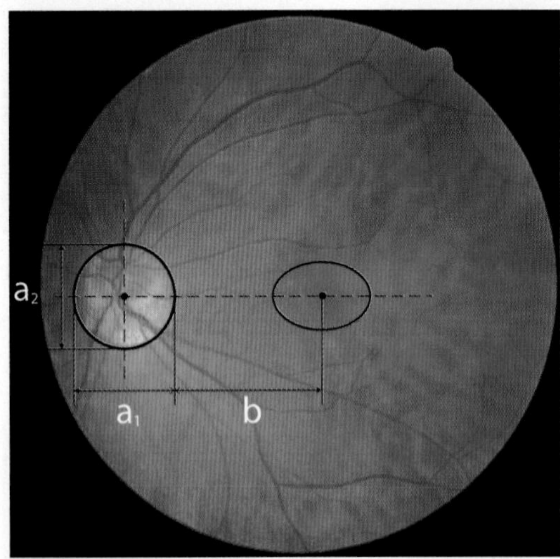

FIGURE 22-10. Optic nerve hypoplasia classification. Photo courtesy of Andrew Gurwood OD, FAAO Artwork courtesy of Susan Doyle.

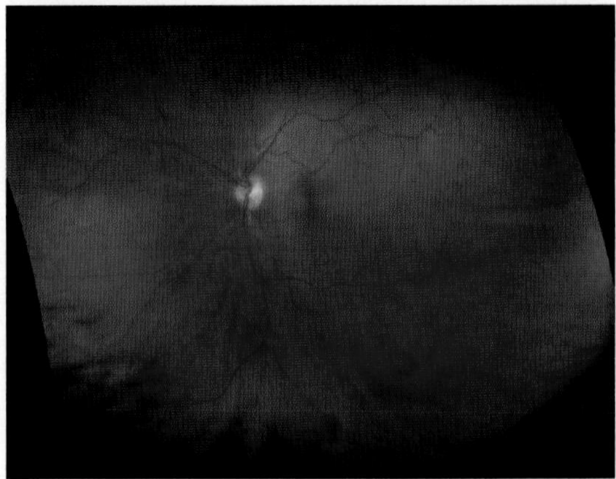

FIGURE 23-4. This picture represents a normal fundus as seen with the Optos "Optomap."

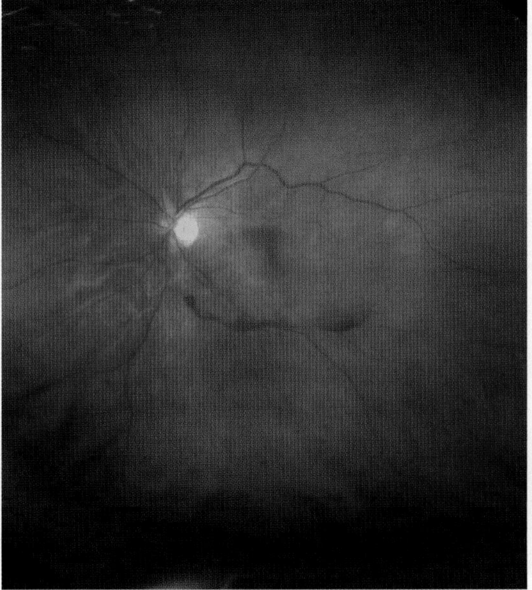

FIGURE 23-5. An Optos image showing a large floater following a complete posterior vitreous detachment.

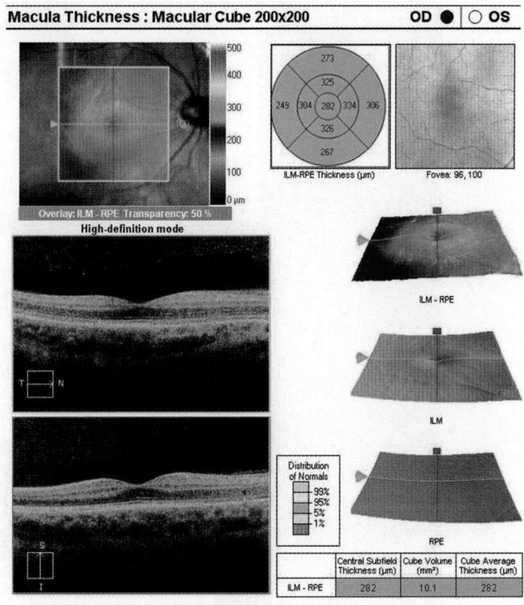

FIGURE 23-6. A normal OCT of the macular region.

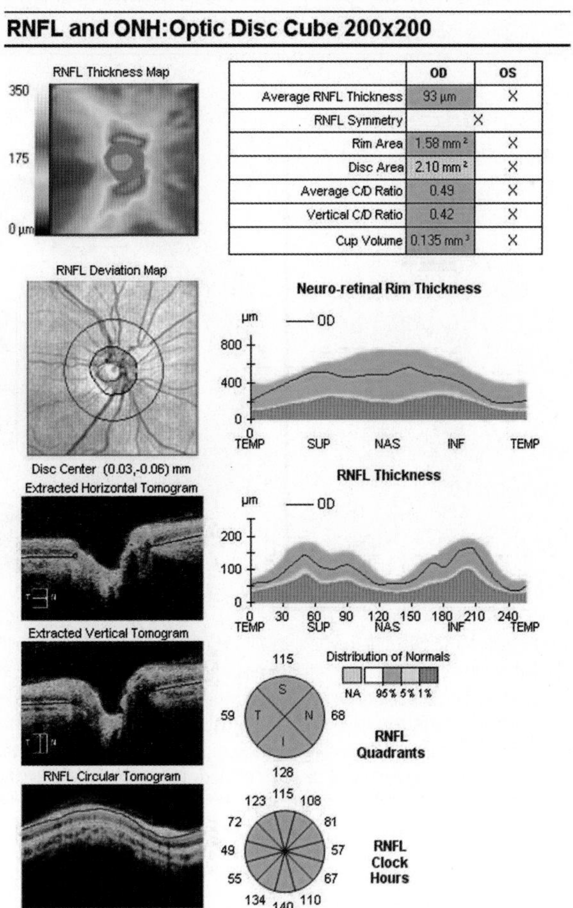

FIGURE 23-7. A normal OCT of the optic nerve head.

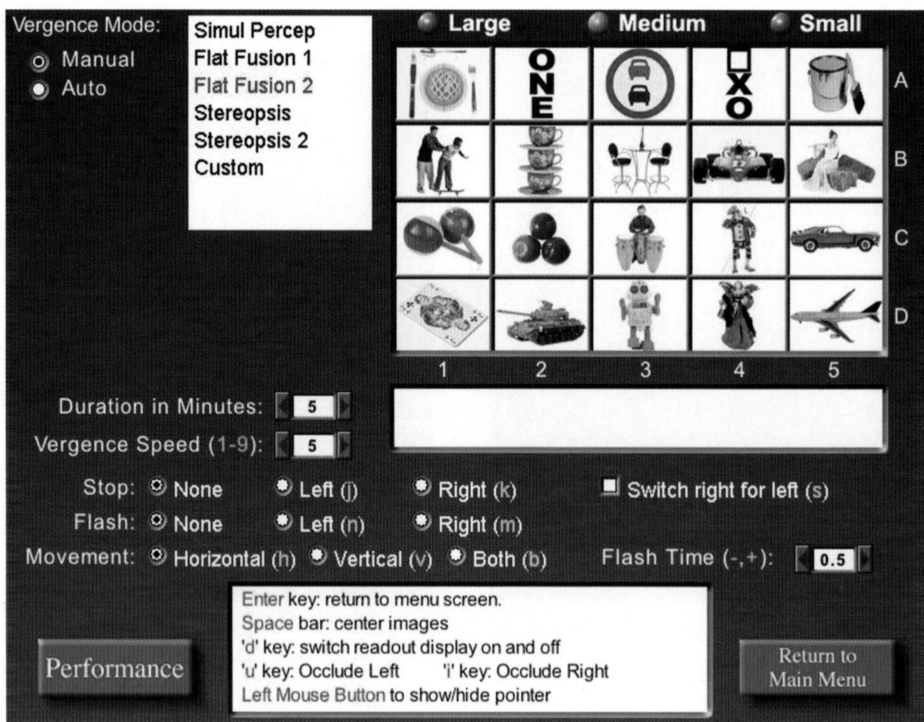

FIGURE 27-2. Computer Orthoptics VTS3 vergence parameters menu. (Image courtesy of HTS Inc.)

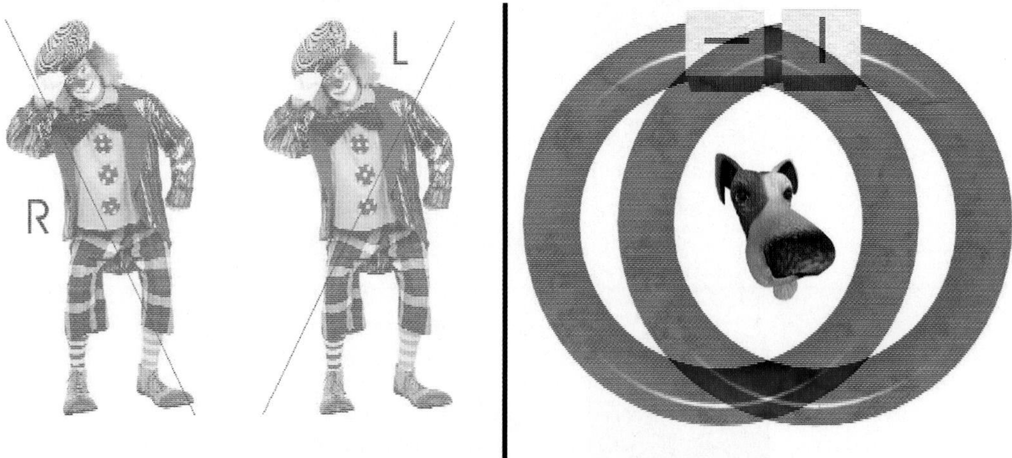

FIGURE 27-3. Depicts computer Orthoptics VTS3 two different targets for improving either fusional amplitudes or stereoscopic appreciation. The target on the left consists of two different dichoptic stimuli that are viewed using liquid crystal glasses to separate the right and left views. The clown on the left is seen by the right eye, while the clown on the right is seen by the left eye. The R and L serve as suppression controls. The eyes are required to converge to see a single, binocular image. Manipulation of the targets is used to train fusion. The target on the right is made up of a central fixation target seen by both eyes (dog) and peripheral rings, which can be separated to created either crossed or uncrossed retinal disparity. Alteration in the separation of the rings results in a change in retinal disparity or stereopsis. (Image courtesy of HTS Inc.)

Betty Thinks Fast
Betty is alone in the house.
She suddenly smells smoke.
She jumps up. She runs out.
She calls 911 from the house
next door.

FIGURE 27-6. This shows sample text for use with the binocular accommodative rock procedure in VisionBuilder. Unlike the conventional Polaroid or Red/Green strips, this random pattern helps deal with suppression better.

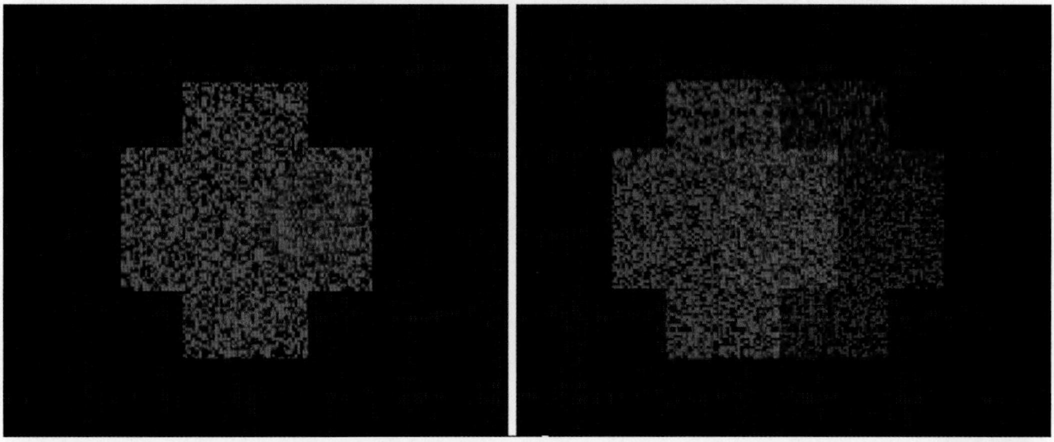

FIGURE 27-7. **A (left):** shows the standard RDS pattern used in VisionBuilder with a cross pattern. Here the circle is shown in the right branch of the cross. **B (right):** shows the RDS displaced with significant base-out demand for glasses with the red lens in front of the right eye.

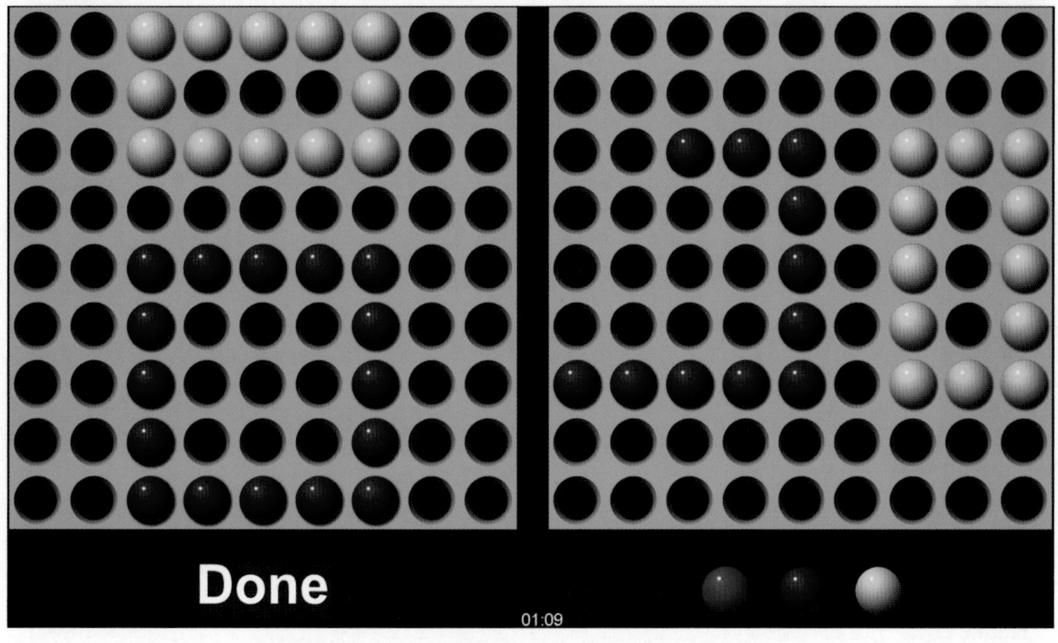

FIGURE 27-9. Pegboard module of the CPT. (Image courtesy of HTS Inc.)

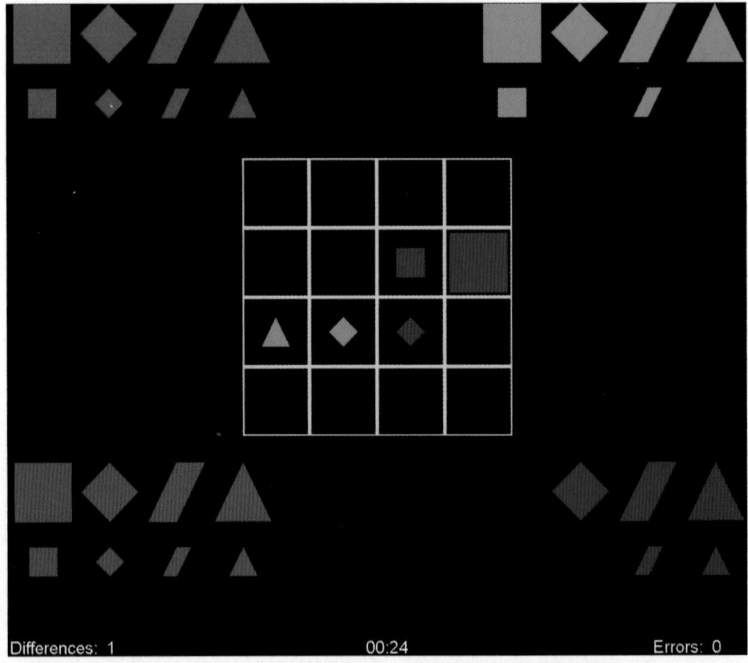

FIGURE 27-10. Visual thinking module of the Computerized Perceptual Therapy (CPT). (Image courtesy of HTS Inc.)

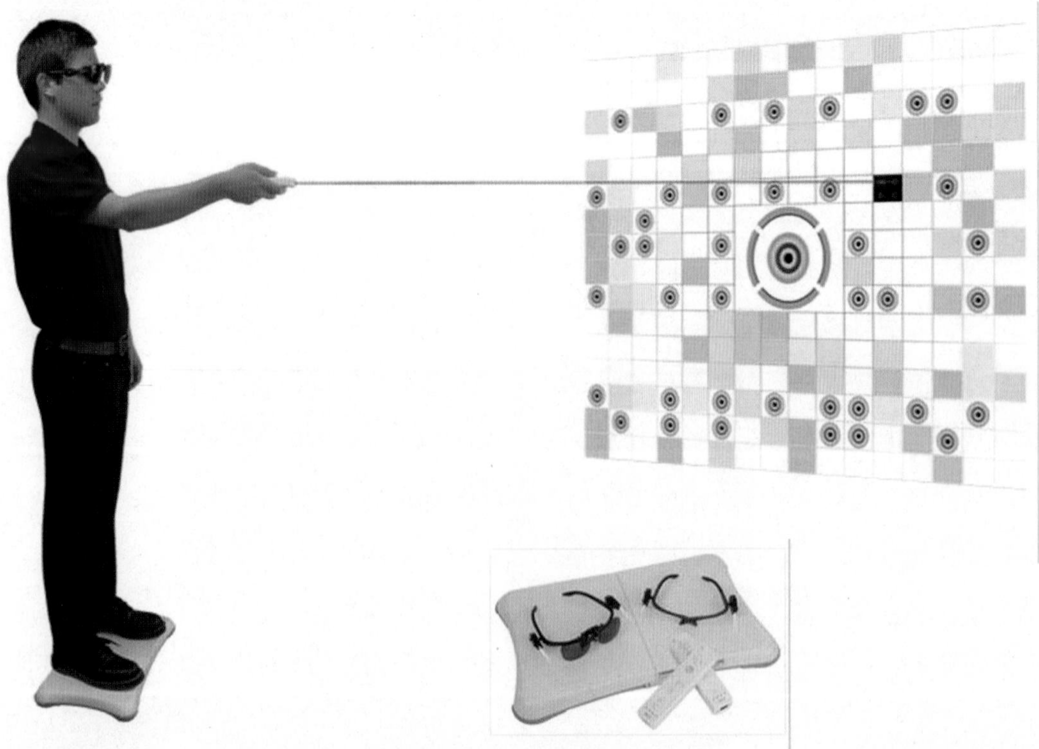

FIGURE 27-13. The NVR employs the use of a remote, balance board, and head sensor in free space. (Image courtesy of HTS Inc.)

CHAPTER 1

Glen T. Steele, OD, FCOVD
Dominick M. Maino, OD, MEd, FAAO, FCOVD-A

The Life Cycle Approach to Care

A considerable amount of our understanding of the world in which we exist becomes known to us through visual processes. Interaction through all of our senses allows each of us to grow and develop in a manner that is meaningful and allows us to function more effectively in our individual cultures. This begins at a very close distance where all sensory and motor processes can be engaged. As the infant develops the need to extend beyond that very close space, the visual process becomes more important and more central to general overall development.

Vision is not a process operating in isolation. It must interact with other sensory and motor processes to reach a level of sophistication expected in today's culture (1). Each infant develops in a unique manner that is dependent on the particular influences of stimulatory and inhibitory actions that are encountered. Thus, a foundation to overall child development is seated in the visual process.

Infancy is a time of great growth but also a time of great vulnerability. Throughout the course of development, the visual process assumes a stronger and more central role when interacting with the world, especially as the need to move to another place in space becomes important.

"Development is a very usable concept—both for theoretic and for practical purposes. It also helps to resolve the artificial distinctions between structure and function" (2). These words regarding child development from Arnold Gesell, MD, stated over 70 years ago, still ring true today. Beginning with conception and continuing throughout the entire life cycle, sensory and motor processes change and evolve at variable times for each of us.

Many of these processes develop quite rapidly while others evolve at a slower rate. It is widely recognized that the most rapid times of growth and development take place in the early years, and this period forms the foundation for continued growth and future development. Development of the human organism begins at conception and only stops at death.

It's been noted that "at any given point in the life span, some abilities are increasing, while others are decreasing. Moreover, the life-span perspective does not posit a specific goal for development, other than successful adaptation to the environment in which a person lives" (3). This statement suggests a unique course of development for each individual that is shaped by physical attributes and responses to the particular environment within which the individual lives—involving both the concepts of nature and nurture. When early disruption of this process occurs, the adverse consequences tend to be greater.

FACTORS INFLUENCING DEVELOPMENTAL DELAY

There are many issues that lead to developmental delay. When an infant does not meet the age-expected developmental milestones, developmental delay is presumed and a course of remediation is often initiated based on the specific presenting signs or symptoms. While the overriding factor is survival, areas that contribute to early development may be neglected or an evaluation postponed; this often includes an assessment of vision. Rarely is vision considered as a contributing factor when developmental delay is suspected. It is critical that all aspects of the process of vision be carefully evaluated when any developmental delay is suspected.

Often, adverse conditions are not diagnosed until the infant is well into the process of development. For instance, increasing research shows the signs and symptoms of autism can potentially be diagnosed before the first birthday (4). An incomplete or inadequate visual looking response is rarely diagnosed during the early evaluations. Any delay in arriving at the correct diagnosis can lead to complications of function and development.

There are a number of conditions that contribute to a diagnosis of developmental delay. During the prenatal period, the mother's activities, stress level, environmental issues, and even the process of birth can be contributing factors. The timing of these potentially adverse factors is often critical.

Prenatal Development Vision is a significant contributor to development with this process beginning prenatally. During pregnancy, the eyes begin as vesicles within days after conception and gradually form into what become the eyes. Early processes of oculomotor and binocular function begin well prior to birth. Any disruption during the early stages of development carries long-term and lasting effects and leads to a greater potential for impairment. Due to the complicated nature of the visual process, the course of vision development is most significantly affected when this disruption occurs early.

The full development of our visual process requires the integration of all sensory and motor abilities. Our ability to see and understand what we see right after birth begins with only a partially developed visual acuity, and immature oculomotor, accommodative, binocular, and visual information processing abilities. The vestibular system at this time is the most developed since it is the only sensory system that is fully myelinated.

Vision and all other sensory–motor systems reciprocally influence each other. As visual skills and visual processing attain a higher level of integration, the visual process will eventually become dominant when interacting with our world. Ornstein (5) remarks that "vision is our most dominant sense, and this is reflected in our own internal hardware, since more of the brain is devoted to processing vision than all the other senses put together."

An example of the importance of multisensory system integration is the development of postural control. Up to the age of 7, vision and motor are used for the development of postural control (6). During this time, the vestibular system is not as important in postural control and appears to be more involved with the basic aspects of arousal. At about the age of 7, the motor and vestibular systems take the lead in the control of posture. This now leaves the visual process available for higher cortical development including cognitive processing. This supports the importance of not only the development of the visual system but also the role of vision in overall child development. Arnold Gesell (7) acknowledges this concept noting, "so integrated are the visual system and the action system that the two should be regarded as inseparable."

It has been noted that "when working well, vision leads and guides in all one does, when not working well, it interferes" (8). This concept reinforces the importance of the visual process in overall development. This suggests that vision emerges as a developmental process and is not fully functional at birth. Some studies advocate that vision is not fully integrated until the teen years or later. During this time frame, the visual process under various stressors, can respond to various stimuli or lack of stimuli and go through a maladaptive process that can result in visual function disorders that affect overall development.

Parental Lifestyle during Pregnancy While many parents, especially mothers, are aware of the need for lifestyle changes necessary during pregnancy, these changes are often not sufficiently followed. The use of alcohol, prescription and recreational drugs, stress, external toxins, and lack of adequate diet are often listed as reasons for complications during pregnancy and delivery. The most frequent immediate outcome is premature birth; however, this may occur even with the strictest adherence to lifestyle changes.

Within the multitude of complications that can occur with prematurity, many visual complications are often present including retinopathy of prematurity, marked refractive conditions, and strabismus. More recent links to environmental factors affecting development include autism and infants on the autism spectrum (9). Care should be taken by the mother to adhere to a healthy lifestyle in order to provide the safest environment for the infant to grow and develop without disruption.

Environmental Factors during Pregnancy It has been shown that adverse emotional and environmental stress faced by the pregnant mother can lead to various complications. Often these adverse stresses continue after birth affecting both mother and child and result in impediments in cognitive, social, and emotional development. Higher levels of stress can create a greater potential for visual complications (10,11). Many of the same outcomes listed above are the result of a compromised environment during pregnancy.

The Process of Birth The birth process as well as pre and post natal factors may lead to problems in overall development. A difficult birth and delivery, failure to thrive, and injury during the birth process, can lead to potential issues and conditions that will impair the developmental process. The APGAR (**A**ppearance (skin color), **P**ulse (heart rate), **G**rimace (reflex irritability), **A**ctivity (muscle tone), and **R**espiration) rating is a guide to the ability of the infant to thrive on its own following delivery. Even at this time in development, any complication often leads to more severe issues throughout the entire life cycle.

Prematurity and Low Birth Weight Premature birth, along with low birth weight, appears to be one of the more significant issues at the time of birth. The complications are far reaching and rarely does the child fully recover. In addition to overall issues related to premature birth and low birth weight, the development of visual function is particularly affected. Visual delays often lead to difficulty in completing even the most basic activities regardless of cultural expectations, and these compromises may be lifelong. Prematurity not only affects individual motor and sensory processes but also influences their ability to become integrated and work as a single unit.

NEWBORN

The visual world of the newborn infant has been described as being a "big, blooming, buzzing confusion." This description likely comes from the casual observation of the apparent vacant stares the baby exhibits in the first few days. This also may be from casual observations of the sporadic nature of the infant's response to attempts at visual stimulation by well-meaning family and professionals.

At birth, all senses respond fully to stimuli regardless of the origin and even the intensity. When sight, sound, touch, movement, and taste are stimulated, the response occurs throughout the full body. Over the course of the first year, the motor and sensory responses begin to differentiate in response and each becomes more distinctive in action. Rather than a full-body stimulation as the infant becomes visually attentive, the body shows a quieting response rather than an excitatory response. Heart rate and respiration rate shows less variability, and general body motor movements become quieter during these short periods of fixation. As vision further develops, more complex targets elicit greater amounts of heart rate change than simpler stimuli (12).

Whereas vision plays a relatively minor role in the world of the newborn infant, by six months it has assumed the position as a dominant sense and forms the basis of later perceptual, cognitive, and social development (13). The role of vision changes very quickly, and the long-term impact of not having vision evolve into the central process inhibits functional development throughout the course of the individual's lifetime. Between birth and 5 weeks, infants prefer to look at faces, and between 7 and 11 weeks, they prefer faces that communicate with them to faces that do not (14–16). Alternatively, when infants prefer geometric patterns to faces, it is reported to be a risk factor for autism (17).

Vision becomes very strongly integrated with other sensory and motor processes. While it is likely that no process can develop in isolation, one process must assume the leading or central role. For instance, in language development, if a child at 10 to 11 months of age develops the ability to follow a caregiver's visual gaze to an object and emit a vocalization, the parent will report the child understands significantly more words at 18 months of age (337 words) than parents of those children who did not correctly follow the caregiver's gaze (195 words) (18). When vision assumes a central role in the process, development progresses on a more appropriate blueprint.

All behavior tends to assume characteristic forms or patterns. Behavior patterns are simply definable formed responses to specific situations (1). Each infant develops a level of sophistication that may vary depending on the need to adapt to the environment or culture in which they live. This sophistication develops in a very distinctive manner for each infant throughout their lifetime, but the beginnings are in very early infancy.

When special needs are encountered during the developmental process, even greater levels of adaptation become necessary. The process of sophistication is altered by such adaptations in addition to the reason for the adaptation in the first place. When the process differs significantly from what would be termed "normal," intervention becomes necessary in order to allow the infant to reach the highest level of function possible. The cost-benefit research shows that for at-risk children, playing catch-up later in life is expensive and inadequate (19). This is not just monetary cost, but physical cost to the child, the family and extended family, and caregivers in general.

DEVELOPMENTAL MILESTONES

Developmental milestones are guidelines used for comparison of the performance of one infant to another throughout the course of development. Most assessments of whether such developmental milestones are met through the first year is most often determined by observing the efficiency the infant has gained in the use of visual function. It has even been proposed that subsequent general intellectual function is associated with the age in which developmental milestones are attained (20).

While important and critical to the process of development, vision is usually given a minor role in this development and is often not a consideration in assessment. The process of vision must become more visible in the assessment of development. Infants must develop the ability to look and sustain fixation in order to most effectively meet the cultural milestones. Gesell has stated, "Vision is a complex sensory–motor response to a light stimulus mediated by the eyes, but involving the entire action system. By this definition, fixation becomes the most basic and, phyletically, the primary visual function" (1,21).

Such importance is also observed when evaluating the motor development of blind infants in activities not perceived to depend on sight. Tröster and Brambring even suggest that "the delay in posture control in blind infants was considered to result from the lower level of motor stimulation due to the lack of sight" (22). Setting aside intelligence, the motor development of blind children becomes a liability as assessment of infant behavior is overwhelmingly based on visual interaction and engagement.

Shelov and Hannemann (23) have listed guidelines for the social and emotional milestones expected at 12 months of age (Table 1.1). Additionally, they also cite the cognitive milestones expected by 12 months, as shown in Table 1.2.

It is clear that the process of vision is intimately involved in each of these milestones and if constrained, the assessment of social and emotional development will be determined to be inadequate for age. Similar milestones are projected throughout the entire course of development. Identifying deviations from these milestones and more closely monitoring the potential for negative impact becomes crucial. It is interesting to note that in Shelov's chapter on vision for parents, he describes quite well the developing process of vision, yet in the chapter on eyes, none of these attributes are recommended for testing.

Early identification and rapid response is a model that should be followed. The process of vision should become increasingly more visible in this model. As the child grows and develops, vision takes a more prominent role and its full capability should be realized.

TABLE 1.1 Guidelines for Social and Emotional Milestones Expected at 12 Months of Age

- Shy or anxious with strangers
- Cries when mother or father leaves
- Enjoys imitating people in his play
- Shows specific preferences for certain people and toys
- Tests parental responses to her actions during feedings
- Tests parental responses to his behavior
- May be fearful in some situations
- Prefers mother and/or regular caregiver over all others
- Repeats sounds or gestures for attention
- Finger-feeds herself
- Extends arm or leg to help when being dressed

Used with permission from Shelov SP, et al. Caring for your baby and young child: birth to age 5. 4th ed. New York: Bantam Books; 2005. p. 247.

TODDLER

Neuroscience confirms that the early years establish the foundation on which later development is built. There is, furthermore, a strong association between children's cognitive skills before they enter kindergarten with achievement in elementary and high school

TABLE 1.2 Cognitive Milestones Expected by 12 Months

- Explores objects in many different ways (shaking, banging, throwing, dropping)
- Finds hidden objects easily
- Looks at correct picture when the image is named
- Imitates gestures
- Begins to use objects correctly (drinking from cup, brushing hair, dialing phone, listening to receiver)

Used with permission from Shelov SP, et al. Caring for your baby and young child: Birth to age 5. 4th ed. New York: Bantam Books; 2005. p. 243.

(24). Thus, it becomes most important to identify conditions that have the potential to impact later development and sophistication as early as possible.

As toddlers begin to expand the world around them, vision takes on a more critical function. Vision must provide guidance in many important areas at this age including locomotion—getting from point A to point B despite any limitations. The practice of near-point activities begins setting the stage for use later in school. Vision is critical in this process and must be assessed to ensure an appropriate course of development. Diagnosis in the earliest stages is crucial to avoid needing "catch-up" attention in the future.

Development is cumulative, and early experiences lay the foundation for all that follows. The toddler uses this foundation to expand movement and exploration and thus begins the need to formulate boundaries—from the basics of hot/cold and hard/soft to the more complex opposites of fast/slow, up/down, yes/no, time/space, etc. If there are either physical or environmental issues that limit such explorations, the child does have sufficient resources to carry forward and operate at higher levels of sophistication.

More efficient and sustained looking develops during this period, which will be especially needed as the child begins to be expected to meet the requirements of the classroom. Getman et al. have described this basic process as the development of reach-grasp-manipulate-release (25). The makeup of this concept includes all visual processes necessary for attention, an attempt at understanding, and the eventual release to the next object that follows. Each of these areas of processing, is important and developing this ability for future use is critical in this particular phase.

By this age, most children who have special needs have already been identified and are receiving care. Unfortunately, many of the visual dysfunctions are not diagnosed and treated due to the pressing needs in other areas. The visual process is often not perceived to be related to these needs, and the importance of the visual process is again minimized.

PRESCHOOL

During the preschool years, children are faced with even more complex issues and tasks. If the child has experienced any disruption of the expected process of development, such complex issues will require more arduous effort to achieve if, in fact, that is possible. More skilled use of motor and sensory processes is required and must be accomplished to lay the foundation for the many complex tasks expected in the school years. Evidence continues to mount substantiating the notion that adult vision is the sum total of the early development plus the organisms adaptation to and utilization of the demands of the particular culture (26). In today's fast-paced culture, it is important for children to have experiences and develop effectiveness of function that prepares them for the rigors of the tasks they will face in school.

Visual functions necessary include sustained ability in oculomotor function, binocular function, and the ability to both sustain and accurately change fixation from one point in space to another. If the child cannot achieve the abilities necessary to perform these functions, whether due to physical limitations or functional limitations, accommodations in school must be considered in order to allow the child to reach the highest level of function. As the expected level of sophistication increases each year, the child must continue this ever-expanding cycle of development in order to accomplish the expected tasks. Any conditions not diagnosed prior to this time allow the child to form adaptations and further delay help in allowing the child to reach maximum potential. As problems persist, more effort is required on the part of the child, parent, and professional to address them.

SCHOOL AGE

The process of vision becomes even more vital as expectations for the school-aged child continue to rise in a very rapid manner. In today's culture, so much more is expected and the preschool years have hopefully prepared the child for the expected onslaught of visual demands in the classroom. This is what the developmental process has been about—to prepare the child for this time period and the ones that follow.

During this age, even more sustained visual effort is required with the complexity and amount increasing throughout each year. Longer hours, smaller print, and fewer pictures on the page necessitate that development of these processes be in place prior to entry into this phase.

These areas are often broken down into definable descriptors for communication but they are not specific causes of any problems. In reality, most descriptors are adaptations to the specific environment rather than a cause of the problem.

When a child is not fully prepared for the rigors of the classroom, some type of remediation and/or accommodation becomes necessary. Determining what accommodation or therapy and whether to place the child in a regular classroom or a self-contained classroom is a decision that should include input from many individuals including family and professionals alike. All involved parties should work for the good of the child. Failure should not be an option.

THE TEENAGER, ADULT, AND SENIOR WITH DISABILITY

Those with disability are living longer, productive lives. Just a few decades ago, children with Down syndrome (DS) often died early from cardiac and respiratory problems. It has been noted that in 1900, children with DS had a life expectancy of 9 to 11 years. Today, these individuals have a life expectancy of >50 years with 10% living to 70 years of age or older (27). Men and women with DS marry (28), go to college (29), and live their lives as fully as possible. Unfortunately, individuals with DS also appear to physically age faster than non-DS individuals which implies age-related eye problems being present earlier in this population, as well as other age-related systemic and cognitive problems (dementia) being of concern at younger ages. Those with cerebral palsy (CP) often have a normal life expectancy as well (30) with many living in their own homes, working, and enjoying recreational activities (31).

In general, almost all of those with disability are leading longer, higher-quality lives. This also means that therapy in all its forms (systemic, neurologic, psychiatric, physical, vocational, and pharmacologic [32]) continues well into adulthood and senior years (33). Older adults with intellectual disabilities (ID), like older adults in general, are at greater risks for falls. Fractures occur up to 3.5 times more frequently in people with ID with prevalence rates of falls among adults with ID ranging from 12% to 61% (34).

A literature search typically shows that there is only limited information on those with disability from a life-cycle approach. A brief description of the more frequently encountered disabilities is discussed below.

High School and the Teen Years The Center for Disease Control notes that teenagers experience many physical, mental, emotional, and social changes. One of the greatest changes is puberty. The onset of puberty for girls results in breast development, pubic area and armpit hair growth, acne, and menstruation. Puberty for males results in the enlargement of the testicles and penis and the growth of hair in the armpits and pubic area. Their muscles also strengthen while their voice deepens and facial hair develops. Acne can become a problem as well.

Teens also continue to develop their own personalities and begin to express their opinions on just about every subject. They become increasingly independent from their parents, show great concern about their body image, and tend to be deeply influenced by their peer group (35). Many of those in high school are preparing for the workforce or for the demands of higher education. All of this also holds true for patients with special needs.

The Teen, Adult, and Senior with Down Syndrome It has been noted that socialization, daily living skills, speech and language skills, literacy, and behavior all tend to improve with age. Children with DS in a mainstreamed classroom show progress in communication skills (expressive language and literacy skills), but this was not true for those in special education classrooms. Mainstreamed DS teens also showed fewer problems with behavior (36). Since children and teens with DS are often taught to read (37), it is important that all learning-related vision problems be assessed and treated as is appropriate (38). This is especially true since it is now known that individuals with DS have accommodative systems that are insufficient for the many tasks these teens need to perform in an academic or school environment (39,40) and that the simple application of multifocal lenses improve not only accommodative function but near-point performance (41–43). Teens with DS often participate in sports activities, including the Special Olympics. Special Olympic research (in conjunction with several other publications) has shown that all athletes with special needs require eye and vision care (44–46). Since teens with DS appear to be vulnerable to peer-interaction emotional abuse, they often have difficulties responding to teen angst and the many emotional situations teens frequently encounter. Many individuals with DS are at risk for potential bodily injury due to atlantoaxial instability and ligamentous laxity disorders as well.

These physical and emotional anomalies can lead to psychiatric issues including depression, anxiety, obsessive–compulsive behaviors, and other mental health problems (47).

During the teenage years, the individual with DS learns how to be independent which prepares them for work and living on their own. They continue to master how to manage their personal daily care needs and do everyday tasks such as washing their clothes, shopping, and cooking. Developing appropriate interactions with the opposite sex and their peers often are challenging for those with disability, as it is for those without disability during these teen years.

Adults with DS can have a variety of illnesses (thyroid disease, diabetes, depression, obsessive–compulsive disorder, hearing loss, atlantoaxial subluxation, and Alzheimer disease) that can affect their abilities to manage their lives and will often need assistance in making plans for long-term housing, estate planning, and other legal arrangements (48). They also require opportunities for social interaction, appropriate exercise, good sleep habits, proper immunizations (flu, pneumonia, hepatitis B, etc.), and antibiotic prophylaxis (needed for dental work [49]).

Seniors with DS have a unique set of requirements for continuing their quality of life. These include all of the noted health issues above combined with the special needs associated with increasing age. Dementia, depression/mental illness, sensory impairments (hearing, vision), and various other biologic changes (women with DS reach menopause 5 to 6 years earlier than non-DS women) are often encountered by those with DS years before non-DS seniors may show these age-related challenges (50).

Cerebral Palsy Individuals with cerebral palsy (CP) often have a much higher cognitive ability than their physical impairments typically imply. Those with severe motor problems can have normal to above normal intelligence, so it is important not to judge the individual by outward appearances. Teens with CP face the same stressors that all teens must deal with and additional ones induced by having a disability. Research notes that interpersonal relationships for teens with CP were few outside of the school environment. They had a tendency not to participate in social activities and the activities they did participate in usually were of a sedentary nature (51). They tend to have various psychological issues, low self-efficacy, and low self-esteem that impair the development of social relationships. At times, overprotecting parents accompanied by the negative attitudes frequently encountered by those with CP also have a negative influence on self-perceived worth of those with CP (52).

Since a high percentage of those with CP will be mainstreamed into regular high schools and participate in an academic program that is as equally demanding as that of their peers, evaluating and treating any learning-related vision problems becomes essential. As is discussed in Chapter 3, Cerebral Palsy, special diagnostic and therapeutic attention to the functional aspects of their oculomotor system, accommodative abilities, binocular vision function, and vision information processing abilities is warranted.

A comprehensive PubMed literature search uncovered little in the way of research concerning the teen years of those with CP. A basic online Internet search returned stories about teens with CP who were skydivers, actors, lawsuit award winners, marathon runners, and other such news stories, but nothing on CP teen development. The lack of available information in this area is not just isolated to those with CP, but is frequently encountered for those with other disabilities as well. The teen years for those with CP results in significant changes, both physical and physiologic, in the maturing individual and can be a challenging time for all.

Adults and seniors with CP experience the same changes we all experience as the years pass. Individuals with CP tend to age prematurely and often experience an increase in back pain, incontinence, muscle contractions, and spasms. They may also note increased oral health problems, increased fatigue/reduced energy levels, gastrointestinal problems, and an increase in general discomfort. Finally, seniors with CP will have less efficient motor control, pain/stiffness/loss of flexibility in joints, and unusually tight muscles (53–55).

Autism Spectrum Disorders Individuals with autism demonstrate many problems with social interaction. These include but are not limited to eye contact, avoidance of social situations, variable speech problems, and intolerance to change. Many of the variable and exaggerated behaviors and emotional aspects of being a teenager are exaggerated for those on the spectrum, but eventually there is usually a return to calmer behavior patterns. A small number of individuals demonstrate significant improvement or regression in their behaviors, however. The stress of the teen years combined with having a disability can lead to an increase in various psychiatric disorders such as anxiety and depression. It should also be noted that teens with autism have higher rates of seizures as well.

Programs for teens with autism should include consistent routines with predictable schedules, small class size, personalized attention, and the teaching of important social skills. These programs will also emphasize communication, as well as daily living skills, with a great deal of hands-on learning in a minimally distractive environment (56–58).

As was seen with other disabilities, there is little in the literature on adults and seniors with autism. Numerous newspapers, magazines, and Web articles time and again pointed out the many resources available for children with autism, but no such resources for these children when they are older (59,60).

CONCLUSION

Unfortunately even for the most frequently encountered disabilities, there does not appear to be a life-cycle approach to care for patients with special needs. There is only limited research in this area and what resources are available are squarely aimed toward children with special needs. Adults and seniors with special needs are all too often ignored and neglected. Hopefully this will change in the not too distant future. The tremendous improvements we have witnessed over the past decades for children with disability should not end with childhood, but be carried on throughout their lifetimes into adulthood and beyond.

REFERENCES

1. Gesell A. Vision its development in infant and child. Santa Ana: Optometric Extension Program Foundation; 1998. p. 7, 106, 110.
2. Gesell A. Developmental pediatrics: its task and responsibilities. Pediatrics. 1947;1:331–6.
3. Uttal D, Perlmutter M. Toward a broader conceptualization of development: the roles of gains and losses across the life span. Dev Rev. 1989;9:101–32.
4. Bhat AN, Galloway JC, Landa RJ. Social and non-asocial visual attention patterns and associative learning in infants at risk for autism. J Child Psychol Psychiatry. 2010;51:989–97.
5. Ornstein R. The right mind-making sense of the hemispheres. Orlando: Houghton Mifflin Harcourt; 1997.
6. Shumway-Cook A, Woollacott M. Motor control theory and practical applications. Philadelphia: Williams and Wilkins; 1995.
7. Gesell A, Ilg FL, Bullis GE. Vision: it's development in infant and child. Santa Ana: Optometric Extension Program; 1998.
8. Streff JW, Gundersen E. Childhood learning journey or race? A parent's and teachers guide. Santa Ana: Optometric Extension Program Foundation; 2004.
9. Hallmayer J, Cleveland S, Torres A, Phillips J, et al. Genetic heritability and shared environmental factors among twin pairs with autism Arch Gen Psychiatry. Available from: http://archpsyc.ama-assn.org/cgi/reprint/archgenpsychiatry.2011.76. Last Accessed July 1, 2011.
10. Excessive stress disrupts the architecture of the developing brain. National Scientific Council on the Developing Child. Cambridge: The Council; 2005. Working Paper No. 3. Available from: http://developingchild.harvard.edu/index.php/resources/reports_and_working_papers/working_papers/wp3/. Last Accessed July 1, 2011.
11. Selye H. The stress of life. New York: McGraw-Hill; 1956.
12. Richards JE, Casey BJ. Heart rate variability during attention phases in young infants. Psychophysiology. 1991;28:43–53.
13. Atkinson J. The developing visual brain. New York: Oxford University Press; 2002.
14. Messinger DS, Mahoor MH, Chow SM, Chn JF. Automated measurement of facial expressions in infant-mother interaction: a pilot study. Infancy. 2009;14:285–305.
15. Colombo J, Mitchell DW. Infant visual habituation. Neurobiol Learn Mem. 2009; 92:225–34.
16. Messinger DS. Positive and negative: infant facial expressions and emotions. Curr Dir Psychol Sci. 2002;11:1–6.
17. Pierce K, Conant D, Hazin R, Stoner R, et al. Preference for geometric patterns early in life as a risk factor for autism. Arch Gen Psychiatry. 2011;68:101–9.
18. Brooks R, Meltzoff A. The development of gaze following and its relation to language. Dev Sci. 2005;8:535–43.
19. Heckman JJ, Gruenwald R, Reynolds A. The dollars and cents of investing early: cost-benefit analysis in early care and education. Zero to Three. 2006;26:10–7.
20. Murray GK, Jones PB, Kuh D, Richards M. Infant developmental milestones and subsequent cognitive function. Ann Neurol. 2007;62:128–36.
21. Meltzoff AN, Moore MK. Newborn infants imitate adult facial gestures. Child Dev. 1983;54:702–9.
22. Trösterm H, Brambring M. Early motor development in blind infants. J Appl Dev Psychol. 1993;14:83–106.
23. Shelov SP, Hannemann RE. Caring for your infant and young child: birth to age 5. 4th ed. New York: Bantam Books; 2005. p. 243, 247, 182–3, 608–99.
24. Executive Summary. Early experiences matter. Zero to Three. Available from: http://main.zerotothree.org/site/DocServer/Policy_Guide.pdf?docID=8401. Last Accessed August 15, 2011.
25. Getman GN, Henry WR, Hendrickson HH, Knight RW. Techniques and diagnostic criteria for the optometric care of children's vision. Duncan: Optometric Extension Program Foundation; 1953.
26. Getman GN. Developmental vision. Optometric Extension Program Foundation; 1951;1:12.

27. Brown R, Taylor J, Matthews B. Quality of life—ageing and Down syndrome. Down Syndr Res Pract. 2001;6:111–6.
28. Brown R. Partnership and marriage in Down syndrome. Down Syndr Res Pract. 1996;4:96–9.
29. Hamill B, Kliewer C. Going to college: the experiences of a young woman with Down syndrome. Ment Retard 2003;41:340–53.
30. Strauss D, Brooks J, Rosenbloom R, Shavelle R. Life expectancy in cerebral palsy: an update 2008. Dev Med Child Neurol. 2008;50:487–93.
31. Anderson C, Mattss E. Adults with cerebral palsy: a survey describing problems, needs, and resources, with special emphasis on locomotion. Dev Med Child Neurol. 2001;43:76–82.
32. Donati RJ, Maino DM, Bartell H, Kieffer M. Polypharmacy and the lack of oculo-visual complaints from those with mental illness and dual diagnosis. Optometry. 2009;80:249–54.
33. Spencer T, Biederman J, Wilens T, Harding M, et al. Pharmacotherapy of attention-deficit hyperactivity disorder across the life cycle. J Am Acad Child Adolesc Psychiatry. 1996; 35:409–32.
34. Hsieh K, Rimmer J. Identification of falls risk in adults with ID. Available from: www.rrtcadd.org/Research/page196/page196.html. Last Accessed August 15, 2011.
35. MedlinePlus Teen Development. Available from: www.nlm.nih.gov/medlineplus/teendevelopment.html. Last Accessed June 6, 2011.
36. Buckley S, Bird G, Sacks B, Archer T. A comparison of mainstream and special education for teenagers with Down syndrome: implications for parents and teachers. Down Syndr Res Pract. 2006;9:54–67.
37. Buckley S, Bird G. Teaching children with Down syndrome to read. Down Syndr Res Pract. 1993;11:34–9.
38. Wesson M, Maino D. Oculo-visual findings in Down syndrome, cerebral palsy, and mental retardation with non-specific etiology. In: Maino D, ed. Diagnosis and management of special populations. St. Louis: Mosby-Yearbook, Inc.; 1995. p. 17–54.
39. Lindstedt E. Failing accommodation in cases of Down's syndrome. A preliminary report. Ophthalmic Paediatr Genet. 1983;3:191–2.
40. Cregg M, Woodhouse JM, Pakeman VH, Saunders KJ, et al. Accommodation and refractive error in children with Down syndrome: cross sectional and longitudinal studies. Invest Ophthalmol Vis Sci. 2001;42:55–63.
41. Nandakumar K, Leat SJ. Bifocals in Down Syndrome Study (BiDS): design and baseline visual function. Optom Vis Sci. 2009;86:196–207.
42. Stewart RE, Woodhouse JM, Trojanowska LD. In focus: the use of bifocals for children with Down's syndrome. Ophthal Physiol Opt. 2005;25:514–22.
43. Al-Bagdady M, Stewart RE, Watts P, Murphy PJ, et al. Bifocals and Down's syndrome: correction or treatment? Ophthalmic Physiol Opt. 2009;29:416–21.
44. Woodhouse JM, Adler P, Duignan A. Vision in athletes with intellectual disabilities: the need for improved eyecare. J Intellect Disabil Res. 2004;48:736–45.
45. Woodhouse JM, Adler PM, Duignan A. Ocular and visual defects amongst people with intellectual disabilities participating in Special Olympics. Ophthalmic Physiol Opt. 2003;23:221–32.
46. Block SS, Beckerman SA, Berman PE. Vision profile of the athletes of the 1995 Special Olympics World Summer Games. J Am Optom Assoc. 1997;68:699–708.
47. Mental Health Issues and Down Syndrome, National Down Syndrome Society. Available from: www.ndss.org/index.php?option=com_content&view=article&id=171%3Amental-health-issues&catid=60%3Aassociated-conditions&Itemid=88&showall=1. Last Accessed June 6, 2011.
48. Smith DS. Health Care management of adults with Down syndrome. Am Fam Phys. 2001;64:1031–9.
49. Chicoine B, McGuire D, Young CV. Promoting health in adults with Down syndrome. Available from: www.dsamn.org/Files/file/adult_issues/AdultHealthCare.pdf. Last Accessed August 15, 2011.
50. Aging and its Consequences for People with Down Syndrome. Available from: www.downsyndromedallas.org/Resource%20Guide/Health%20PDF/aging%20&%20consequences.pdf. Last Accessed August 15, 2011.
51. Blum RW, Resnick MD, Nelson R, St Germaine A. family and peer issues among adolescents with spina bifida and cerebral palsy. Pediatrics. 1991;88:280–5.
52. Wiegerink DJ, Roebroeck ME, Donkervoort M, Stam HJ, et al. Social and sexual relationships of adolescents and young adults with cerebral palsy: a review. Clin Rehabil. 2006;20:1023–31.
53. Turk MA, Overeynder JC, Janicki MP, editors. Uncertain future—aging and cerebral palsy: clinical concerns. Albany: New York State Developmental Disabilities Planning Council; 1995. Available from: http://www.rrtcadd.org/Resource/Interest/CP/assets/future.pdf. Last Accessed August 15, 2011.
54. Haak P, Lenski M, Hidecker MJ, Li M, et al. Cerebral palsy and aging. Dev Med Child Neurol. 2009;51:16–23.
55. Turk M. Health, mortality, and wellness issues in adults with cerebral palsy. Dev Med Child Neurol. 2009;51:24–9.
56. LaZebrik C, Koegel L. Growing up on the spectrum: a guide to life, love, and learning for teens and young adults with autism and Asperger's. New York: Penguin Group; 2010.
57. White SW, Koenig K, Scahill L. Social skills development in children with autism spectrum disorders: a review of the intervention research. J Autism Dev Disord. 2007;37:1858–68.
58. Rogers SJ. Interventions that facilitate socialization in children with autism. J Autism Dev Disord. 2000;30:399–409.
59. Cooney B. The older autistic. What happens when they grow up? Available from: http://today.uchc.edu/headlines/2007/jul07/autistic.html. Last Accessed August 15, 2011.
60. Greenfeld K. Growing old with autism. Available from: www.time.com/time/magazine/article/0,9171,1898322,00.html. Last Accessed August 15, 2011.

CHAPTER 2

Charles G. Connor, OD, PhD, FAAO

Genetics

Genetics is the study of heredity. Heredity is the passing on of characteristics, such as eye color, from one generation to the next. The eye care professional is concerned with the tendency to develop certain ocular diseases as a result of inheritance. This chapter discusses genetic anomalies that cause traits characteristic of those exhibited by individuals with special needs. Many medical disorders have now been shown to have a genetic basis as a result of advanced molecular techniques. Genetic alterations leading to disease are present at birth, but many are not clinically manifested until later in life, with some never presenting clinically. It is vital that all health care providers understand the language of genetics so they can communicate appropriately with their patients. They also need to recognize the possibility of a genetic disorder in an individual or family so they can provide genetic counseling.

BASIC OVERVIEW OF GENETICS

The basic units of heredity are the genes. A gene is a segment of deoxyribonucleic acid (DNA) that codes for the structure of a polypeptide (an amino acid chain). In humans, genes vary in size from a few hundred DNAs to more than 2 million bases. The Human Genome Project has estimated that humans have about 30,000 genes (1). The vast majority of these are located in the cell nucleus, but are also present in the mitochondria of the cells. Genes are responsible for structural proteins, enzymes, hormones, and cell membrane receptors. Genes regulate the proteins and enzymes that guide development. Altered genes may therefore have effects on function and developmental outcomes.

Genes are arranged in a linear fashion on a chromosome. Chromosomes are packaged, threadlike structures that are composed of DNA and proteins. That DNA–protein complex is referred to as chromatin, while histones are proteins involved in the organization of DNA. The normal human chromosome number is 46. Chromosomes occur in pairs with one member of the pair coming from the mother and the other from the father. This is referred to as a diploid genome. There are 22 pairs of autosomes (nonsex chromosomes) and a pair of sex chromosomes. The sex chromosomes present in a normal female are two X chromosomes (XX). The sex chromosomes present in the normal male are one X chromosome and one Y chromosome (XY). The egg and sperm cells each contain one member of a chromosome pair, for a total of 23 chromosomes (22 autosomes and 1 sex chromosome) (1).

Geneticists can map the location of a particular gene on a chromosome. One type of map uses the cytogenetic location to describe a gene's position. The cytogenetic location is based on a distinctive pattern of bands created when chromosomes are stained. It is a combination of numbers and letters that provide a gene's "address" on a chromosome. The first number or letter used to describe a gene's location represents the chromosome number. Therefore, chromosomes 1 through 22 (the autosomes) are designated by their chromosome number, and the sex chromosomes are designated by X or Y. The gene's location on the chromosome is further defined based on its position relative to the centromere. The chromosome is divided into two sections (arms) based on the location of a narrowing (centromere), which is the region that joins two sister chromatids (two identical copies of a single chromosome). By convention, the shorter arm is called p, and the longer arm is called q. The chromosome arm is the second part of the gene's address. The position of a gene is based on a distinctive pattern of light and dark bands that appear when the

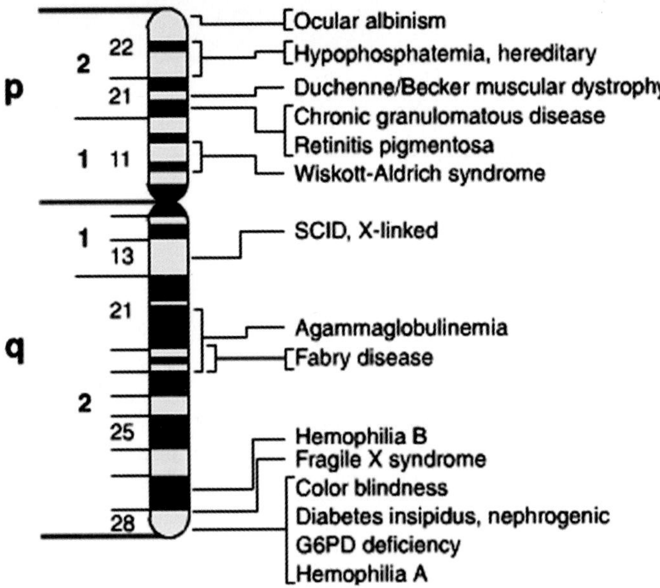

FIGURE 2-1. An example of the gene connected to Fragile X syndrome. (From Rubin R, Strayer DS. Rubin's pathology. Clinicopathologic foundations of medicine. 5th edition. Baltimore: Lippincott Williams & Wilkins; 2008.)

chromosome is stained in a certain way. The position is usually designated by two digits (representing a region and a band), which are sometimes followed by a decimal point and one or more additional digits (representing subbands within a light or dark area). The number indicating the gene position increases with distance from the centromere (1). For example, the gene connected to fragile X syndrome maps to the X chromosome Xq27.3. This represents region 2 position 27 on the long arm of the X chromosome (2) (Figure 2-1).

MUTATION

A mutation is a permanent change in the DNA sequence. All genetic variation originates from the process known as mutation. Mutations in a gene's DNA sequence can alter the amino acid sequence of the protein encoded by the gene. If a gene mutates, it may pass on a trait (phenotype) that is different from the original trait encoded by that gene. Gene mutations occur by inheriting them from a parent or acquiring them during an individual's lifetime. Mutations can affect either germline cells (cells that produce sperm and egg) or somatic cells (all cells other than germline cells). Mutations in somatic cells can lead to cancer and are thus of significant clinical concern. This chapter's focus, however, is directed primarily to germline mutations, because they can be transmitted from one generation to the next (3).

GENETIC DISORDERS

The genes involved in normal development code for numerous different products. These products include hormones and their receptors, DNA transcription factors, components of the extracellular matrix, enzymes, transport systems, as well as other critical proteins. Each of these genetic mediators is expressed in combinations of spatially and temporally overlapping patterns that control different developmental aspects. Mutations in the genes involved in development are a common cause of human birth defects (3).

Genetic disorders may result from a single-gene trait, a chromosomal defect, or may be multifactorial. Most genetic diseases are familial, or hereditary, which means they are passed on from parent to child in the egg or sperm, and are caused by changes in the DNA sequence that alters the expression of a single-gene product. Because of redundancy in the genetic code, not all mutations result in problems. Some genetic disorders are due to chromosomal rearrangements. The rearrangements result in deletion or duplication of a group of closely linked genes. Mistakes also occur during meiosis or mitosis and this can result in an abnormal number of chromosomes (4) (Figure 2-2).

In the case of a genetic disorder carried by a dominant gene, only one parent needs to carry the abnormal gene to give rise to the disease. An example of this is Marfan syndrome, a connective tissue disease. The basic biochemical abnormality in Marfan

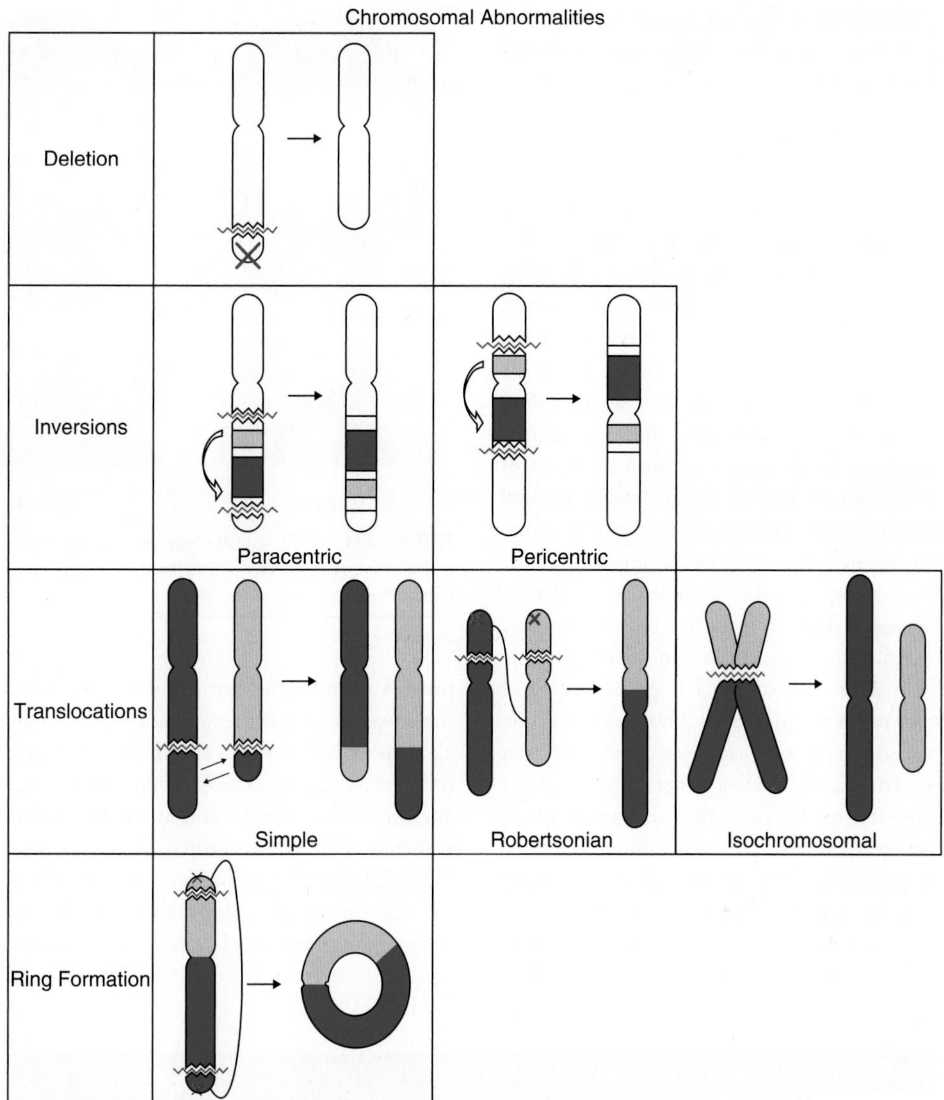

FIGURE 2-2. Common chromosomal abnormalities.

syndrome affects fibrillin I, an extracellular matrix protein. These microfibrils form the scaffolding for the deposition of elastin and are considered integral components of elastic fibers. People with Marfan syndrome are tall, thin, have heart defects, and can have a subluxated lens due to weakened zonules (5). In contrast, an individual must inherit an abnormal gene from both parents to give rise to an autosomal recessive disease.

Fragile X syndrome is the most common cause of inherited mental retardation in both males and females. It is an X-linked recessive disorder associated with what appears to be a fragile site on an arm of the X chromosome. In males, it also causes enlarged testes, hyperactivity, mitral valve malfunction, high forehead, and enlarged jaw and ears. X-linked recessive inheritance occurs when a mutation occurs in a gene on the X chromosome. This causes the phenotype to be expressed in males with only one abnormal X chromosome because they lack a second copy of the genes to replace the missing genes, but females must inherit two abnormal chromosomes to exhibit the disease because they have two X chromosomes (3) (see Chapter 5, Fragile X syndrome).

Multifactorial disorders, which can affect up to approximately 10% of the population, are more complex. Multifactorial disorders are those involving a number of genes or genetic influences combined with environmental factors. They may be polygenic (caused by multiple genes), or they may be the result of an inherited tendency toward a disorder that is expressed following exposure to certain environmental factors. A combination of factors is required for the problem to be present, whether at birth or later in life.

Frequently, the predisposing factors of a disorder, such as atherosclerosis (heart and vascular disease), certain cancers (e.g., breast cancer), or schizophrenia (a psychiatric disorder), include a familial tendency. This means that family members have an increased risk of developing the disorder, but not every family member will have the disease. Common examples of multifactorial disorders include cleft palate, congenital hip dislocation, congenital heart disease, type 2 diabetes mellitus, anencephaly, and hydrocephalus. These disorders tend to be limited to a single, localized area. The same defect is likely to recur in siblings, but there is no increased risk of occurrence of other defects (1).

Cleft lip with or without cleft palate is one of the most common birth defects. The incidence varies among ethnic groups, ranging from 3.6 per 1,000 live births among Native Americans to 2.0 per 1,000 among Asians, 1.0 per 1,000 among people of European ancestry, and 0.3 per 1,000 among Africans.

Developmentally, the defect has its origin at about the 35th day of gestation when the frontal prominences of the craniofacial structures fuse with the maxillary process to form the upper lip. This process is under the control of many genes, and disturbances in gene expression at this time may result in cleft lip with or without cleft palate (Figure 2-3). The defect may also be caused by teratogens (e.g., rubella, anticonvulsant drugs) and is often encountered in children with chromosomal abnormalities (3). See Table 2.1 for other examples of genetic disorders.

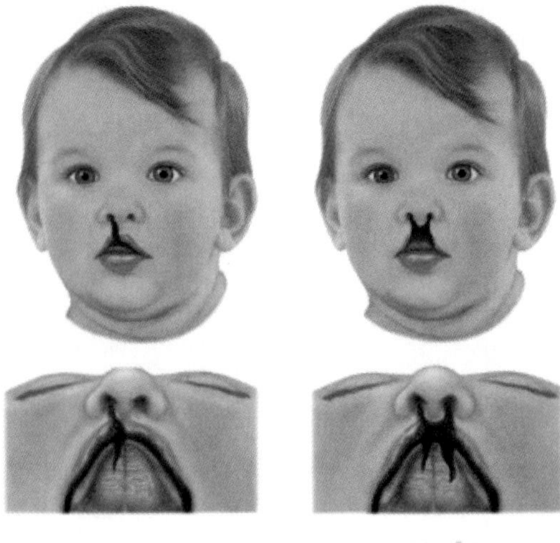

FIGURE 2-3. Cleft lip and cleft palate. (From Porth CM. Porth pathophysiology concepts of altered health states. 8th ed. Philadelphia: Lippincott Williams & Wilkins, 2008.)

Chromosomal abnormalities are responsible for a significant fraction of genetic diseases, occurring in about 1 of every 150 live births. They are the leading

TABLE 2.1 Summary of Common Genetic Disorders

Single-gene Disorders	**Dominant Inheritance**	**Recessive Inheritance**
Autosomal disorders	Adult polycystic kidney disease	Cystic fibrosis
	Huntington chorea	Phenylketonuria
	Familial hypercholesterolemia	Sickle cell anemia
	Marfan syndrome	Tay-Sachs disease
X-linked disorders	Fragile X syndrome	Color blindness
		Duchenne muscular dystrophy
		Hemophilia A
Chromosomal Disorders	**Disorder**	
Chromosome deficiency	Monosomy X (Turner syndrome)	
Chromosome excess	Trisomy 18 (Edwards syndrome)	
	Trisomy 21 (Down syndrome)	
	Polysomy X (Klinefelter syndrome)	
Multifactorial Disorders		
Anencephaly	Clubfoot	Myelomeningocele
Cleft lip and palate	Congenital heart disease	Schizophrenia

known cause of mental retardation and pregnancy loss. Chromosomal abnormalities are seen in 50% of first-trimester and 20% of second-trimester spontaneous abortions. Thus, they are an important cause of morbidity and mortality (3).

Chromosomal anomalies usually result from an error during meiosis. Meiosis results in egg and sperm cells, which have half the number of chromosomes, 23 instead of the normal 46. If DNA fragments are displaced or lost during the process of meiosis, the genetic information becomes altered. During meiosis, genes are often redistributed during the process of "crossover" in which chromosomes may swap portions. There may be an error in chromosomal duplication or reassembly, resulting in abnormal placement of part of the chromosome (a translocation), altered structure (deletion), or an abnormal number of chromosomes; this change is reflected in the expression of genes in the child. These birth defects are more common when the mother is over age 35. New research has also identified a higher risk in children of older fathers (3).

Down syndrome is an example of a trisomy, in which there are three copies of chromosome 21 rather than two, so it is called trisomy 21. Therefore, an individual with Down syndrome has 47 chromosomes. This anomaly may be spontaneous or result from exposure to a damaging substance. A less common form of Down syndrome exists in which a part of chromosome 21 is attached to another chromosome (translocation) (see Chapter 4, Down syndrome). The trisomy 21 change has marked effects throughout the body. Monosomy X, or Turner syndrome, occurs when only one sex chromosome, the X chromosome, is present. Thus, only 45 chromosomes are present, resulting in a variety of physical abnormalities and lack of ovaries. In Klinefelter syndrome or polysomy X, an extra X chromosome is present (XXY), resulting in a total of 47 chromosomes in each cell. Not all males show signs and are diagnosed, but typically, testes are small and sperm are not produced. Other common chromosomal abnormalities occur when parts of chromosomes are rearranged or lost during replication (1).

GENETIC DISORDERS OF PATIENTS WITH SPECIAL NEEDS

Spina bifida is part of a group of birth defects called neural tube defects. The neural tube is the embryonic structure that eventually develops to become the baby's brain and spinal cord, as well as the tissues that enclose them. Normally, the neural tube forms early in pregnancy and closes by the 28th day after conception. In babies with spina bifida, a portion of the neural tube fails to develop or close properly, causing defects in the spinal cord and in the bones of the spine. Spina bifida occurs in various forms of severity. When treatment for spina bifida is necessary, it involves surgery, although such treatment does not always completely resolve the problem.

The exact cause of spina bifida remains a mystery. No one knows what disrupts complete closure of the neural tube, causing a malformation to develop. Researchers suspect genetic, nutritional, and environmental factors play a role. Studies indicate that insufficient intake of folic acid, a common B vitamin, in the mother's diet is a key factor in causing spina bifida and other neural tube defects (1) (see Chapter 7, Oculovisual Abnormalities Associated with Rare Neurodevelopmental Disorders).

Williams syndrome is characterized by mild to moderate intellectual disability or learning problems, unique personality characteristics, distinctive facial features, and cardiovascular problems. It affects an estimated 1 in 7,500 to 20,000 people. It is caused by the deletion of genetic material from a specific region of chromosome 7. The deleted region includes more than 25 genes. Most cases of Williams syndrome are not inherited, but occur as random events during the formation of reproductive cells. In a small percentage of cases, people with Williams syndrome inherit the chromosomal deletion from a parent with the condition (4) (see Chapter 7, Oculovisual Abnormalities Associated with Rare Neurodevelopmental Disorders).

Lowe syndrome is also known as oculocerebrorenal syndrome of Lowe (OCRL). It is a rare, multisystem, X-linked recessive disorder that is characterized by the presence of developmental abnormalities involving the eyes, brain, and kidneys. The prevalence of Lowe syndrome is very low, at about 1 in 200,000 to 500,000 births. Due to the X-linked recessive inheritance pattern, the vast majority of patients are males, with few case reports of affected females. Most of the affected females have X autosomal translocations (a translocation between an X chromosome and an autosomal chromosome) involving the OCRL1 locus, which permits full expression of the Lowe syndrome phenotype. Lowe syndrome is caused by inherited mutations in the OCRL gene, mapped to chromosome Xq26.1, which encodes the OCRL1 protein. Because of this defective gene, an essential enzyme called PIP2-5-phosphatase is not produced (loss of function mutation). Although it has been known for many years that the mutation of OCRL1 causes Lowe syndrome, we still know relatively little about what the protein actually does inside the cell. Corrective contact lenses or glasses, with or without eye patches, are required to manage the visual deficits caused by cataracts and strabismus (4) (see Chapter 7, Oculovisual Abnormalities Associated with Rare Neurodevelopmental Disorders).

CRANIOFACIAL GENETIC DISORDERS

Craniofacial genetic disorders represent a group of malformations in the growth of the skull and facial bones that deforms the patient's appearance. These abnormalities are present at birth and will present with numerous variations. Some can be mild but many require reconstructive surgery. These conditions received little medical research attention until recently, due to major advances in genetics. Although, several thousand distinct syndromes have been reported, their rarity means that the average optometrist will not encounter the vast majority of them. It is noteworthy that more than half of all birth defects are associated with some form of craniofacial malformation. The National Institute of Dental and Craniofacial Research reports orofacial clefts alone occur in approximately 1 in 700 live births and affect more than 6,800 infants every year in the United States.

Craniofacial disorders can be understood by first looking at fetal development. In the first 2 months of pregnancy, tissues from each side of a fetal head and neck grow toward one another and fuse at the centerline. These tissues are known as the pharyngeal, or branchial arches. They form the crucial bones, skin, nerves, muscle, and other features of the head and neck. These pairs of tissue are composed of six separate arches (Figure 2-4).

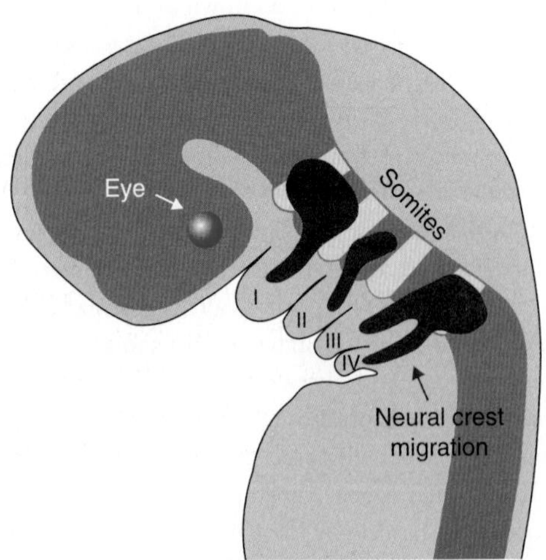

FIGURE 2-4. Pharyngeal, or branchial, arches form the crucial bones, skin, nerves, muscle, and other features of the head and neck.

The first arches produce the lower jaw, two bones in the middle ear, and nerves and muscles for chewing. The second arches give rise to the nerves and muscles of facial expression, one bone in the middle ear, most of the outer ear, and parts of the bone above the larynx (voice box). The third arches produce the nerves for swallowing and the rest of the bone above the larynx. The remaining arches give rise to the nerves for the vocal cords and other nerves and cartilage in the neck (6).

Several of the cranial nerves are associated with the branchial arches and craniofacial function. The trigeminal nerve (V) provides sensory innervation for the face and lining of the nose and mouth and motor innervation for the muscles of mastication. The facial nerve (VII) supplies motor function for the muscles of facial expression. The glossopharyngeal nerve (IX) supplies sensory function for the posterior third of the tongue, the pharynx, and the middle ear. The vagus nerve (X) has a wide array of functions both in the head and in the thorax and abdomen, including the regulation of heart rate, peristalsis, and speech. The hypoglossal nerve (XII) supplies motor function to the tongue. Most cranial nerves are of mixed sensory and motor function. The cell bodies of the motor neurons of the cranial nerves reside in the Central nervous system (CNS), like any other motor neurons, and they arise in the basal plate of the CNS. The sensory neurons are derived from the neural crest and/or placodes.

Anything that disrupts this process—whether in the production, growth, or movement of key cells in the arches—will cause parts of the face to develop abnormally. The problem may occur in both sides of the face, in which case it is considered a "symmetrical" condition, or predominantly on one side, when it is considered "asymmetrical," or uneven. Children with these disorders often have ear abnormalities and an underdeveloped lower jaw (6). Table 2.2 lists some of the more common conditions as well as the associated mutation and incidence (see Chapter 7, Oculovisual Abnormalities Associated with Rare Neurodevelopmental Disorders).

TABLE 2.2 Summary of Craniofacial Genetic Disorders

Syndrome Name	*Damaged Gene (Location)*	Damaged Protein	Type of Mutation	Incidence
Pfeiffer	FGFR1 (8p12) or FGFR2 (10q26)	Fibroblast Growth Factor Receptor 1 or 2	Gain of function (Pro252Arg on FGFR1 or change in number of Cys on FGFR2)	1 in 100,000
Apert	FGFR2 (10q26)	Fibroblast Growth Factor Receptor 2	Gain of function (Ser252Trp or Pro253Arg)	1 in 65,000
Crouzon	FGFR2 (10q26) or FGFR3 (4p16.3)	Fibroblast Growth Factor Receptor 2 or 3	Gain of function (various point mutations on FGFR2 or Ala391Glu on FGFR3)	1 in 60,000
Treacher-Collins	TCOF1 (5q32-q33.1)	Treacle Protein	Various insertions or deletions	1 in 40,000–70,000
Pierre Robin	COL11A2 (6p21.3)	Pro-alpha2(XI) Chain (a component of type XI collagen)	Loss of function (Gly955Glu)	1 in 8,500
DiGeorge	Many, including TBX1 & COMT (22q11.2)		Deletion	1 in 4,000
Goldenhar	Undetermined			1 in 3,500–25,000

Data from Traboulsi E. A Compendium of inherited disorders and the eye. Oxford: Oxford University Press; 2005.

EPIGENETICS

Epigenetics examines the effects of environmental factors on gene expression. The field of epigenetics is the study of inherited changes in a phenotype (physical trait) arising without change in the DNA sequence. In essence, this is non-DNA sequence–related heredity. It is an area of intense research in modern medicine because it may help to explain the connection between an individual's genetic background, the environment, aging, and disease (7). The epigenetic state will vary among tissues and change during a lifetime, while the DNA sequence remains essentially the same throughout life. The epigenetic change, which is often exposure induced, creates a physical trait (phenotype) that does not follow the classical genetic inheritance rules of Mendel, where inheritance of traits is either dominant or recessive. In Mendelian genetics, both parental copies are equally likely to contribute to the outcome. All epigenetic phenomena are characterized by chemical modifications to DNA. Adding methyl groups to the DNA changes its molecular appearance and structure and thus alters gene expression. The impact of this epigenetic modification (imprinting) of a gene copy depends only on which parent it was inherited from. For some imprinted genes, the cell only uses the copy from the mother to make proteins, and for others only that from the father. It is thought epigenetic modification expands the capacity of the genome for diversity of expression (8).

It was previously thought that genetic information was inherited through DNA only, but epigenetic studies show that parental experiences are passed on to offspring through these epigenetic tags. Identical twins illustrate the epigenetic process. They are from the same fertilized egg and include the same epigenetic tags. Over time, the twins' environments will diverge, resulting in individual epigenetic tags to form for each twin. These differences contribute to that which makes them observably different when they become older. Epigenetic tag differences can have such an impact on the twins that one will develop a disease, while the other does not (9).

Epigenetic tags provide a cellular memory for transcriptional control in all cell types of higher organisms. The molecular basis for many epigenetic changes seems to be the methylation of cytosines (C) in the DNA. This is a covalent addition of a methyl (CH_3) group to the nucleotide cytosine. The methylation of cytosine near the promoter region of a gene prevents transcription. This means a heavily methylated gene is permanently inactivated. Each cell type and tissue has its own methylation pattern, keeping some genes functional and others permanently inactivated. Certain environmental and dietary factors such as smoking have been linked to abnormal changes in epigenetic pathways in experimental and epidemiologic studies (10).

The human diploid genome has the advantage of having a backup for nearly every gene. Unfortunately, this does not hold true for imprinted genes. Sexual reproduction yields offspring with two copies of the same gene, one from each parent, but in an epigenetic phenomenon known as genomic imprinting, one copy of certain genes is turned on or off, depending on which parent contributed it. Imprinted genes are stamped by patterns of DNA methylation or histone modification during gamete formation, and their activation or inactivation is then passed on to offspring. The term "imprinting" refers to the fact that some chromosomes, segments of chromosomes, or some genes, are stamped with a "memory" of the parent from whom it came, such that in the cells of a child it is possible to tell which chromosome copy came from the mother (maternal chromosome) and which copy came from the father (paternal chromosome). The disadvantage to this imprinting process is that only one defective gene is necessary to yield the phenotypic defects if the mutation occurs in the turned-on gene because there is no compensation from the silenced copy on the other chromosome (7–11).

Many imprinted genes are involved in growth; therefore, imprinted genes likely play a major role in the development of cancer and other conditions in which cell and tissue growth are abnormal. Imprinted genes in which the copy from the mother is turned on (maternally expressed) usually suppress growth, while paternally expressed genes usually stimulate growth. In cancer, some tumor suppressor genes are actually maternally expressed genes that are mistakenly turned off, preventing the growth-limiting protein from being made. Likewise, many oncogenes (growth-promoting genes) are paternally expressed genes for which a single dose of the protein is just right for normal cell proliferation. However, if the maternal copy of the oncogene loses its epigenetic marks and is turned on as well, uncontrolled cell growth can result. For example, in the collection of birth defects known as Beckwith-Wiedemann syndrome (chromosome 11) abnormal epigenetics leads to abnormal growth of tissues, overgrowth of abdominal organs, low blood sugar at birth, and cancers (7).

Imprinted genes are especially sensitive to environmental signals because of the single-copy expression. Appropriate expression of imprinted genes is important for normal development. For example, a small deletion of part of the long arm of chromosome 15 results in Prader-Willi syndrome if the single copy of chromosome 15 is inherited from the mother, and Angelman syndrome if the chromosome is inherited from the father. This chromosomal region has different

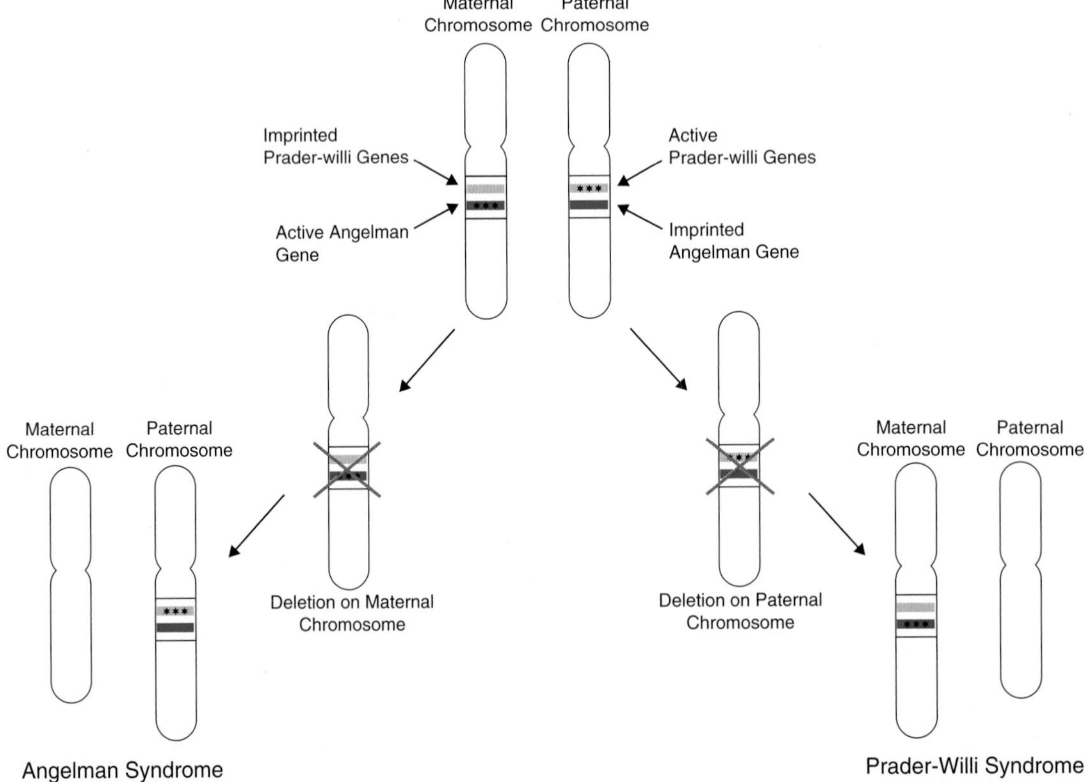

FIGURE 2-5. Genes associated with Angelman and Prader-Willi syndromes.

methylation patterns depending on whether it comes from the sperm or the egg. Prader-Willi is characterized by an uncontrollable appetite for food, among other things. Angelman has been called the happy puppet syndrome because of the associated jerky movements and happy, laughing demeanor (Figure 2-5). These conditions are described in greater detail in later chapters and other texts and papers (11–15).

CONCLUSION

This is a very exciting time in medical genetics where we can approach diagnosis, treatment, and management of disorders from a genetics perspective. The main goal of genetics is to determine the role of genetic variation and mutation in the etiology of clinical conditions. This chapter presented the genetics underpinnings of many conditions the optometrist may encounter with those who have special needs.

Genetics education and research regarding the eye and vision problems of those with special needs is vital to prepare primary care providers for the impact of ongoing rapid advances in genomics and those who require our expertise (16). It is hoped that this knowledge will increase optometrists' comfort with diagnosis, treatment, and counseling about genetic diseases.

ACKNOWLEDGMENT *I would like to thank Christie Puglis for all of her assistance in editing this chapter and the creation of figures.*

REFERENCES

1. Porth GM, Matfin G. Pathophysiology: concepts of altered health states. 8th ed. Philadelphia: Lippincott Williams & Wilkins; 2008. p. 160.
2. Rubin R, Strayer DS. Rubin's pathology. Clincopathologic foundations of medicine. 5th ed. Baltimore: Lippincott Williams & Wilkins; 2008. p. 214.
3. Jorde LB, Carey JC, Bamshad, MJ. Medical genetics. 4th ed. Philadelphia: Mosby Elsevier; 2010. p. 27–31.
4. Traboulsi EI. A Compendium of inherited disorders and the eye. New York: Oxford University Press; 2005. p. 197–8.
5. Pyeritz RE. Inherited diseases of connective tissue. In: Goldman L, Ausiello D, editors. Cecil medicine. 23rd ed. Philadelphia: Saunders Elsevier; 2007. p. 1983–5.
6. Bogart BI, Ort V. Elsevier's integrated anatomy and embryology. Philadelphia: Elsevier; 2007. p. 319.
7. Feinberg AP. Epigenetics at the epicenter of modern medicine. JAMA. 2008;299:1345–50.
8. Westman JA. Medical genetics for the modern clinician. Baltimore: Lippincott Williams & Wilkins; 2006. p. 46–9.
9. Poulsen P, Esteller M, Vaag A, Fraga MF. The epigenetic basis of twin discordance in age-related diseases. Pediatr Res. 2007;61:38R–42R.
10. Wilkins JF, Haig D. What good is genomic imprinting: the function of parent-specific gene expression. Nat Rev Genet. 2003;4:359–68.
11. Kumar V, Abbas AK, Fausto N, Mitchell RN. Robbins basic pathology. 8th ed. Philadelphia: W.B. Saunders Company; 2007. p. 251.
12. Wesson M, Maino D. Oculo-visual findings in Down syndrome, cerebral palsy, and mental retardation with non-specific etiology. In: Maino D, editor. Diagnosis and management of special populations. St. Louis: Mosby-Yearbook, Inc.; 1995. p. 17–54.
13. Maino DM, Maino JH, Cibis GW, Hecht F. Ocular health anomalies in patients with developmental disabilities. In: Maino, D editor. Diagnosis and management of special populations. St. Louis: Mosby-Yearbook, Inc.; 1995. p. 189–206.
14. Libov A, Maino D. Prader-Willi syndrome. J Am Optom Assoc. 1994;65:355–9.
15. Schneider B, Maino D. Angelman syndrome. J Am Optom Assoc. 1993;64:502–6.
16. Sands W, Taub M, Maino D. Limited research and education on special populations in optometry and ophthalmology. Optom Vis Dev. 2008;39:60–1.

CHAPTER 3

Marc B. Taub, OD, MS, FAAO, FCOVD
Ashley Reddell, OD

Cerebral Palsy

INTRODUCTION

Cerebral palsy (CP) was first described by Dr. William James Little, an orthopedic surgeon in 1862. Dr. Little described CP as a motor disorder resulting from a nonprogressive (static) insult to the developing brain (1). In 2004, an international workshop convened to reassess the definition and classification of CP. From this meeting emerged the following definition:

> *Cerebral Palsy describes a group of disorders of the development of movement and posture, causing activity limitation that is attributed to non-progressive disturbances that occurred in the developing fetal or infant brain. The motor disorders of cerebral palsy are often accompanied by disturbance of sensation, cognition, communication, perception, and/or behavior, and/or by a seizure disorder (2).*

The diagnosis of CP is based on a clinical assessment and not laboratory testing or neuroimaging. CP has a substantial impact on families' well-being and societal healthcare costs.

Cerebral palsy is classified into three physiologic and three anatomical subtypes. The physiologic subtypes are spastic, dyskinetic (also known as athetoid), or ataxic (3). Each subtype is thought to affect different brain areas leading to the varied manifestations. Spastic CP represents the majority of cases (70%–80%) and results in stiffness of muscles due to damage specifically to the brain's periventricular white matter (3,4). Affecting 10% to 15% of patients, dyskinetic CP is associated with damage to the basal ganglia, causing uncontrolled, slow, writhing movement. Ataxic CP, characterized by difficulty with balance and coordination due to cerebellar damage, affects <5% of people with CP (Table 3.1).

The three anatomical subtypes are hemiplegia, diplegia, and quadriplegia (5). Hemiplegia affects 20% to 30% of patients resulting in dysfunction of one side of the body (4). Diplegia refers to reduced abilities in the lower or upper limbs with the lower extremities being affected with much greater frequency (60%–70%). The most severe anatomical dysfunction is quadriplegia, which affects all four limbs and the trunk (10%–15%). When both the physiologic and anatomical subtypes are considered, spastic hemiplegia is the most common manifestation (4,6) (Table 3.2).

Beyond the main physiologic and anatomical subtypes, researchers have further classified CP patients according to gross motor abilities. The Gross Motor Function Classification System (GMFCS) was introduced in 1997 by Palisano et al. (7) with the purpose of classifying the abilities and limitations in gross motor function of children with CP. Previous classification systems had limited documentation and uniformity and were based on norms for children without motor impairments (8). Without a consistent classification system, prognosis and parent education were challenging and usually made based on the clinician's past experience instead of statistical trends. The GMFCS was designed for children with CP between 2 and 12 years of age, with description age brackets from 1 to 2, 2 to 4, 4 to 6, and 6 to 12 years of age (7–10). The system has five levels that describe differences in self-initiated movement ability (Table 3.3).

The GMFCS has proven to be a reliable and repeatable diagnostic tool in assessing gross motor ability and a valuable prognostic indicator. Clinicians should be cautioned not to use GMFCS data to withhold therapies from patients after a certain age, but rather as a prognostic guide. With successful therapy, a patient can make gains in activities of daily living and quality-of-life indicators (5,8–14).

TABLE 3.1 Physiologic Classifications of Cerebral Palsy

Subtypes	Prevalence	Characteristics
Spastic	70%–80%	Stiffness of muscles; damage to periventricular white matter
Dyskinetic/athetoid	10%–15%	Uncontrolled, slow writhing movement; damage to basal ganglia
Ataxic	<5%	Difficulty with balance and coordination; damage to cerebellum
Mixed		Blend of two or more of the above forms

From Thorogood C, Alexander M. Cerebral palsy. Available from: http://emedicine.medscape.com/article/310740-overview. Last Accessed on August 28, 2010.

A 2002 population-based study by Kennes et al. (15) compared eight functional health status domains to the GMFCS to investigate potential correlations between other neurodevelopmental disorders that are comorbid with CP and the GMFCS levels. The eight areas of measure included mobility, dexterity, speech, vision, hearing, cognition, emotion, and pain (14,15). A statistically significant association was found between the GMFCS levels and the functional limitations of mobility, dexterity, speech, and vision (15). Low correlations were found with hearing and cognition. Neither emotion nor pain was associated with the degree of functional limitation as described by GMFCS. A National Institutes of Health (NIH) cross-sectional designed study similarly found that the probability of debilitating visual deficits was greater in children with higher GMFCS scores (3,5,11).

Incidence/Prevalence The prevalence of CP in developed countries is 1 to 2 per 1,000 live births (16). Variation of prevalence depending upon geography has been found (China 1.6 per 1,000 [17], United States [Mississippi] 2.12 per 1,000 [18], Australia 2.0–2.5 per 1,000 [19]). Taking into account all live births, the prevalence of CP has been stable for decades. The prevalence of CP among low-birth-weight children is higher than normal birth weight children (20). Children of 32 to 42 weeks gestation with a birth weight for gestational age below the 10th percentile are four to six times more likely to have CP than are children between the 25th and 75th percentile (21). Among low birth weight and preterm infants, the prevalence of CP increased after the introduction of neonatal care and has begun to decrease in the past decade (16).

A study performed in the United Kingdom (UK) investigating CP from 1976 to 1999 found the rate among children with birth weights <2,500 g was significantly higher (16 per 1,000 live births) than for normal weight children (1.2 per 1,000 live births) (22). From 1964 to 1993, the incidence of CP in low birth weight children (<1,500 g) rose from 29.8 to 74.2 per 1,000. In comparison, for those weighing between 1,500 and 2,499 g, the incidence rose from 3.9 to 11.5 per 1,000 (17).

In examining the numbers in greater detail, between the years 1983 and 1995, the incidence of CP increased for those weighing <1,000 g to 90 per 1,000 in 1987 to 1989. This number decreased to 57 per 1,000 in 1993 to 1995. Among infants weighing 1,000 to 1,500 g, the rate rose to 77 in 1987 to 1989 and fell to 40 in 1993 to 1995 (23,24).

TABLE 3.2 Anatomical Classifications of Cerebral Palsy

Subtypes	Prevalence	Characteristics
Hemiplegia	20%–30%	Affecting RIGHT or LEFT side of body
Diplegia	30%–40%	Affecting UPPER or LOWER extremities (usually lower)
Quadriplegia	10%–15%	All four limbs and trunk are affected.

From Thorogood C, Alexander M. Cerebral palsy. Available from: http://emedicine.medscape.com/article/310740-overview. Last Accessed on August 28, 2010.

TABLE 3.3 Gross Motor Function Classification System

Level	Functional Capability/Limitation
1	Walks without assistance; limited advanced motor skills
2	Walks without assistance; limited advanced walking
3	Walks with assistance walking device
4	Self-mobility with a transporter
5	Self-mobility with a transporter; severely limited

A second study over a longer time frame showed the same trend. In 1979, the CP rate for infants weighing 1,000 to 1,499 g at birth was approximately 180 per 1,000, which decreased to 50 per 1,000 live births in the early 1990s onward (22).

Between 1966 and 1989, there was an 18% increase (32% to 50%) in the proportion of low birth weight infants among all children with CP (25). Newborns weighing <2,500 g now make up half of all CP cases and a little over half of the most severe cases. Despite being at a greater risk of developing CP, smaller birth weight babies are less likely to develop the most severe forms of motor involvement (22).

A social class gradient in the prevalence of CP overall as well as the hemiplegia and diplegia subtypes has been documented. In normal birth weight children with CP, there is a strong association with social class (26,27). The lower the socioeconomic class, the higher the prevalence of CP.

Etiology Two classifications exist to document the etiology of CP. The etiologies can be classified according to timing of onset or the actual cause. If using a time-based system, the categories are prenatal, perinatal, and postnatal (28,29). An alternative classification by actual cause is categorized by congenital or acquired. Development, malformations, and syndromes are considered congenital, while trauma, infection, hypoxia, ischemia, and TORCH infections would be cataloged as acquired (29).

Among the risk factors in the prenatal time period is intrauterine infection (29,30). This is considered to be the most important prenatal factor in the pathogenesis of CP in low birth weight children. In full-term infants, the relative risk (a ratio of the probability of the event occurring in the exposed group versus a nonexposed group) of intrauterine infection for CP is 4.7 and in preterm infants, 1.9 (31–33). The relative risk (34) of CP increases approximately fourfold in low birth weight infants with a neonatal history of sepsis (35). Along with other risk factors such as death of a co-twin, placental abruption, and cerebral ischemia, infection is thought to trigger a cytokine cascade resulting in damage to the brain (36).

Reported perinatal risks for CP include neonatal convulsions, birth asphyxia, instrument-assisted delivery, neonatal jaundice, antepartum hemorrhage, and neonatal infection (37). The role of asphyxia as a risk factor for CP is controversial (28). Some reports indicate that asphyxia is a minimal risk factor, while others report that it is the likely cause in one-third of term CP children (38). Despite the reduction in the rate of birth asphyxia from 40 per 100,000 to 11 per 100,000 in 1996, no associated reduction in the prevalence or incidence of CP has been seen (39).

Multiple gestations are also a risk factor (40). The prevalence is 12.6 in twins and 44.8 in triplets. From 1971 to 1997, there was an increase in the rate per live births in triplets as compared to single births (26.6 vs. 1.6) (41). The live birth of a co-twin of a fetus that died in utero is also at increased risk for CP. The prevalence is 95 to 167 per 1,000 in same-sex births and 21 to 29 per 1,000 in different sex births (42,43). Low Apgar scores at 5, 10, and 20 minutes are also strongly associated with CP (44–46).

Periventricular leukomalacia (PVL) is one of the most common underlying causes of CP in preterm infants but accounts for a fraction of infants born at term. Periventricular leukomalacia is a white matter lesion in premature infants that results from hypotension, ischemia, and coagulation necrosis at the border of deep penetrating arteries of the middle cerebral artery. It is the most common ischemic brain injury in premature infants (47). The risk of PVL is higher with a delivery at a very low gestational age and maternal or placental infection (48,49).

Approximately 10% of children who have CP acquire the disorder after birth although the figures are higher in underdeveloped countries. Acquired CP results from brain damage in the first few months or years of life. The most common causes of postnatal CP include brain infections, such as bacterial meningitis or viral encephalitis, and traumatic brain injury secondary to a motor vehicle accident, a fall, or child abuse (50).

Review of Systems Patients with CP suffer impairment to most body systems. By definition, the motor system is affected but many of the sensory systems are also impacted including hearing and vision (28,29). Using validated instruments to assess quality of life (QOL), it has been determined that children with CP report similar QOL to children not affected and that the QOL is not worse with greater levels of functional impairment (51). Health-related QOL, which takes into account areas such as self-care, mobility, and communication, is influenced by the severity of impairment (52).

Feeding, nutrition, and growth issues are of greatest concern in children with the most severe forms of CP. Approximately 30% of children with severe CP are undernourished (53). Although the leading cause appears to be poor nutrition due to a pseudobulbar palsy, the delays in growth appear to be multifactorial. Pseudobulbar palsy occurs when the connections from the cerebral cortex are disrupted without intrinsic damage to the brain stem or cranial nerves. Symptoms include poor coordination of sucking, swallowing, chewing, speaking, and using the tongue (29). A secondary side effect of pseudobulbar palsy is drooling, which occurs in up to 30% of children with CP. This can lead to aspiration, skin irritation, and articulation difficulties (54).

Sleep disorders are common in children with CP and occur in up to 50% of patients who have a visual impairment. These children often have fragmented sleep and might awaken several times per night. It is thought that visual impairment diminishes a child's ability to perceive and interpret cues for synchronizing their sleep with the environment. Melatonin, a natural compound, has shown positive effects in up to 80% of children with CP (55).

As expected, those with CP have a lower level of physical fitness compared to age-matched peers (56). Adults suffer from physical fatigue in greater amounts (57), while diplegic children have higher fat percentage and are hypoactive when compared to healthy children (58). Children and adolescents also have subnormal values for peak anaerobic power and muscular endurance of the upper and lower limbs (59). Associated motor impairments often lead to other impairments of the musculoskeletal system, especially in those that fall into the spastic category.

Bladder and bowel dysfunction is common as well. Constipation results from multiple factors including poor feeding, reduced water intake, and immobility (29). There is an increased risk of urinary incontinence, urgency, and infection (60). Almost one-quarter of children and adolescents have primary incontinence. These symptoms correlate with lower cognition and greater severity of motor deficits (61). Communication skills, an ability to go to the bathroom promptly, and managing clothing are barriers in attaining continence in this population (29).

Orthopedic anomalies are common as developing bones grow in the direction of the forces put upon them by the stress on the body. These anomalies are more common in the more severe forms of CP such as quadriplegia. Manifestations include progressive joint fractures, shortened muscles, hip or foot deformities, scoliosis, and fracture (29).

The prevalence of cognitive impairment associated with CP is directly related to the severity of the condition (62) and increases when epilepsy or cortical abnormalities are associated (29). While the most common type of CP (spastic diplegia) is characterized by normal cognition (62), only 40% of those with hemiplegic CP have normal cognition (59,63). In severely disabled children, 97.7% suffer from profound mental impairment (64). Since 1976, the prevalence of severe intellectual disability has decreased significantly (65).

Upwards of 36% of children have epilepsy, and onset will occur in 70% within the first year of life (66). The frequency of seizures has been found to decrease after the age of 16 (28). All types of epilepsy occur, but generalized and partial epilepsy are the most common types (67). Epilepsy can be an indicator of the severity of the neurologic or cortical insult and is most common among those with hemiplegia and quadriplegia (68). Antiepileptic medication has been used successfully to control seizures in this population (52,69).

Behavior problems are five times more likely in children with CP compared to children with no known health problems. Attention deficit hyperactivity disorder, dependency, being headstrong, and hyperactivity generally are more common in this population (70).

A hearing assessment is recommended routinely for all children with global developmental delay including CP. If not diagnosed early on, hearing loss can interfere even further with development. Upwards of 60% of those with CP have sensorineural hearing loss. This is two times more commonly found to occur bilaterally versus unilaterally. Approximately 45% of cases with hearing loss are associated with intellectual disability. These patients can be treated successfully with hearing aids or cochlear implants (71).

Visual Findings Multiple investigative studies have demonstrated that the CP population is more likely to have deficient visual skills than the general population (5,14,72–78). Common visual anomalies include strabismus, amblyopia, visual field defects, saccadic and pursuit dysfunction, accommodative insufficiency, and reduced visual-perceptual abilities (Table 3.4). The most common type of ametropia in a study of 50 children with CP by Ghasia et al. (5) was low to moderate hyperopia with high myopia being found in severe CP cases. Of the patients evaluated who were between levels 3 and 5 on the GMFCS (Table 3.3), ≥70% lacked any form of binocularity. Children with CP were found to have a mean acuity

TABLE 3.4 Ocular Findings Associated with CP

Optic atrophy
Strabismus
Amblyopia
Cortical visual impairment
Nystagmus
Refractive error
Visual field defect
Oculomotor dysfunction
  Pursuit and saccadic dysfunction
Accommodative dysfunction
Perceptual deficiency

of approximately two Snellen-equivalent lines worse than found in age-matched, normal children (14). On an object recognition test performed by children with CP, Stiers et al. (79) found >70% to have a specific visual-perceptual impairment. Kozeis et al. (75) examined 105 children with CP and found 49.53% to have reduced accommodative amplitude and 54.3% to have some form of strabismus. Peripheral visual field defects were found in 19%, while abnormal fundoscopic findings (i.e., optic atrophy) were seen in 10.47%. Lagunju and Oluleye (80) found approximately 14% of their study group of 149 CP patients suffered from cortical blindness, optic atrophy, and/or strabismus. Regardless of intelligence, the visual deficits alone can lead to reduced reading success. Vision care can play a critical role in the day-to-day functional abilities of these patients.

EXAMINATION ELEMENTS

Medical History Although knowing a CP patient's anatomical and physiologic classification may not specifically change the vision specialist's treatment strategy, it can enhance communication among the multidisciplinary health care team. As the GMFCS has gained international usage when describing ambulation abilities, it is important that optometrists apply it. Knowing that the patient is a level 5, for example, tells the clinician that there is a higher likelihood of visual deficits (i.e., decreased VA) (3,5,11). As visually guided motor therapy is often part of an optometric vision therapy program, being aware of the motor potential from a patient's GMFCS level can shape the prognostic picture. The lower the GMFCS ability, the more focus should be placed on improving success with activities of daily living as large gains in motor ability are less likely.

Visual Acuity Assessing visual acuity in children and adults with CP can be challenging, especially those patients at higher levels on the GMFCS (14). Reduced mental capacity, speech impairments, and reduced gaze control may impede accurate testing. Several studies have shown significant variation in the ability to obtain visual acuity measurement with routine methods, like Snellen acuity. Kozeis et al. (75) studied 105 children aged 6 to 15 with severe intellectual disability who were all able to complete the acuity testing protocol. Katoch et al. (81) found that only 22% of 200 children aged 8 months to 21 years were able to have recorded Snellen acuities. Yet in a third study by da Cunha Matta et al. (82), 100 of 123 children with CP aged 4 to 12 were able to perform the testing.

In looking more closely at testing performed by Kozeis et al. (75), 170/210 (81%) eyes recorded Snellen acuity at 20/40 or better. In contrast, 34 eyes recorded Snellen acuity of 20/60 or worse. This differs in comparison to the acuity levels from the study by Katoch et al. (81), which found that 27/44 (61%) had acuity better than 20/40.

In 2009, Ghasia et al. (14) examined 76 children to determine the probability of obtaining quantitative visual acuities in CP children with different levels of motor dysfunction. Compared to age-matched norms, the CP group averaged two lines worse in Snellen-equivalent acuities. Of the CP children tested, logMAR acuities were obtainable in 88% with either spatial-sweep visually evoked potentials (SSVEPs) or optotypes. A correlation was found between reduced levels of visual acuity and increased deficits on the GMFCS, but logMAR acuities were still obtainable in 56% of children with the most severe disease (11,14).

As optotypes require a verbal or motor response, SSVEPs circumvent this problem (14). The use of the SSVEP for the measurement of visual acuity in these patients allows for more precise and reliable data collection and should be used if readily available (11).

Refractive Error Several studies have documented the distribution and prevalence of different types and levels of refractive errors (76,83). Hyperopia, myopia, and astigmatism have been shown to occur in greater amounts versus the general population. Kozeis et al. (75) showed that the prevalence of hyperopia and astigmatism was over ten times greater versus the non-CP population. In that study, the amount of hyperopia and astigmatism ranged from +1.00 to +6.50 and −1.00 to −4.50, respectively.

Stereopsis Stereopsis assessment may result in similar limitations when a verbal or motor response is required. The use of an optokinetic nystagmus drum can be a helpful tool in evaluating whether gross stereopsis is present or not. The drum should be used to measure nasal to temporal and temporal to nasal tracking abilities in each eye. It has been postulated that symmetry between these measurements is indicative of a gross level of stereoscopic vision (83).

In using the Lang stereo test, which does not require the patient use of polarized lenses, 14.28% children presented with a gross degree of stereopsis ranging between 1,200 and 550 seconds disparity. In contrast, 85.29% of children demonstrated an absence of any level or stereopsis. This can be in part correlated to the high amount of strabismus found in patients with CP (75).

Strabismus The high incidence of strabismus in children with CP has been well established. It is reported to be between 39% and 50% (81,82,84,85) and is evenly distributed between esotropia and exotropia across CP types Kozeis et al. (75) found an esotropia range of 25 to 40 Δ base out and an exotropia range of 30 to 45 Δ base in. Erkkila et al. (86) observed that esotropia presented in a higher degree in those with quadriplegic CP. Alternating strabismus is found in greater amounts versus those considered to be unilateral.

Accommodation Saunders et al. (73) evaluated the near-pupillary response in comparison to dynamic retinoscopy (Knott retinoscopy) as a measure of accommodative ability in children with CP. Pupillary response was classified as normal, reduced, or absent by subjective observation. The researchers discovered that patients with reduced or absent pupillary responses demonstrated significantly lower accommodative ability as measured with dynamic retinoscopy. Although not a replacement for more formal accommodative testing, the near-pupillary response can provide another insight into the functional level of CP patients.

McClelland et al. (3) examined 90 children and found that 57.6% demonstrated an accommodative lag outside of normal limits at one or more distances. The greatest accommodative deficits were associated with more severe motor and intellectual impairments. They also found that the subjects with dyskinetic (or athetoid) CP had significantly more reduction than the spastic CP subtype. Leat (87) and Kozeis et al. (75) reported that 42% and 49.53% of patients in their studies had reduced amplitude of accommodation as measured with dynamic retinoscopy. Approximately 16% of subjects in the later study required plus correction ranging between +1.50 and +2.00 for reading. It is essential that a thorough accommodative evaluation is performed on all patients with CP to best determine the appropriate lens management.

Perceptual Abilities In a retrospective study, Orbitus et al. (74) evaluated 70 children, 36 of which had CP, with both a visual-perceptual and cognitive assessment. They compared visual perceptual testing (L94 visual perceptual battery) to the performance age obtained on nonverbal intelligence subtests. Of the areas tested, the visual-matching task was found to be the easiest, while the identification of objects using visual imagery and visual–spatial orientation manipulation were the most difficult. Of the patients found to have a perceptual visual impairment, 62% had CP.

Similar perceptual deficits have been repeatedly found in other research studies (75,76). In a study of 33 subjects with CP, Barca et al. (88) found that 25% of children failed testing in the area of visuocognitive skills, 69% failed visuoperceptual tests, and 60% failed visuospatial tasks. Visuospatial neglect has been documented to occur on both the left and right side (82). Perceptual testing may be challenging due to motor skill limitations, but an optometric vision therapy assessment can include nonmotor perceptual testing appropriate for the patient's cognitive level.

Oculomotor In assessing gross smooth pursuits using a technique similar to the Northeastern State University College of Optometry (NSUCO) oculomotor test, Da Cunha Matta et al. (82) showed that 25.9% (29/112) of subjects demonstrated dysfunction. Deficiency ranged from interruption to asynchronism. Smooth pursuit dysfunction was associated with the presence of strabismus, nystagmus, and visual field defects.

Jackson et al. (89) in a study of 131 consecutive patients with CP identified pursuit (smooth) and saccadic (jumping between fixation points) deficits in 85% (94 patients) and 80% (88 patients), respectively. The most common pursuit deficits were initiation of movement (45%, 42 cases) and problems with the amplitude of the eye movement not matching the velocity of the target. Vertical pursuits were affected in a greater number of patients (70%, 66 cases) in comparison to horizontal pursuits (41%, 39 cases). Sixty-five percent (57 cases) had increased saccadic latency and 63% (55 cases) had hypometric saccades. Vertical saccades were affected more commonly (79%, 70 cases) in comparison to horizontal saccades (42%, 36 cases).

One hundred and five CP children with IQ levels between 70 and 100 were evaluated by Kozeis et al. (77) using the Developmental Eye Movement (DEM) Test to evaluate reading eye movements. Only 19% were found to have normal function, while 20.9% exhibited purely oculomotor dysfunction. Perceptual/automaticity problems were found in 32.4%, and 27.7% had a combined oculomotor and perceptual/automaticity problem. According to the authors, "Eye tracking skills are very important in reading. A harmonic pattern of eye movement is needed for reading to be effective." As such, it is appropriate to include the Developmental Eye Movement and/or NSUCO oculomotor tests as part of the visual evaluation of the patient with CP.

Visual Fields The assessment of visual field function may be hampered by an inability to understand or cooperate with tests. Porro et al. (90) examined 24 children with spastic hemiplegia aged 1 to 10 years using Goldmann perimetry and confrontation techniques. Only four patients were able to perform Goldmann perimetry, while 18 children were found to have visual field defect using the confrontation technique. Jacobson et al. (91), using the same two techniques, investigated 29 children with unilateral CP. Eighteen children had subnormal visual field function. Patients identified as having more severe defects were detected with both techniques, but those with relative defects on Goldmann perimetry had normal results when tested with the confrontation technique. Guzzetta et al. (92) used an arc perimeter and a white ball to evaluate 47 children aged 8 months to 4 years 4 months. Abnormal visual field function was found in 16 children. When 16 of the children were tested using the confrontation technique, only two were abnormal. Kozeis et al. (75) differentiated between peripheral and central field loss in their investigation. They found 19.05% and 3.8% of patients to have peripheral and central defects, respectively. The peripheral defect was typically identified as a left temporal hemianopia sparing the central field while the central defects were paracentral scotomas in the absence of underlying maculopathy.

Ocular Pathology The incidence of ocular pathology in patients with CP is higher than in the general population. The incidence of nystagmus ranges from 5.5% to 49%. Jackson et al. (89) identified eight types of nystagmus in a study group of 131 consecutive CP patients. The most common were latent nystagmus associated with infantile strabismus (37%), congenital conjugate horizontal nystagmus (22%), and rotary nystagmus (17%). The study also identified that 14% of patients had trouble generating voluntary conjugate gaze manifesting as gaze apraxia or palsy. In contrast, Katoch et al. (81) and Pennefather (93) identified only 5.5% and 16.7% of their study groups as having nystagmus.

Retinal and optic nerve changes are also found in greater numbers. Optic nerve atrophy, which is described in detail in Chapter 22, Diagnosis and Treatment of Commonly Diagnosed Ocular Health Anomalies has been identified in 10.47% to 16.5% of patients (81,93). Diffuse and temporal disc pallor is most commonly identified. Retinopathy of prematurity (ROP), which is covered in greater detail in Chapter 22, Diagnosis and Treatment of Commonly Diagnosed Ocular Health Anomalies, is found in significantly greater amounts in patients with CP. In a study of 558 children born before 32 weeks gestation, 54 were diagnosed with CP. Retinopathy of prematurity was identified in eight children (14.8%) with CP in comparison to eight (1.6%) without CP (93).

CONCLUSION

As optometrists, we play a critical role in the care of patients with CP. It is important that we know the details concerning each case due to the large variability of the disorder. Knowing each patient's physiologic and anatomical type as well as his/her level on the GMFCS can affect treatment, patient education, and prognosis. Most importantly, by communicating more effectively with the multidisciplinary health care team, we set our patient up for superior outcomes.

REFERENCES

1. Shevell MI, Bodensteiner JB. Cerebral palsy: defining the problem. Semin Pediatr Neurol. 2004;11(1):2–4.
2. Bax M, Goldstein M, Rosenbaum P, et al. Proposed definition and classification of cerebral palsy. Dev Med Child Neurol. 2005; 47:571–6.

3. McClelland JF, Parkes J, Hill N, et al. Accommodative dysfunction in children with cerebral palsy: a population-based study. Invest Ophthalmol Vis Sci. 2006;47(5):1824–30.
4. Thorogood C, Alexander M. Cerebral palsy. Available from: http://emedicine.medscape.com/article/310740-overview. Last Accessed on August 28, 2010.
5. Ghasia F, Brunstrom J, Gordon M, et al. Frequency and severity of visual sensory and motor deficits in children with cerebral palsy: gross motor function classification scale. Invest Ophthalmol Vis Sci. 2008;49(2):572–80.
6. Wichers MJ, Odding E, Stam HJ, et al. Clinical presentation, associated disorders and aetiological moments in cerebral palsy: a Dutch population-based study. Disabil Rehabil. 2005; 27(10):583–9.
7. Palisano R, Rosenbaum P, Walter S, et al. Development and reliability of a system to classify gross motor function in children with cerebral palsy. Dev Med Child Neurol. 1997;39: 214–23.
8. Palisano R, Hanna SE, Rosenbaum PL, et al. Validation of a model of gross motor function for children with cerebral palsy. Phys Ther. 2000;80(10):974–85.
9. Rosenbaum P, Walter SD, Hanna SE, et al. Prognosis for gross motor function in cerebral palsy: creation of motor development curves. JAMA. 2002;288(11):1357–63.
10. Morris C, Bartlett D. Gross motor function classification system: impact and utility. Dev Med Child Neurol. 2004; 46:60–5.
11. da Costa MF, Rios Salomao S, Berezovsky A, et al. Relationship between vision and motor impairment in children with spastic cerebral palsy: new evidence from electrophysiology. Behav Brain Res. 2004;149(2):145–50.
12. Himmelmann K, Beckung E, Hagberg G, et al. Gross and fine motor function and accompanying impairments in cerebral palsy. Dev Med Child Neurol. 2006;48(6):417–23.
13. Beckung E, Hagberg G. Neuroimpairment, activity limitations, and participation restrictions in children with cerebral palsy. Dev Med Child Neurol. 2002;44(5):309–16.
14. Ghasia F, Brunstom J, Tychsen L. Visual acuity and visually evoked responses in children with cerebral palsy: Gross Motor Function Classification Scale. Br J Ophthalmol. 2009; 93:1068–72.
15. Kennes J, Rosenbaum P, Hanna SE, et al. Health status of school-aged children with cerebral palsy: information from a population-based sample. Dev Med Child Neurol. 2002;44(4):240–7.
16. Paneth N, Hong T, Korzeniewski S. The descriptive epidemiology of cerebral palsy. Clin Perinatol. 2006;33:251–67.
17. Liu JM, Li S, Lin Q, et al. Prevalence of cerebral palsy in China. Int J Epidemiol. 1999;28:949–54.
18. Haerer AF, Anderson DW, Schoenberg BS. Prevalence of cerebral palsy in the biracial population of Copiaj County, Mississippi. Dev Med Child Neurol. 1984;26:195–9.
19. Reddihough DS, Collins KJ. The epidemiology and causes of cerebral palsy. Aust J Physiother. 2003;49:7–12.
20. Platt MJ, Cans C, Johnson A, et al. Trends in cerebral palsy among infants of very low birthweight (<1500 g) or born prematurely (<32 weeks) in 16 European centres: a database study. Lancet. 2007;369:43–50.
21. Jarvis S, Glinianaia SV, Torrioli MG, et al. Cerebral palsy and intrauterine growth in single births: European collaborative study. Lancet. 2003;362:1106–11.
22. Surman G, Hemming K, Platt MJ, et al. Children with cerebral palsy: severity and trends over time. Paediatr Perinatal Epidemiol. 2009;23:513–21.
23. Grether JK, Nelson KB. Possible decrease in prevalence of cerebral palsy in premature infants. J Pediatr. 2000;136:133.
24. Surman G, Newdick H, Johnson A. Cerebral palsy rates among low-birthweight infants fell in the 1990s. Dev Med Child Neurol. 2003;45:456–62.
25. Pharoah PO, Platt MJ, Cooke T. The changing epidemiology of cerebral palsy. Arch Dis Child Fetal Neonatal Ed. 1996;75:F169–73.
26. Dowding VM, Barry C. Cerebral palsy: social class differences in prevalence in relation to birthweight and severity of disability. J Epidemiol Community Health. 1990;44:191–5.
27. Dolk H, Pattenden S, Johnson A. Cerebral palsy, low birthweight and socio-economic deprivation: inequalities in a major cause of childhood disability. Paediatr Perinat Epidemiol. 2001;15:359–63.
28. Odding E, Roebroek ME, Stam HJ. The epidemiology of cerebral palsy: incidence, impairments and risk factors. Dis Rehab. 2006;28(4):183–91.
29. Jan MSS. Cerebral palsy: comprehensive review and update. Ann Saudi Med. 2006;26(2):123–32.
30. Stelmach T, Kallas E, Pisarev H, et al. Antenatal risk factors associated with unfavorable neurologic status in newborns and at 2 years of age. J Child Neurol. 2004;19(2):116–22.
31. Wu YM, Colford JM Jr. Chorioamnionitis as a risk factor for cerebral palsy. JAMA. 2000;284:1417–24.
32. Wu YM, Escobar GJ, Grether JK, et al. Chorioamnionitis and cerebral palsy in term and near-term infants. JAMA. 2003;290:2677–84.
33. Schendel DE, Schuchat A, Thorsen P. Public health issues related to infection in pregnancy and cerebral palsy. Ment Retard Dev Disabil Res Rev. 2002;8:39–45.
34. Sistrom CL, Garvan CW. Proportions, odds, and risk. Radiology. 2004;230(1):12–9.
35. Wheather M, Rennie JM. Perinatal infection is an important risk factor for cerebral palsy in very-low-birthweight infants. Dev Med Child Neurol. 2000;42:364–7.
36. O'Shea TM, Dammann O. Antecedents of cerebral palsy in very-low-birthweight infants. Clin Perinatol. 2000;27:285–302.
37. Suvanand S, Kapoor SK, Reddaiah VP, et al. Risk factors for cerebral palsy. Indian J Pediatr. 1997;64:677–85.
38. Pschirrer ER, Yeomans ER. Does asphyxia cause cerebral palsy? Semin Perinatol. 2000;24:215–20.
39. Nelson K, Grether J. Causes of cerebral palsy. Curr Opin Pediatr. 1999;11:487–96.
40. Pharoah PO, Cooke T. Cerebral palsy in multiple births. Arch Dis Child Neonatal. 1996;75:F174–7.
41. Keith LG, Oleszczuk JJ, Keith DD. Multiple gestation: reflection on epidemiology, causes and consequences. Int J Fertil Womens Med. 2000;45:206–14.
42. Pharoah PO, Adi Y. Consequences of in-utero death in twin pregnancy. Lancet. 2000;355:1597–602.
43. Pharoah PO. Cerebral palsy in the surviving twin associated with infant death of the co-twin. Arch Dis Child Fetal Neonatal Ed. 2001;84: F111–6.
44. Van de Riet JE, Vandenbussche FP, Le Cessie S, et al. Newborn assessment and long-term adverse outcome: a systematic review. Am J Obstet Gynecol. 1999;1980:1024–9.

45. Moster D, Lie RT, Irgens LM, et al. The association of Apgar score with subsequent death and cerebral palsy: a population-based study in term infants. J Pediatr. 2001;138:798–803.
46. Jacobsson B, Hagberg G, Hagberg B, et al. Cerebral palsy in preterm infants: a population-based case-control study of antenatal and intrapartal risk factors. Acta Paediatr. 2002; 92:946–51.
47. Available from: http://emedicine.medscape.com/article/975728-overview. Last Accessed on September 14, 2010.
48. Leviton A, Paneth N. White matter damage in preterm newborns—an epidemiological perspective. Early Hum Dev. 1990; 24:1–22.
49. Zupan V, Gonzalez P, Lacaze-Masmonteil T, et al. Periventricular leukomalacia: risk factors revisited. Dev Med Child Neurol. 1996;38:1061–7.
50. United Cerebral Palsy of the Mid-South. Available from: http://www.ucp.org/ucp_localsub.cfm/143/15533#causes. Last Accessed on January 12, 2011.
51. Dickinson HO, Parkinson KN, Ravens-Seiberer U, et al. Self-reported quality of life of 8012 year old children with cerebral palsy. A cross-sectional European study. Lancet. 2007; 369:2171–8.
52. O'Shea TM. Diagnosis, treatment and prevention of cerebral palsy. Clin Obstet Gynecol. 2008;51(4):816–28.
53. Jan MMM, Shaabat AO. Clozabam for the treatment of intractable childhood epilepsy. Saudi Med J. 2000;21(7):622–4.
54. Siegel L, Klingbeil M. Control of with transdermal scopolamine in a child with cerebral palsy. Dev Med Child Neurol. 1991; 33:1010–4.
55. Jan MMS. Melatonin for the treatment of handicapped children with severe sleep disorder. Pediatr Neurol. 2000;23(3):229–32.
56. van den Berg-Emons HJG, van Baak MA, Speth L, et al. Physical training of school children with spastic cerebral palsy: effects on daily activity, fat mass and fitness. Int J Rehabil Res. 1998; 21:179–94.
57. Jahnsen R, Villien L, Stanghelle JK, et al. Fatigue in adults with cerebral palsy in Norway compared with the general population. Dev Med Child Neurol. 2003;45:296–303.
58. van den Berg-Emons HJG, Saris WH, de Barbanson DC, et al. Daily physical activity of school children with spastic diplegia and healthy control subjects. J Pediatr. 1995; 127:578–84.
59. Unnithan VB, Clifford C, Bar-Or O. Evaluation by exercise testing of the child with cerebral palsy. Sports Med. 1998; 26:239–51.
60. Dormans J, Pellegrino L. Caring for children with cerebral palsy: a team based approach. Baltimore: Paul H. Brookes Publishing Co.; 1998. p. 533.
61. Rojjen LEG, Postema K, Limbeek J, Kuppevelt HJM. Development of bladder control in children and adolescents with cerebral palsy. Dev Med Child Neurol. 2001;43:103–7.
62. Russman BS, Aschwal S. Evaluation of the child with cerebral palsy. Semin Pediatr Neurol. 2004;11(1):47–57.
63. Frampton I, Yude C, Goodman R. The prevalence and correlates of specific learning difficulties in a representative sample of children with hemiplegia. Br J Educ Psychol. 1998;68:39–51.
64. Nakada Y. An epidemiological survey of severely mentally and physically disabled children in Okinawa. Brain Dev. 1993; 15:113–8.
65. Rumeau-Rouquette C, Grandjean H, Cans C, et al. Prevalence and time trends of disabilities in school-age children. Int J Epidemiol. 1997;26:137–45.
66. Zafeiriou D, Kontopoulos E, Tsikoulas I. Characteristics and prognosis of epilepsy in children with cerebral palsy. Epilepsy Cerebral Palsy. 1999;14:289–93.
67. Bruck I, Antoniuk SA, Spessato A, et al. Epilepsy in children with cerebral palsy. Arq Neuropsiquiatr. 2001;59:35–9.
68. Fennell EB, Dikel TN. Cognitive and neuropsycological functioning in children with cerebral palsy. J Child Neurol. 2001; 16:58–63.
69. Hassan A, Jan MMS, Shaabat AO. Topiramate for the treatment of intractable childhood epilepsy Neurosciences. 2003; 8(4):233–s6.
70. McDermott S, Coker AL, Mani S, et al. A population-based analysis of behavior problems in children with cerebral palsy. J Pediatr Psychol. 1996;21:447–63.
71. Morales AC, Azuara BN, Gallo TJ, et al. Sensorineural hearing loss in cerebral palsy patients. Acta Otorrinolaringol Esp. 2006; 57(7):300–2.
72. Guzzetta A, Mercuri E, Cioni G. Visual disorders in children with brain lesions: visual impairment associated with cerebral palsy. Eur J Paediatr Neurol. 2001;5:115–9.
73. Saunders K, McClelland J, Richardson P, et al. Clinical judgment of near pupil responses provides a useful indicator of focusing ability in children with cerebral palsy. Dev Med Child Neurol. 2008;50:33–7.
74. Orbitus E, Lagae M, Casteels I, et al. Assessment of cerebral visual impairment with the L94 visual perceptual battery: clinical value and correlation with MRI findings. Dev Med Child Neurol. 2009;51:209–17.
75. Kozeis N, Anogeianaki A, Mitova DT, et al. Visual function and visual perception in cerebral palsied children. Ophthalmic Physiol Opt. 2007;27:44–53.
76. Stiers P, Vanderkelen R, Vanneste G, et al. Visual-perceptual impairment in a random sample of children with cerebral palsy. Dev Med Child Neurol. 2002;44:370–82.
77. Kozeis N, Anogeianaki A, Mitova DT, et al. Visual function and execution of microsaccades related to reading skills, in cerebral palsied children. Int J Neurosci. 2006;116:1347–58.
78. Ross L, Heron G, Mackie R, et al. Reduced accommodative function in dyskinetic cerebral palsy: a novel management strategy. Dev Med Child Neurol. 2000;42:701–3.
79. Stiers P, De Cock P, Vandenbussche E. Impaired visual perceptual performance on object recognition task in children with cerebral visual impairment. Neuropediatrics. 1998; 29:80–8.
80. Lagunju IA, Oluleye TS. Ocular abnormalities in children with cerebral palsy. Afr J Med Med Sci. 2007;36:71–5.
81. Katoch S, Devi A, Kulkarni P. Ocular defects in cerebral palsy. Indian J Ophthal. 2007;55:154–6.
82. Da Cunha Matta AP, Nunes G, Rossi L, et al. Outpatient evaluation and ocular motility in 123 children with cerebral palsy. Devel Rehab. 2008;11:159–65.
83. Tychsen L. Motion sensitivity and the origins of infantile strabismus. In: Simons K, editor. Early visual development, normal and abnormal. New York: Oxford University Press; 1993. p. 364–87.
84. Lo Cascio GP. A study of vision in cerebral palsy. Am J Optom Physiol Opt. 1977;54:332–7.

85. Pigassou-Albouy R, Fleming A. Amblyopia and strabismus in patients with cerebral palsy. Ann Ophthal. 1975;7:382–7.
86. Erkkila H, Lindberg L, Kallio AK. Strabismus in children with cerebral palsy. Acta Ophthal Scand. 1996;74:636–8.
87. Leat SJ. Reduced accommodation in children with cerebral palsy. Ophthalmic Physiol Opt. 1996;16:385–90.
88. Barca L, Cappelli FR, Di Giulio P, et al. Outpatient assessment of neurovisual functions in children with cerebral palsy. Res Dev Dis. 2010;31:488–95.
89. Jackson J, Castelberry C, Galli M, et al. Cerebral Palsy for the pediatric eye care team-Part II: Diagnosis and treatment of ocular motor defects. Am Orthop J. 2006;56:86–96.
90. Porro G, van Nieuwenhuzien O, Wittebol-Post D, et al. Visual functions in congenital hemiplegia. J Neuroophthalmol. 1999; 21:59–68.
91. Jacobson L, Rydberg A, Eliasson AC, et al. Visual field function in school-aged children with spastic unilateral cerebral palsy related to different patterns of brain damage. Dev Med Child Neurol. 2010;52:e184–.
92. Guzzetta A, Fazzi B, Mercuri F, et al. Visual function in children with hemiplegia in the first years of life. Dev Med Child Neurol. 2001;43:321–9.
93. Pennefather PM, Tin W. Ocular abnormalities associated with cerebral palsy after preterm birth. Eye. 2000;14:78–81.

CHAPTER 4

J. Margaret Woodhouse, PhD, BSc, FSMC
Dominick M. Maino, OD, MEd, FAAO, FCOVD-A

Down Syndrome

Patients with special needs, including those with Down syndrome (DS), should be treated as individuals by all health care professionals. Stereotypes and generalizations should be avoided. Recognition that there are frequently encountered systemic, cognitive, psychiatric, physical, and oculovisual characteristics that aid in understanding of their strengths and weaknesses is important. This helps us not only in conducting a successful examination but also in determining the best and most appropriate treatment options.

Down syndrome was one of the first developmental disabilities to be recognized as a syndrome (Langdon Down in 1866) and is a frequently encountered cause of intellectual and physical disability in the infant. Initially the syndrome could only be diagnosed solely on the physical findings. The two major characteristics of DS are an upward slanting of the temporal palpebral fissures and a significant presence of epicanthal folds, so this is why DS was initially referred to as mongolism. This term is now considered archaic with DS or trisomy 21 being used in the literature.

Currently 1/691 babies are born each year with DS, and more than 400,000 individuals with DS live in the United States. Down syndrome occurs in all races and at all economic levels. As the mother's age increases, the likelihood of having a baby with DS also increases, but since younger women have higher fertility rates, 80% of children with DS are born to females <35 years of age. The life expectancy of those with DS is currently 60, which has increased significantly from a life expectancy of 25 years in 1983 (1–3).

ETIOLOGY

Down syndrome is an inherited, genetic anomaly that usually involves chromosome number 21. There are three possible causes of DS. These are

1. ***Trisomy 21*** (94%): There are three instead of two 21st chromosomes. This results in 47 chromosomes being present.
2. ***Translocation*** (5%): A portion of a 21st chromosome breaks off and is reattached to other chromosomes (chromosome 14 is usually involved, a 14/21 translocation). Down syndrome individuals with a translocation etiology have a normal complement of 46 chromosomes.
3. ***Mosaicism*** (1%): In mosaicism, some cells have the normal complement of 46 chromosomes while other cells have 47.

Those individuals with translocation and mosaicism etiologies will display many of the characteristics of trisomy 21, but often in a less pronounced manner (4).

REVIEW OF SYSTEMS

A review of systems should include questions and assessments of the general overview of the patient's health, skin, head (eyes, ears, nose, throat), and neck, as well as the respiratory, cardiovascular, gastrointestinal, and urinary systems. Questions concerning potential problems involving the musculoskeletal system, neurologic system, hematologic anomalies, endocrine system, and the presence of any psychiatric illnesses or concerns should be reviewed as well.

Since social skills and receptive language are usually well developed in people with DS, we should expect appropriate interactions with most of these patients. It should be noted that expressive speech and language skills can be relatively poor. Speech production is often delayed or unclear and lags behind receptive language skill levels. It is unfortunately easy to underestimate the intellectual capacity of the patient if he or she cannot talk in a way that is readily comprehensible to us. Many children with DS learn sign language at a young age to assist in their speech development (e.g., Makaton,* SignAlong†). Health care providers should consider learning at least some appropriate sign vocabulary, so that our patients can participate more actively in the eye and vision examination process. As is seen with Fragile X syndrome (Chapter 5), Autism (Chapter 8) can be a comorbid finding in those with DS. If the patient has this dual diagnosis, this will likely alter the approach to patient care.

Hearing impairment is also frequently present in those with DS. This will add to difficulties in speech production. In addition, auditory processing tends to be relatively slow. The slower auditory processing combined with the frequently encountered hearing impairment associated with DS should be compensated by using short, concrete, polite commands that break a complex instruction set into small manageable parts. We need to wait for our patient to absorb each part of our request before we continue. For example, "Please sit in the chair, put your glasses on, and look at the letters on the wall" would change to "Please sit in the chair." Only when the patient is seated comfortably do we proceed to the next step: "Please put on your glasses." We should be guided by the language the parent uses. If the child does not respond appropriately, do not necessarily change the wording used, as this can confuse the child. Simply repeat the instruction, with added visual clues (e.g., use pointing to the eye chart along with the verbal instructions).

People with DS are described as visual learners with their visual skills usually more advanced than their auditory skills. Demonstrating what you would like them to do (e.g., miming putting on glasses), pointing to the letters on the wall, and using pictures to illustrate the steps in the examination can facilitate their understanding of what is required.

When we measure visual acuity, our standard procedure is to begin with a large target and quickly proceed to smaller targets, until the patient cannot recognize the optotype. We force the patient to fail. This procedure works well with most typical children who are motivated and love to show how good their eyes are. The more difficult the task becomes, the harder the child will try. Children with DS are usually sensitive to failure and behave quite differently. Generally, the more difficult the task becomes, the less inclined the child with DS is to try and the more likely he or she is to become distracted or uncooperative. Our methodology of visual acuity assessment requires adaptation for a child with DS. The practitioner needs to progress more gradually, using plenty of easy targets to build confidence. Optometrists need to use significant amounts of praise throughout the examination. We might consider interspersing the difficult tasks with easier ones. And it is important to always end on a good note, with the final task being successful, by going back to a really easy optotype.

Overall, a person with DS processes information and reacts to this information more slowly than an individual without DS. An examination can take longer, so we should schedule these patients appropriately. However, if the patient requires primarily objective examination procedures (5), the evaluation time could be quite brief. Trying to rush a person with DS is often counterproductive since he or she may become confused and frightened during the assessment. Another strategy if necessary is to reappoint the patient to complete the evaluation on another day. (see Chapter 16, Comprehensive Examination Procedures)

OCULOVISUAL ANOMALIES

Refractive Errors Moderate to high refractive errors are much more common in people with DS than in the general population. The reported prevalence depends upon the criteria used. One study that used a control (non-DS) group reported hypermetropia ≥ +2.00 D in 62% (DS) and 16% (non-DS) and myopia ≤ 0.50 D in 8% and 17.2% among 77 children with DS and 151 controls respectively (6). Figure 4-1 shows the distribution of spherical refractions among children and young people.

Astigmatism is also more prevalent. Akinci et al. used a criterion of ≥1.00 DC and reported a prevalence of 60% of the population showing astigmatism in DS compared to only 25% in controls. The prevalence of this astigmatism increases with age (5). This increase was almost entirely due to the development of oblique astigmatism, which was most frequently seen among the older children and adults (7–9).

Since infants with DS have a similar refractive distribution to typically developing infants, the high prevalence of refractive errors in DS is thought to be a failure of emmetropization (10). Refractive errors increase with age among children with DS, while the overall distribution widens,

*See http://www.makaton.org/about/resources.htm for additional information.

†See http://www.signalong.org.uk/.

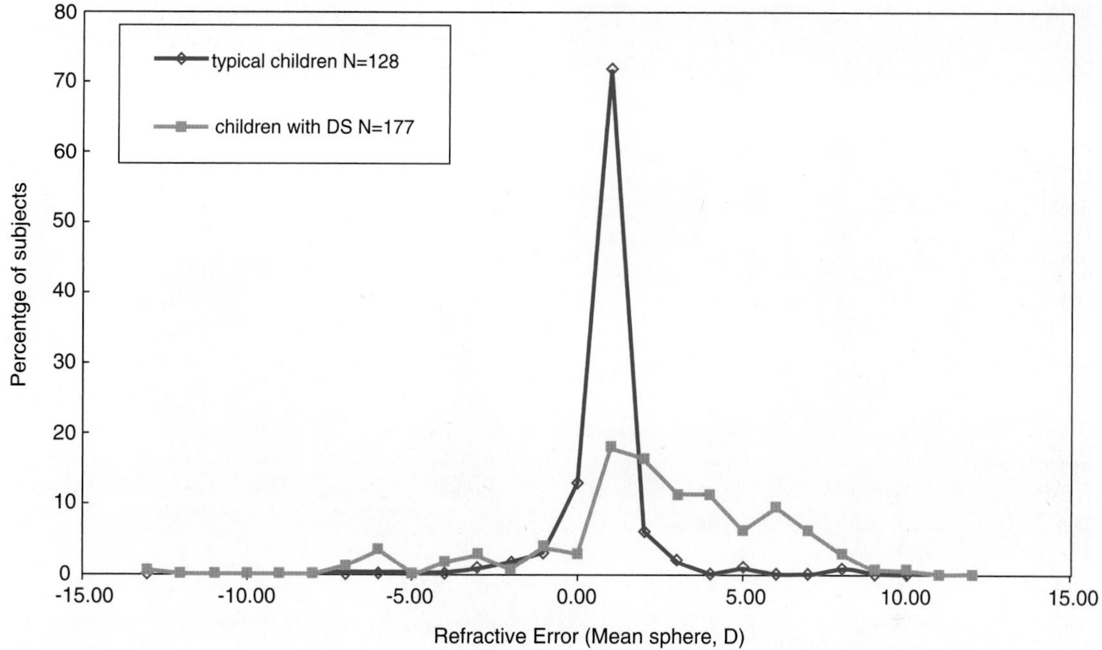

FIGURE 4-1. Distribution of Refractive Error in Control Children (Aged 4–18 Years) and in Children and Young People with DS (Aged 2–25 Years). (Control data courtesy of Julie McLelland and Kathryn Saunders, DS data from Mohammad Al-Bagdady and J Margaret Woodhouse.)

rather than narrows, as it does in children without DS (6,11,12). Biometric measures of the eyes in children with DS show that, as noted for typical children, axial length is related to refractive error. However, the etiology of the emmetropization failure remains a mystery.

Clinical Implications The above prevalence and refractive error distribution (see Figure 4-1) show that hypermetropia is common in DS—more common, in fact, than emmetropia. The average patients with DS will be hypermetropic. The failure in emmetropization indicates that a prescription given to correct hyperopia is often warranted. Most experienced eye care practitioners tend to prescribe spectacles at younger ages for children with DS than for typical children.

Accommodation Studies have shown that children with DS frequently have a deficit in accommodation. This was first proposed by Lindstedt (13) who reported that visual acuity was poorer for near targets than for distance ones. Subsequent measures with dynamic retinoscopy confirmed that 55% to 68% of children with DS have a significant lag of accommodation (14,15) (Figure 4-2). It is important to note that the above measures of accommodation in DS were taken when the subjects' refractive errors were corrected with spectacles. This means that the majority of children with DS are out of focus for near tasks, even when wearing their spectacles. Even more intriguing are the reports that the accommodative lag remains the same for hypermetropic children when they wear their distance spectacle correction. This means that the children relax their accommodation to maintain an out-of-focus error for near tasks. This implies that the accommodative deficit is not due to early presbyopia or an inability to control accommodation, but rather these children appear to have an accommodative anomalous "set point" (13).

Because of their clinical experience, optometrists have recommended using bifocals for children with DS for decades in the United States. Only recently has the research caught up to the clinician and provided evidence that bifocal lenses are a successful intervention for the accommodative deficit present (16,17). Children with DS tolerate the lenses well and *perform significantly better* on school tasks (18). An added positive outcome is that a proportion of these individuals (around 40%) learn how to use their own accommodation accurately while wearing the bifocals. This may allow the individual with DS to be able to return to single-vision lenses at some point (19). This could

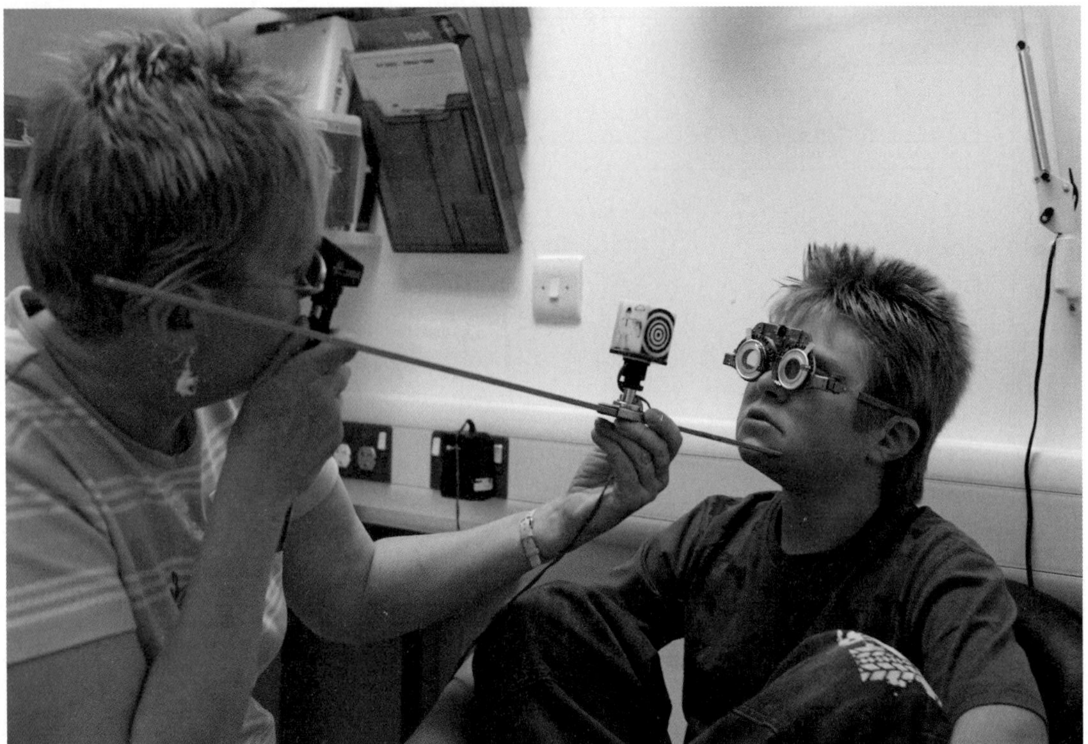

FIGURE 4-2. The Measurement of Accommodation by Dynamic Retinoscopy. Oliver is wearing his distance correction and attending to a detailed picture on the self-illuminated cube. Dr. Woodhouse is recording the position of the retinoscopy neutral point. In Oliver's case, the neutral point is significantly behind the target.

also indicate that a program of active optometric vision therapy emphasizing accommodative activities could be beneficial as well, although at this time no studies have been conducted to suggest this.

Clinical Implications If a child with DS has an accommodative deficit, it appears that smaller amounts of hypermetropia are more detrimental than for a typical child. All practitioners should prescribe for lower levels of hypermetropia and not undercorrect a hyperopic prescription for a child with DS. The correction of only the distance refractive error should be considered insufficient for children (or adults) with DS, since this single-vision solution may not meet the needs for completing near tasks successfully. We must assess and record accommodative function as routinely as we assess and record anomalies of refractive error and eye health. Correcting any deficit present with appropriate spectacles for both distance and near tasks is mandatory for those with DS.

As with typical children, bifocals should be fitted high, with the segment top bisecting the pupil. This bifocal placement may be modified if a deficit of head, neck, and trunk control due to hypotonia interferes with overall function and mobility. Flat top bifocals afford minimum jump and a wide field of view through the segment (Figure 4-3). There are as yet no reports of the use of varifocals for children with DS, but currently there are no reasons known for practitioners to automatically discount their use. Since with these progressive addition lenses the peripheral distortion induced by the manufacturing process may interfere with function, it is important to monitor the child's use of and adaptation to these lenses. All children should also be prescribed polycarbonate lenses for appropriate protection against injury. The use of two pairs of glasses (one for distance and the other for near) is often inappropriate for children with intellectual disability unless it has been shown to be beneficial for specific tasks.

Facial Characteristics and Dispensing Spectacles Children with DS are usually smaller than their age-matched non-DS peers. As far as spectacle fitting is concerned, this does not translate to simply using frames designed for young

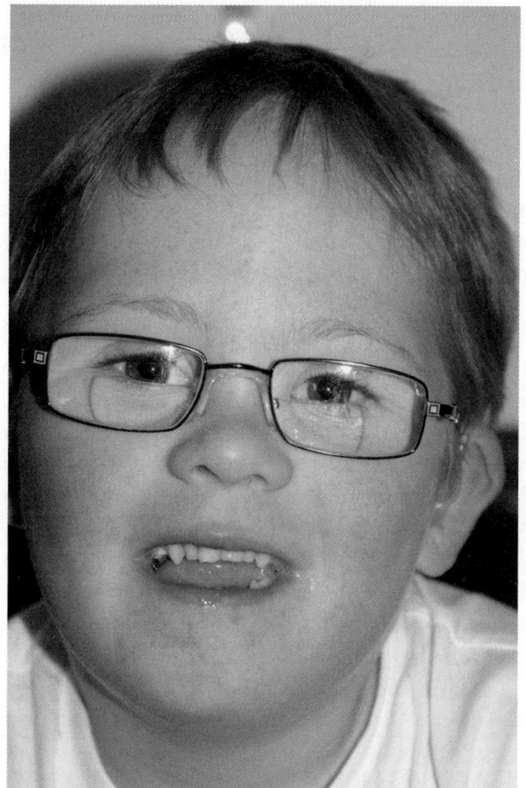

FIGURE 4-3. Five-year-old James has been wearing bifocals on a full-time basis since he was 2 years old.

children. Compared to typical children, young children with DS tend to have a larger head width and older children a shorter interpupillary distance with all ages having a shorter front-to-bend distance (distance from frame's temple joint to the bend of the temple). Bridge projection is particularly small in children with DS. Thus, frames designed for typical children may require substantial modification to fit a child with DS. As practitioners, we must be prepared to put in the time and effort to achieve a good and comfortable fit so our patients can wear and benefit from the spectacles. Frames designed specifically for children with DS are available[‡] and discussed in Chapter 25, Optometric Management of Functional Vision Disorders.

Strabismus Strabismus, or squint, is much more common in children with DS than in typical children. The prevalence has been reported as being between 29% and 42% (5,10,14). All authors agree that esodeviations are much more common than exodeviations and that alternating squints occur more readily than in the general population. There is not necessarily the same association between hypermetropia and strabismus as exists for non-DS children. Children with DS are at risk of strabismus irrespective of their refractive error (10). The strabismus appears to be of a functional etiology and very amenable to treatment by nonsurgical intervention (11).

Clinical Implications Children with DS should be monitored for strabismus whatever their refractive error. In alternating squints, amblyopia is much less likely and patching should be avoided. For children with amblyopia, a shortened patching schedule, as supported by current amblyopia treatment research, may be appropriate. Since those with DS appear to have sensitivity to cycloplegic agents and because of their systemic cardiac and respiratory problems, using atropine in the treatment of amblyopia in this population may not be desirable. This caveat is not universally accepted by all, however. You should also use some caution when instilling eye drops in your patients' eyes and avoid hyperextending the neck because of the possibility of causing an atlantoaxial dislocation (20).

Visual Acuity and Contrast Sensitivity Both visual acuity and contrast sensitivity are poorer in people with DS even in the absence of refractive errors or other ocular defects (21–23). Both of these functions appear equivalent to typical children at early ages but plateau at a younger age in DS, so that the deficits in visual acuity and contrast sensitivity increase with age. Among older children who would normally be expected to score 0.1 LogMAR (20/20 or 6/6) in acuity, a recent study reported an average acuity score of 0.42 LogMAR (20/53 or 6/16) among 14 children with DS wearing appropriate refractive corrections (23).

These deficits are not attributable to low confidence or poor compliance with testing (18). These factors can of course contribute to reduced visual acuity and contrast sensitivity if the practitioner uses inappropriate procedures. The etiology of the poor vision is yet to be established, although at least where acuity is concerned, optical factors appear to be implicated (24).

Clinical Implications As mentioned earlier, the practitioner should ensure that the testing procedure is right for the child (and the test used recorded with

[‡]For additional information concerning frames please go to http://www.specs4us.com/index.html.

appropriate notation concerning its result reliability). School staff, teachers/educators, and all who care for the patient should be made aware of any deficit in vision, and advice should be given on modifications to learning materials and if adaptations are needed when engaging in various activities (physical education, reading, etc.). For example, a child with DS may find it much easier to write in pen rather than pencil, or the teacher may need to make sure that the lines on the paper are readily visible. Text used for reading may need to be enlarged as well.

It is important that any difficulties a child experiences in school give rise first of all to the question, "Does the child have single, clear, comfortable, binocular, and pathology-free vision?" Only when that has been answered in the affirmative should the teacher ask, "Is the intellectual disability causing the problem?"

Blepharitis All eye care practitioners are familiar with this common condition of the lid margins. Up to 47% of those with DS have been noted to have blepharitis. The management of blepharitis should be aggressive with appropriate follow-up given (25). (Management is discussed in Chapter 22, Diagnosis and Treatment of Commonly Diagnosed Ocular Health Anomalies.)

Cataract Congenital cataract, although rare in DS, occurs more commonly than in the general population (26). Among older children and adults, the prevalence is difficult to establish. This is partly due to differences among studies in the criteria used for reporting cataract and also due to the differences in the age range of groups studied. As with the non-DS population, the prevalence of cataract increases with age. There is general agreement that cataracts appear earlier in people with DS. In the general population of 45- to 64-year-olds, the prevalence of cataract is 2% to 8%; in DS, it has been reported as 17% (27). One suggestion for the cause of the high prevalence of cataract in DS is the increased concentration of free radicals due to augmented enzyme activity associated with the trisomy (28). Although the research on this varies, if free radicals due to increased enzyme activity are causative for cataracts, then nutritional supplementation for people with DS may be beneficial in reducing cases of cataract (25,29). There are few long-term studies that have assessed outcomes for postcataract surgery for those with DS. At least one 25-year follow-up study involving 25 infants notes that complications such as glaucoma, a large-magnitude myopic shift, posterior capsular opacification, and retinal detachments may be more frequently encountered (30).

Keratoconus Keratoconus is a degenerative condition of the cornea in which the cornea thins and steepens. The prevalence is approximately 0.05% in the general population, but in those with DS, it may occur in 15% to 30% of individuals (22,31). The condition begins during adolescence and usually stabilizes by the late twenties. It leads to myopia and high amounts of astigmatism and distorted vision that cannot be satisfactorily corrected with spectacles, leading to permanent visual impairment. It is usually well managed in the general population with contact lenses, and practitioners should not discount contact lenses on the grounds of an individual having DS. There are cases of people with DS wearing contact lenses very successfully (Figure 4-4). However, if contact lenses are not offered or not successful, the condition can be visually disabling.

Until recently, the only medical treatment for keratoconus has been corneal transplants in the late stages of the disease. There has, therefore, been no urgency for early diagnosis of the condition. Now there are therapies becoming available that can halt progression of the disease and prevent further deterioration of vision, if applied in the early stages (Chapter 22, Diagnosis and Treatment of Commonly Diagnosed Ocular Health Anomalies). It is increasingly important that keratoconus be diagnosed early. And therein lays a challenge. A keratoconic cornea is thinner and steeper than a normal cornea and with an increasing likelihood of irregular astigmatism. In DS, the cornea is, on average, thinner and steeper than

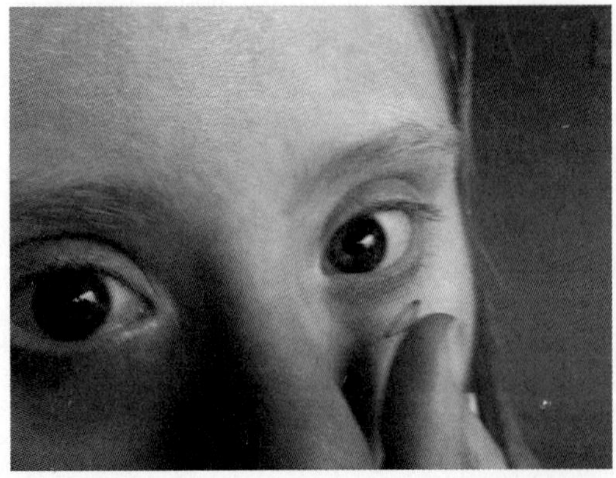

FIGURE 4-4. Charlotte, who is now 18, is a successful contact lens wearer for her keratoconus.

in the general population, and regular astigmatism is prevalent. In young people with DS (14 to 26 years) the average corneal thickness is 480 μm and with keratometry readings noted as 46.39 D, compared with 550 μm and 43.41 D in the non-DS population (32). It is also noted that for therapy to be viable, it must be instituted before the cornea thins to <400 μm. Early diagnosis, then, is more urgent than for a non-DS individual. When those who wore PMMA hard contact lenses developed keratoconus, a suggested etiology was the mechanical rubbing of the contact lens and the cornea. It has been speculated that if blepharitis results in an individual with DS constantly rubbing the eyes, in conjunction with the noted corneal structural changes associated with DS, then this may be a possible etiology for the development of keratoconus. This association of eye rubbing and keratoconus has not been noted in some non-DS populations, however (33).

Nystagmus The most recent reports of the prevalence of nystagmus in DS range from 10% to 22% (7,34,35). In the general population, the prevalence is around 0.001%. Only one study appears to have classified the type of nystagmus present, with a latent/manifest latent nystagmus being the most commonly encountered form. This study only had seven individuals, however.

Clinical Implications Nystagmus should be taken every bit as seriously in a patient with DS as in a nondisabled patient. Too often the nystagmus is considered as part of DS and the inevitable visual impairment neglected. Any patient with nystagmus should be supported by available local resources (e.g., visual impairment teachers in education) regardless of the associated condition. If the nystagmus appears to be acquired and not congenital, a comprehensive neurologic evaluation should be considered.

Brushfield Spots These spots are discrete areas of hypoplasia in the peripheral iris that appears as pale spots. They are frequently seen in young children with DS, even more so for children with light irides, and usually disappear with age. They are of no visual consequence whatsoever and are given unwarranted attention in older texts about DS (along with slanting palpebral fissures). Some parents notice the spots and ask about them, so practitioners should be aware of their presence and provide reassurance to concerned parents.

Fundus Appearance The fundus can have an unexpected appearance in patients with DS. Practitioners who lack experience working with patients who have DS need to be aware of this, in order to determine normality from abnormality. In general, blood vessels tend to bifurcate early at the optic nerve head, and there are more blood vessels on the fundus surface. A recent study reported an average of 15 vessels in young people with DS compared with 11 in controls. Further, the disc is slightly larger in those with DS, even when the eyes are matched for axial length (38). It has also been noted that retinal pigment epithelial disturbances are often seen at the disc margins (2). Peripapillary atrophy is very common. Fundus pigmentation is lessened, which gives the eyes in patients with DS a myopic appearance irrespective of the refractive error (31). Figure 4-5 shows the fundus appearance of one young people with DS who are both low hyperopes.

CONCLUSION

The familiar ophthalmic disorders of refractive error and strabismus are frequently seen in those with DS. In addition, defective accommodation, which is often overlooked in children with DS, has a very high prevalence. Because DS is associated with intellectual disability, visual difficulties may not be reported by the patient. This decrease of reported symptoms by patients with special needs has been noted in other populations as well (39). All too often, when a person struggles to carry out a task, caregivers, teachers, and health care providers may assume that the problem reflects the intellectual disability rather than decreased visual function. It is essential that all people with DS are provided frequent eye and vision examinations. Those with DS have a high incidence of visually disabling pathology and functional anomalies that if diagnosed and treated early will lead to an improvement in the person's quality of life. The need for eye care for this population remains lifelong.

The eye care practitioner should become familiar with the particular strengths and challenges of those with DS and modify the usual eye examination routine as is required (4). There is no reason why an eye examination and its often quality of life improving outcomes should not be as successful for a patient with DS as it is for the non-DS individual.

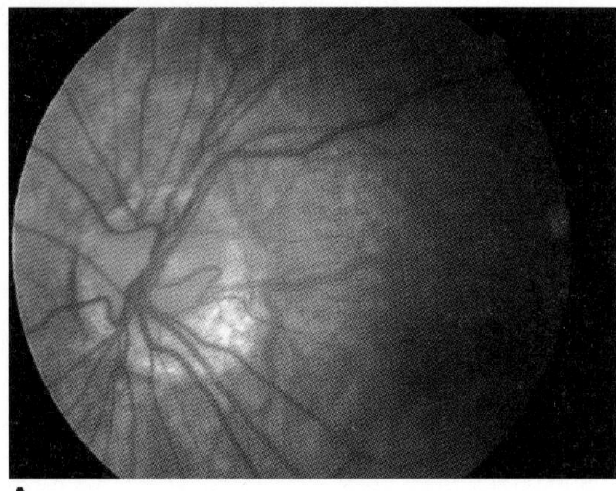
A

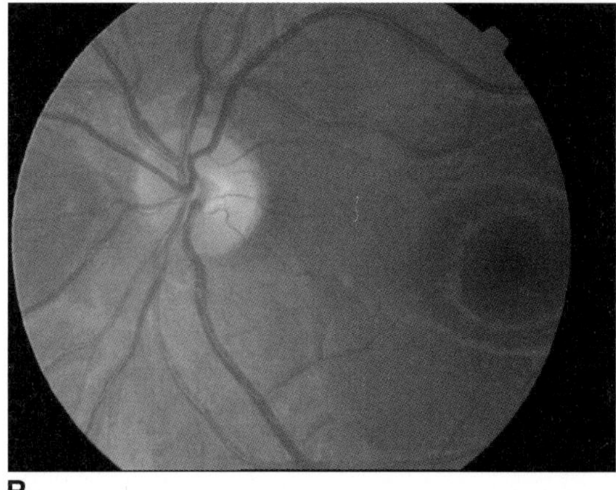
B

FIGURE 4-5. The fundus of **(A)** a young person with DS and **(B)** a control. Both subjects have low hypermetropia (See also Color Section).

REFERENCES

1. National Down Syndrome Society. Available from: www.ndss.org/index.php?option=com_content&view=article&id=54&Itemid=74. Last Accessed June 6, 2011.
2. About Down Syndrome. Available from: www.about-down-syndrome.com/down-syndrome-statistics.html. Last Accessed August 7, 2011.
3. National Down Syndrome. Available from: Society.www.ndss.org/index.php?option=com_content&view=article&id=54&Itemid=74. Last Accessed June 6, 2011.
4. Wesson M, Maino D. Oculo-visual findings in Down syndrome, cerebral palsy, and mental retardation with non-specific etiology. In: Maino D, editor. Diagnosis and management of special populations. St. Louis, MO: Mosby-Yearbook, Inc.; 1995. p. 17–54.
5. Schlange D, Maino D. Clinical behavioral objectives: assessment techniques for special populations. In: Maino D, editor. Diagnosis and management of special populations. St. Louis, MO: Mosby-Yearbook, Inc.; 1995. p. 151–88.
6. Arsen Akinci, MD; Ozgur Oner, MD; Ozlem Hekim Bozkurt, MD; Alev Guven, MD; Aydan Degerliyurt, MD; Kerim Munir, MD, MPH, DSc. Refractive errors and strabismus in children with Down syndrome: a controlled study. J Pediatr Ophthalmol Strabismus. 2009;46:83–6.
7. Al-Bagdady M, Murphy P, Woodhouse JM. Development and distribution of refractive error in children with Down's syndrome. Br J Ophthalmol. 2011;95:1091–7.
8. Doyle SJ, Bullock J, Gray C, Spencer A, Cunningham C. Emmetropisation, axial length, and corneal topography in teenagers with Down's syndrome. Br J Ophthalmol. 1998;82:793–6.
9. Little JA, Woodhouse JM, Saunders KJ. Corneal power and astigmatism in Down syndrome. Optom Vis Sci. 2009; 86:748–54.
10. Woodhouse JM, Pakeman VH, Cregg M, Saunders KJ, Parker M, Fraser WI, Sastry P, Lobo S. Refractive errors in young children with Down syndrome. Optom Vis Sci 1997;74:844–51.
11. Cregg M, Woodhouse JM, Stewart RE, Pakeman VH, Bromham NR, Gunter HL, Trojanowska L, Parker M, Fraser WI. Development of refractive error and strabismus in children with Down syndrome. Invest Ophthalmol Vis Sci. 2003; 44:1023–30.
12. Haugen OH, Hovding G, Lundstrom I. Refractive development in children with Down's syndrome: a population based, longitudinal study. Br J Ophthalmol. 2001;85:714–19.
13. Lindstedt E. Failing accommodation in cases of Down's syndrome. A preliminary report. Ophthal Paediatr Genet. 1983;3:191–2.
14. Cregg M, Woodhouse JM, Pakeman VH, Saunders KJ, Gunter HL, Parker M, Fraser WI, Sastry P. Accommodation and refractive error in children with Down syndrome: cross sectional and longitudinal studies. Investigative Ophthalmol Vis Sci. 2001;42:55–63.
15. Haugen OH, Hovding G. Strabismus and binocular function in children with Down syndrome: A population-based, longitudinal study. Acta Ophthalmol Scand. 2001;79:133–9.
16. Nandakumar K, Leat SJ. Bifocals in Down Syndrome Study (BiDS): design and baseline visual function. Optomet Vis Sci. 2009;86:196–207.
17. Nandakumar K, Leat SJ. Bifocals in children with Down syndrome (BiDS)—visual acuity, accommodation and early literacy skills. Acta Ophthalmol. 2010;88:e196–e204.
18. Stewart RE, Woodhouse JM, Trojanowska LD. In focus: the use of bifocals for children with Down's syndrome. Ophthalmic Physiol Opt. 2005;25:514–22.
19. Al-Bagdady M, Stewart RE, Watts P, Murphy PJ, Woodhouse JM. Bifocals and Down's syndrome: correction or treatment? Ophthalmic Physiol Opt. 2009;29:416–21.
20. Nucci P, de Pellegrin M, Brancato R. Atlantoaxial dislocation related to instilling eyedrops in a patient with Down's syndrome. Am J Ophthalmol. 1996;122:908–10.
21. Courage ML, Adams RJ, Hall EJ. Contrast sensitivity in infants and children with Down syndrome. Vision Res. 1997;37:1545–55.
22. Courage ML, Adams RJ, Reyno S, Kwa PG. Visual acuity in infants and children with Down syndrome. Dev Med Child Neurol. 1994;36:586–93.

23. John FM, Bromham NR, Woodhouse JM, Candy TR. Spatial vision deficits in infants and children with Down syndrome. Invest Ophthalmol Vis Sci. 2004;45:1566–72.
24. Little JA, Woodhouse JM, Lauritzen JS, Saunders KJ. The impact of optical factors on resolution acuity in children with Down syndrome. Invest Ophthalmol Vis Sci. 2007;48:3995–4001.
25. Shapiro M, France T. The ocular features of Down's syndrome. Am J Ophthalmol. 1985;99:659–63.
26. Kallen B, Mastroiacovo P, Robert E. Major congenital malformations in Down syndrome. Am J Med Genet. 1996;65: 160–6.
27. Puri BK, Singh I. Prevalence of cataract in adults Down's syndrome patients aged 28 to 83 years. Clin Pract Epidemiol Ment Health. 2007;3:26–9.
28. Cengiz M, Seven M, Suyugul N. Antioxidant system in Down syndrome: a possible role in cataractogenesis. J Genet Couns 2002;13:339–42.
29. Ellis JM, Hooi KT, Gilbert RE, Muller DPR, Henley W, Moy R, Pumphrey R, Ani C, Davies S, Edwards V, Green H, Salt A, Logan S. Supplementation with antioxidants and folinic acid for children with Down's syndrome: randomized controlled trial. Br Med J. 2008;336:594–7.
30. Gardiner C, Lanigan B, O'Keefe M. Postcataract surgery outcome in a series of infants and children with Down syndrome. Br J Ophthalmol. 2008;92:1112–6.
31. Hestnes A, Sand T, Fostad K. Ocular findings in Down's syndrome. J Ment Defic Res. 1991;35:194–203.
32. Haugen OH, Hovding G, Eide GE. Biometric measurements of the eyes in teenagers and young adults with Down syndrome. Acta Ophthalmol Scand. 2001;79:616–25.
33. Millodot M, Shneor E, Albou S, Atlani E, Gordon-Shaag A. Prevalence and associated factors of keratoconus in Jerusalem: a cross-sectional study. Ophthalmic Epidemiol. 2011;18: 91–7.
34. Kim JH, Hwang J-M, Kim HJ, Yu YS. Characteristic ocular findings in Asian children with Down syndrome. Eye. 2002;16:710–4.
35. Tsiaras WG, Pueschel S, Keller C, Curran R, Giesswein S. Amblyopia and visual acuity in children with Down's syndrome. Br J Ophthalmol. 1999;83:1112–4.
36. Ahmad A, Pruett RC. The fundus in mongolism. Arch Ophthalmol. 1976;94:772–6.
37. Williams EJ, McCormick AQ, Tischler B. Retinal vessels in Down's syndrome. Arch Ophthalmol. 1973;89:269–71.
38. Ji P, Woodhouse JM, Watts PO, Morgan JE. Properties of the fundus and optic disc in children with Down syndrome. Invest Ophthalmol Vis Sci. 2005;46:E-Abstract 4116.
39. Donati RJ, Maino DM, Bartell H, Kieffer M. Polypharmacy and the lack of oculo-visual complaints from those with mental illness and dual diagnosis. Optometry. 2009;80: 249–54.

CHAPTER 5

Elizabeth Berry-Kravis, MD, PhD
Dominick M. Maino, OD, MEd, FAAO, FCOVD-A

Fragile X Syndrome

INTRODUCTION AND INCIDENCE

Fragile X syndrome (FXS) is the most frequently encountered inherited cause of intellectual disability (ID) and the most common known genetic cause of autism (accounting for 3%–6% of those with autism). This disorder has an estimated frequency of about 1/2,500 to 1/4,000 (1,2). Males typically display mild to moderate ID, although the level of functioning can vary from intelligence quotients (IQs) in the normal range to severe impairment (3–6). Females typically present with learning disabilities (LD) (especially math disabilities and nonverbal LD) although approximately 25% have ID (3–6). Physical features (5,6) of FXS include prominent ears, macrocephaly, a long face, midfacial hypoplasia, a high arched palate, and loose connective tissue leading to hyperextensible joints, flat feet, and soft velvety skin over the palms. Macroorchidism (enlarged testes) is present in most adult males although this may not be obvious before puberty. Medical problems (5,6) frequently include recurrent ear infections, strabismus, mitral valve prolapse, and seizures.

Males with FXS have characteristic behavioral features including hyperactivity, impulsivity, attention problems, and hyperarousal to sensory stimuli, as well as mood lability and anxiety. Other common behaviors noted are shyness, self-talk, hand flapping, hand biting, and autistic features such as poor eye contact and perseverative language and behavior (3–7). Anxiety disorders are frequently seen in both males and females including generalized anxiety with multiple areas of difficulty such as selective mutism, separation anxiety, and various phobias (3–7). Aggression occurs in at least 30% to 50% of males, most commonly in adolescence.

Females exhibit less frequent but more variable involvement with regard to physical features and medical problems. They often have attention problems, impulsivity, and executive function deficits even when IQ is in the normal range (3–6). Shyness, phobias, and social deficits are also present (3,5,6).

GENETIC ETIOLOGY AND CELLULAR MECHANISMS

Fragile X syndrome results from a trinucleotide (cytosine, guanine, guanine, or CGG) repeat expansion mutation of >200 repeats (full mutation) in the promoter of the Fragile X mental retardation 1 (*FMR1*) gene. This leads to methylation and transcriptional silencing of the *FMR1* promoter and consequent absence or significant reduction of expression of the gene product, fragile X mental retardation protein (FMRP). Fragile X mental retardation protein is an mRNA-binding protein involved in the dendritic transport, localization, and translational regulation of up to several hundred mRNAs coding for key synaptic proteins. Hence, FMRP is thought to regulate translation at the dendrite in response to neural activation, thereby modulating synaptic plasticity and dendritic morphology (8,9).

The *FMR1* full mutation is always inherited from the mother, who may carry a full mutation, or a smaller FMR1 expansion with 55 to 200 repeats (normal is <45), termed a premutation. The premutation can be inherited in families for many generations before expanding to the full mutation. It is not associated with *FMR1* methylation, loss of FMRP expression, or typical FXS, but can be associated with fragile X–associated tremor/ataxia syndrome (FXTAS, about 50% of premutation carriers, predominantly males) (10) or fragile X–associated primary ovarian insufficiency (FXPOI, about 20% of premutation carrier females) (11). Some premutation carriers have subtle evidence of features that overlap those seen in

FXS including emotional problems (anxiety, social deficits, obsessive thinking, and/or depression) (10). A small subgroup of carriers with a larger premutation have mild cognitive disorders and various features of FXS, likely due to mild reduction of FMRP levels observed with large premutation alleles (10).

Because *FMR1* is located on the X chromosome, females with a full mutation are variably affected and typically less affected than males. Severity of cognitive impairment and behavioral symptoms in females with FXS and the full mutation is inversely related to the activation ratio for the normal *FMR1* allele and the level of FMRP. Likewise in males with a full mutation and mosaicism for an unmethylated allele, severity of the cognitive disorder is related to the percent of methylated DNA and the amount of reduction of FMRP levels (12).

Because of the complex inheritance patterns of *FMR1* and multiple potential conditions (termed Fragile X–associated disorders [FXD], which includes FXS, FXTAS, and FXPOI) that may be segregating in FXS families, genetic counseling is recommended whenever any FXD is diagnosed (3,5,6). For families with a child with FXS, or known carrier females, reproductive and family planning options include prenatal testing by amniocentesis or chorionic villus sampling, in vitro fertilization followed by preimplantation genetic diagnosis, egg donation, and adoption.

MEDICAL ISSUES AND TREATMENT

In addition to the cognitive and behavioral deficits that are the main features of FXS, there are a number of medical problems associated with FXS in males that may require monitoring and management. These include gastroesophageal reflux and failure to thrive in early infancy, recurrent otitis media, and sinusitis. Other systemic anomalies include eye and vision problems, mitral valve prolapse, seizures, sleep disorders, orthopedic issues, and dental malocclusions (3,5,6). These problems occur more frequently in FXS than in the general population, and many are thought to be due to mild dysfunction of connective tissue. Most of the medical problems described in males with FXS have also been seen in females, although their presence is much more variable.

Gastrointestinal Clinically significant symptoms of gastroesophageal reflux are reported in 31% of infants with FXS, and some of these infants show signs of failure to thrive (5,6). If FXS is diagnosed in infancy, these symptoms should be screened carefully, diagnostic studies performed, and treatment with antacids and thickened feeds implemented, if needed.

Ear/Nose/Throat Recurrent otitis media is seen in about 60% of boys with FXS (5,6). To avoid fluctuating conductive hearing loss, which might add to language and cognitive deficits, it is essential to monitor and manage this problem aggressively with prophylactic antibiotics and myringotomy tubes if hearing loss is documented. Predisposition to otitis media in FXS is thought to be due to poor drainage of the middle ear, likely related to the facial structure and a more collapsible eustachian tube. Recurrent sinusitis has been reported in 23% of males with FXS. This may also be related to facial structure and can require prophylactic antibiotics or surgical drainage (5,6).

Orthopedic Abnormalities Flexible pes planus (flat feet), excessive joint laxity, and scoliosis are the most common orthopedic problems in FXS (5,6). Treatment of pes planus with a foot orthosis or shoe inserts may result in improved gait pattern and shoe wear for some patients.

Hypotonia and Motor Incoordination Hypotonia is frequent and varies in severity from normal tone to very low tone, and can affect feeding and swallowing (5). This problem is managed with an individualized therapy program involving physical, occupational, and speech/feeding therapy. Hypotonia improves with age, evolving into a centrally mediated coordination and praxis disorder involving both gross and fine motor functions (5). Fine motor incoordination negatively affects daily functioning, and occupational therapy is required to improve fine motor skills and facilitate adaptive strategies at home and at school. In conjunction with the occupational therapist, optometrists may want to initiate a program of optometric vision therapy to improve hand–eye coordination, oculomotor, and other functional visual skills as well.

Cardiac Abnormalities Mitral valve prolapse has been reported in 22% to 77% of adult males with FXS (5,6) along with other findings of mild aortic and pulmonary root dilatation, and tricuspid septal leaflet prolapse. These findings are much less common in children with FXS (10%), suggesting that they develop during adolescence and early adulthood, and can lead to valvular insufficiency. All children with FXS should have careful cardiac auscultation during each examination, followed by echocardiography if a click or a murmur is present.

Sleep Problems Sleep problems are extremely common in children with FXS (13) and in most cases probably result from poor sleep regulation and difficulty maintaining sleep. In cases with suspicious events associated with sleep disruption, nocturnal seizures should be ruled out. Sleep apnea, snoring, congestion, and mouth breathing are common complaints. Obstructive apnea may be due to oromotor hypotonia, floppy connective tissue blocking the airway, or problems with secretion clearance. Tonsillectomy and/or adenoidectomy may resolve symptoms in these individuals. In patients with difficulty falling asleep and midnight awakenings, melatonin treatment can be quite helpful.

Obesity A subgroup of males with FXS has hyperphagia and obesity beginning in early to midchildhood, with a physical phenotype similar to Prader-Willi syndrome (PWS), but with negative molecular testing for 15q11 abnormalities. This is described as the Prader-Willi phenotype (PWP) of FXS (14). Treatment for children with FXS, obesity, and the PWP includes consultation and follow-up with a dietitian, regular physical exercise, environmental modifications such as locking the kitchen or cupboards, and intensive dietary programs such as those developed for PWS (3). Aggressive screening and treatment of complications of obesity such as hypertension, type II diabetes, dyslipidemias, and obstructive sleep apnea is required. Additionally, psychopharmacologic and anticonvulsant medications that are less likely to precipitate weight gain should be utilized.

Seizures Seizures occur in about 15% of males and 6% to 8% of females (15). In general, the risk of epilepsy onset appears to be highest in childhood. The peak incidence of epilepsy occurs between the ages of 4 to 10 years (15). Many individuals also have abnormal electroencephalography findings without apparent overt epileptic seizures. Electroencephalography abnormalities frequently appear to resemble those observed in childhood epilepsy with centrotemporal spikes (16,17) with complex partial seizures being the most common seizure type (15–17). A wide range of seizure types has been reported in FXS, however, and simple partial, febrile convulsions, and generalized tonic clonic seizures can occur. Status epilepticus has been reported, but is relatively rare (16).

The majority of individuals show resolution of their epilepsy during childhood (15,17). Although the type of seizures do not seem to predict seizure remission, the centrotemporal spikes pattern appears to be an excellent prognostic factor for remission of epilepsy. A presence of seizures seems to be an indicator of an increased risk for autism in FXS (15).

When treatment is required (typically after two clinical seizures have occurred), seizures in FXS are for the most part easily controlled with a single anticonvulsant medication (3,5,15,17). Since FXS is associated with hypotonia, loose connective tissue, and cognitive and behavioral problems, all of these issues should be taken into account when considering choice of medication. Side effects that exacerbate hypotonia, clumsiness, cognitive dulling, and daytime sedation are particularly undesirable. Historically, most individuals with FXS have been well controlled with carbamazepine or valproic acid with fairly limited side effects. More recently, lamotrigine (Lamictal), oxcarbazapine (Trileptal), zonisamide (Zonegran), and levetiracetam (Keppra) have proven to be effective potential anticonvulsant choices and have the advantage of minimal cognitive side effects. Since managing dental issues in these children can be difficult, phenytoin is avoided due to the side effects of gum hypertrophy and tissue overgrowth. Phenobarbital and gabapentin should also be avoided because they exacerbate behavioral problems. It has been noted that on occasion levetiracetam may worsen irritability and aggressive behavior as well. As a wide range of anticonvulsants with good safety profiles are now available, individuals who are not attaining control or are having a significant side effect should be switched to reasonable alternative preparations. It should also be noted that though immunizations may be given at a time of risk for individuals predisposed to seizures, the epilepsy or autism risks are not a contraindication to a standard immunization schedule.

Ocular, Visual, and Vision Information Processing For more than two decades, clinical studies have noted an increased presence of eye and vision problems in those with FXS when compared to the general population with 25% or more having significant oculovisual anomalies (18–24). Initially, it was noted that strabismus could be found in 30% to 50% of the population, but later prospective studies noted a lower, but still significant incidence of 8% (25). The true prevalence at different ages awaits further studies currently in progress. Most studies showed that esotropia was more prevalent than exotropia with up to 70% of those with strabismus having esotropia. Maino et al. noted that this strabismus did not appear to be accommodative in nature (20). Although the etiology of the strabismus is unknown, research on the *Xenopus laevis* (an African clawed frog) shows that the loss of *FMR1* or *FXR1* (a highly homologous fragile X–related gene) results in abnormal eye and neural crest development (26). This could play a role in the high incidence of strabismus in the FXS population.

Significant refractive error has also been reported with one study finding up to 59% of the eyes evaluated showing hyperopia of +1.00 D or greater, 17% myopia of −1.00 D or greater, and 22% with at least 1.00 D of astigmatism (20). Another study noted that 17% of the sample had significant refractive errors (25). The assessment of visual acuity in this population often proves to be quite challenging. Those that can be evaluated should show age-expected levels of visual acuity unless the individual has other complicating factors such as nystagmus.

There have been no studies that have assessed functional vision attributes such as the lag, facility, amplitude and/or stability of accommodation, or near point of convergence. Nor has stereopsis, positive and negative fusional ranges or fusion facility been determined. Objective assessments of oculomotor skills (pursuits, saccades) have also not been reported in the literature. A few case reports hint that these areas may also be adversely affected in the FXS (20,24). The color vision abilities of individuals with FXS appear unaffected (27). The presence of any consistent ocular health anomalies has not been reported.

Initially, case studies noted vision information processing problems that included mild to severe dysfunctions in visual motor integration, laterality/directionality, visual figure ground, visual closure, visual form constancy, visual memory, and visual sequential memory. Later studies have shown that full mutation female carriers performed more poorly in visual–motor processing and on various subtests of the test of visual-perceptual skills (24,28). This impairment in visual motion processing indicates that various neurologic functions of the parietal lobe are affected. Abnormal magnocellular input into the lateral geniculate nucleus (LGN) appears to account for this deficit. Research also suggests that the loss of a single-gene product, FMRP, in these individuals results in an abnormal neurological and anatomical morphology of the LGN and a visual deficit of the magnocellular pathway (29,30). The processing of visual information, visual perception, and related areas needs additional research before we will be able to fully understand the diagnostic and treatment needs of those with FXD.

Fragile X individuals share many traits with those on the autistic spectrum. Although our knowledge of the etiology of FXS is fairly well understood, that cannot be said for autism (31). The sharing of traits between autism and FXS may be due to similar anatomical and physiological changes (32) within the brain of the two disorders, but additional research needs to be completed in this area for confirmation.

The diagnosis and management of oculovisual anomalies of those with FXS may require similar approaches as those used for children on the autism spectrum (33,34). Information on how to diagnose the eye and vision problems of special populations can be found in multiple sources (35–37), including Chapter 16, Comprehensive Examination Procedures.

Cognitive Function and Educational Interventions Children with FXS are typically identified due to presentation due to delays in development and speech. As soon as the diagnosis is made, the child should be referred to early intervention to maximize developmental potential. The average IQ for males is 40 to 50 (3,5,6), with an adult mental age of about 5 to 6 years, and adaptive and achievement skills somewhat higher than IQ measures. Intelligence quotient may measure higher in young boys and decline during midchildhood due to poor acquisition of abstraction and complex processing skills relative to typically developing children (5,6). Males have a characteristic cognitive profile with strengths in receptive vocabulary, grammatical structure, visual memory, simultaneous processing, experiential learning, and imitation. Weaknesses are seen in auditory processing, sequential processing, and mathematical and quantitative skills. Other weaknesses noted include abstraction, visuospatial and constructional ability, as well as working memory, executive function, attention, coordination, and praxis (5,38). Females have similar patterns of strengths and weaknesses, but these are quantitatively not as severe. The average IQ in females is about 80. Females can have a normal IQ but demonstrate executive or nonverbal LD. Knowledge of the FXS characteristic cognitive profile allows educational programming to be tailored to enhance learning by capitalizing on strengths (e.g., visual presentation of information and instructions, reading programs based on visual memory instead of phonics) and minimize weaknesses (e.g., one auditory direction at a time, minimize distractions, assistive technology for writing) (36). In addition, speech therapy, occupational therapy, optometric vision therapy, and a socialization program with social skills training should be part of the supportive programming throughout the school years for children with FXS.

Behavioral Problems and Treatment The behavioral phenotype of FXS involves multiple domains of dysfunction, many of which can be ameliorated with supportive medical treatment. Most of the experience with medication use in FXS described in this section is from medication surveys and clinical experience. There is a tremendous need for controlled trials to confirm efficacy and safety, particularly for long-term use.

Autistic Features Many boys with FXS (50%–90%) display autistic behavioral patterns, particularly avoidant and anxious behaviors. Approximately 18% to 36% meet formal criteria for autistic disorder (4), and approximately 43% to 67% of individuals have an autism spectrum disorder (ASD) (4). The percentage of ASD in females, however, is lower (20%–23%) (4). Patterns of social deficits may differ somewhat from those with autism even in FXS individuals who meet the criteria for ASD. Individuals with FXS often have strong social interest, but high levels of social anxiety, deficits in peer entry, and poor understanding of social cues.

Autism is a major concern in FXS because it is associated with more severe impairment of social interactions and lower cognitive ability, academic achievement, adaptive behavior, and language ability than what is seen with FXS without autism or ASD alone (4). Although, we do not know why some individuals with FXS also have autism and others do not, it has been suggested there may be secondary gene effects additive to the *FMR1* mutation that lead to the development of autism (4).

Attention Deficit Hyperactivity Disorder Symptoms Relative to other genetic conditions or to individuals with nonspecific ID, the prevalence of Attention Deficit Hyperactivity Disorder (ADHD) symptoms in children with FXS is higher. In addition to behavioral intervention and individualized therapies, stimulants have been shown to improve symptoms of ADHD in FXS (3,7,39). These studies indicate that stimulants are the most frequently used class of medication in boys with FXS (3,7), helping up to 70% of the patients (7).

Treatment of ADHD symptoms in younger children (<5 years) is particularly challenging. Stimulants may induce irritability and other behavioral problems in these young children, so other nonstimulant medications may be used (3,7,40). Alpha-adrenergic agonists, including clonidine or guanfacine, appear to be helpful in 60% to 70% of patients (3,7,38) and seem to be most effective for hyperactivity and overstimulation in younger children or those more neurologically involved who do not do well with stimulants (7,39). Clonidine can also be beneficial for those who have sleep disturbances.

Anxiety Symptoms Selective serotonin reuptake inhibitors (SSRIs) can be helpful more than 50% of the time in relieving anxiety and related problems (4,41). Activation can occur with SSRIs in approximately 20% of individuals (40) manifested by restlessness, mood changes, and disinhibited behaviors including aggression. Fluoxetine may be the most activating and is not the SSRI of choice for hyperactive patients, but can be useful for individuals with social anxiety, autism, or selective mutism (3,7). Selective serotonin reuptake inhibitors can lead to suicidal ideation in depressed patients (although never reported in FXS), so careful monitoring of the patient for mood changes is justified (3).

Aggression and Mood Instability Antipsychotics are used in a clinical setting to target irritability, aggression, mood instability, and perseverative behaviors in both males and females. In a study of a large FXS clinical population, about 80% of individuals with FXS responded to at least one antipsychotic, without side effects requiring withdrawal (3,7). Risperidone (Risperdal) has been the most frequently used antipsychotic and is effective clinically with high response rates for aggressive behavior in older males, and other irritable, aberrant, and undesired behaviors in young boys with autistic traits (7). This is consistent with the finding that risperidone is safe and effective in several double-blind, placebo-controlled trials in individuals with autism who did not have FXS (3), and is now approved by the Federal Drug Administration for treatment of irritability in ASD. More recently, aripiprazole (Abilify) is emerging as the first-choice atypical antipsychotic in FXS, with the highest overall response rate for an individual antipsychotic (~71%), and it presents only a slight concern about weight gain than for risperidone (3,7). Because of its unique pharmacological profile, aripiprazole targets multiple behavior difficulties in FXS including distractibility, anxiety, mood instability, aggression, and aberrant social behaviors.

This medication can be associated with agitation, however. Aripiprazole has also shown effectiveness for irritable behavior in autism and is now approved by the FDA for that indication, and has been shown to show efficacy in FXS in an open label trial (42).

Progress toward Targeted Treatments

Current treatment for FXS is supportive; however, in the past decade, the study of the neurobiology and synaptic mechanisms in FXS has led to identification of dendritic and synaptic targets for therapy directed at the underlying disorder (3,4,7,43). These treatments would be expected to compensate for dysregulation of neural mechanisms brought about by absence of FMRP. Treatment mechanisms proposed to act to reverse excessive dendritic signaling or its downstream consequences in neurons include (a) reducing activity in pathways that transduce signals from group 1 mGluRs or other Gq-linked receptors to the dendritic translational machinery, (b) reducing activity of individual proteins regulated by FMRP, (c) increasing surface AMPA receptors and activity, (d) modifying activity of other receptors/proteins that regulate synaptic activity, and (e) blocking translation of mRNAs regulated by FMRP using antisense technology (4,42). Many of these treatment strategies, particularly mGluR5 blockers, have shown striking reversal of phenotypes in the FXS model mouse and fly and have moved to early-stage human trials (42,44–48). Current ongoing trials involve mGluR5 blockers and gamma-aminobutyric acid agonists, both of which have shown improvement in symptoms in subgroups of patients with FXS (42,46,47).

CONCLUSION

As noted above, the eye care professional should be aware that individuals with FXD have numerous systemic, neurological, psychological, behavioral, oculovisual, and vision information processing dysfunctions. They are often prescribed medications that have potential unwanted ocular side effects. The most frequently reported side effects for many of the drugs discussed include decreased or blurred vision (near or far), visual hallucinations/disturbance, decreased accommodation, and irregularities of the eyelid and/or conjunctiva. All health care providers should know that patients with special needs often do not communicate complaints that would indicate a vision problem or other ocular anomalies induced by medication (49) and be vigilant for unwelcomed outcomes of various treatment regimens. Examination strategies should take into account the various systemic, neurological, psychological, and behavioral anomalies seen in this population, so that the ocular, visual, and vision information processing dysfunctions can be diagnosed and treated in an appropriate manner.

REFERENCES

1. Hagerman PJ. The fragile X prevalence paradox. J Med Genet. 2008;45:498–9.
2. Turner G, Webb T, Wake S, Robinson H. Prevalence of fragile X syndrome. Am J Med Genet. 1996;64:196–7.
3. Hagerman RJ, Berry-Kravis E, Ono MY, Tartaglia N, Lachiewicz A, Kronk B, et al. Advances in the treatment of fragile X syndrome. J Pediatr. 2009;123:378–90
4. Wang LW, Berry-Kravis E, Hagerman RJ. Fragile X: leading the way for targeted treatments in autism. Neurotherapeutics. 2010;7:264–74.
5. Berry-Kravis E, Grossman AW, Crnic LS, Greenough WT. Fragile X syndrome. Curr Pediatr. 2002;12:316–24.
6. Hagerman RJ. Physical and behavioral phenotype. In: Hagerman RJ, Hagerman PJ, editors. Fragile X syndrome: diagnosis, treatment and research. 3rd ed. Baltimore: The Johns Hopkins University Press; 2002. p. 3–109.
7. Berry-Kravis E, Potanos K. Pschopharmacology in fragile X syndrome—present and future. Ment Retard Dev Disabil Res Rev. 2004;10:42–8.
8. Bagni C, Greenough WT. From mRNP trafficking to spine dysmorphogenesis: the roots of fragile X syndrome. Nat Rev Neurosci. 2005;6:376–87.
9. Bassell GJ, Warren ST. Fragile X syndrome: loss of local mRNA regulation alters synaptic development and function. Neuron. 2008;60:201–14.
10. Berry-Kravis E, Abrams L, Coffey S, Hall D, Greco C, Gane L, et al. Fragile X-associated tremor/ataxia syndrome (FXTAS): clinical features, genetics and testing guidelines. Mov Disord. 2007;22:2018–30.
11. Sullivan AK, Marcus M, Epstein MP, Allen EG, Anido AE, Paquin JJ, et al. Association of FMR1 repeat size with ovarian dysfunction. Hum Reprod. 2005;20:402–12.
12. Loesch DZ, Huggins RM, Hagerman RJ. Phenotypic variation and FMRP levels in fragile X. Ment Retard Dev Disabil Res Rev. 2004;10:31–41.
13. Kronk R, Bishop EE, Raspa M, Bickel JO, Mandel DA, Bailey DB Jr. Prevalence, nature, and correlates of sleep problems among children with fragile X syndrome based on a large scale parent survey. Sleep. 2010;33:679–87.
14. Nowicki ST, Tassone F, Ono MY, Ferranti J, Croquette MF, Goodlin-Jones B, et al. The Prader-Willi phenotype of fragile X syndrome. J Dev Behav Pediatr. 2007;28(2):133–8.
15. Berry-Kravis E, Raspa M, Loggin-Hester L, Bishop E, Holiday D, Bailey D. Epilepsy in fragile X syndrome: characteristics and co-morbid diagnoses. Am J Intellect Dev Disabil. 2010;115:461–72.
16. Musumeci SA, Hagerman RJ, Ferri R, Bosco P, Dalla Bernardina B, Tassinari CA, et al. Epilepsy and EEG findings

in males with fragile X syndrome. Epilepsia. 1999;40(8): 1092–9.

17. Berry-Kravis E. Epilepsy in fragile X syndrome. Dev Med Child Neurol. 2002;44:724–8.
18. Storm RL, PeBenito R, Ferretti C. Ophthalmologic findings in the fragile X syndrome. Arch Ophthalmol. 1987 Aug; 105(8):1099–102.
19. Maino D, Schlange D, Maino J, Caden B. Ocular anomalies in fragile X syndrome. J Am Optom Assoc. 1990;61:316–23
20. Maino D, Wesson M, Schlange D, Cibis G, Maino J. Optometric findings in the fragile X syndrome. Optom Vis Sci. 1991;68:634–40.
21. Maino D, King R. Oculo-visual dysfunction in the Fragile X syndrome. In: Hagerman R, McKenzie P, editors. International Fragile X Conference Proceedings. Dillon: Spectra Publishing Co.; 1992. p. 71–8.
22. Martinez S, Maino D. A comprehensive review of the Fragile X syndrome: oculo-visual, developmental, and physical characteristics. J Behav Optom. 1993;4:59–64. Available from: http://www.oepf.org/jbo/journals/4% to 3%20Martinez,%20 Maino.pdf.
23. Dibler LB, Maino DM. Martin-Bell phenotype, Fragile X syndrome, and the very low birth weight child: the differential diagnosis. J Optom Vis Dev. 1994;233–46.
24. Amin V, Maino D. The Fragile X female: visual, visual perceptual, and ocular health anomalies. J Am Optom Assoc. 1995;66(5):290–5.
25. Hatton DD, Buckley E, Lachiewicz A, Roberts J. Ocular status of boys with fragile X syndrome: a prospective study. J AAPOS. 1998 Oct;2(5):298–302.
26. Gessert S, Bugner V, Tecza A, Pinker M, Kühl M. FMR1/ FXR1 and the miRNA pathway are required for eye and neural crest development. Dev Biol. 2010 May 1;341(1):222–35.
27. Finucane BM, Jaeger E, Dunn E, Scott CI Jr. Study of color vision in fragile X syndrome. Am J Med Genet. 1992 Jan 15;42(2):184–6.
28. Block SS, Brusca-Vega R, Pizzi WJ, Berry-Kravis E, Maino DM, Treitman T. Cognitive and visual processing skills and their relationship to mutation size in full and permutation female fragile X carriers. Optom Vis Sci. 2000;77(11):592–9.
29. Kogan CS, Boutet I, Cornish K, Zangenehpour S, Mullen KT, Holden J, et al. Differential impact of the FMR1 gene on visual processing in fragile X syndrome. Brain. 2004;127:591–601.
30. Kogan CS, Bertone A, Cornish K, Boutet I, Der Kaloustian VM, Andermann E, et al. Integrative cortical dysfunction and pervasive motion perception deficit in fragile X syndrome. Neurology. 2004;63:1634–9.
31. Maino DM, Viola, SG, Donati R. The etiology of autism. Optom Vis Dev. 2009:(40)3:150–6 Available from: http://www.covd.org/Portals/0/Article_Etiology%20of%20Autism.pdf.
32. Viola SG, Maino DM. Brain anatomy, electrophysiology and visual function/perception in children within the autism spectrum disorder. Optom Vis Dev. 2009;40(3):157–63. Available from: http://www.covd.org/Portals/0/Article_Children_ASD.pdf.
33. Coulter RA. Understanding the visual symptoms of individuals with autism spectrum disorder (ASD). Optom Vis Dev. 2009;40(3):164–75. Available from: http://www.covd.org/Portals/0/Article_UnderstandingVisualSymp.pdf.
34. Torgerson NG. Insights into optometric evaluations of patients on the autism spectrum. Optom Vis Dev. 2009;40(3): 176–83. Available from: http://www.covd.org/Portals/0/Article_InsightsDiagnosis.pdf.
35. Schlange D, Maino D. Clinical behavioral objectives: assessment techniques for special populations. In: Maino D, editor. Diagnosis and management of special populations. St. Louis: Mosby-Yearbook, Inc.; 1995. p. 151–88.
36. Maino DM, Maino JH, Cibis GW, Hecht F. Ocular health anomalies in patients with developmental disabilities. In: Maino D, editor. Diagnosis and Management of Special Populations. St. Louis: Mosby-Yearbook, Inc.; 1995. p. 189–206.
37. Maino D. Overview of special populations. In: Scheiman M, Rouse M, editors. Optometric management of learning related vision problems. St. Louis; Mosby Inc.: 2006. p. 85–106.
38. Braden ML. Academic interventions. In: Hagerman RJ, Hagerman PJ, editors. Fragile X syndrome: diagnosis, treatment and research. 3rd ed. Baltimore: The Johns Hopkins University Press; 2002. p. 428–64.
39. Hagerman RJ, Murphy MA, Wittenberger MD. A controlled trial of stimulant medication in children with the fragile X syndrome. Am J Med Genet. 1988;30:377–92.
40. Hagerman RJ, Riddle JE, Roberts LS, Brease K, Fulton M. A survey of the efficacy of clonidine in fragile X syndrome. Dev Brain Dysfunct. 1995;8:336–44.
41. Hagerman RJ, Fulton MJ, Leaman A, Riddle J, Hagerman K, Sobesky W. A survey of fluoxetine therapy in fragile X syndrome. Dev Brain Dysfunct. 1994;7:155–64.
42. Erickson CA, Stigler KA, Posey DJ, McDougle CJ. Aripiprazole in autism spectrum disorders and fragile X syndrome. Neurotherapeutics. 2010;7:258–63.
43. Berry-Kravis E, Knox A, Hervey C. Targeted treatments for fragile X syndrome. J Neurodev Disord 2011;3:193–210.
44. Berry-Kravis E, Krause SE, Block SS, Guter S, Wuu J, Leurgans S, et al. Effect of CX516, an AMPA-modulating compound, on cognition and behavior in fragile X syndrome: a controlled trial. J Child Adolesc Psychopharmacol. 2006;16:525–40.
45. Berry-Kravis E, Sumis A, Hervey C, Nelson M, Porges SW, Weng N, et al. Open-label treatment trial of lithium to target the underlying defect in fragile X syndrome. J Dev Behav Pediatr. 2008;29:293–302.
46. Paribello C, Tao L, Folino A, Berry-Kravis E, Tranfaglia M, Ethell I, et al. Open-label add-on treatment trial of minocycline in fragile X syndrome. BMC Neurol. 2010;10:91.
47. Berry-Kravis E, Hessl D, Coffey S, Hervey C, Schneider A, Yuhas J, et al. A pilot open label, single dose trial of fenobam in adults with fragile X syndrome. J Med Genet. 2009;46:266–71.
48. Jacquemont S, Curie A, des Portes V, Berry-Kravis E, Hagerman RJ, Ramos F, Cornish K, He Y, Paulding C, Torrioli MG, Neri G, Chen F, Hadjikhani N, Martinet D, Meyer J, Beckman JS, Delenge K, Brun A, Bussy G, Gasparini F, HIlse T, Floesser A, Branson J, Bilbe G, Johns D, Gomez-Mancilla B. Epigenetic modification of the FMR1 gene in fragile X patients leads to a differential response to the mGluR5antagonist AFQ056. Sci Trans Med 2011;3:64ra1.
49. Donati RJ, Maino DM, Bartell H, Kieffer M. Polypharmacy and the lack of oculo-visual complaints from those with mental illness and dual diagnosis. Optometry. 2009;80:249–54.

CHAPTER 6

Karen A. Kehbein, OD
Marc B. Taub, OD, MS, FAAO, FCOVD

Intellectual Disability of Unknown Etiology

INTRODUCTION

In the past, unacceptable terms such as terms idiot, imbecile, mental retardation, or retarded have been used historically in the literature to describe individuals with intellectual and developmental delay. More recently, the term "intellectual disability" has come into the vernacular. In this chapter, we discuss the history of ID including the various definitions as well as its incidence and prevalence. We also review the more frequently utilized tests that are used to determine developmental levels and intelligence and the related visual issues.

DEFINITION OF INTELLECTUAL DISABILITY

Classification systems emerged because of a need to determine the different causes of and ways to help individuals with ID. Throughout the 19th and 20th centuries, researchers worked to create a classification system for ID. Many of these early classification systems used the mental age of an individual but did not specify any adaptive behavior characteristics (1).

One of the early definitions was created by the Committee on Classification of the Feebleminded, which is formly known as the American Association on Mental Retardation (AAMR) and is now known as the American Association of Intellectual and Developmental Disability (AAIDD). This original definition divided individuals into four categories based on mental age: feebleminded, moron, imbecile, and idiot (1). Since the development of this 1910 definition, the intelligence quotient (IQ) has replaced mental age as an indicator of a person's level of intelligence. In 1961, the AAIDD created the following definition: *Mental Retardation refers to sub-average general intellectual functioning that originates during the developmental period (age 16) and is associated with impairment in adaptive behavior.* This definition allowed for the classification of mental retardation based on intelligence level as well as adaptive behavior ability.

At least four classification systems now exist that define ID. These differ in the emphasis placed upon intelligence versus adaptive behavior. The four systems are the International Classification of Diseases (ICD-10), the Diagnostic and Statistical Manual of Mental Disorders (DSM-IVTR), the AAIDD definition, Classification and Systems of Supports, and the International Classification of Functioning, Disability, and Health (ICF).

The ICD-10 definition says, *Mental retardation is a condition of arrested or incomplete development of the mind, which is especially characterized by impairment of skills manifested during the development period, which contribute to the overall level of intelligence, i.e. cognitive, language, motor and social abilities (2).*Additionally, the definition continues to recognize that adaptive behavior is impaired but to varying degrees. The ICD-10 definition has the following six categories: mild mental retardation, moderate mental retardation, severe mental retardation, profound mental retardation, other mental retardation, and unspecified mental retardation (2). Table 6.1 compares the first four categories. The "other mental retardation" category is used when typical means of assessing ID cannot be used, such as in the case of blind, deaf, or severely behaviorally disturbed individuals. The "unspecified mental retardation category" is used when evidence of mental retardation is insufficient to assign an individual to one of the other categories.

TABLE 6.1 ICD-10 Categories of Mental Retardation

Category	IQ	Etiology	Achievement	Also known as
Mild	50–69	Etiology known in a minority of cases	Full independence in self-care and domestic skills; specially designed education programs to develop skills; may have emotional or social immaturity	Feeblemindedness, moron, mild mental abnormality
Moderate	35–49	Organic etiology known in majority of cases	May need supervision of self-care and motor skills; limited school progress but some learn basic reading, writing, and counting	Imbecility, moderate mental subnormality
Severe	20–34	Organic etiology known in majority of cases	Most have marked degree of motor impairment; possible maldevelopment of the central nervous system	Severe mental subnormality
Profound	Under 20	Organic etiology known in most cases	Most are immobile, incontinent; only capable of rudimentary forms of nonverbal communication; epilepsy and visual and hearing impairments are common	Idiocy, profound mental subnormality

The DSM-IVTR definition of ID uses the following three criteria (3):

1. An IQ of approximately 70 or below on an individually administered IQ test (or clinical judgment of ID in the case of infants)
2. Deficits or impairments in adaptive functioning in at least two of the following areas: communication, self-care, home living, and social/interpersonal skills, as well as the use of community resources, self-direction, functional academic skills, and the areas of work, leisure, health, and safety
3. Onset before age 18 years

As with the ICD-10 definition, the DSM-IVTR also has the categories of mild, moderate, severe, and profound mental retardation with roughly the same IQ levels. The DSM-IVTR definition is the one most commonly used in the United States when classifying mental disorders (1).

The third classification system is that used by the AAIDD. The 2002 AAIDD definition states, *Mental retardation is an intellectual disability characterized by significant limitations, both in intellectual function and adaptive behavior expressed in conceptual, social and practical adaptive skills. The disability originates before age 18 (4).* The AAIDD definition focuses on the needs of an individual and the methods for improving functioning. Thus, this definition is useful in conjunction with either the ICD-10 or DSM-IVTR definitions.

As with the AAIDD definition, the ICF system classifies the intellectual functioning of an individual. This system is intended to be used with the ICD-10 or DSM-IV definition to provide a comprehensive diagnosis for a person with ID that includes IQ, etiology, achievement ability, and the level of intellectual functioning.

PREVALENCE/INCIDENCE OF INTELLECTUAL DISABILITY

Numerous studies have attempted to assess the prevalence of ID in industrialized countries, and several have attempted to determine the prevalence of ID in developing nations as well. Determining the prevalence of ID in a country can be a difficult task since many factors need to be considered. These factors can include the IQ cutoff used and the characteristics of the population sampled (institutionalized vs. living with family, rural vs. urban, etc.)

The World Health Organization suggests that the prevalence rate of ID is between 1% and 3% of the population (5). When just looking at moderate, severe, and profound ID, prevalence has been documented as 0.3% (5). The prevalence in developing nations is thought to be higher than in industrialized nations due to increased potential for injury or lack of oxygen at birth, as well as early childhood brain infections.

Within the United States, the prevalence is suggested to be 12 per 1,000 children (6). When separated by IQ level, it is 8.4 per 1,000 for mild ID (IQ 50–70) and 3.6 per 1,000 for severe ID (IQ lower than 50). This prevalence for severe ID is comparable to the average prevalence of 3.8 per 1,000 found in a literature review (7). The same literature review found an average prevalence for mild ID to be 29.8 per 1,000. This rate is higher than that found in the population, but this literature review included an age range of 5 to 19 years of age. The assessment of mild ID may not be made until an individual reaches maturity, which would allow for a higher prevalence in the age range just noted as compared to a study only looking at 10-year-old children (7).

When comparing ID among races within the United States, the prevalence rate of severe ID is two times higher in African Americans (AA) than in Caucasians. In those with mild ID, the ratio is higher, 2.7:1 (6). This increase may be due in part to socioeconomic factors in addition to the Anglocentrism in the IQ test (6). When the cutoff IQ score is raised to 75, the percentage of AA children diagnosed as having ID is 18.4% while the percentage is 2.6% of Caucasians (8).

Males tend to show a higher prevalence of ID than females with ratios ranging from 1.3:1 to 2.1:1. This difference may be related to X-linked genetic disorders (see Chapter 5, Fragile X syndrome). Additionally, more males tend to be referred for psychometric testing which can cause an increased prevalence because of referral bias (6).

FREQUENTLY PERFORMED TESTS

The diagnosis of developmental delay is an important topic for many health care providers to address. This affects 10% to 15% of young children (9,10) and is significantly higher among children who live in poverty (11,12). As studies have shown that early diagnosis and intervention can have an affect on long-term academic and behavioral outcomes, the importance of having easy-to-use tools that provide a quality assessment is crucial (13–15). In 2006, the American Academy of Pediatrics issued a policy statement recommending the systematic developmental screening in primary care by using a validated tool with children 9, 18, and 30 months of age (16).

While tests like the Wechsler Scales of Intelligence put an actual value on intelligence, for a younger population, there are evaluations that allow parents to compare how their child is developing in relation to other children. The Parent Evaluation of Developmental Status (PEDS) and Ages and Stages Questionnaires (ASQ) are two of the more commonly performed tests. These tests are both general developmental screening tools, but represent different approaches to gathering parent observations on children's development (17) (Table 6.2).

The PEDS is a validated 10-item parent questionnaire that addresses developmental concerns in children from birth through 8 years of age. It is a simple test that can be used across social class and cultures as it is validated in both English and Spanish. Two of the questions ask about general concerns while the remaining eight target specific areas of development (18). Questions cover many areas of concern including speech, hearing, gross and fine motor skills, behavior, and learning. The score sheet is used to indicate whether a concern is predictive or nonpredictive of the occurrence of further developmental issues. Based on the results, a pathway of care including (a) the need for referral, (b) a second screening, (c) counseling to monitor development, including behavior and academic progress, or (d) no action can be determined (19). The test takes approximately 2 to 5 minutes to complete and is written at a fifth-grade reading level (18). The PEDS has a sensitivity and specificity of 79% and 80%, respectively (20), and shows varied results in comparison with other developmental screening tools (16,17,20–22).

The ASQ, a screening test developed by the University of Oregon's Center on Human Development, is a series of age-based, parent-completed

TABLE 6.2 Comparison of the PEDS and ASQ

Characteristic	PEDS	ASQ
Approach	Parent developmental concerns	Parents provide general information concerning child's skills
Areas addressed	Speech, hearing, gross and fine motor skills, behavior, learning	Communication, gross motor, fine motor, problem solving, personal–social
Number of questions	10 questions	30 questions
Response options	no/yes/little	yes/sometimes/not yet
Time to screen	5 min of parent time	10–15 min of parent time
Age validation	Birth to 8 y	1 mo to 5 y

questionnaires (16,23–25). There are 21 questionnaires at prescribed intervals to provide the closest chronologic age assessment. Adaptation can be made based on prematurity. It is designed to identify infants and children who have developmental delays or disorders in order to assess the need for intervention (25). It consists of 30 questions about children's skills in five areas of development and yields a simple pass/fail score. The five domains include communication, gross motor, fine motor, problem solving, and personal–social. Ages and Stages Questionnaires is validated in children age 1 month to 5 years of age (23–25). Ages and Stages Questionnaires has moderate to good sensitivity (0.70–0.90) and specificity (0.76–0.91) (25).

The Kaufman Brief Intelligence Test (K-BIT) is a screening designed to provide an estimate of cognitive ability in individuals aged 4 to 90. It can be administered by psychologists and trained laypersons and takes approximately 15 to 30 minutes. A verbal and nonverbal estimate as well as a composite estimate of cognitive ability is determined (26,27).

The K-BIT is composed of two subtests, vocabulary and matrices. The vocabulary subtest is composed of expressive vocabulary and definition sections. The expressive vocabulary section requires the subject to name objects shown in pictures. The definition section, which is only administered to patients 8 years or older, requires the subject to provide a word based on two clues: a phrase describing the word and a partial spelling of the word. The Matrices subtest requires the subject to solve multiple-choice analogies that, in general, requires the recognition of relationships among visual stimuli, both meaningful and abstract. The questions become more difficult as the test advances (26). It has been shown to be a valid estimate of intelligence in a wide variety of patient populations, including students referred for poor performance in academics, incarcerated juvenile delinquents, children with traumatic brain injury, youth in psychiatric hospitals, as well as those children and adolescents that have no disability (27).

The gold standard test and the ones that are most familiar within the health care community and to the public are the various tests collectively known as the Wechsler Scales of Intelligence (25,28–35). These include the Wechsler Intelligence Scales for Children (WISC-IV), Wechsler Adult Intelligence Scale (WAIS-IV), and the Wechsler Preschool and Primary Scale of Intelligence (WPPSI-III). The WISC-IV is used for those 6 to 16, the WAIS-IV for those 16 to 89, and the WPPSI-III for those 2.5 to 7 years of age. These tests purport to measure the individual's IQ and the age level at which they function. Keep in mind that due to random factors, IQ scores can fluctuate about 5 points week to week and can often change by 10 points or more over a period of years (30). Optometric vision therapy, which will be discussed in Chapter 25, Optometric Management of Functional Vision Disorders Plasticity, has been shown to impact the IQ (36).

The WISC-IV (revised 2003) consists of 15 subtests and yields four composite indexes and an overall IQ (31–35). Table 6.3 shows an overview of the tested areas as well as the subtests that make up each composite index. The standardization sample is a national, stratified, random sample consisting of 2,200 children and adolescents from the United States between the ages of 6 and 16 years. There were 200 children in each of the 11 age groups with an equal number of boys and girls in each group. Stratification by age, race/ethnicity, geographic location, and parental education was based in the US census survey in March 2000 (33). Reliability is excellent. Internal consistency as reported in the Technical Manual for the Full-Scale Intelligence Quotient (FSIQ) ranges from 0.96 to 0.97 and the four-index test–retest reliabilities range from 0.79 to 0.89. Over a 9-week interval, the FSIQ increased on average 5.6 points, and an increase ranging from 2.1 to 7.1 was found on the indexes. This practice effect must be taken into account if a retest is performed soon after initial testing (28).

This version is different from the previous version in several ways. The WISC-III, which consisted of 10 core subtests, provided a verbal intelligence quotient (VIQ), a performance intelligence quotient (PIQ), and an FSIQ. The VIQ and PIC have been eliminated, five new subtests added, and factor-based indexes are provided along with an FSIQ. Keep in mind that due to these significant changes, previous performance on the WISC-III cannot be generalized to the WISC-IV, despite claims (35).

The WAIS-IV (revised 2008) is similar to the WISC-IV. There are four indexes with 15 core subtests, and an FSIQ is determined. The validity is considered high (0.98) and similar practice effects as found with the WISC-IV exist. These changes are statistically significant and have clinical implications. It can be difficult to assess whether real improvement is occurring or whether the change is related to the practice effect (28).

TABLE 6.3 Description of the WISC-IV

Variable	Subtests Included	What Does It Measure?
Verbal comprehension index	Vocabulary Similarities Comprehension Information Word reasoning[a]	Verbal concept formation • Assesses ability to listen to a question, draw upon learned information from both formal and informal education, reason through an answer and express thoughts out loud
Perceptual reasoning index	Block design Picture concepts[a] Matrix reasoning[a] Picture completion	Nonverbal and fluid reasoning • Assesses ability to examine a problem, draw upon visual–motor and visual skills, organize thoughts, create solutions, and then test them.
Working memory index	Digit span Letter-number sequencing[a] Arithmetic	Working memory • Assesses the ability to memorize new information, hold it in short-term memory, concentrate and manipulate the information to produce some result or reasoning process.
Processing speed index	Coding Symbol search Cancellation[a]	Processing speed • Assesses the ability to focus attention and scan, discriminate between and sequentially order visual information

[a]Represents a new subtest in WISC-IV.

The WPPSI-III contains 14 subtests that can be combined to measure VIQ, PIQ, processing speed quotient, general language composite, and an FSIQ. Testing in this age group can be tenuous, as environmental factors can influence the results to a greater degree versus older children and adolescents. Also, the test scales expect increases in IQ in sudden increments every 2 to 3 months (37).

VISUAL SYSTEM COMPLICATIONS

Individuals with ID often rely heavily on their visual systems to communicate and interact with their surroundings. Within the population of individuals with ID, various visual dysfunctions are often diagnosed (refractive errors, strabismus, amblyopia, and other vision function and eye health conditions) that interfere with development and overall quality of life.

When reviewing the prevalence of oculovisual conditions within the population of those with ID, many factors can affect the findings. First, individuals with ID may have other disabilities that can affect the visual system (i.e., Down syndrome (DS), tuberous sclerosis, and Fragile X syndrome. See Chapters 4, Down syndrome and 5, Fragile X Syndrome) (38,39). Additionally, visual impairments can result from etiologies or damage to the cerebral visual system (39). Furthermore, individuals with ID may be less likely to recognize or effectively communicate their visual difficulties, resulting in an underdiagnosis of many visual conditions (40).

The overall prevalence of visual system complications in those with ID ranges from 28% to 92% based on the population studied and the inclusion criteria used (38,39). In the population of individuals with ID and DS, the prevalence of visual impairment increases compared to those individuals without DS (40). Additionally, as the age of an individual or severity of ID increases, so does the prevalence of visual impairment (41). In individuals without DS, the degree of ID shows a better correlation with increased prevalence of visual impairment, whereas those with DS have a better correlation between the age of the individual and increased prevalence of visual impairment (39).

When looking at the ability to obtain a normal level of visual acuity, one study found that 88% and <60% of individuals with mild and severe ID, respectively, were able to obtain good visual acuity. No estimate of visual acuity could be made for many of the individuals with profound ID (38).

Refractive errors range from high hyperopia to high myopia, with many individuals showing emmetropia (38). In a screening of 146 adults (ages 19–62) with moderate ID, myopia (32%) was the most common ocular finding (42). Additionally, 18% had astigmatism. The prevalence of hyperopia was not noted.

Reduced binocularity and strabismus are also common, with a prevalence ranging from 19% to

84% (38,39,42). In a study of adults with severe and profound ID, 84% were unable to use both eyes to maintain binocularity. The main cause was strabismus and amblyopia (39). Another study found that 25% and 60% of individuals with mild and profound ID showed strabismus. That study also found that those with more mild forms of ID were likely to have an esodeviation, whereas those with more severe forms of ID showed an exodeviation (38).

Ocular health abnormalities also occur in greater amounts in those with ID. The most common condition in one study was an abnormality of the crystalline lens, including cataracts, with a reported prevalence of around 20%. Most of those individuals had not received any treatment related to the cataracts. Other notable ocular abnormalities include optic nerve atrophy, keratopathy, and glaucoma (38,42).

Regular vision examinations for individuals with ID are important. This population is less likely to be able to effectively communicate with their caregivers if they are experiencing a visual complication. Studies have found that only 30% of individuals with ID who were found to have a visual system complication had a previous diagnosis of a visual problem and over 80% of the problems were unknown to the caregivers (38,39). After receiving treatment, many individuals with ID showed an improved ability to identify objects and people as well as improved gross motor and fine motor movement. In addition, challenging behaviors such as temper tantrums decreased (38).

CONCLUSION

Performing a comprehensive vision examination on patients with ID may be difficult. However, because of the many potential oculovisual problems noted in those with ID (43–45), it is critical that eye care professionals fully assess (46) the patient's visual system (see Chapter 16, Comprehensive Examination Procedures) and provide intervention when possible (see Chapter 25, Optometric Management of Functional Vision Disorders). This may include glasses, optometric vision therapy, medical intervention, or surgery when appropriate. Once the examination has been completed and the suitable treatment begun, we can improve an individual's performance during his daily activities, which will have a significant and positive effect on the patient's quality of life.

REFERENCES

1. Harris JC. Intellectual disability: Understanding its development, causes, classifications, evaluation, and treatment. North Carolina: Oxford University Press; 2005. p. 42–78.
2. World Health Organization Staff. ICD-10 Classification of mental and behavioral disorders. Clinical descriptions and diagnostic guidelines. New York: World Health Organization; 1992. p. 225–31.
3. First M. Diagnostic and statistical manual of mental disorders. 4th ed. Washington: American Psychiatric Association; 2000.
4. Luckasson R. Mental retardation: definition, classification, and systems of supports. 10th ed. Washington: American Association on Mental Retardation; 2002.
5. The World Health Report 2001 Available from: http://www.who.int/whr/2001/en/whr01_ch2_en.pdf. Last Accessed on December 9, 2010.
6. Murphy CC, Yeargin-Allsopp M, Decouflé P, et al. The Administrative Prevalence of Mental Retardation in 10-Year-Old Children in Metropolitan Atlanta, 1985 through 1987. Am J Public Health. 1995;85(3):319–23.
7. Roeleveld N, Zielhuis GA, Gabreels F. The prevalence of mental retardation: a critical review of recent literature. Dev Med Child Neurol. 1997;39:125–32.
8. McMillan DL, Greshman FM, Siperstein GN. Conceptual and psychometric concerns about the 1992 AAIDD definition of mental retardation. Am J Ment Retard. 1993;98:325–35.
9. Boyle CA, Decoufle P, Yeargin-Allsopp M. Prevalence and health impact of developmental disabilities in US children. Pediatrics. 1994;93:399–403.
10. Yeargin-Allsopp M, Boyle C. Overview: the epidemiology of neurodevelopmental disorders. Ment Retard Dev Disabil Res Rev. 2002;8:113–6.
11. Drews CD, Yeargin-Allsopp M, Decoufle P, et al. Variation in the influence of selected socio-demographic risk factors for mental retardation. Am J Public Health. 1995;85:329–34.
12. Stevens GD. Gradients in the health status and developmental risks of young children: the combined influences of multiple social risk factors. Matern Child Health J. 2006;10:187–99.
13. Anderson LM, Shinn C, Fullilove MT, et al. The effectiveness of early childhood development programs: a systematic review. Am J Prev Med. 2003;24:32–46.
14. Berlin LJ, Books-Gunn J, McCarton C, et al. The effectiveness of early intervention: examining risk factors and pathways to enhanced development. Prev Med. 1998;27:238–45.
15. Hill JL, Brooks-Gunn J, Waldfogel J. Sustained effects of high participation in an early intervention for low-birth-weight premature infants. Dev Psychol 2003;39:730–44.
16. American Academy of Pediatrics, Council on Children with Disabilities, Section on Developmental Behavioral Pediatrics, Bright Futures Steering Committee, Medical Home Initiatives for Children with Special Needs Project Advisory Committee. Identifying infants and young children with developmental disorders in the medical home: an algorithm for developmental surveillance and screening. Pediatrics. 2006;118:405–20.
17. Sices L, Stancin T, Kirchner L, et al. PEDS and ASQ developmental screening tests may not identify the same children. Pediatrics. 2009;124:640–7.

18. Schonwald A, Huntington N, Chan E, et al. Routine developmental screening implemented in urban primary care settings: more evidence of feasibility and effectiveness. Pediatrics. 2009;123:660–8.
19. Davies S, Feeney H. A pilot of the parent's evaluation of developmental status tool. Community Pract. 2009;82;29–31.
20. Theeranate K, Chuengcitraks S. Parent's Evaluation of Developmental Status (PEDS) detects developmental problems compared to the Denver II. J Med Assoc Thai. 2005;88: S188–S191.
21. Glascoe FP. Parents' concerns about children's development: prescreening technique or screening test? Pediatrics. 1997;99:522–8.
22. Glascoe FP, MacLean WE, Stone WL. The importance of parent's concerns about their child's behavior. Clin Pediatr. 1991;30:8–14.
23. Jee S, Szilagyi M, Ovenshire C, et al. Improved detection of developmental delays among young children in foster care. Pediatrics. 2010;125:282–9.
24. Elbers J, Macnab A, McLeod E, et al. The ages and stages questionnaires: feasibility of use as a screening tool for children in Canada. Can J Rural Med. 2008;13:9–14.
25. Spies RA, Carlson JF, Geisinger KF. Mental measurements yearbook. 18th ed. Lincoln: University of Nebraska Press; 2010. pp. 10–15, 684–90.
26. Grados JJ, Russo-Garcia KA. Comparison of the Kaufman brief intelligence test and the Wechsler intelligence scale for Children-Third edition in economically disadvantaged African American Youth. J Clin Psychol. 1999;55:1063–71.
27. Chin CE, Ledesma HML, Cirino PT et al. Relation between the Kaufman Brief Intelligence Test and the WISC-III scores in children with RD. J Learn Disabil. 2001;34:2–8.
28. Groth-Marnat G. Handbook of psychological management. 5th ed. Hoboken: John Wiley and Sons; 2009. pp. 119–81.
29. Flanagan DP, Kaufman AS. Essentials of WISC-IV assessment. 2nd ed. Hoboken: John Wiley and Sons; 2009.
30. Intelligence Testing. www.psychologicaltesting.com/1qtest.htm. Last Accessed 12/10.
31. Niolon R. History of the WISC-IV. Available from: www.pschpage.com/learning/library/intell/wisciv_hx.htm. Last Accessed 12/10.
32. Ryan JJ, Glass LA, Brown CN. Administration time estimates for the Wechsler Intelligence scale for Children-IV Subtests, Composites and Short Forms. J Clin Pshychol. 2007;63:309–18.
33. Brooks BL. Seeing the forest for the trees: prevalence of low scores on the Wechsler Intelligence Scale for Children, Fourth Edition (WISC-IV). Psychol Assess. 2010;22:650–6.
34. Sandu IK. The Wechsler Intelligence Scale for Children, Fourth Edition (WISC-IV). Available from: www.brainy-child.com/expert/WISC_IV.shtml Last Accessed 12/10.
35. Ryan JJ, Glass LA, Bartels KM. Stability of the WISC-IV in a sample of elementary and middle school children. App Neuropsychol. 2010;17:68–72.
36. Silverman LK. Diagnosing and treating visual perceptual issues in gifted children. J Optom Vis Dev. 2001;32: 153–76.
37. Sandu IK. The WPPSI-III. Available from: www.brainy-child.com/expert/WPPSI-III.shtml. Last Accessed 12/10.
38. McCulloch DL, Sludden PA, McKeown K, et.al. Vision care requirements among intellectually disabled adults: a residence-based pilot study. J Intellect Disabil Res. 1996;40(2): 140–50.
39. van den Broek EGC, Janssen CGC, van Ramshorst T, et al. Visual impairments in people with severe and profound multiple disabilities: an inventory of visual functioning. J Intellect Disabil Res. 2006;50(6):470–5.
40. Donati RJ, Maino DM, Bartell H, Kieffer M. Polypharmacy and the lack of oculo-visual complaints from those with mental illness and dual diagnosis. Optometry. 2009;80(5): 249–54.
41. Warburg M. Visual impairment in adult people with intellectual disability: literature review. J Intellect Disabil Res. 2001;45(5):424–38.
42. Isralowitz R, Madar M, Reznik A. Vision needs of people with intellectual disability in residential facilities and community-based homes for independent living. Disabil Rehabil. 2005; 27(23):1451–3.
43. Wesson M, Maino D. Oculovisual findings in Down syndrome, cerebral palsy, and mental retardation with non-specific etiology. In: Maino D, editor. Diagnosis and management of special populations. St. Louis: Mosby-Yearbook, Inc.; 1995. p. 17–54.
44. Maino DM, Maino JH, Cibis GW, Hecht F. Ocular health anomalies in patients with developmental disabilities. In: Maino D, editor. Diagnosis and management of special populations. St. Louis: Mosby-Yearbook, Inc.; 1995. p. 189–206.
45. Viola SG, Maino DM. Brain anatomy, electrophysiology and visual function/perception in children within the autism spectrum disorder. Opt Vis Dev. 2009;40(3):157–63.
46. Schlange D, Maino D. Clinical behavioral objectives: assessment techniques for special populations. In: Maino D, editor. Diagnosis and management of special populations. St. Louis: Mosby-Yearbook, Inc.; 1995. p. 151–88.

CHAPTER 7

Daniel E. Smith, OD, FAAO

Oculovisual Abnormalities Associated with Rare Neurodevelopmental Disorders

RARE NEURODEVELOPMENTAL DISORDERS

Anomalies preventing normal structural architecture and/or neurologic capability of the central nervous system (CNS) are collectively referred to as neurodevelopmental disorders. When studying these disorders, the underlying mutation of specific genes may be clearly defined; however, those factors responsible for preventing their normal expression are still widely unknown. Because the eyes and visual system are the direct extension of the developing CNS, brain impairment holds tremendous implication in eye health and vision function. It is generally accepted that the earlier the anomaly occurs in the embryologic sequence, the greater potential for catastrophic structural defect. Rather than provide an exhaustive list of potential etiologies, this chapter briefly describes several neurodevelopmental disorders and their respective varying degrees of ocular or orbital involvement. A summary of these and other conditions are listed in Table 7.1. (Table 7.1)

Aicardi Syndrome Aicardi syndrome is a genetic anomaly involving either the dysgenesis or possibly agenesis of the corpus callosum. There are 3000 cases reported cases worldwide, 900 of those in the United States (1). The corpus callosum is the large white matter neurologic tract comprised of interhemispheric neurons allowing the right and left cerebral hemisphere of the human brain to coordinate their activities. Children with this malformation are thought to follow an X-linked inheritance pattern, therefore affecting females predominantly. However, there are cases of males, namely, those with Klinefelter syndrome, reported to demonstrate the same chromosomal mutation and phenotype (2).

Systemically, individuals with Aicardi syndrome appear to be developmentally normal at birth up to 3 months of age. However, normal milestones are interrupted by infantile spasms, epileptic-like seizures, vertebral malformations, and mental retardation. Other common systemic signs may include hydrocephalus and head deformities such as plagiocephaly and occipital flattening (3).

Ophthalmologic associations reported include microphthalmia, myokymia, optic nerve colobomas, optic nerve hypoplasia, and diminished pupillary responses. One classic feature is the presence of large multiple chorioretinal lacunae that appear to be more associated with a deficiency of the retinal pigment epithelium and choroid rather than the neurosensory retina itself (3).

Treatment for both systemic and ophthalmologic issues primarily involves intervention protocols. Neurologic consults are indicated for the seizure management, while developmental delays are typically monitored by the child's developmental pediatrician. Optometric management would include comprehensive evaluations with dilated fundus examinations to monitor any retinal changes as well as to maximize visual acuity through spectacle prescription and/or occlusion therapy.

Alport Syndrome Alport syndrome is characterized by end-stage kidney disease, hearing loss, and vision disturbances. Because the kidney, ear, and eye all rely on structurally sound basement membrane systems for adequate functioning, any mutation in genes that synthesize collagen, as those implicated in Alport syndrome, will cause negative effects. The filtration system of the kidney cannot filter waste, consequently allowing blood and protein to spill into the urine. The continued irregular synthesis of

TABLE 7.1 Rare Neurodevelopmental Disorders

Syndrome	Etiology	Systemic Manifestation	Ophthalmic Manifestation
Aicardi syndrome	Dysgenesis of the corpus callosum	Infantile spasms, epileptic-like seizure, occipital flattening, mental retardation	Chorioretinal lacunae, optic nerve colobomas, optic nerve hypoplasia
Alport syndrome	Irregular synthesis of collagen	End-stage kidney failure, hearing loss	Fleck retinal dystrophy, anterior lenticonus, corneal dystrophy, cataracts
Angelman syndrome	Deletion of maternal genetic material on chromosome 15	Mental and physical delay, happy demeanor, seizures	Strabismus, hypopigmentation of the choroid
Batten-Mayou syndrome	Autosomal recessive disorder resulting in accumulation of lipid	Loss of motor control, deficits intellect	Lipofuscin accumulation in retina, optic atrophy, macular pigment
Behçet disease	Postulated to be episodic hyperactivity of immune system	Mouth/genital ulcers, folliculitis, erythema nodosum	Uveitis, cataract, optic atrophy, macular edema
Behr syndrome	Autosomal recessive disease resulting in progressive deterioration of the nervous system	Reduction in coordination, spastic paraplegia, hand tremor, and mental deficiency	Optic atrophy, retrobulbar neuritis, nystagmus
Branchial arch syndromes	Disruption of neural crest cell migration	Craniosynostosis, dysgenesis of mandible, ear, soft palate	Strabismus, proptosis from poorly formed orbits, coloboma of eyelid
Cerebral palsy	Disorder of movement and posture secondary to damage to motor control connections	Varying degrees of hypotonicity, neurologic impairment	Strabismus, nystagmus, optic nerve pallor, cataracts, myopia
Cerebro-oculo-facial syndrome	Autosomal recessive disorder resulting in defective swallowing mechanism	Microcephaly, hypotonia, osteoporosis	Microphthalmia, involuntary eye movements, congenital cataracts, blepharophimosis
Charcot-Marie-Tooth syndrome	Genetic anomaly resulting in progressive muscular atrophy	Small muscle atrophy (hands) progressing to larger muscle groups (leg), cramps	Nystagmus, diminished visual acuity
CHARGE syndrome	Common mutation on chromosome 8 resulting in association of multiple systemic defects	Cardiac defects, atresia of nasal choanae, delay in physical growth, genital/urinary tract anomalies, deafness	Bilateral retinal coloboma involving the optic nerve, strabismus, amblyopia
Cri-du-chat syndrome	Deletion of short arm of chromosome 5	Characteristic cry like that of a crying cat secondary to laryngeal defect, mental retardation, micrognathia	Strabismus, hypertelorism, slanting of palpebral fissures
Dandy-Walker syndrome	Absence of the cerebellar vermis and dilation of fourth ventricle	Hydrocephalus, scoliosis, diminished tendon reflexes	Papilledema often seen with hydrocephalus ptosis and strabismus secondary to cranial nerve palsy
de Lange syndrome	Mutation in genes responsible for chromosomal adhesions	Growth retardation with facial and skeletal changes, upper limb abnormalities, and hirsutism	Long eyelashes, ptosis telecanthus, alternating exotropia
Down syndrome	Triplicate 21st chromosome	Congenital heart defects, short limbs, protruding tongue, simian crease	Epicanthal folds, upslanting palpebral fissure, high refractive error, strabismus, keratoconus, blepharitis
Dubowitz syndrome	Unknown etiology	Microcephaly, triangular face, hormone deficiency	Strabismus, ptosis, telecanthus, epicanthal folds

Ehlers-Danlos syndrome	Genetic or nutritional defects that have altered the biosynthesis of collagen	Highly flexible fingers, stretchy skin, bruising, arthralgia, scoliosis	Lens subluxation, palpebral skin laxity, keratoconus myopia, blue sclera, and angioid streaks
Fetal alcohol syndrome	CNS damage secondary to alcohol crossing the blood–brain barrier	Low birth weight, microcephaly, flat philtrum, cognitive deficits	Telecanthus, strabismus, optic nerve hypoplasia, ptosis, microphthalmia
Fragile X syndrome	Gene (FMR1) on the X chromosome fails to allow protein synthesis necessary for neural development.	Long face, low-set ears, flexible joints, mental retardation	Strabismus, astigmatism, amblyopia
Gaucher disease	Lysosomal storage disease	Hypertonia, dysphagia, laryngeal spasm, hepatosplenomegaly	Strabismus, gaze palsies corneal clouding, pinguecula
Hunter syndrome	Mucopolysaccharidosis II—Lysosomal storage disease	Enlarged forehead, abdominal hernia, enlarged tongue, occipital flattening	Corneal clouding, pigmentary degeneration of the retina, optic atrophy
Hurler syndrome	Mucopolysaccharidosis I—Lysosomal storage disease	Enlarged forehead, abdominal hernia, enlarged tongue, occipital flattening	Corneal clouding, pigmentary degeneration of the retina, optic atrophy
Lowe syndrome	Abnormal protein transport within cellular membranes	Renal disease, hypotonia, respiratory disorders, mental retardation	Bilateral congenital cataracts, glaucoma, corneal keloids, strabismus
Prader-Willi syndrome	Deletion of paternal genetic material on chromosome 15	Obesity, hypotonia, short stature, learning disability	Strabismus, almond-shaped palpebral fissures, myopia
Rett syndrome	Mutation of binding protein (MECP2) that alters the development of gray matter	Deficits in motor control and communication skills, observable hand-wringing behavior	Difficulty maintaining eye contact
Spina bifida	Incomplete closure of embryonic neural tube	Spinal cord cysts, posterior meningocele hydrocephalus, deformity of hips and legs	Papilledema, nerve palsies, nystagmus, optic atrophy
Stickler syndrome	Defective biosynthesis of collagen	Midface hypoplasia with possible cleft palate, joint hypermobility, audiologic defects	Myopia, retinal detachments, vitreous anomalies
Williams syndrome	Vast deletion of genes on chromosome 7	Elf-like facial features, cheerful demeanor, mental retardation, hypotonia, cardiac disease	Infantile esotropia, anomaly in visual–spatial relationship

collagen causes the scarring of the kidney and eventually failure. Hearing loss is usually classified as a high frequency loss and usually present before the third decade of life (4).

Multiple ocular features are noted in this syndrome. Approximately 85% of individuals will have a fleck dystrophy of the retina resulting from the aforementioned breakdown of retinal basement membrane (4). Anterior lenticonus, a bulging of the anterior surface of the intraocular lens, occurs in 25%, and posterior polymorphous dystrophy of the cornea is rare. Other ophthalmic findings reported include iris atrophy, cataracts, posterior lenticonus, and abnormalities of the retinal fluorescein angiogram, electroretinogram, and electrooculogram (4).

Treatment consists of addressing the individual symptoms, dialysis for the kidney failure, and hearing devices for deafness, if necessary. Visual needs typically consist of glasses or contact lenses for refractive changes and/or surgical removal of damaged intraocular lenses. Currently, there is no treatment for the retinal compromise (5).

Angelman Syndrome Angelman syndrome is a disorder involving mutation or deletion of the maternal genetic contribution to a segment of chromosome 15. Marked by both mental and physical delays, these patients' characteristic clinical findings include an individual with a happy demeanor, laughter, and puppet-like hand/arm movements (Figure 7-1). Seizures, mental retardation, and speech impairment are also important diagnostic criteria. In order to eliminate the use of antiquated and stigmatizing terminology, children with Angelman syndrome are sometimes referred to as "Angels" considering both the syndrome name as well as the individual's happy appearance. These individuals have also been referred to as having the "happy puppet syndrome."

There are few publications stating common visual manifestations in individuals with Angelman syndrome. Of those reported, strabismus was a commonly shared diagnosis. Others include hypopigmentation of the choroid (6). Surgery or optometric vision therapy for the strabismus would be determined by the prognosis of the outcome. Photochromic spectacle lenses are warranted if the lack of choroidal pigmentation produces complaints of photosensitivity.

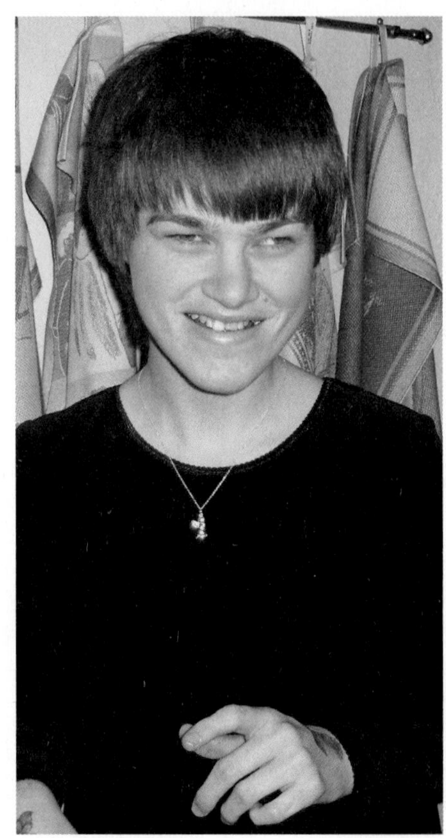

FIGURE 7-1. Happy demeanor and strabismus in a young female with Angelman syndrome. (Photo courtesy of Angelman Syndrome Foundation.)

Batten-Mayou Disease Batten-Mayou, also known as juvenile neuronal ceroid lipofuscinosis disease, is a condition where an early-onset deterioration of visual acuity is often the first sign of the disease and useful in initial diagnosis. Considered to be a deficiency in lipid metabolism, Batten-Mayou is an autosomal recessive disorder resulting in the abnormal accumulation of fat, or lipofuscin, within the body tissue. Full course of the disease exhibits a vast deficiency of the CNS manifested by loss of motor control as well as deficits in intellect (7).

Visual prognosis in those with Batten-Mayou is devastating. Vision loss has been reported as early as 4 years of age due to the lipid buildup in the inner retinal layers and pigmented epithelium. In addition to the retinal changes, optic atrophy and macular pigmentary changes result in an extinguished electroretinogram.

Unfortunately there is no treatment for Batten-Mayou, and average life expectancy is under 30 years. With the age of the patient in mind, palliative care consisting of low vision consultation should be considered throughout the progression of the disease (7).

Behçet Disease Commonly characterized as a vasculitis, the underlying cause of this disorder is still unknown. Episodic hyperactivity of the immune system appears to produce areas of inflammation involving the vascular system. If left untreated, these areas of vasculitis often lead to clinically significant ulcerations of the mouth and genitals (8). In addition to the oral and genital ulcers, it is common to appreciate skin lesions such as folliculitis and erythema nodosum. An infectious component is suspected in Behçet disease, but has yet to be confirmed (9). While rare in the United States, Behçet's is common in Middle Eastern and Asian men, which could be an indication of the etiology being linked to a warm or tropical environment (10).

Multiple ocular findings present in Behçet disease. A high incidence of panuveitis, cataract, and optic atrophy has been demonstrated in retrospective studies. Additional visually related issues include isolated posterior and anterior uveitis, posterior synechiae, vitreous condensation from chronic vitritis, branch retinal vein occlusion, macular edema, and neovascularization of the disk (11).

Current treatment is to reduce the areas of inflammation by use of medications known to suppress parts of the immune system. These medications include oral or ophthalmic prednisone, methotrexate, and/or cyclophosphamide (8,10). Because this disorder is a potentially fatal disease, and the immune-suppressing drugs commonly used in its management can have serious side effects, it is imperative that this condition be managed by qualified physicians.

Behr Syndrome First reported in the early 1900s, Behr syndrome is an autosomal recessive disease characterized by progressive atrophy of the neurologic system. The mechanism was reported to be associated with an anomaly within the pyramidal tracts. Pyramidal tracts are defined as "A major pathway of the CNS, originating in the sensorimotor areas of the cerebral cortex and generally descending through the brain stem to the spinal cord. The fibers of the pyramidal tract transmit motor impulses that function in the control of voluntary movement (12)." Early impairment of this neurologic system is first noted in infancy or early childhood and is characterized by a generalized reduction in coordination and blurred vision. As the degeneration continues, systemic findings progress to spastic paraplegia, mental deficiency, hand tremors, and unusual reflexes such as a positive Babinski sign.

Vision potential is impaired due to atrophy of the optic nerves. Given the reduction of acuity, and the continued loss of voluntary muscle control, nystagmus is also diagnostic in those with Behr syndrome. Retrobulbar neuritis is reported but as with many signs associated with Behr, its distinction is unclear. Management of these conditions includes palliative care as well as consultation with a low vision specialist to determine the efficacy of magnification devices.

Currently, there is no treatment to suspend or repair the atrophy to the neurologic system appreciated in Behr syndrome; however, some therapy is offered to alleviate hand tremors (13).

Branchial (Pharyngeal) Arch Syndromes: Apert Syndrome, Crouzon Syndrome, Goldenhar Syndrome, Pfeiffer Syndrome, Treacher Collins Syndrome When observing the developmental sequence of vertebrates, branchial arches are credited as the initial collection of embryonic cells that result from the invasion of neural crest cells migrating to those parts of the embryo to eventually derive the head and neck. These arches serve as the beginning point for a multitude of craniofacial structures, therefore disruption in their development results in easily appreciated malformations. These malformations include incomplete formation of the ear, soft palate and mandible (specifically Goldenhar and Treacher Collins), a peaked head, and webbed fingers and toes. This disruption is thought to occur primarily due to specific mutations in those genes responsible for fibroblast growth factor receptors (14).

What makes Crouzon, Pfeiffer, or Apert disorders clinically significant is the fact that they involve craniosynostosis, or early fusion of the cranial sutures, which can result in pressure on the developing brain and consequential mental retardation (14). Since there are multiple sutures, the growth pattern of the skull is determined by which fuse or are unable to expand.

Craniofacial deformities are commonly responsible for shallow or poorly formed orbits. As a result,

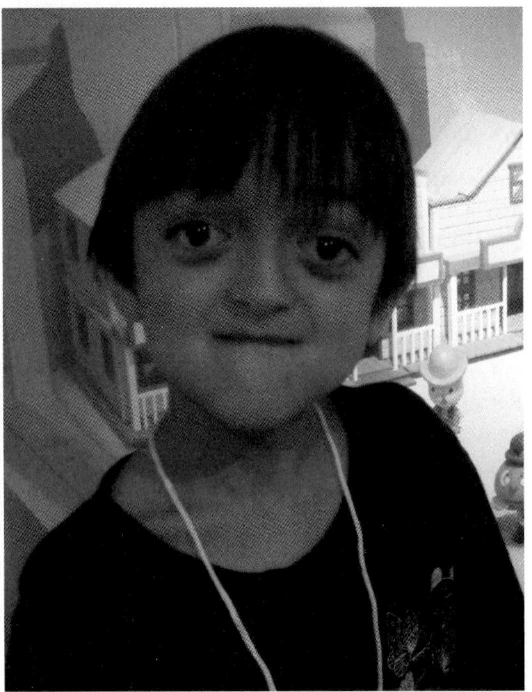

FIGURE 7-2. Crouzon syndrome demonstrating craniofacial deformity with poorly formed orbits resulting in proptosis. (Photo courtesy of FACES: The National Craniofacial Association.)

ophthalmic manifestations primarily include proptosis and strabismus (Figure 7-2). Surgical restoration of the cranial sutures and craniofacial deformities is needed prior to any consideration of surgery for eye misalignment. Coloboma of the eyelid is a common finding in both Treacher Collins and Goldenhar. Typically, the upper eyelid is affected in Goldenhar and the lower in Treacher Collins. If symptomatic, the colobomas may be surgically closed in the event of ectropion, trichiasis, and/or ocular surface desiccation.

CHARGE Syndrome With an incidence of only 1:10,000, CHARGE syndrome is surprisingly well known. This is likely due to the unusual distinguishable clinical features noted in the newborns. Historically, CHARGE was referred to as an "association" of the following anomalies: ***C***oloboma of the eyes, ***H***eart defects, ***A***tresia of the nasal choanae, ***R***etardation of physical growth or development, ***G***enital and/or urinary tract anomalies, and ***E***ar defects/deafness. Not until genetic testing demonstrating a common mutation on chromosome 8 in the majority of individuals with this association was CHARGE considered a syndrome (15). However, diagnosis remains largely the responsibility of the clinician due to genetic testing ability to identify only two-thirds CHARGE patients and the variation of their clinical presentation (16).

The most distinguished ocular feature of CHARGE syndrome is bilateral chorioretinal colobomas involving the optic nerve. Given this feature, it is not uncommon to have significant deficits in visual acuity that respond poorly, if at all, to amblyopic therapy. Other ocular complications noted in literature include anisometropia, myopic astigmatism, visual field defects that correlate to the loss of neurologic tissue and restriction of elevation when the eye is in the adducted position, suggesting an acquired Brown syndrome (17). Management from an eye care provider would be to compensate for any refractive error need, amblyopic treatment utilizing optometric vision therapy (occlusion, low vision devices), as well as annual eye health examinations.

Attention to each of the clinical anomalies must be given when deciding on the appropriate management. It is evident that multiple disciplines are necessary to provide adequate care to ensure maximum health. Consultation with a developmental pediatrician for referrals to ENT, eye care professionals, cardiologists, urologists, and geneticists is imperative.

Ehlers-Danlos Syndrome Collagen is comprised of fibrous proteins that are used as supporting tissue in tendons, ligaments, cornea, skin, muscle, and bone providing tissue strength and elasticity. Its production is dependent on a particular arrangement of amino acids. Connective tissue disorders, of which Ehlers-Danlos is included, are the result of nutritional or genetic defects that have altered the biosynthesis of collagen, therefore negatively affecting its integrity. Individuals who have Ehlers-Danlos manifest signs that are caused by flawed collagen production, including highly flexible fingers, loose joints prone to subluxation, stretchy skin, and easy bruising are all such findings. Medical associations include cardiac effects such as dysautonomia, arthralgia, otosclerosis, and scoliosis (18).

With respect to the eye, it is not uncommon to find a laxity of the palpebral skin secondary to the loss of collagenous tensile strength. Corneal tissue is thin and susceptible to keratoconus (19). Laxity of zonular strength is responsible for lens subluxation. Axial elongation results because of the thinning of the sclera. As a result, the sclera may yield a blue color as choroidal pigment is visible through the tissue. In addition to the blue sclera, increased axial length will cause a myopic shift in refractive error and potential breaks in the choroidal tissue known as angioid streaks (20).

Management is supportive. Specialist care involving cardiology, physical therapy, and orthopedics are all indicated. Routine eye exams monitoring refractive changes, compromise in corneal health, lens positioning, and retinal health are recommended at least annually.

Fetal Alcohol Syndrome Fetal alcohol syndrome is the result of permanent CNS damage secondary to alcohol crossing the placental barrier during pregnancy. Once contributed primarily to the amount of ingested alcohol, additional liable factors now include the type of alcohol consumed and gestational age of the fetus at the time of exposure. In addition to adverse anatomical effects such as low birth weight and craniofacial anomalies including microcephaly and a flat philtrum, alcohol exposure is known to create a variety of cognitive and functional disabilities. The incidence of fetal alcohol syndrome is estimated around 1.9:1,000 worldwide and thought to be the leading cause of mental retardation in the United States (21).

Common ophthalmic manifestations include telecanthus, strabismus, optic nerve hypoplasia, and ptosis. Treatments sought for these conditions would include surgical and/or optometric vision therapy for correction of the strabismus if binocularity function can be restored or levator tuck if the ptotic eyelid is blocking the visual axis creating an amblyogenic threat. If optic nerve hypoplasia is present, poor visual acuity is expected and a low vision evaluation is indicated. Lastly, perceptual testing/therapy is performed to address vision information processing deficits such as visual memory.

Lowe Syndrome Lowe syndrome manifests as developmental anomalies of the eye, brain, and kidney. Complications noted in all three of these areas are referred to as oculocerebrorenal syndrome and are required for appropriate diagnosis. First reported in 1952, Lowe syndrome has an incidence of about 1:500,000 and is found only in males (22).

The mechanism behind this disorder involves the mutation of the OCRL1 gene. Because of the mutation, an enzyme (PIP2–5) needed for normal cytoskeleton development and transport of protein within the cellular membranes is absent. As a result, complications such as renal disease, hypotonia, respiratory disorders, and mental retardation are noted during the first few months of life (22). Behavioral issues also affect a high percentage of children with Lowe syndrome. Aggressiveness, irritability, anger, and obsessive–compulsive behavior are common (23).

Dense bilateral congenital cataracts are the hallmark ophthalmic finding in Lowe syndrome. The cataracts are typically derived early in prenatal development and result from abnormal formation and degeneration of the posterior lens fibers. Characteristics of the cataracts in Lowe syndrome have been reported as disciform and located in either the anterior or posterior lens. Therefore, specific location of the lenticular defects is not required for diagnosis (24). Glaucoma is found in 50% to 60% of patients with Lowe syndrome. It is typically diagnosed within the first year of life and may or may not be associated with buphthalmos. Early surgical intervention is usually indicated for both the cataracts and glaucoma. Also specific to this disease, in about 25% of patients, is the formation of conreal keloids that are not caused by an earlier injury. Strabismus is also reported (23).

Mucopolysaccharidoses: Hurler Syndrome (MPS I), Hunter Syndrome (MPS II), Sanfilippo Syndrome (MPS III) Diseases involving abnormal carbohydrate metabolism are collectively known as mucopolysaccharidoses (MPS). As a whole, occurring in only about 1:20,000 live births, it is a rare group of inherited diseases that result from the accumulation of complex carbohydrates (glycosaminoglycans) within the lysosome organelles of the cells responsible for building connective tissue (24). Without the appropriate enzyme necessary for the breakdown of these carbohydrates, organ systems are altered and unable to function normally. Currently, the MPS are divided into seven (MPS I–VII) groups each based on their own enzyme deficiency.

Common systemic findings among the MPS involve course facial features, including a prominent forehead, depressed nasal bridge, enlarged tongue, and flat face (Figure 7-3). Organs such as the liver, heart, and spleen are often larger than normal, airways may become obstructed and joints are often stiff and limited in motion. Inguinal and umbilical hernias are reported, and progressive deterioration of mental capacity affecting gait, hearing, and speech are expected (25).

Mucopolysaccharide deposition in the cornea is common among individuals with Hurler

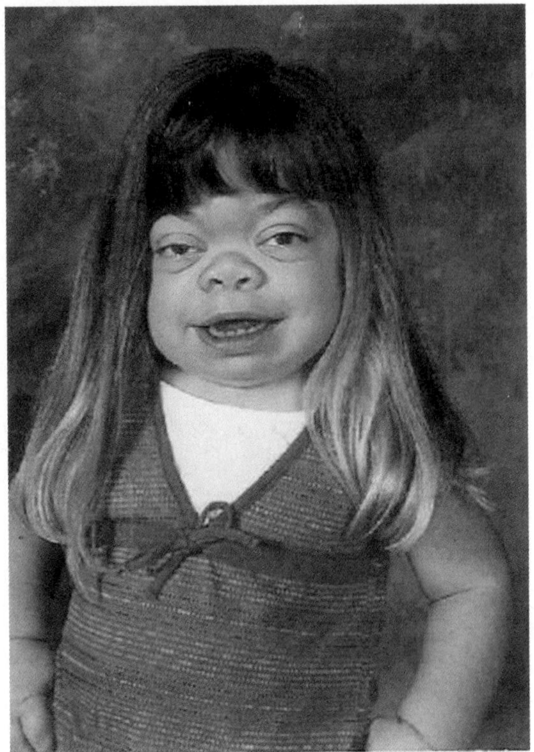

FIGURE 7-3. Young female with characteristic prominent forehead and depressed nasal bridge commonly noted in Hurler syndrome (MPS I). (Photo courtesy of The National MPS Society.)

syndrome (MPS I). However, this clinical finding is absent in Hunter (MPS II) and Sanfilippo (MPS III) syndromes (25). Additional ocular findings include pigmentary degeneration of the retina, attenuation of retinal vasculature, scleral thickening, and optic atrophy (26).

Treatment regimen depends on the type of MPS diagnosed, yet all require multidiscipline approach (25). Management strategies range from palliative care to the use of gene therapy. Presently, there is some utilization of enzyme replacement therapy for MPS I, and while this has proven successful in reducing symptoms, there has been no cure to date. The prevention of amblyopia is indicated when corneal deposition is dense enough to cause a decline in visual acuity. Depending on the severity of the corneal clouding, refractive correction, optometric vision therapy, penetrating keratoplasty, or a combination of these treatments may be warranted. Annual comprehensive eye examinations including patient counseling and consultation with a low vision specialist may also be necessary (25).

Prader-Willi Syndrome Prader-Willi syndrome, often regarded as the sister syndrome to Angelman, is the partial deletion of chromosome 15 on the paternal side. With an incidence of 1:15,000, its systemic manifestation by adulthood includes hypotonia, obesity, learning disabilities, and short stature (27). These individuals will eat nonstop if allowed to do so and will then demonstrate all of the health issues frequently associated with obesity. However, with early intervention and the use of growth hormone therapy, many of these clinical characteristics are negligible or they do not develop (Figure 7-4A,B). Similar to Angelman syndrome, strabismus is the most commonly reported ophthalmic sign. Less noted are the almond-shaped palpebral fissures and myopia (28).

Rett Syndrome Although often included within the autism spectrum disorder category, some experts believe that Rett syndrome is different enough from autism to be considered as a separate entity. It has been confused with Angelman syndrome, however. Rett syndrome is a mutation on the X chromosome, specifically the methyl CpG–binding protein 2 (MECP2), which alters the development of brain gray matter. As a result, significant deficits of motor control, sensory input, and autonomic function are appreciated. Clinical presentation is most typical in females due to the location on the X chromosome, though rare cases are reported in males (28). Incidence is thought to be about 1:15,000 female births (29).

A child with Rett syndrome may appear developmentally normal at birth, until about 6 to 18 months of life when delays in neurologic function become evident. Regression in neurologic development is noted by a loss of communication skills, declining motor control, missed milestones such as head circumference, and an observable hand-wringing/washing behavior (28,29).

A review of the current literature regarding ophthalmic manifestations of this syndrome is sparse. Unlike other neurodevelopmental disorders, Rett syndrome does not manifest with any particularly common ocular pathology. Difficulty in maintaining eye contact has been reported, but is commonly attributed to apraxia, or lack of motor control (30).

Spina Bifida The accurate development of the CNS is contingent on the complete closure of the embryonic neural tube. Without this closure, vertebrae and meninges needed to surround and protect

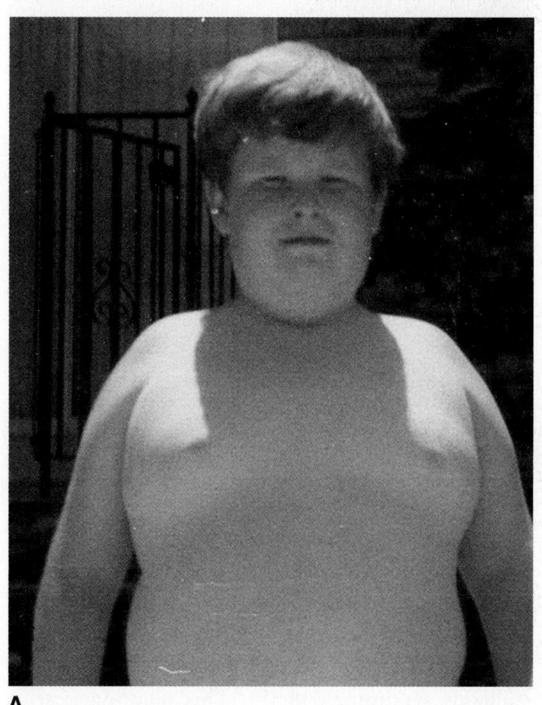

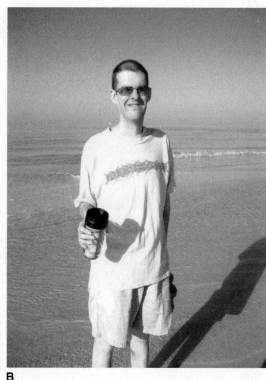

A B

FIGURE 7-4. **A:** Young male exhibiting early weight gain in children with Prader-Willi syndrome. **B:** Same male as **(A)** 30 years after early intervention and growth hormone therapy. (Photos courtesy of Prader-Willi Syndrome Association.)

the spinal cord remain undeveloped and unfused. This opening in the vertebrae may allow a portion of the spinal cord to protrude and become exposed making it susceptible to damage. Spina bifida is an example of this incomplete closure and can present in many degrees of severity depending on the displacement of the spinal cord. Surgical closure of the opening is required, but functional damage that occurred prior to treatment cannot be restored (6,30).

Common manifestations of spina bifida include spinal cord cysts, posterior meningocele, and hydrocephalus. Complications from these presentations will include pain, loss of muscle tone, and deformity of the hips and legs. An increase of intracranial pressure secondary to hydrocephalus is common in children with this condition because of the downward displacement of the cerebellum into the foramen magnum preventing normal flow of cerebrospinal fluid. Surgical implantation of a ventriculoperitoneal shunt is indicated to prevent neurologic damage resulting from the elevated intracranial pressure (31).

Research has identified several ophthalmic associations secondary to the increase in intracranial pressure associated with spina bifida. Conditions such as fourth cranial nerve palsy, nystagmus, papilledema, and optic atrophy have been reported. Dysfunction of ventriculoperitoneal shunts are also implicated in the acute onset of strabismus and other motility disorders. Due to the chance of optic atrophy, conservative follow-up on these patients is necessary (32).

Stickler Syndrome With an estimated prevalence of 1:8,000 newborns, Stickler syndrome is another genetic mutation that ultimately affects the biosynthesis of collagen. Like many collagenopathies, these mutations can affect multiple genes creating a range of signs and symptoms. Some individuals have no signs/symptoms and those that do vary from subtle to profound. Characteristic findings include craniofacial defects (midface hypoplasia, flattened bridge of nose, and cleft palate), arthropathy (joint hypermobility and precocious osteoarthritis), audiologic deficits (sensorineural and conductive loss), and ophthalmologic involvement (myopia, retinal detachment, and vitreous anomalies) (33) (Figure 7-5A,B).

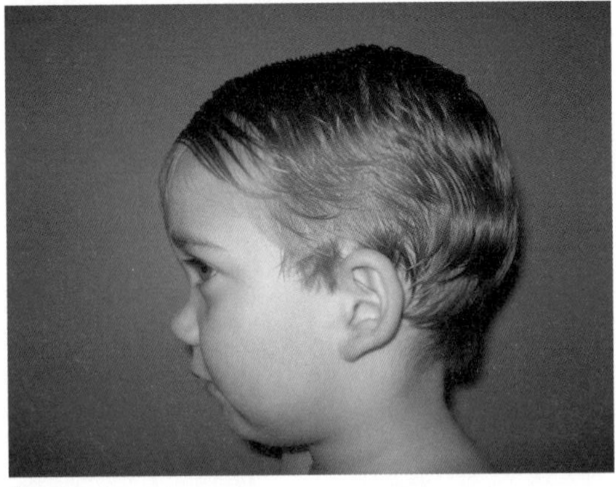

A

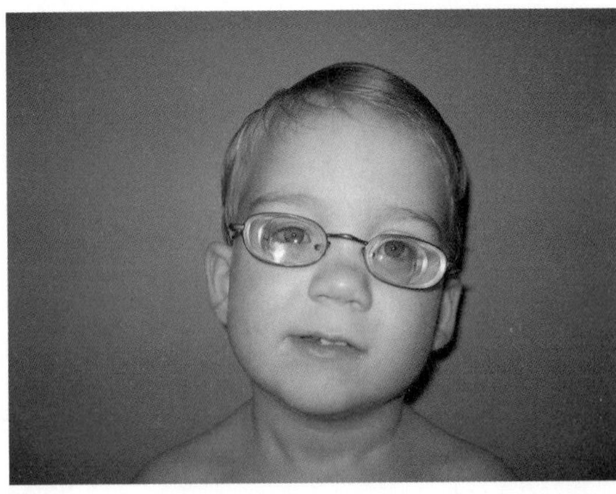

B

FIGURE 7-5. **A:** A young male with midface hypoplasia and flattened bridge of nose commonly associated with Stickler syndrome. **B:** Same young male shown in **(A)** wearing high myopic correction associated with Stickler syndrome. (Photo courtesy of Stickler Involved People.)

Though clinical diagnostic criteria have not been clearly established, ophthalmic findings are common in individuals with Stickler's syndrome. A clinically significant finding for Stickler syndrome is myopia >3 diopters in the infant. Accepting that the refractive error of an infant is generally hyperopic, any degree of myopia is suspicious. Additional ocular findings include anomalies such as vitreal veils or folds in the retrolental space, or less commonly, thickened wax-like bundles throughout the posterior vitreal cavity (34). The degeneration of retinal tissue leading to retinal holes, tears, or detachments is related to the compromised collagen synthesis. Cataracts and glaucoma are both commonly reported in literature (35,36).

The treatment for Stickler syndrome should include genetic counseling due to the syndrome's wide variability. Conservative follow-up schedules should be administered to those who are considered "at risk." Therefore, comprehensive eye examinations are performed at least annually, and more frequently in the presence of glaucoma, cataracts, or chorioretinal changes. Referral to the appropriate vision specialist is indicated.

Williams Syndrome Williams syndrome is a genetic disorder involving the vast area of deletion of approximately 26 genes on chromosome 7. Because of this deletion, the phenotype of Williams can vary. However, consistent clinical findings of mental retardation, hypotonia, and cardiac anomalies persist. The most notable characteristics of Williams syndrome are the elf-like facial features and the cheerful demeanor they possess (Figure 7-6). The Incidence of Williams is only 1:15,000 (37).

Developmental issues arise because of abnormalities noted in the cerebellum, right parietal cortex, and left frontal cortical regions. Anomalies in these areas would explain problems with environmental visual–spatial relationships noted in individuals with Williams syndrome (38,39). This may manifest as

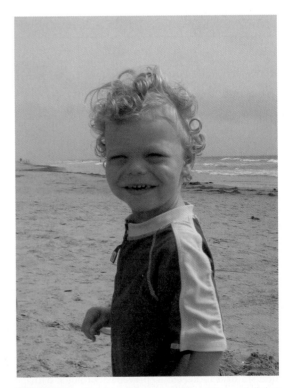

FIGURE 7-6. Cheerful demeanor, hypopigmentation, and distinct facial features shown in a young male with Williams syndrome. (Photo courtesy of Williams Syndrome Association.)

deficits in visual memory when trying to copy words or figures to paper, or difficulty arranging material on spaces like a desktop. In addition, a connection to infantile esotropia is also suspected. In those with esotropia, dissociated vertical deviations and oblique dysfunctions were reported (40). Presently, no cure exists, however, specific therapies are indicated to improve existing skills. Speech therapy may be utilized for verbal strengthening, strabismus surgery for the esotropia, and optometric vision therapy/physical therapy for visual–spatial issues (41).

CONCLUSION

Individuals with various neurodevelopmental disorders often exhibit multiple functional, perceptual, and pathologic disorders with which the optometrist should not only be familiar, but they should also understand the underlying anatomical, physiologic, genetic, and neurologic anomalies associated with these special needs patients (42). Children with disabilities should have every opportunity to grow and develop into adults with the highest quality of life possible. Ensuring that children have single, clear, comfortable, binocular, and pathology-free vision is an important part of the overall care of individuals with neurodevelopmental disorders (43).

REFERENCES

1. Kroner BL, Preiss LR, Ardini MA, Gaillard WD. Aicardi syndrome. J Child Neurol. 2008;23:531–5.
2. Zubairi MS, Carter RF, Ronen GM. A male phenotype with Aicardi syndrome. J Child Neurol. 2009;24:204–7.
3. Walsh FB. Clinical neuro-ophthalmology: the essentials. 2nd ed. Philadelphia: Lippincott Williams & Wilkins; 2008. p. 88–9.
4. Colville DJ, Savige J. Alport syndrome. A review of the ocular manifestations. Ophthalmic Genet. 1997;18:161–73.
5. McCarthy P, Maino D. Alport syndrome: a review. Clin Eye Vis Care. 2001;12:139–50.
6. Schneider BB, Maino DM. Angelman syndrome. J Am Optom Assoc. 1993;64:502–6.
7. Seeliger M, Ruther K, Apfelstedt-Sylla E, et al. Juvenile neuronal ceroid lipofuscinosis (Batten-Mayou) disease. Ophthalmologic diagnosis and findings. Ophthalmologe. 1997;94:557–62.
8. Johns Hopkins Vasculitis Center. http://vasculitis.med.jhu.edu/typesof.behcets.html. Last Accessed November 3, 2010.
9. Yanagihori H, Oyama N, Nakamura K, et al. Role of IL-12B promoter polymorphism in Adamantiades-Behcet's disease susceptibility: an involvement of Th1 immunoreactivity against Streptococcus Sanguinis antigen. J Invest Dermatol. 2006;126:1534–40.
10. Behcet's Disease. Medline Plus. National Institute of Health. Available from: http://www.nlm.nih.gov/medlineplus.behcetssyndrome.htm. Last Accessed December 21, 2010.
11. Citirik M, Berker N, Songur MS, et al. Ocular findings in childhood-onset Behcet disease. J AAPOS. 2009;13:391–5.
12. The American Heritage Dictionary of the English Language. 4th ed. Boston: Houghton Mifflin; 2000.
13. Sheffler RN, Zlotogora J, Elpeleg ON, et al. Behr's syndrome and 3-methylglutaconic aciduria. Am J Ophthalmol. 1992;114:494–7.
14. Craniofacial Anomalies Causes by Altered Branchial Arch Morphogenesis. Institute of Dental and Craniofacial Research. National Institute of Health. Available from: http://www.nidcr.nih.gov/DataStatistics/SurgeonGeneral/sgr/chap3.htm. Last Accessed July 1, 2010.
15. Vissers LE, van Ravenswaaij CM, Admiraal R, et al. Mutations in a new member of the chromodomain gene family cause CHARGE syndrome. Nat Genet. 2004;36:955–7.
16. Zenter GE, Layman WS, Martin DM, et al. Molecular and phenotypic aspects of CHD7 mutation in CHARGE syndrome. Am J Med Genet. 2010;152A:674–86.
17. McMain K, Blake K, Smith I, et al. Ocular features of CHARGE syndrome. J AAPOS. 2008;12:460–5.
18. Beighton P, De Paepe A, Steinmann B, Tsipouras P, Wenstrup RJ. Ehlers-Danlos syndromes: revised nosology, Villefranche, 1997. Ehlers-Danlos National Foundation (USA) and Ehlers-Danlos Support Group (UK). Am J Med Genet. 1988;77:31–7.
19. May MA, Beauchamp GR. Collagen maturation defects in Ehler-Danlos keratopathy. J Pediatr Ophthalmol Strabismus. 1987;24:78–82.
20. Green WR, Friedman-Kien A, Banfield WG. Angioid Streaks in Ehler-Danlos Syndrome. Arch Ophthalmol. 1966;76: 197–204.
21. Abel RL, Sokol RJ. Incidence of fetal alcohol syndrome and economic impact of FAS-related anomalies: drug alcohol syndrome and economic impact of FAS-related anomalies. Drug Alcohol Depend. 1987;19:51–70.
22. Loi M. Lowe syndrome. Orphanet J Rare Dis. 2006;1:16.
23. Amira A. Oculocerebrorenal dystrophy. eMedicine. WebMD, http://emedicine.medscape.com/article/946043-overview. Last Accessed November 20, 2010.
24. Tripathi RC, Cibis GW, Tripathi BJ. Pathogenesis of cataracts in patients with Lowe's syndrome. Ophthalmology. 1986;93:1046–51.
25. Defendi GL. Mucopolysaccharidosis Type III. eMedicine. WebMD, http://emedicine.medscape.com/article/948540-overview. Last Accessed November 1, 2010.
26. Roy FH. Ocular syndromes and systemic diseases. 3rd ed. Philadelphia: Lippincott Williams & Wilkins; 2002. p. 571–2.
27. Prader-Willi Syndrome. Mayoclinic.com. Mayo Clinic. Available from: http://www.mayoclinic.com/health/prader-willi-syndrome/DS00922. Last Accessed October 21, 2010.
28. Libov A, Maino D. Prader-Willi syndrome. J Am Optom Assoc. 1994;65:355–9.
29. About Rett Syndrome. International Rett Syndrome Foundation. p. 2008. Available from: http://www.rettsyndrome.org/about-rett-syndrome.html. Last Accessed October 21, 2010.
30. Rett Syndrome Fact Sheet. National Institute of Neurological Disorders and Stroke. National Institute of Health. Available

from: http://ninds.nih.gov/disorders/rett/detail_rett.htm. Last Accessed December 15, 2010.

31. Segawa M. Visual child neurology. Rinsho Shinkeigaku. 2003;43:739–43.
32. Foster MR. Spina bifida. eMedicine. WebMD. Available from: http://www.emedicine.com/orthoped/TOPIC557.HTM. Last Accessed January 6, 2011.
33. Gaston H. Ophthalmic complications of spina bifida and hydrocephalus. Eye (Lond). 1991;5:279–90.
34. Robin NH, Moran RT, Warman M. Stickler syndrome. GeneReviews. Available from: http://www.ncbi.nlm.nih.gov/books/NBK1302/#stickler. Last Accessed November 1, 2010.
35. Snead MP, Yates JR. Clinical and molecular genetics of Stickler syndrome. J Med Genet. 1999;36:353–9.
36. Seery CM, Pruett RC, Liberfarb RM, Cohen BZ. Distinctive cataract in the Stickler syndrome. Am J Ophthalmol. 1990;110: 143–8.
37. Ziakas NG, Ramsay AS, Lynch SA, et al. Stickler's syndrome associated with congenital glaucoma. Ophthalmic Genet. 1998;19:55–8.
38. Martens MA, Wilson SJ, Reutens DC. Research review: Williams syndrome: a critical review of the cognitive, behavioral, and neuroanatomical phenotype. J Child Psychol Psychiatry. 2008;49:576–608.
39. Cozolino L. The neuroscience of human relationships: attachment and the developing social brain. New York, NY. W W Norton & Co. 2006. p.289–91.
40. Hirota H, Matsuoka R, Chen X, et al. Williams syndrome deficits in visual spatial processing linked to GTF2IRD1 and GTF2I on chromosome 7q11.23. Genet Med. 2003;5:311–21.
41. Kapp ME, von Noorden GK, Jenkins R. Strabismus in Williams syndrome. Am J Ophthalmol. 1995;120:266–7.
42. Maino DM, Maino JH, Cibis GW, et al. Ocular health anomalies in patients with developmental disabilities. In: Maino D, editor. Diagnosis and management of special populations. St. Louis: Mosby-Yearbook, Inc.; 1995. p. 189–206. Reprinted Optometric Education Program Foundation, Santa Anna, CA. 2001.
43. Maino D. Overview of special populations. In: Scheiman M, Rouse M, editors. Optometric management of learning related vision problems. St. Louis: Mosby Inc.; 2006. p. 85–106.

CHAPTER 8

Rachel Anastasia Coulter, OD, FAAO, FCOVD

Autism

AUTISM: DEFINITIONS AND CATEGORIES

Autism is a group of developmental brain disorders characterized by problems in social interaction, communication, and sensory processing, as well as repetitive, stereotyped behaviors (1–3). Symptoms usually start before age 3 years and vary greatly from individual to individual. Autism spectrum disorder (ASD) refers to three conditions: autistic disorder (classic autism), Asperger syndrome, and pervasive developmental disorder not otherwise specified (PPD-NOS). Another term sometimes used, Pervasive Developmental Disorders (PPD) includes the three conditions of ASD (autistic disorder, Asperger syndrome, and PPD-NOS) as well as childhood disintegrative disorder (CDD) and Rett syndrome (2,4). All of the PDD conditions share core deficits of social and communication impairment and unusual behaviors but differ in symptom severity, onset, and progression as well as some physical characteristics.

Individuals with autistic disorder show signs before the age of 3 years. Social interaction impairment manifests as decreased eye contact, little facial expression, an inability to develop peer relationships, and a lack of social or emotional reciprocity (meaning the individual does not return social and emotional gestures). Communication deficits appear as a delay developing spoken language, an inability to carry on a conversation, use of stereotyped, repetitive, or idiosyncratic language, and limited ability for make-believe or pretend play. Repetitive, stereotyped behavior patterns include difficulty in transitioning to new activities, continued repetitive motor actions, preoccupation with an object's parts rather than its intended purpose, and restricted, abnormal focus of interest (4–6). Individuals with PDD-NOS have some, but not all, of the characteristics of autistic disorder. Symptoms are milder or onset after age 3 years (4). Individuals with Asperger syndrome have normal or above intelligence, acquire language early, and speak fluently (4,5). These individuals, however, struggle to interact socially due to inability to read nonverbal cues, problems in sharing and interpreting others' emotions, and overfocusing on very narrow topics of interest (4).

Childhood disintegrative disorder and Rett syndrome are rare and more severe. Individuals with CDD develop normally for at least 2 years. After an initial period of normal development, they experience severe regressions and significant loss of previously acquired skills in expressive or receptive language, social abilities or adaptive behavior, bowel or bladder control, play, or motor skills. Autistic behaviors also emerge (4). Individuals with Rett syndrome show early milestones that are grossly normal. Development then plateaus and regression occurs at 6 to 30 months of age (4). Communication and socialization skills deteriorate. Individuals develop an unsteady gait and stereotypic hand movements and have difficulty in the regulation of breathing. Rett syndrome occurs only in females. Transmission is by X-linked dominance.

PREVALENCE/INCIDENCE

The Center for Disease Control and Prevention reports that the prevalence for ASD is between 1 in 80 and 1 in 240, averaging 1 in 110 children in the United States (7). Since ASD is four times more common in boys than in girls, the prevalence for boys is approximately 1 out of 70. Autism spectrum disorder is found in children of all races and nationalities (8,9).

This prevalence rate is markedly higher than was reported 15 to 20 years ago (8,10). The increase has been a source of debate in the scientific community and general public. ASD was redefined in 1994, when the Diagnostic and Statistical Manual of

Mental Disorders broadened the diagnostic criteria including more individuals in the classification (9). Other factors contributed to more individuals being diagnosed. Parent and advocacy groups worked to increase public awareness and media coverage of the condition increased. The provision of educational and medical services under the diagnosis ultimately resulted in more individuals diagnosed with an ASD. Training programs for physicians, psychologists, educators, and other specialists to detect and diagnose ASD increased (9,10). Since all of these factors had some impact, much deliberation occurred as to whether the increase in new cases was a real increase in the number of individuals manifesting ASD characteristics or was the result of reclassification (11).

Studies of the increase in ASD incidence have differed in their conclusions. A study of data from a national special education database found that the increase in autism prevalence paralleled the change in diagnostic criteria, eventually stabilizing (12). A study of prevalence in four areas of the United States found that the increase could be partially attributed to better access to services and improved diagnostic capabilities but that a real increase could not be ruled out (13). Studies of the Center for Disease Control's tracking system, a telephone survey of parents, and a population-based study suggested the reported prevalence might actually be an underestimate (14–16).

ETIOLOGY

The exact cause of autism is unknown. Evidence suggests that autism is linked to a complex interaction between environmental stressors, genetic mutations, and biologic factors including inflammatory processes (17,18). Scientific evidence does not support a link between autism and the measles–mumps–rubella (MMR) vaccine or Thimerosal, a vaccine preservative (19–25). The association began after Wakefield and colleagues published a study in the Lancet in 1998 implying a link between the MMR vaccine, gastrointestinal symptoms, and autism (26). The study was later discredited for multiple reasons (27). Wakefield had undisclosed financial conflicts of interest and selected subjects whose parents were involved in lawsuits against immunization manufacturers. Eventually, Wakefield was found guilty of dishonesty by Britain's General Medical Council. In 2004, 10 of the 13 original authors retracted support for the article. In 2010, the Lancet retracted the study (27). In the last decade, at least 20 higher-quality studies of large numbers of children evaluating data from many countries failed to show any link between the MMR vaccine and autism (28,29). These studies included a cohort study of more than 500,000 children followed over years, a case–control study of 1,294 autistic and 4,469 nonautistic children, and time-series analyses. All showed no connection between the start of MMR immunization and the onset of autism and no relationship between vaccination rates and autism (30–35).

MEDICAL CONDITIONS ASSOCIATED WITH ASD

Though the exact cause of autism is unknown, some medical conditions have been associated with ASD. Fragile X syndrome, discussed in greater detail in Chapter 5, Intellectual Disabilities of Unknown Etiology, is a genetically transmitted X-linked dominant disorder with reduced penetrance (36). Characteristics of Fragile X syndrome include mental retardation, macrocephaly, hypotonia, and joint hyperextensibility (5). Only 3% to 4% of individuals with ASD test positively for Fragile X syndrome by DNA testing (5). Tuberous sclerosis is a genetically transmitted dominant disorder with half of cases representing new mutations (5,37). This neurocutaneous disorder is characterized by café au lait macules, axillary freckling, and ocular Lisch nodules and is found in 1% to 4% of the ASD population (5,37). Angelman syndrome, discussed in Chapter 7, Oculovisual Abnormalities Associated with Rare Neurodevelopmental Disorders, is a rare neurodevelopmental disorder linked to a deletion of the ubiquitin-protein gene (UBE3A) (38). Angelman syndrome is characterized by severe mental retardation, hypotonia, seizures, ataxia (lack of coordination of muscle movement), and a happy temperament (5).

RISK FACTORS

Risk of autism increases when a sibling has a PDD, when parents are older than 35 years of age, and when the mother has a history of autoimmune diseases such as rheumatoid arthritis or celiac disease (39–43). Low birth weight, prematurity, and breech birth are associated with an increased risk of autism; however, the association is believed to be one of shared etiology rather than a cause–effect relationship (44,45).

IMPACT ON THE FAMILY

Clinicians working with patients with ASD should realize that though one family member has a diagnosis of ASD, the impact of living with ASD extends throughout the family. Studies show that the demands and stress of living with a family member who has ASD is greater than that experienced by living with a family member who has mental retardation, another developmental problem or a chronic medical condition. Stress from caring for a child with ASD throughout the life span can result in adverse financial pressure, decreased employment opportunities, increased risk of physical impairment, and decreased quality of life (46–53). Social support and other positive coping responses have been shown to moderate stress levels (54).

Siblings are also greatly impacted by the demands of living with a family member with ASD. Parents tend to overestimate the sibling's understanding of the disorder's impact (55).

Siblings may be at greater risk for developing more behavior problems including attention difficulties, conduct problems and poorer socialization abilities (56,57). A goal in working with families with a developmentally challenged family member is to shift the balance from vulnerability to resilience. Family strengths that support resilience include close family relationships, good communication and problem-solving abilities, friendliness, helpfulness, and the ability to obtain support from friends, teachers, and extended family members (54,57).

GENERAL/CONSTITUTIONAL

Primary Care and the Patient with Autism

Children with autism have more outpatient visits, physician visits, and medication prescribed than children in general. Physician visits for children with autism require more time than for other children (58). Not surprisingly, annual medical expenditures for individuals with ASD are on average seven times higher than those without ASD (59).

Physicians often feel unprepared to care for individuals with autism due to lower overall self-perceived competency and a need for education on how to care for children with autism (60). Physicians who are more prepared attribute their abilities to more experience with patients with ASD (greater number of patient visits), having a friend or relative with autism, and previous training on how to care for patients with autism (60). Partnering with families can facilitate the patient care process. A variety of strategies can be used including sharing information in advance of the appointment, preparing the child for the visit, bringing a bag of toys or books to entertain or sensory items to alleviate fidgeting, scheduling at optimal times, and planning for time demands (61).

Medical conditions are common in ASD. The social and communication problems of autism make patient care more difficult (62). A child with autism who is ill may not be able to communicate his symptoms, but may show behavioral changes including irritability, withdrawal, decreased cooperation, or decreased appetite (62). Treatment of medical conditions is critical as it improves the quality of life for individuals with ASD and their families (63,64). In addition to routine preventative care and treatment of acute illness, a variety of chronic medical conditions co-occur including sleep disturbances, gastrointestinal problems, seizures, and anxiety (65,66). Individuals with ASD are also increased risk for obesity and acute injury. Americans face an epidemic of obesity and individuals with ASD face increased risk. Motor planning and social and cognitive challenges often make exercise and recreation activities more difficult. In addition, the side effects of medications commonly taken include weight gain (67).

Individuals with ASD have higher rates of acute injury as indicated by higher rates of emergency department and hospital admission. They are more likely to have head, face, and neck injuries and to be treated for poisoning or self-inflicted injury (68). High school students with autism who participate in interscholastic sports leagues are more likely to experience sports-related injuries (69).

REVIEW OF SYSTEMS

Skin Specific to individuals with ASD is a concern regarding skin picking, a self-injurious behavior, in which one scratches or gouges of one's own skin using fingers or tools. Skin picking can result in severe tissue damage, scars, and infections and can create social, mental health, and functional problems. Treatment consists of cognitive–behavioral treatments and pharmacologic management of associated compulsiveness, anxiety, and depression (70).

Eyes/Ears/Nose/Mouth/Throat

Eyes Most research focusing on vision and ocular health in individuals with ASD preceded the change in the diagnostic criteria of 1994. As of 2010, two studies on individuals diagnosed since 1994 were published. Their results differ. A vision-screening study reported by Milne et al. (71) in 2009 compared 51 individuals with ASD and 44 typically developing individuals aged 8 to 18 years old in the United Kingdom. Measures included visual acuity, stereoacuity, prism bar convergence and divergence, ocular motility by extraocular muscle testing, cover test for presence of strabismus, and optokinetic response. Results suggest that most vision measures, including visual acuity, are unaffected in ASD, but convergence may be reduced. In contrast, Adams et al. reported vision-screening results of 44 individuals aged 3 to 22 years old in 2010. Using measures of visual acuity, alignment, stereoacuity, refractive error, contrast sensitivity, and Vernier acuity, they found that 3-to-6-year-olds showed moderate deficits in visual acuity, Vernier acuity, stereoacuity, and ocular alignment. Those in the older group, aged 7 to 22 years, performed even more poorly, showing significant deficits in visual acuity, Vernier acuity, stereoacuity, and ocular alignment (72). Studies of cohorts of patients with autism diagnosed before the diagnostic criteria changed suggest that saccades and pursuits are poorer in these patients than in typically developing patients (73).

Ocular Injury and Ocular Health Conditions

Special concerns for individuals with ASD regarding ocular injury emphasize the need for an objective examination and consideration of eye protection. Two cases of children with ASD presenting with recurrent corneal metallic foreign bodies are reported. The foreign bodies were obtained through the extensive use of a therapeutic home swing that was suspended by a metallic tether. Protective eyewear worn during swinging prevented further recurrences (74).

Optic neuropathy secondary to poor diet is a concern. Three cases of children with ASD presenting with partially reversible optic neuropathy secondary to dietary vitamin B_{12} deficiency have been reported. These cases manifested as gradual visual loss as the result of severe food selectivity manifested as not eating animal products in the diet and outright food refusal (75). Clinicians should inquire about nutrition and food intake in the history.

Dental Individuals with autism are at increased risk for oral health problems due to their sensory sensitivities, communication deficits, and diet. These conditions include widespread caries, advanced periodontitis, bruxism (teeth grinding), oral–facial pain, and xerostomia, that is, a dry mouth due to a lack of saliva (often a side effect of medication). Dental prevention and treatment efforts may be less successful resulting in increased severity. Increased risk of dental caries occurs due to perseverating on foods with high sugar and refined carbohydrates. Limited self-cleansing action of the mouth can occur due to poor tongue and cheek coordination. Poor oral hygiene due to the individual's increased sensitivity and resistance and parents' and caretakers' attention to other care priorities also can contribute to dental caries. Poor nutrition resulting in insufficient levels of vitamins, minerals, and folate necessary for red blood cell production may contribute to a higher incidence of anemia and increased gingivitis in these patients. Increased mouth trauma is noted due to a higher occurrence of accidents (76).

Respiratory The most significant respiratory problems associated with autism are those of Rett syndrome. These include breathing irregularities, episodes of apnea, and hyperventilation (4).

Gastrointestinal Gastrointestinal symptoms are common (77). Research indicates that 24% of individuals with ASD have a history of at least one chronic gastrointestinal symptom. The most common symptoms are diarrhea (17%), constipation (8.8%), reflux/vomiting (6.6%), abdominal pain (2.1%), and gas (1.5%) (77). Due to the communication deficits of ASD, symptoms may present as changes in behavior: screaming, whining, or sobbing for no reason, delayed echolalia that includes a reference to pain or the stomach (e.g., child says, "Does your tummy hurt?" echoing what mother may have said to child in the past), constant eating/drinking/swallowing, mouthing behaviors such as chewing on clothes, leaning one's abdomen against or over furniture, agitation including jumping up and down or pacing, an unexplained increase in repetitive behavior, increased irritability, sleep disturbance, aggression, and self-injurious behaviors (78). Pediatric guidelines for diagnostic evaluation of abdominal pain, chronic constipation, and gastroesophageal reflux disease can help to determine when gastrointestinal symptoms are self-limited or when additional evaluation is warranted (79). Neurobehavioral differences may contribute to constipation and feeding issues as much as gastrointestinal etiology (80). Depending on the type and severity of the problem, treatments include all or some of the following: dietary interventions, behavioral interventions focused on feeding and diet, nutritional supplements, and medications that address gastrointestinal disorder (e.g., gastroesophageal reflux) (81).

Potential links between the immune and gastrointestinal systems and the brain are an area of interest in autism (82). The "leaky gut" theory hypothesizes that altered intestinal permeability in individuals with ASD allows increased passage of food-derived peptides through damaged gut mucosa. Abnormal peptide passage from the intestine to the circulatory system results in immune dysfunction and excess opiate activity in the central nervous system. Under this theory, altered microflora in the gut contributes to increased intestinal permeability. Treatment of recurrent otitis media by antibiotics decreases healthy bacteria normally found in the gut. Probiotics, supplements that restore healthy bacterial population, can be used to offset gut permeability (82).

Scientific support for the "leaky gut" theory is limited. One study of 25 children who had autism and GI symptoms found that 76% have altered intestinal permeability, measured by lactulose-to-mannitol recovery ratios. Other research does not confirm the presence of abnormal opioid peptid circulation in individuals with ASD or that a "leaky gut" contributes to the underlying brain changes or behaviors manifesting as autism (83–85).

Nutrition In individuals with ASD, nutrition is linked to not just gastrointestinal problems, but also dental problems, behaviors, and other medical problems, such as optic neuropathy. Nutritional status can be adversely impacted by gastrointestinal symptoms, food allergies, metabolic abnormalities, and/or preexisting nutrient deficiencies and nutrition-related medication side effects (86). Eating behaviors commonly found in autism such as pica (eating nonfood items) and food selectivity (eating the same food much of the time) can adversely impact nutritional status (86–88). Sensory processing differences including hyper- and hyposensitivities to taste and smell that may result in specific food cravings or food avoidance.

Studies comparing the nutritional status of children with ASD with typical peers have diverged in their findings but identified some areas of concern. Children with ASD who showed feeding symptoms from 15 months of age consumed less vegetables and fruit but also less sweets and soft drinks (89). A study focusing on the impact of risperidone (an antipsychotic used to treat aggression in autism) on nutritional status found great variability at baseline, with some individuals having very low levels of calcium, pantothenic acid, and vitamin K (90). In contrast, other research found children with ASD were more likely to have a significantly greater intake of all nutrients including protein, carbohydrates, niacin, thiamine, riboflavin, calcium, phosphorus, and iron. This occurred, because the parent or caretaker believed that diet was linked to behavior and made a substantial effort for the child to eat better diet (91).

Many individuals with autism are on a gluten-free, casein-free diet (GFCF) (92). The diet eliminates gluten in wheat and other grains as well as food starches, malt and some flavorings, and casein, a protein found in milk, cheese, cream, yogurt, and other dairy products. The GFCF diet is used as a treatment to decrease hypersensitivities to gluten and casein and the associated immune reaction. Under the leaky gut theory, it also decreases opioid production and behaviors linked to autism. Research has not validated the leaky gut hypothesis, nor has it confirmed that the GFCF diet decreases problematic behaviors associated with autism (93). Studies have shown that children with ASD have an elevated immune response to dietary proteins associated with wheat, dairy, and soy than typical children (93,94). The GFCF diet in combination with food selectivity, digestive problems, decreased exercise, and decreased vitamin D can increase risk for thinner, less dense bones when compared with a group of boys the same age who do not have autism (94).

Genitourinary Girls with autism are more likely to present with behavioral issues related to the onset of menstruation than girls with other developmental disabilities (95).

Neurologic/Psychiatric Individuals with autism often have co-occurring neurologic and psychiatric problems. Epilepsy is common occurring in 11% to 39% of these patients (96). The onset of epilepsy peaks during two periods: before age 5 years and during adolescence. Children with ASD who have severe cognitive or motor impairment are at higher risk of epilepsy than those who are less impaired.

Sleep disturbances, manifest as difficulty going to sleep and night waking, occur in 44% to 83% of children and adolescents with autism (97,98). The cause of sleep disturbance is unknown, although theories include gastrointestinal problems or diminished melatonin production.

Psychiatric problems such as mood disorder and aggression behaviors occur in 32% of children (98). Other common co-occurring psychiatric diagnoses include specific phobias, attention deficit hyperactivity disorder, obsessive–compulsive disorder, anxiety disorders, and major depression (96,99).

Chronic pain is an issue in some individuals with autism. Case reports of two adolescents evaluated on medical consult for pain management found that both had had signs and symptoms consistent with pervasive developmental or autistic disorder. Review of medical records and parental interviews suggested that health care professionals did not identify the need for evaluation of these characteristics or consider them relevant in management of chronic pain (100).

Allergic/Immunologic/Lymphatic/Endocrine

Allergic disorders are at least as prevalent in ASD children as in the general population. Multiple research studies have identified abnormalities in both adaptive and innate immunity in patients with ASD (4). Allergic disorders may be underdiagnosed and undertreated due to the communication challenges and behaviors associated with ASD. Chronic inflammatory conditions can present as neuropsychiatric symptoms. In these cases, behavioral symptoms improve with medical management (101).

TREATMENT

Rehabilitation Treatment and Therapies

Treatment for autism is an intensive, comprehensive process involving a multidisciplinary team of professionals and the child's whole family (102,103). Experts agree intervention should begin as soon as a diagnosis of autism is considered and that most individuals with autism respond to highly structured, specialized programs (102,103). Effective treatment programs consist of many hours per week of therapy designed to reach specific behavioral, developmental, and educational goals (103). Treatment may occur in a preschool or school settings, therapy centers, or the child's home.

Many different therapies and approaches to treatment exist. Professionals new to learning about autism treatment may be overwhelmed by the "alphabet soup" of acronyms that refer to different approaches (applied behavior analysis [ABA], verbal behavior [VB], developmental individual difference relationship based [DIR], relationship development intervention [RDI], Picture exchange communication system [PECS]). Therapies differ in the research support for their efficacy. The intervention with the most substantial research support for autism is ABA (5,102).

Given the complexity of autism, a child's challenges often require more than only one therapy (103). Each challenge must be considered, evaluated, and targeted with an appropriate therapy. No therapy works for every child. What works for a child at one time may not work later (102). The ability, experience, and approach of the therapist can be critical to the effectiveness of the intervention. Families have strong preferences for treatment choice based on their experience, belief system, and parenting style. Though it is not possible to describe each and every therapy, a summary of therapies commonly used to treat autism is provided in Table 8.1 (104-114).

Educational Interventions In addition to teaching traditional academic skills, an effective educational program targets the core deficits of autism. Model programs have been described using behavior analytic, developmental, and structured teaching. The American Academy of Pediatrics (AAP) Council on Children with Disabilities (COCWD) has identified core elements of effective programs for early childhood (104):

- Intensive levels of intervention using systematically planned, developmentally appropriate activities to target objectives and that include active engagement of the child for at least 25 hours per week, 12 months per year
- Low student-to-teacher ratio that provides adequate time for individualized and small group instruction to target individualized goals
- Inclusion of a family component including a parent training program
- Opportunities for meaningful interaction with typically developing peers
- Ongoing measurement, documentation, and review of child's progress in mastering educational objectives; appropriate revision of goals and program based on review
- Use of high levels of structure including a predictable routine, visual activity schedules, and defined physical boundaries in classroom to minimize distractions
- Opportunities and strategies to promote generalization
- Assessment-based curricula that promote the development of functional, spontaneous communication; social skills including joint attention, imitation, reciprocal interaction, initiation, and

TABLE 8.1 Autism Treatments, Therapies, and Educational Interventions (104–114)

Category	Treatment	Core Principles	Implementation
Behavioral approach	Applied behavior analysis (ABA)	Scientific approach focused on principles of how learning takes place; positive behaviors are rewarded and undesired behaviors are decreased; based on the work of Lovaas	• Intervention designed by qualified, well-trained behavior analysts • Traditionally emphasized compliance, imitation, and receptive language; modified to incorporate other aspects of behavior • Detailed assessment of learner • Selection of meaningful goals for learner • Objectives for skills that are broken into small steps • Learner is given many opportunities to acquire skills • Ongoing collection of data and analysis to measure learning and to troubleshoot • Emphasis on skills for learners to become independent • Planned opportunities to use skills in new settings to promote generalization • Parent training and meetings with family
	Pivotal response treatment (PRT)	Used to teach language, decrease disruptive or self-stimulatory behavior, and increase social, communication, and academic skills by emphasizing acquisition of critical/pivotal behaviors that impact a wide range of uses	• Implemented by psychologists, special education teachers, speech therapists trained in PRT • Does not use preset curricula; curricula is child directed to determine activities used • Program includes language, play, social skills, and family routines • Tasks are varied; return to mastered tasks to increase retention • Purposeful attempts to communicate are rewarded
	Verbal behavior (VB)	Like ABA, uses behavior analysis to teach language skills; emphasizes acquisition of expressive language before receptive language and function of language over form	• Provided by VB-trained psychologists, special education teachers, speech therapists, other providers • Based on Skinner's analysis of teaching language and shaping behavior • Considers what child wants, then teaches the child how to request by gesture then by sign language/verbal expression; request rewarded to reinforce • Operant for labeling an object "tact"; "mand" (using language) more important than "tact" (knowing language) • Other parts of language, "intraverbals" include answers to w-questions (Who? What? When? Where? Why?) as well as something not physically present are reinforced by social reinforcement

Developmental approaches	Developmental individual difference relationship model (DIR)/"floortime"	Greenspan and Weider's clinical model of a relationship-based developmental approach; adult can help child expand circles of communication by meeting the child at his or her developmental level, building on the child's strengths and supporting child's ability to expand capabilities; Floortime refers to interaction in which adult gets down on floor to engage child in earlier levels; program also includes semi-structured play, and motor and sensory play	• Floortime-trained psychologists, special education teachers, speech therapists, occupational therapists, and other providers incorporate techniques in clinical practice and train parent and caregivers
			• Does not separate or focus on one area (speech, motor, or cognitive skills), instead addresses areas through synthesized emphasis on emotional development
			• First six levels include
			  • Co-regulation
			  • Engagement
			  • Affect-based two-way communication
			  • Behavioral organization/problem solving
			  • Creating and elaborating via symbolic play
			  • Emotional thinking, logical, abstract

(*Continued*)

TABLE 8.1 Autism Treatments, Therapies, and Educational Interventions (104–114) *(Continued)*

Category	Treatment	Core Principles	Implementation

	Relationship development intervention (RDI)	Gutstein's model is a cognitive-based developmental approach; model is based on parent-provided treatment to develop "dynamic intelligence"; goal is to improve individual's quality of life by helping them improve social skills, adaptability, and self-awareness	• RDI-certified consultant provides training and guidance to parents, teachers
			• Parents provide primary treatment to child
			• Children begin working one-on-one with parent, with mastery move to dyad
			• Focuses on child's current development, while systematically teaching skills and child's competency, focusing on the child's current developmental level of functioning
			• Six objectives:
			  • Emotional referencing
			  • Social coordination
			  • Declarative language
			  • Flexible thinking
			  • Relational information processing
			  • Foresight and hindsight

Educational interventions	Treatment and education of autistic and related communication handicapped children (TEACCH)	Special education program based on "structured teaching"; designed to use relative strength of students with autism to process visually while instilling skills	• TEACCH-trained psychologists, special education teachers, speech therapist, and others • Uses a highly structured environment and visual supports to support completion of tasks
	Learning experiences—an alternative program for preschoolers and parents (LEAP)	Comprehensive inclusive preschool program	• Includes aspects of behavioral analysis, but primarily a developmentally based approach • Curriculum aims to develop social and emotional growth, enhance language and communication abilities, increase independence in play and work, promote choice making, improve ability to make transitions, develop overall cognition and physical activities • Typical classroom includes a teacher and teacher assistant for a class of 10 typically developing children and 3–4 children with autism • Play skills are facilitated by using peer models and by prompting, fading, and reinforcing target behaviors • Includes a parent-training program to promote gains to home and community
	Social communication, emotional regulation, implementing transactional supports (SCERTS®) model	Educational model that is comprehensive, team based, and multidisciplinary	• SCERTS-trained special education teachers, speech therapist provide approach in a school-based setting • Incorporates practices from other approaches including PRT, DIR, RDI, TEACCH, and Social Stories • Promotes child-initiated communication in everyday activities • Emphasizes child-developing ability to learn and apply a range skills in a variety of settings with a variety of partners
Communication	Speech and language therapy	Addresses communication challenges in receptive and expressive language	• Licensed speech and language pathologist provides evaluation and therapy • Program is based on individual needs and goals • A variety of techniques, programs may be implemented • Goals may include increasing use of verbal language, sign language, PECS, or a communication device • May also address problems in language comprehension, pragmatics (social rules of a language)
	Picture exchange communication system (PECS)	Learning system that allows children with little or not verbal ability to communicate using pictures; can be used at home, in the classroom, or in a variety of settings	• A therapist, teacher, or parent helps the child acquire vocabulary and to express desires, observations, or feelings by using pictures consistently • Beginning level teaches child to exchange a picture for desired object • With progress, child uses pictures and symbols to create sentences • PECS builds understanding of language that can promote verbal expression as well

Other therapies	Social skills	Promotes acquisition of knowledge of social rules and expectations and how to successfully navigate social situations	• Social workers, psychologists, occupational therapists, and speech/language therapists who specialize in people with autism • Uses techniques and practice activities such as using scripts, group conversations games, and social activities needed to interact socially • Objectives may range from basic skills (such as remembering to make eye contact) to complex and subtle skills (like completing a job interview)
	Occupational therapy	Goal of occupational therapy is for individual to gain independence and increase function by developing cognitive, physical, and motor skills needed for appropriate play, learning, and day-to-day living	• Licensed occupational therapist provides evaluation and therapy • Evaluates child's development and identifies psychological, social, and environmental factors • Program may include independent dressing, feeding, grooming, toileting, as well as social, fine motor, and perceptual skills • Creates strategies and tactics to learn tasks at home, in school, and other settings
	Sensory integration (SI) therapy	Targets problems in ability to process information through senses (touch, movement, smell, taste, vision, and hearing), integrate with prior information, and to make meaningful response; also targets ability to attend to information and regulate systems	• Licensed occupational therapists, physical therapists, and speech and language pathologists certified in SI provide evaluation and intervention; neuropsychologists and physicians certified in SI may provide evaluation • In addition to therapy, intervention may include supports to enhance sensory processing, regulation and attention
	Physical therapy	Addresses problems with movement that cause functional limitations including motor skills such as sitting, walking, running, and jumping and poor muscle tone, balance, and coordination	• Certified physical therapist provides services • Evaluates abilities and developmental level of child • Creates program to target deficient areas; intervention can include assisted movement, various forms of exercise, and orthopedic equipment
	Auditory integration (AIT)	Also called sound therapy; used to treat children difficulties in auditory processing or sound sensitivity	• Treatment provided by certified provider usually a speech pathologist, audiologist, or occupational therapist • Treatment involves patient listening to electronically modified music through headphones during multiple sessions • Different methods including Tomatis, Berard, Samonas, and others
	Inclusion	Children with disabilities placed with neurotypical children to maximum extent possible in schools, organizations, and recreation activities	• Provides more opportunities for social interaction • Promotes relationship development with typical peers • Provides exposure to role models, language, age-appropriate routines and activities
	Social stories	Developed by Carol Gray to teach students social rules of behavior; Provide support for addressing problematic situations	• Presented as stories and scripts specific to person to address problematic situations • Stories constructed with three types of sentences: perspective, descriptive, and directive • Individual reads story or is read to immediately before targeted event • Goal is to improve behavior, reduce frustration and anxiety
Biomedical treatments	Immunoregulatory interventions	Dietary restriction of food allergens—GFCF diet, specific carbohydrate diet (SC)	• GFCF eliminates foods containing gluten or casein including wheat, dairy products, malt, whey, others • SC eliminates complex carbohydrates such as grains, corn, wheat, and rice and most sugar as well as lactose containing foods (milk); yogurt is allowed

(Continued)

TABLE 8.1 Autism Treatments, Therapies, and Educational Interventions (104–114) *(Continued)*

Category	Treatment	Core Principles	Implementation
		Immunoglobulin	• Intravenous administered, immunoglobulin administered over multiple administrations to target immunologic abnormalities and behaviors linked to these abnormalities
		Antiviral agents	• Used to treat chronic viral infections
	Gastrointestinal treatments	Digestive enzymes	• Target underlying gastrointestinal dysfunction, including malabsorption and incomplete breakdown of ingested proteins • Used to assist digestive process and remove toxic compounds
		Antifungal agents	• Antifungals such as Nystatin and Diflucan are used to inhibit the growth of or kill yeast, particularly, *Candida,* in the gut
		Probiotics	• Beneficial microorganisms that assist vitamin utilization, help to break down sugars, assist the body's immune process, correct pH, and prevent the growth of harmful bacteria such as clostridium
		Dietary supplements	• Act by modulating neurotransmission, through immune factors or epigenetic gene expression mechanisms • Supplements may include vitamin A, C, B_{12}, B_6, magnesium, dimethylglycine, trimethylglycine, omega-3 fatty acids, minerals, others
	Detoxification	Chelation	• Chelating agents such as dimercaptosuccinic acid (DMSA) used to remove mercury, lead, and other heavy metals
	Oxygen perfusion	Hyperbaric oxygen therapy (HBOT)	• A hyperbaric chamber, a pressurized, oxygen-filled room or enclosure, provides a large concentration of oxygen to the body • Theorized to reduce inflammation and hypoperfusion of oxygen in the brain and to stimulate tissue regeneration

self-management; functional adaptive skills; cognitive skills such as symbolic play and perspective taking; traditional academic skills
- Application of scientifically supported strategies to decrease maladaptive behaviors
- Immediate entry into program when a diagnosis of ASD is considered rather than waiting for a diagnosis to be made

Some educational interventions identified as model programs are included in Table 8.1.

Biomedical Biomedical therapies consist of a wide range of therapies including pharmacologic management of symptoms associated with autism as well as regimens targeting faulty immunoregulatory processes, addressing gastrointestinal problems, or detoxifying the body from toxic substances. The project, Defeat Autism Now (DAN!), created by the Autism Research Institute, disseminates a common protocol to treat autism based on a biomedical approach (113). Defeat Autism Now practitioners include medical doctors in the areas of psychiatry, neurology, immunology, allergy, biochemistry, genetics, and gastroenterology as well as chiropractic doctors, naturopathic and homeopathic practitioners, nurse practitioners, and nutritionists. Biomedical treatments commonly used are summarized in Table 8.1.

Medications Medications are not curative but may be used to help decrease problematic symptoms and to increase desired behaviors. Symptoms that may be targeted by medications include hyperactivity, short attention and impulsivity, repetitive thoughts and compulsive behaviors, stereotyped movements, anxiety, irritability, depressed mood, aggression, sleep disturbance, and motor planning issues. Table 8.2 provides a summary of medications used to treat symptoms of autism as well as their trade and generic names, mechanisms, effects, and side effects (104,115).

TABLE 8.2 Medications Used to Manage Associated Symptoms Found in ASD (104,115)

Class of Medication	Trade Name (Generic Name)	Mechanism	Effects of Medication	Side Effects
Serotonin reuptake inhibitors (SSRIs)	Prozac (fluoxetine) Paxil (paroxetine) Luvox (fluvoxamine) Zoloft (sertraline) Celexa (citalopram) Lexapro (escitalopram)	Block serotonin transport back into presynaptic neuron results in increased serotonin in synapse	Decrease obsessive–compulsive disorder behaviors, anxiety, depression, perseveration, stereotypical behaviors Increase sociability	Sleep disturbance, hyperactivity aggression
Dopamine antagonists	Risperdal (risperidone)	Mixed serotonin and dopamine antagonist	Decrease self-injurious behavior, stereotyped movements, mania, and aggression	Sedation weight gain dyskinesias (diminished voluntary movement, presence of involuntary movements)
Neuroleptics	Abilify (aripiprazole)	Dopamine partial agonist and serotonin antagonist	May stabilize mood Increase social interaction	Headache anxiety insomnia (may interact with other meds, esp. SSRIs) tardive dyskinesia (involuntary, repetitive tic-like movements primarily in facial muscles) weight gain but less than risperidone
Tricyclic antidepressants	Tofranil (imipramine) Norpramine (desipramine) Anafranil (clomipramine)	Blocks reuptake norepinephrine (NE) and serotonin in presynaptic neuron	Increase attention, social skills Decreases impulsivity, activity, depression	Dry mouth, dizziness, drowsiness, irritability possible cardiac
Alpha 2 agonists	Catapres (clonidine) Tenex (guanfacine)	Stimulation of central alpha 2 receptor reducing sympathetic nerve impulses	Increase attention Decrease hyperactivity, tics	sedation depression

(Continued)

TABLE 8.2 Medications Used to Manage Associated Symptoms Found in ASD (104,115) *(Continued)*

Class of Medication	Trade Name (Generic Name)	Mechanism	Effects of Medication	Side Effects
Beta-blockers	Inderol (proplanolol)	Blocks betareceptor on postsynaptic neuron	Reported to reduce severe and treatment-resistant aggressiveness and self-injurious behavior	decreased blood pressure, pulse
Dopamine/ norepinephrine enhancers	Dopamine only Short acting: • Ritalin (methylphenidate) Long acting: • Concerta • Metadate CD • Ritalin SR • Ritalin LA (all are trade names for methylphenidate) Dopamine and norepinephrine Short acting: • Dexedrine (dextroamphetamine) • Adderall (amphet-amine and dextroamphetamine) Long acting: • Dexedrine Spansules (dextroamphetamine) • Adderall XR (amphetamine and dextroamphetamine) • Wellbutrin (bupropion) Norepinephrine primarily • Strattera (atomoxetine)	Enhance dopamine (+/– NE) release into synapse Block dopamine reuptake into presynaptic neuron Result in increased dopamine in synapse	Increased attention Decreased activity	decreased appetite decreased sleep
Anticonvulsants	Depakote (Valproic acid) Tegretol (carbamazepine) Trileptal (oxcarbazepine) Neurontin (gabapentin) Lamictal (lamotrigine) Topamax (topimarate) Tiagabine (gabitrol)	Decreases abnormal electrical activity in the brain	Decrease aggression, irritability, emotional lability	Sleepiness, dizziness liver, bone marrow toxicity (valproic acid) Carbamazepine may be associated with Stevens–Johnson syndrome
Opioid antagonist	Depade, (naltrexone)	Blocks action of endogenous opioids at opiate receptors	Possibly decreases hyperactivity and restlessness	Unknown
Cholinesterase inhibitor	Aricept (donepezil)	Increases concentrations of acetylcholine in brain	Improved expressive language Possibly improved receptive language Improved motor function Improved social skills	GI complaints, sleep disturbance, mild irritability, aggression, mania
N-methyl D-aspartate (NMDA) antagonist	Namenda (Memantine)	Acts on the glutamatergic system blocking NMDA receptors	May improve frontal lobe function including increase attention Decrease perseveration Improve motor planning	Minor to none

Complementary and Alternative In addition to the biomedical interventions summarized in Table 8.1, many complementary and alternative therapies are used in the treatment of autism. Surveys of parents of children with autism found that 52% to 92% reported using at least one complementary or alternative therapy (111,112). For a more detailed discussion of specific therapies, see Chapter 26, Complementary and Alternative Approaches.

CONCLUSION

Autism is a group of complex developmental brain disorders. Approximately 1 in 110 children is diagnosed with autism. The cause of autism is unknown. Research indicates that both genetics and environmental factors contribute, and inflammatory processes may play a role. Research does not support vaccination as a cause of autism. The core deficits of autism in the areas of social and communication as well as sensory sensitivities impact preventative care as well as diagnosis and management of health problems. Successful management of the patient with ASD should also focus on family members including parents and siblings. Treatments for autism include those based on behavioral, developmental, and biomedical approaches. Applied behavior analysis has the strongest research support. The majority of parents of children with autism use at least one therapy categorized as complementary or alternative medicine.

REFERENCES

1. Levy SE, Mandell DS, Schultz RT. Autism. Lancet. 2009;374:1627–38.
2. National Institute of Child Health and Development. Autism spectrum disorders. Available from: http://www.nichd.nih.gov/health/topics/asd.cfm. Last Accessed November 26, 2010.
3. Autism Speaks. What is autism? Available from: http://www.autismspeaks.org/whatisit/index.php. Last Accessed November 26, 2010.
4. Hollander E, Kolevzon A, Coyle J, editors. Textbook of autism spectrum disorders. Washington: American Psychiatric Publishing; 2011.
5. Johnson CP, Myers SM; the Council of Children with Disabilities. Identification and evaluation of children with autism spectrum disorders. Pediatrics. 2007;120:1183–215.
6. American Psychiatric Association. The diagnostic and statistical manual of mental disorders. 4th ed. Washington: American Psychiatric Publishing, Inc.; 2000.
7. Centers for Disease Control and Prevention. Data & statistics. Available from: http://www.cdc.gov/ncbddd/autism/data.html. Last Accessed November 13, 2010.
8. Yeargin-Allsopp M, Rice C, Karapurkar T, et al. Prevalence of autism in a US metropolitan area. JAMA. 2003;289:49–55.
9. Fombonne E, Simmons H, Ford T, et al. Prevalence of pervasive developmental disorders in the British nationwide survey of child; mental health. J Am Acad Child Adolesc Psychiatry. 2001;40:820–7.
10. Rutter M. Incidence of autism spectrum disorders: changes over time and their meaning. Acta Paediatr. 2005;94:2–15.
11. Chakrabarti S, Fombonne E. Pervasive developmental disorders in preschool children: confirmation of high prevalence. Am J Psychiatry. 2005;162:1133–41.
12. Newschaffer CJ, Falb MD, Gurney JG. National autism prevalence trends from United States Special Education Data. Pediatrics. 2005;e277–82.
13. Rice C, Nicholas J, Baio J, et al. Changes in autism spectrum disorder prevalence in 4 areas of the United States. Disabil Health J. 2010;186–201.
14. Autism and Developmental Disabilities Monitoring Network Surveillance Year 2006 Principal Investigators. Prevalence of Autism Spectrum Disorders—Autism and Developmental Disabilities Monitoring Network, United States, Centers for Disease Control and Prevention. Available from: http://www.cdc.gov/mmwr/preview/mmwrhtml/ss5810a1.htm. Last Accessed November 13, 2010.
15. Kogan MD, Blumberg SJ, Schieve LA, et al. Prevalence of parent-reported diagnosis of Autism Spectrum Disorder among children in the US, 2007. Pediatrics. 2009;124:1395–403.
16. Posserud M, Lundervold AJ, Gillberg C. Autistic features in a total population of 7–9-year-old children assessed by the AAAQ (Autism Spectrum Screening Questionnaire). J Child Psychol Psychiatry. 2006;47:167–75.
17. Muhle R, Trentacoste SV, Rapin I. The genetics of autism. Pediatrics. 2004;113:e472–86.
18. Altevogt BM, Hanson SL, Leshner AI. Autism and the environment: challenges and opportunities for research. Pediatrics. 2008;121:1225–9.
19. Price CS, Thompson WW, Goodson B, et al. Prenatal and infant exposure to thimerosal from vaccines and immunoglobulins and risk of autism. Pediatrics. 2010;126:656–64.
20. Kemp ML, Hart MB. MMR vaccine and autism: is there a link? JAAPA. 2010;23:48,50.
21. Allan GM. The autism-vaccine story: fiction and deception? Can Fam Phys. 2010;56:1013.
22. Fombonne E, Zakarian R, Bennett A, Meng L, McLean-Heywood D. Pervasive developmental disorders in Montreal, Quebec, Canada: prevalence and links with immunizations. Pediatrics. 2006;118(1):e139–50.
23. Hviid A, Stellfeld M, Wohlfahrt J, et al. Association between thimerosal-containing vaccine and autism. JAMA. 2003;290:1763–6.
24. Andrews N, Miller E, Grant A, et al. Thimerosal exposure in infants and developmental disorders: a retrospective cohort study in the United Kingdom does not support a causal association. Pediatrics. 2004;114:584–91.
25. Verstraeten T, Davis RL, DeStefano F, et al. Safety of thimerosal-containing vaccines: a two-phased study of computerized

health maintenance organization databases. Pediatrics. 2003; 112:1039–48.

26. Wakefield AJ, Murch SH, Anthony A, et al. Ileal-lymphoid-nodular hyperplasia, non-specific colitis, and pervasive developmental disorder in children. Lancet. 1998;351:637–41.
27. Eggertson L. Lancet retracts 12-year-old article linking autism to MMR vaccines. Can Med Assoc J. 2010;182:e199–200.
28. DeStefano F. Vaccines and autism: evidence does not support a causal association. Clin Pharmacol Ther. 2007;82:756–9.
29. Hornig M, Briese T, Buie T, et al. Lack of association between measles virus vaccine and autism with enteropathy: a case-control study. Available from: http://www.plosone.org/article/info%3Adoi%2F10.1371%2Fjournal.pone.0003140. Last Accessed February 26, 2011.
30. Madsen KM, Hviid A, Vestergaard M, et al. A population-based study of measles, mumps, and rubella vaccination and autism. N Engl J Med. 2002;347:1477–82.
31. Smeeth L, Cook C, Fombonne E, et al. MMR vaccination and pervasive developmental disorders: a case-control study. Lancet. 2004;364:963–9.
32. Taylor B, Miller E, Lingam R, et al. Measles, mumps, and rubella vaccination and bowel problems or developmental regression in children with autism: population study. Br Med J. 2002;324:393–6.
33. Taylor B, Miller E, Farrington CP, et al. Autism and measles, mumps, and rubella vaccine: no epidemiological evidence for a causal association. Lancet. 1999;353:2026–9.
34. Dales L, Hammer SJ, Smith NJ. Time trends in autism and in MMR immunization coverage in California. JAMA. 2001;285:1183–5.
35. Kaye JA, del Mar Melero-Montes M, Jick H. Mumps, measles, and rubella vaccine and the incidence of autism recorded by general practitioners: a time trend analysis. Br Med J. 2001;322:460–3.
36. Garber KB, Visootsak J, Warren ST. Fragile X syndrome. Eur J Hum Genet. 2008;16:666–72.
37. Wiznitzer M. Autism and tuberous sclerosis. J Child Neurol. 2004;19:675–9.
38. Peters SU, Beaudet AL, Madduri N, Bacino CA. Autism in Angelman syndrome: implications for autism research. Clin Genet. 2004;66:530–6.
39. Lauritsen MB, Pedersen CB, Mortensen PB. Effects of familial risk factors and place of birth on the risk of autism: a nationwide register-based study. J Child Psychol Psychiatry. 2005;46:963–71.
40. Durkin MS, Maenner MJ, Newschaffer CJ, et al. Advanced parental age and the risk of autism spectrum disorder. Am J Epidemiol. 2008;168:1268–76.
41. Croen LA, Najjar DV, Fireman B, et al. Maternal and paternal age and risk of Autism spectrum disorder. Arch Pediatr Adolesc Med. 2007;161:334–40.
42. Reichenberg A, Gross R, Weiser M, et al. Advancing paternal age and autism. Arch Gen Psychiatry. 2006;63:1026–32.
43. Atladóttir H, Pedersen MG, Scient C, et al. Association of family history of autoimmune diseases and Autism spectrum disorders. Pediatrics. 2009;124:687–94.
44. Bilder D, Pinborough-Zimmerman J, Miller J, et al. Prenatal, perinatal and neonatal factors associated with Autism spectrum disorders. Pediatrics. 2009;1293–300.
45. Schendal D, Bhasin TK. Birth weight and gestational age characteristics of children with autism, including a comparison with other developmental disabilities. Pediatrics. 2008;121:1155–64.
46. Schieve LA, Blumberg SJ, Rice C, et al. The relationship between autism and parenting stress. Pediatrics. 2007;119:S114–21.
47. Myers BJ, Mackintosh VH, Goin-Kochel RP. My greatest joy and my greatest heart ache: parents' own words on how having a child in the autism spectrum has affected their lives and their families' lives. Res Autism Spectr Disord. 2009;3:670–84.
48. Kayfitz AD, Gragg MN, Orr R. Positive experiences of mothers and fathers of children with autism: positive experiences of mothers and fathers of children with autism. J Appl Res Intellect Disabil. 2010;23:337–43.
49. Mugno D, Ruta L, D'Arrigo VG, et al. Impairment of quality of life in parents of children and adolescents with pervasive developmental disorder. Health Qual Life Outcomes. 2007;5:22.
50. Blacher J, McIntyre LL. Syndrome specificity and behavioural disorders in young adults with intellectual disability: cultural differences in family impact. J Intellect Disabil Res. 2005;3:184–98.
51. Kogan MD, Strickland BS, Blumberg SJ, et al. A national profile of the health care experiences and family impact of Autism Spectrum Disorder among children in the United States, 2005–2006. Pediatrics. 2008;122:e1149–58.
52. Montes G, Halterman JS. Association of childhood Autism spectrum disorders and loss of family income. Pediatrics. 2008;121:e821–6.
53. Sharpe DL, Baker DL. Financial issues associated with having a child with Autism. J Fam Econ Issues. 2007;28:247–64.
54. Pottie CP, Ingram KM. Daily stress, coping, and wellbeing in parents of children with autism: a multilevel modeling approach. J Fam Parenting. 2008;22:855–64.
55. Glasberg BA. The development of siblings' understanding of Autism spectrum disorders. J Autism Dev Disord. 2000;30:143—56.
56. Hastings RP. Brief report: Behavioral adjustment of siblings of children with autism. J Autism Dev Disord. 2003;33:99–104.
57. Schunterman P. Sibling experience: growing up with a child who has pervasive developmental disorder or mental retardation. Harv Rev Psychiatry. 2007;15:93–108.
58. Liptak GS, Stuart T, Auinger P. Health care utilization and expenditures for children with autism: data from U.S. national samples. J Autism Dev Disord. 2006;36:871–9.
59. Shimbakuro TT, Grosse SD, Rice C. Medical expenditures for children with an autism spectrum disorder in a privately insured population. J Autism Dev Disord. 2008;38:546–52.
60. Golnik A, Ireland M, Wagman-Borowsky I. Medical homes for children with autism: a physician survey. Pediatrics. 2009;123:966–71.
61. McGinnis K. Close encounters of the medical kind: when kids with autism or other developmental disabilities visit the doctor. Exceptional Parent. 2009;39:48–51.
62. Volkmar FR, Weisner LA. Healthcare for children on the Autism spectrum. Bethesda: Woodbine House, Inc.; 2004.
63. Bauman ML. Medical comorbidities in autism: challenges to diagnosis and treatment. Neurotherapeutics. 2010;7:320–7.

64. Coury D, Jones NE, Klatka K, et al. Health care for children with autism: the Autism Treatment Network. Curr Opin Pediatr. 2009;21:828–32.

65. Myers SM, Johnson CP; Council of Children with Disabilities. Management of children with Autism spectrum disorders. Pediatrics. 2007;120:1162–82.

66. Carbone PS, Farley M, Davis T. Primary care for children with autism. Am Fam Phys. 2010;15:453–60.

67. Curtin C, Anderson SE, Must A. The prevalence of obesity in children with autism: a secondary data analysis using national representative data from the National Survey of Children's Health. BMC Pediatr. 2010;10:11.

68. McDermott S, Zhou L, Mann J. Injury treatment among children with autism or pervasive developmental disorder. J Autism Dev Disord. 2008;38:626–33.

69. Ramirez M, Yang J, Bourque L, et al. Sports injuries to high school athletes with disabilities. Pediatrics. 2009;123:690–6.

70. Lang R, Didden R, Machalicek W, et al. Behavioral treatment of chronic skin-picking in individuals with developmental disabilities: a systematic review. Res Dev Disabil. 2010;31:304–15.

71. Milne E, Griffiths H, Buckley D, Scope A. Vision in children and adolescents with Autism spectrum disorder: Evidence for reduced convergence. J Autism Dev Disord. 2009;39:965–75.

72. Adams RJ, Dove CN, Drover JR, et al. Optics and spatial vision in children and young adults with Autism spectrum disorder. J Vis. 2010;10:464.

73. Coulter RA. Understanding the visual symptoms of individuals with Autism spectrum disorder. Optom Vis Dev. 2009;40:164–5.

74. Kehat R, Bonsall DJ. Recurrent corneal metallic foreign bodies in children with autism spectrum disorders. J Am Assoc Pediatr Ophthalmol Strabismus. 2009;13:621–2.

75. Pineles SL, Avery RA, Liu GT. Vitamin B12 optic neuropathy in autism. Pediatrics. 2010;126:e967–s70.

76. Waldman HB, Perlman SP, Wong A. Providing dental care for the patient with autism. Calif Dent Assoc J. 2008;36:663–70.

77. Molloy CA, Manning-Courtney P. Prevalence of chronic gastrointestinal symptoms in children with Autism and Autism spectrum disorders. Autism. 2003;7:165–71.

78. Buie T, Fuchs GJ, Furuta GT, et al. Recommendations for evaluation and treatment of common gastrointestinal problems in children with ASDs. Pediatrics. 2010;S19–29.

79. Buie T, Campbell DB, Fuchs GJ, et al. Evaluation, diagnosis, and treatment of gastrointestinal disorders in individuals with ASDs: a consensus report. Pediatrics. 2010;125:S1–18.

80. Ibrahim SH, Voigt RG, Katusic SK, et al. Incidence of gastrointestinal symptoms in children with autism: a population-based study. Pediatrics. 2009;124:680–6.

81. Coury D. Medical treatment of autism spectrum disorders. Curr Opin Neurol. 2010;23:131–6.

82. Horvath K, Perman JA. Autism and gastrointestinal symptoms. Curr Gastroenterol Rep. 2002;4:251–8.

83. Murch S. Diet, immunity and autistic spectrum disorders. J Pediatr. 2005;582–4.

84. Cass H, Gringas P, March J, et al. Absence of urinary opioid peptides in children with autism. Arch Dis Child. 2006;93:745—s50.

85. Elder JH, Shankar M, Shuster J, et al. The gluten-free, casein-free diet in autism: results of a preliminary double blind clinical trial. J Autism Dev Disord. 2006;36:413–20.

86. Geraghty ME, Depasquale GM, Lane AE. Nutritional intake and therapies in autism: a spectrum of what we know. Infant Child Adolesc Nutr. 2010;2:62–9.

87. Bandini LG, Anderson SE, Curtin C, et al. Food selectivity in children with autism spectrum disorders and typically developing children. J Pediatr. 2010;157:259–64.

88. Cornish E. Gluten and casein-free diets in autism: a study of the effects on food choice and nutrition. J Hum Nutr Diet. 2002;15:261–9.

89. Emond A, Emmett P, Steer C, et al. Feeding symptoms, dietary patterns and growth in young children with Autism spectrum disorders. Pediatrics. 2010;126:e337–42.

90. Lindsay RL, Arnold LE, Aman MG, et al. Dietary status and impact of risperidone on nutritional balance in children with autism: a pilot study. J Intellect Dev Disabil. 2006;31:204–9.

91. Lockner DW, Crowe TK, Skipper BJ. Dietary intake and parents' perception of mealtime behaviors in preschool-age children with autism spectrum disorder and in typically developing children. J Am Diet Assoc. 2008;108:1360–3.

92. Jyonouchi H. Food allergy and Autism spectrum disorders: Is there a link? Curr Allergy Asthma Rep. 2009;9:194–201.

93. Dietary intervention for young children with autism, University of Rochester Medical Center. Available from: http://www.urmc.rochester.edu/childrens-hospital/developmental-disabilities/Research/dietary-intervention.cfm. Last Accessed December 24, 2010.

94. Hediger ML, England LJ, Molloy CA, et al. Reduced bone cortical thickness in boys with autism or autism spectrum disorder. J Autism Dev Disord. 2008;38:848–56.

95. Burke LM, Kalpakjian CZ, Smith YR, et al. Gynecologic issues of adolescents with Down syndrome, autism and cerebral palsy. J Pediatr Adolesc Gynecol. 2010;23:11–5.

96. Scarpinato N, Bradley J, Kurbjun K, et al. Caring for the child with an autism spectrum disorder in the acute care setting. J Spec Pediatr Nurs. 2010;15:244–54.

97. Krakowiak P, Goodlin-Jones B, Hertz-Picciotto I, et al. Sleep problems in children with autism spectrum disorders, developmental delays, and typical development: a population-based study. J Sleep Res. 2008;197–206.

98. Cortesi F, Giannotti F, Ivanenko A, et al. Sleep in children with autistic spectrum disorder. Sleep Med. 2010;11:659–64.

99. Chalfant A, Rapee R, Carroll L. Treating anxiety disorders in children with high functioning Autism spectrum disorders: a controlled trial. J Autism Dev Disord. 2007;37:1842–57.

100. Bursch B. Chronic pain in individuals with previously undiagnosed autistic spectrum disorders. J Pain. 2004;5:290.

101. Jyonouchi H. Autism spectrum disorders and allergy: observation from a pediatric/immunology clinic. Exp Rev Clin Immunol. 2010;6:397–411.

102. Treating autism. Autism speaks. Last accessed December 25, 2010.

103. Thomas KC, Morrissey JP, McLaurin C. Use of autism-related services. J Autism Dev Disord. 2007;37:818–29.

104. Myers SM, Johnson CP; the Council on Children with Disabilities. Management of children with autism spectrum disorders. Pediatrics. 2007;120:1162–82.

105. Autism Society of America. Autism treatments. Available from: http://www.wrightslaw.com/info/autism.methods.compare.pdf. Last accessed December 24, 2010.
106. Greenspan S, Wieder S. Engaging autism. Cambridge: Da Capo Lifelong Books; 2006.
107. The Gray Center. Social stories. Available from: http://www.thegraycenter.org/social-stories/what-are-social-stories. Last accessed December 26, 2010.
108. Simpson RL, de Boer-Ott SR. Autism spectrum disorders: interventions and treatments for children and youth. Thousand Oaks: Corwin Press; 2005.
109. Levy SE, Hyman SL. Novel treatments for autistic spectrum disorders. Ment Retard Dev Disabil Res Rev. 2005;11:131–42.
110. Odom SL, Boyd A, Hall LJ, et al. Evaluation of comprehensive treatment models for individuals with Autism spectrum disorders. J Autism Dev Disord. 2010;40:425–36.
111. Hanson E, Kalish LA, Bunce E, et al. Use of complementary and alternative medicine among children diagnosed with Autism spectrum disorder. J Autism Dev Disord. 2007;37:628–36.
112. Autism Research Institute. [Internet]. San Diego, CA. The Autism Research Institute and Defeat Autism Now: who we are and what we do. Available from: http://www.autism.com/ed_aridan.asp. Last accessed January 1, 2011.
113. Adams JB. Summary of biomedical treatments for autism. Available from: http://www.autism.com/pdf/providers/adams_biomed_summary.pdf. Last Accessed January 1, 2011.
114. Bennett M, Mitchell S, Neuman T, et al. Hyperbaric oxygen therapy and neurological disease. Undersea Hyperb Med. 2010;37:371–3.
115. Robinson R. Autism spectrum disorders: medication management. Presented at: DIR Institute, July 2009; Monterey, CA.

CHAPTER 9

Mary Bartuccio, OD, FAAO, FCOVD
R. Terry Browning, PhD
Angela C. Howell, OD

Attention Deficit Hyperactivity Disorder (ADHD)

Attention deficit hyperactivity disorder (ADHD), first described by G.F. Still in 1902 (1), is a neurologic disorder that manifests as three patterns of behavior: inattention, hyperactivity, and impulsivity (2–4). In the 1960s, ADHD became a distinct entity in Diagnostic and Statistical Manual of Mental Disorder (DSM). In the next decade, the American Psychiatric Association established guidelines for diagnosing both ADHD (with hyperactivity) and attention deficit disorder (ADD) (without hyperactivity). In 1987, ADD was renamed ADHD (5). Today, this disorder often is first seen in childhood and is listed under the designation of "Disorders Usually First Diagnosed in Infancy, Childhood or Adolescence" in the Diagnostic and Statistical Manual of Mental Disorders, Fourth Edition, Text Revision (DSM IV-TR) (2).

Current descriptions of ADHD in the DSM IV-TR include three major subtypes. The ADHD predominantly inattentive type (ADHD-IT) is the most common type and is mainly characterized by difficulty with inattention and concentration. The ADHD predominantly hyperactive–impulsive type (ADHD-HI) includes individuals typically found to have difficulty mainly with hyperactivity and impulsivity. Finally, the ADHD combined type (ADHD-CT) describes those with characteristics of both (6,7).

Attention deficit hyperactivity disorder is a combination of behavior patterns that are exhibited throughout the day and must persist for more than 6 months (2,8). In the school setting, these behaviors may exhibit themselves in a child that shows difficulty maintaining attention, acting impulsively, and having a higher baseline level of activity to a degree that is beyond the typical level for their age or gender (9). It is widely recognized that during development, ADHD behaviors often negatively affect students in both home and school settings and may seriously impact social, emotional and cognitive functioning as well (7,10).

Students with ADHD may show great difficulty managing school expectations in the classroom as well as during transitions and in larger settings (e.g., cafeteria, gymnasium) within school. In the classroom, these students may interrupt the teacher more frequently, interfering with the concentration of other students and the teacher's ability for overall instruction. They often have difficulty staying seated and may gain negative attention with these movements. By nature, the attention issues associated with the disorder may interfere with the patient's ability to concentrate, thereby also interfere with their own academic progress (9). This issue is addressed in greater detail later in this chapter.

A Global ADHD Working Group, comprised of both researchers and experienced clinicians, was created to evaluate the current research and best practices for working with and treating those with ADHD. This group was convened to gain consensus of current thought globally. One initial concern was the recognition of the underdiagnosis and poor recognition of the condition and how these factors negatively affect receipt of treatment. This problem was seen across many countries. The group also affirmed and recognized ADHD as a viable disorder that is present across people groups and cultures worldwide and has global implications for diagnosis and treatment (10).

Health professionals are constantly altering the diagnostic criteria for this condition. Historically, patients with this condition were diagnosed with attention deficit, ADD, hyperkinetic disorder (HKD or HD) or hyperactivity. The common term used today in the United States is ADHD, while in the

United Kingdom, professionals refer to this condition as HKD or HD. In the United States, children with ADHD are diagnosed using the DSM-IV criteria, while in the United Kingdom, the ICD-10 criteria is used (10). The criteria for this diagnosis continue to evolve as research furthers our understanding of this condition.

The Global ADHD Group cites the ICD-10 (used internationally) prevalence rate as 1% to 3% and the DSM-IV criteria rate as 4% to 8%. There is an emphasis that large portions of those with the disorder may remain without adequate treatment even in the lower estimate (10,11). Other studies estimate the prevalence to be 4.1% of children aged 7 to 9 years. Males are affected at a rate of two to three times greater than females (12,13). Other studies suggest that ADHD has been found to affect 4% to 12% of school-aged children (12–14).

While changes in symptoms may be seen over a patient's life span, about 50% of adolescents with ADHD continue to struggle with this condition as an adult. This disorder has been found to be present in 1.5% to 3% of adults (15). Clinicians who ordinarily work with older patients should also be familiar with this condition, as it is sometimes first recognized and diagnosed in adulthood (2).

ETIOLOGY

The investigation of the etiology of ADHD has branched into several major directions but no clear origin has been found. Support for a genetic influence has expanded in recent years. These findings are based in the discovery of neuroanatomical differences in the prefrontal cortex in those with ADHD (16). In 2004, the Global ADHD Working Group highlighted both genetic factors (10). Single-gene effects have not been documented but some potential genes have been identified.

Much of the genetic interest has been focused on dopaminergic systems. One factor is that dopaminergic acting drugs (e.g., methylphenidate) are found to be useful in the treatment of ADHD. The frontal striatal areas of the brain have been implicated in ADHD through the use of positron emission tomography (PET) and magnetic resonance imaging (MRI), since both areas have dopaminergic influence on brain activity. Meta-analysis of studies questions the strength of this relationship (17,18). Further research includes numerous systems including genes related to serotonin transporter coding (19).

Other brain structures that have been found to be important in ADHD have been studied by using MRI which show that children with ADHD have demonstrated atypical function in the prefrontal cortex, striatum, and cerebellum (20). Inhibition and attention have long been studied and linked to ADHD. More recent data reveals differential morphology in the ADHD brain within these structures (21). Lennert and Martinez-Trujillo (22) have recently isolated neurons in the primate dorsolateral prefrontal cortex, which filter out visual distracters so that the brain can pay more attention to desired visual stimuli. They postulate that these neurons help orchestrate important cognitive functions by reducing brain clutter (22).

Evidence of prenatal factors is seen with the maternal use of drugs and alcohol. Environmental toxins such as lead may be a factor. Environmental factors such as the classroom set up and how undesired behavior is dealt with at home and school are more likely to affect the expression of the disorder rather than be causative (9).

Prenatal factors that affect the development of the brain and are therefore linked as risk factors for ADHD include nicotine and use of alcohol by the mother during pregnancy (10). Daley also described a division of biologic and environmental factors involved in the etiology of ADHD. Environmental factors would include parenting, the home, child–peer relationships, and nutritional aspects such as diet (18).

DIAGNOSIS OF ADHD

Daley (18) reviewed over 50 years of literature and found that the current ADHD diagnosis shares symptoms with earlier designations including minimal brain dysfunction, hyperactive child syndrome, and ADD with or without hyperactivity (23). The common areas shared include impulsivity, inattention, and motor restlessness. Onset of ADHD symptoms is first seen mainly during either the preschool or early elementary years (9,24). In diagnosing ADHD, the health care practitioner should be aware that typical child development could produce symptoms similar to ADHD. No clear biologic markers exist presently and therefore, the diagnosis is made based on the presence of symptoms. Behavioral symptoms indicated in both the World Health Organization International Classification of Diseases (ICD-10) (25) and the DSM-IV-TR (2) are similar. A variety of behavioral questionnaires, including the Connors Parent Rating Scale, are available to quantify the symptoms.

These questionnaires are distributed to parents and teachers so the overall picture of the child's behavior at school and home can be assessed as observed by the people closest to the child. Once symptoms are established, the practitioner needs to follow the criteria listed in DSM IV-TR (Table 9.1) to make the final diagnosis. The use of the Test of Variable Attention, a computer-based program, is useful but has been shown to overestimate the prevalence of ADHD (26).

A thorough physical examination by a medical doctor as well as a behavioral/psychological evaluation is required to determine comorbid conditions. In particular, a mental health professional that is familiar with ADHD should be involved in making the diagnosis. Since there is a high incidence of visual problems associated with ADHD, a comprehensive eye exam is essential to rule out visual disorders including, but not limited to,

TABLE 9.1 DSM-IV-TR: Diagnostic Criteria for ADHD

Inattention:

At least six of the following often apply:
- Fails to pay close attention to details or makes careless errors in schoolwork, work, or other activities
- Has trouble keeping attention on tasks or play
- Doesn't appear to listen when being told something
- Neither follows through on instructions nor completes chores, schoolwork, or jobs (not because of oppositional behavior or failure to understand)
- Has trouble organizing activities or tasks
- Dislikes or avoids tasks that involve sustained mental effort (e.g., homework, schoolwork)
- Loses materials needed for activities (e.g., assignments, book, pencils, tools, toys)
- Easily distracted by extraneous stimuli
- Forgetful

Hyperactivity–Impulsivity

At least six of the following often apply:
- Squirms in seat or fidgets
- Inappropriately leaves seat
- Inappropriately runs or climbs (in adolescents or adults, there may be only a subjective feeling of restlessness)
- Has trouble quietly playing or engaging in leisure activity
- Appears driven or "on the go"
- Talks excessively

Impulsivity
- Answers questions before they have been completely asked
- Has trouble waiting for his or her turn
- Interrupts or intrudes on others

Additional Criteria
- Symptoms must be present in at least two types of situations (e.g., school, work, or home)
- The disorder impairs school, social or occupational functioning
- The symptoms do not occur solely during a pervasive developmental disorder or psychotic disorder (including schizophrenia)
- The symptoms are not better explained by a mood, anxiety, dissociative, or personality disorder

Associated Features

Learning problem
Hyperactivity

American Psychiatric Association. Diagnostic and statistical manual of mental disorders, 4th ed, Text revision (DSM-IV TR). Washington: American Psychiatric Association; 2000, used with permission of American Psychiatric Publishing, Inc.

convergence insufficiency, accommodative dysfunctions and ocular motor dysfunction (27,28).

DIFFERENTIATING ADHD FROM OTHER DISORDERS

Many studies have shown a high correlation of symptoms in children with ADHD and other neuropsychiatric disorders (29) (Table 9.2). There has also been a strong link between learning disabilities (in particular, reading disorder) and ADHD (30).

A more complex picture of ADHD has also been proposed with evidence that additional diagnoses are much more common than previously described. Oppositional defiant disorder (ODD) is the most common. It is estimated that 60 % of children with ADHD have ODD and 20% have a conduct disorder (CD) as co-morbid factors. (4,31). Additionally, risk of other psychiatric disorders (e.g., bipolar, anxiety disorders) is also seen to be more prevalent in those with ADHD and combined oppositional or CD (32). Oppositional defiant disorder is described as a "recurrent pattern of negativistic, defiant, disobedient, and hostile behavior directed at an authority figure that persists for at least six months" (2). Conduct disorder is a repetitive and persistent pattern of behavior in which the basic rights of others or major age-appropriate societal norms or rules are violated (2). Conduct disorder can be described as childhood-onset type if one of the criteria is present before the age of 10 years. If the onset is later, CD becomes characterized as adolescent-onset CD. With additional complications of these comorbid disorders, it becomes even more important that clinicians understand how the course and treatment of these conditions are affected (4).

OCULOVISUAL ANOMALIES

Attention deficit hyperactivity disorder has been associated with visual disorders. Granet et al. (27) found a threefold greater incidence of ADHD among patients with convergence insufficiency (CI) ... and a threefold greater incidence of CI in the ADHD population. Other research has shown that "school-aged children with symptomatic accommodative dysfunction or CI, have a higher frequency of behaviors related to school performance and attention as measured by the Connors Parent Rating Scale-Revised Short Form (CPRS-R:S) (33). This study was consistent with the work of Farrar et al. (34) and Damari et al. (35) who both documented the association of ADHD with CI and accommodative dysfunction. Farrar et al. (34) documented the most significant visual symptoms often found in children with ADHD (Table 9.3). Furthermore, the coexistence of ocular motor, binocular, and

TABLE 9.2 Neuropsychiatric Disorders Associated with ADHD

Name of the disorder
1. Oppositional Defiant disorder
2. Conduct disorder
3. Depression and anxiety
4. Bipolar disorder
5. Tics disorder (Tourette syndrome)
6. Obsessive–compulsive disorder
7. Substance use disorder
8. Developmental coordination disorder
9. Autism spectrum disorder
10. Cerebral palsy
11. Fragile X
12. The 22q11 deletion syndrome (CATCH-22 syndrome)

Adapted from Gillberg C, Gillberg IC, Rasmussen P, et al. Co-existing disorders in ADHD-implications for diagnosis and intervention. Eur Child Adolesc Psychiatry. 2004;13:I/80–I/92.

TABLE 9.3 The Most Significant Visual Symptoms Often Found in Children with ADHD

Visual symptoms associated with ADHD
1. Blur when looking at near
2. Words run together when reading
3. Dizzy/nausea when reading
4. Skips/repeats line when reading
5. Difficulty copying from blackboard
6. Poor hand–eye coordination
7. Clumsy, knocks things over
8. Difficulty completing assignments on time
9. Poor use of time
10. Does not make change ($) well
11. Always I can't before trying
12. Loses belongings/things
13. Forgetful/poor memory

Adapted from Farrar R, Call M, Maples WC. A comparison of the visual symptoms between ADD/ADHD and normal children. Optometry. 2001;72:441–51.

accommodative dysfunctions with ADHD has been shown to produce greater visual symptoms in these children (34). It is important to note that some ADHD medications have been found to affect accommodation (36) and therefore should be closely monitored in routine eye exams.

Interventions and Treatment While this disorder can present at any age, this section focuses on interventions and treatment in younger patients. Demands in school settings change from having an individual teacher in elementary school to multiple teachers with differing expectations in higher education. Academic subjects become progressively difficult in content and workload. Additionally, children face more and more complicated schedules in school, as they begin to develop long-term academic and career goals. The student with ADHD may have a problem looking beyond short-term goals. Additionally, difficulty with social relationships may also be exacerbated in the middle and high school years again as peer relationships become more complex (9). Finally, ADHD is not simply a parenting issue. While parenting programs may be helpful, they are not the sole answer. Be mindful that this disorder is not a response to poor parenting skills or purely related to environmental factors (e.g., poverty).

DuPaul and White also discussed the evidence that ADHD is not a learning disability (LD), though there might be overlap in needs seen with the two conditions; that is, the behaviors that are seen in LD and ADHD are similar. They state that about 25% of those who have an ADHD diagnosis have the additional diagnosis of LD.

Multifaceted interventions are recommended often including behavioral and environmental interventions as well as potential medication needs (9). In the school setting, the term interventions is more likely to describe those academic, environmental, and behavioral factors that are designed to help the student cope in the classroom. A functional behavioral assessment and behavioral plan is often recommended to support and encourage as well as to decrease problem behavior. School-wide plans may are of assistance, but classroom and personal plans are necessary to establish good functioning in the school. Also, treatment both in and out of the school can involve psychotropic medications, psychosocial (e.g., counseling, parenting workshops), as well as behavioral interventions.

In any disorder that affects a child's behavior adversely at home and school, a functional behavioral assessment helps clarify behavior that should be addressed. A functional analysis of behavior and corresponding individualized behavioral support plan should help tailor interventions to the needs of the student and family. Early identification can help to give needed support to help the student, parents, and teachers who work with them. Those with milder forms of ADHD generally function well with this behavioral support.

ADHD AND MEDICATIONS

Behavior management medications are frequently used to manage ADHD. In the 1930s, amphetamines were first discovered to be an effective treatment for this disorder and continue to be the mainstay of treatment (5). Many different categories of medication have been used in Food and Drug Administration (FDA)-approved and off-label treatments. Off-label treatments are defined as using an approved medication to treat a nonapproved condition, or using the medication to treat a child younger than approved by the FDA.

Categories of medication to treat ADHD include stimulants, antidepressant, antianxiety, antiepileptic, antipsychotic, antihypertensive, anticonvulsant, mood stabilizers, and norepinephrine reuptake inhibitors. A one-size-fits-all approach does not apply to children and different medications and combinations of drugs may be needed to achieve the best outcome. A customized treatment plan must be formed with careful observation of behavior by parents and physicians.

The most commonly used category of medication is the stimulant group. The mechanism of action is to stimulate the central nervous system thereby allowing concentrated focus of attention. Stimulant medications come in different forms, such as pill, capsule, liquid, or skin patch. Some medications come in short-acting, long-acting, or extended-release varieties (37) (Table 9.4).

Of the medications listed, Concerta, Adderal XR, Vyvanse, and Focalin XR were among the top 200 products in the market by sales for 2009 (38). Antidepressant medications that include serotonin selective reuptake inhibitors have been the most commonly prescribed medications in those with autism. Fluoxetine (Zoloft), paroxetine (Paxil),

TABLE 9.4 Stimulant Group

Trade Name	Generic Name	Approved Age
Adderall	Amphetamine	3 and older
Adderall XR	Amphetamine (extended release)	6 and older
Concerta	Methylphenidate (long acting)	6 and older
Daytrana	Methylphenidate patch	6 and older
Desoxyn	Methamphetamine hydrochloride	6 and older
Dexedrine	Dextroamphetamine	3 and older
Dextrostat	Dextroamphetamine	3 and older
Focalin (XR)	Dexmethylphenidate	6 and older
Metadate CD/ER	Methylphenidate (extended release)	6 and older
Methylin	Methylphenidate	6 and older
Ritalin (SR/LA)	Methylphenidate	6 and older
Strattera	Atomoxetine	6 and older
Vyvanse	Lisdexamfetamine dimesylate	6 and older

and citalopram (Celexa) are effective in managing preservative behaviors such as compulsions, stereotypies, and self-injurious behavior (39). Using antidepressants to treat ADHD and behaviors associated with autism is off-label but commonly practiced. Dopamine blockers such as atypical antipsychotics, clozapine, risperidone (Risperdal), olanzapine, quetiapine, and ziprasidone, have been observed to alleviate symptoms such as hyperactivity, stereotypical behaviors, aggression, and self-injury (40). Common side effects of medications used in the treatment of ADHD are listed in Table 9.5.

OTHER INTERVENTIONS

Behavioral interventions are be used to target behaviors at individual, class-wide, or school-wide levels. Behavioral intervention plans target particular behaviors in terms of antecedents (what has gone before) and consequences. These plans are applicable in both home and school settings. Good communication may help the plan to be successful. Self-monitoring and self-evaluations can also be useful and helpful in those with less severe symptoms (9). Contracts should be made with the student by family and/or school staff.

The National Association of School Psychologists (NASP) in a 2003 position statement states that "effective interventions should be tailored to the unique strengths and needs of every student" (41). They list specific areas such as classroom modifications designed to improve work output and focus as well as the social areas of adjustment. Behavioral support systems are another strong area and may include a functional behavioral assessment to systematically study the child's behavior. From this information, a behavioral intervention plan that is specific to the child can be developed. Direct instruction may be designed with specific study strategies that are designed to help generalize the skills to broader natural settings for the child (41).

Family involvement is essential as parents are the primary experts and know their child best. Therefore, methods that support parents at home are essential to help all those involved with the child as we develop supports that can be meshed with school and the broader community settings. Having a case manager or central person that integrates information can help to coordinate implementation of the efforts and to evaluate how effective the interventions have been in meeting needs and goals.

School staff should have specific training in the management of the classroom for children with attention problems to help to develop targeted strategies and monitor behavioral interventions. Similarly, other medical and community service agencies that are involved should be included in collaborative efforts. Finally, NASP recommends that students who are helped through these interventions appreciate and develop their own talents and abilities.

National Association of School Psychologists and other organizations also acknowledge that medication may be necessary and helpful to compliment these interventions. The decision to involve medication lies primarily with the parents and should be considered as a part of a complete program that includes those

TABLE 9.5 Common Behavior Medications

Class	Drugs	Benefit	Side Effects
Antipsychotic or neuroleptics	Haldol Mellarill Stelazine Thorazine	Reduce agitation, anxiety aggression, hyperactivity, stereotypic and self-stimulatory behaviors, and temper outbursts	Addiction **Blurred vision** Dyskinesia Psychosis Sedation Tremors
Typical neuroleptics	Abilify Clozaril Geodon Risperdal Seroquel Zyprexa	Reduce aggression, agitation, self-injurious behaviors	Agitation Increased appetite Lowers white blood cell count Tardive dyskinesia
Antidepressants	Anafranil Celexa Elavil Lexapro Luvox Paxil, Prozac Tofranil Wellbutrin Zoloft	Raise serotonin levels Reduce anxiety Reduce obsessive–compulsive and ritualistic behaviors	Arrhythmias **Blurred vision** Constipation Dry mouth Dizziness Hyperactivity and impulsivity Lowered threshold for seizures Sleep disturbances
Antianxiety agents	Ativan Buspar Klonapin Valium Xanax	Reduce anxiety	**Abnormal eye movements** Crying Disinhibition Irritability
Stimulants	Adderal Cylert Datrona patch Dexedrine Focalin Ritalin	Affect dopamine Improve focus and regulation Monitor arousal system Decrease impulsivity	Depression Increase in perseveration and repetitive behaviors Irritability Palpitations Sleep disturbance
Antihypertensives	Clonodine Tenex	Calm and improve sleep Decrease hyperactivity and impulsivity	Irritability Lower blood pressure Sedation
Anticonvulsants/mood stabilizers	Depakote, Dilantin Keppra Phenobarbitol Tegretol Trileptal	Calm behavior Lessen mood swings Lessen outbursts	Affects kidney function **Vision impairments such as rapid eye movements**
Norepinephrine reuptake inhibitor	Strattera	Reduces inattention, hyperactivity, and impulsivity	Possibly bipolar disorder

Source: Lemer P. Envisioning a bright future. Santa Ana: Optometric Extension Program Foundation; 2008, used with permission of the Optometric Extension Program Foundation.

interventions mentioned above. Close communication is also recommended to help problem solve and provide for better overall effectiveness. Finally, the monitoring and communication of behavioral and academic data to the medical team should further extend effective collaboration (41).

Guidelines for the treatment of school-age children with ADHD have been described by the American Academy of Pediatrics, which includes use of DSM-IV, with observation and information from parents and teachers. These guidelines describe ADHD as a chronic disorder and also recommend both medication and behavioral–psychosocial interventions in an overall treatment regimen (42).

Guidelines developed by experts state that a behavioral-psychosocial-combined treatment may be effective as a "first-level" treatment for some situations (e.g., milder forms of ADHD, younger children, families who prefer to avoid medications, comorbid social skills deficits) (43). Root and

Resnick (42) also describe medication and psychosocial treatment as the first-line treatment for most applications including more severe cases, where family is more severely affected and other problems (e.g., aggression) are present. Other indications for this combined treatment include situations where change is needed more urgently, for all older-age groups beyond preschool, and when other comorbid disorders are present (24).

CONCLUSION

Attention deficit hyperactivity disorder is a commonly seen neurobiologic disorder that affects both younger and older individuals. The disorder may manifest in three different ways as described by the APA diagnostic manual. While genetic and biologic factors have been identified and described, more research in these areas is needed. The best practice of treatment for those with ADHD currently indicates both psychological treatment in combination with medical and pharmaceutical intervention. Since many conditions may be comorbid in a patient with ADHD, a multidisciplinary team, including physician, mental health specialist, eye care profession, and many support services, is essential in the management of these patients.

REFERENCES

1. Still GF. Some abnormal psychical conditions in children. Lancet. 1902;1:1008–12, 1010–77; 82:1163–8.
2. American Psychiatric Association. Diagnostic and statistical manual of mental disorders. Text revision (DSM-IV TR). 4th ed. Washington: American Psychiatric Association; 2000.
3. American Academy of Pediatrics. Clinical practice guidelines: diagnosis and evaluation of the child with attention-deficit/hyperactivity disorder. Pediatrics. 2000;105:1158–70.
4. Connor DF, Steeber J, Mc Burnett KA. Review of attention-deficit/hyperactivity disorder complicated by symptoms of oppositional defiant disorder or conduct disorder. J Dev Behav Pediatr. 2010;31:427–40.
5. Barkley RA. Attention deficit hyperactivity disorder: a handbook for diagnosis and treatment. New York: The Guilford Press; 1998.
6. Wolraich ML, Hannah J, Baumgaertel A, Feurer ID. Examination of DSM-IV criteria for attention deficit/hyperactivity disorder in a county-wide sample. J Dev Behav Pediatr. 1998;19:162–8.
7. American Academy of Pediatrics. Clinical practice guideline: diagnosis and evaluation of the child with attention-deficit/hyperactivity disorder. Pediatrics 2000; 105:1158–1770.
8. Richman JE. Overview of attention and learning. In Scheiman M, Rouse, M. Optometric Management of Learning-Related Vision Problems. 2nd ed. Philadelphia, PA: Mosby Inc. 2006, 121–64.
9. DuPaul GP, White GP. Counseling 101 Column. An ADHD primer. Principal Leadership Magazine. 2004;5(2). Available from: www.nasponline.org/resources/principals/nassp_adhd.aspx. Last Accessed May 15, 2011.
10. Remschmidt, H. (2005). Global consensus on ADHD/HKD. European Child & Adolescent Psychiatry, 14(3), 127–137.
11. Barkley RA. International consensus statement on ADHD. Clinical Child and Family Psychological Review. 2002;5(2): 89–111.
12. Barbaresi WJ. How common is attention deficit disorder? Incidence in a population-based birth cohort in Rochester, Minnesota. Arch Pediatr Adolesc Med. 2002;156:217–24.
13. Biederman J, Spencer TJ, Wilens T, Greene R. Attention-deficit/hyperactivity disorder. In: Gabbard GO, editor. Treatment of psychiatric disorders. 3rd ed. Washington: American Psychiatric Publishing; 2001. p. 145–76.
14. Lerner JW. Learning disabilities: theories, diagnosis and teaching strategies. 9th ed. Boston: Houghton Mufflin; 2003.
15. Silver L. Attention deficit/hyperactivity disorder. A clinical guide to diagnosis and treatment for health and mental health professionals. 3rd ed. Washington: American Psychiatric Publishing, Inc.; 2004.
16. Arnsten AFT, Berridge CW, McCracken JT. The neurobiological basis of attention-deficit/hyperactivity disorder. Prim Psychiatry. 2009;16:47–54.
17. Puper-Oakil D, Wohl M, Mouren MC, Verpillat P, et al. Meta-analysis of family-based association studies between the dopamine transporter gene and attention deficit hyperactivity disorder. Psychiatr Genet. 2005;15:53–9.
18. Daley D. Attention deficit hyperactivity disorder: a review of the essential facts. Child: Care Health Dev. 2006;32:193–204.
19. Manor I, Eisenberg J, Tyano S, Sever Y, et al. Family-based association study of the serotonin transporter promoter region polymorphism (5-HTTLPR) in attention deficit hyperactivity disorder. Am J Med Genet. 2001;105:91–5.
20. Castellanos FX, Acosta MT. Syndrome of attention deficit with hyperactivity as the expression of an organic functional disorder. Revista de Neurologia. 2002;35:1–11.
21. Semrud-Clikeman M, Steingard RJ, Filipek P, Biederman J, et al. Using MRI to examine brain behavior relationships in males with attention deficit disorder with hyperactivity. J Am Acad Child Adolesc Psychiatry. 2000;39:477–84.
22. Lennert T, Martinez-Trujillo J. Strength of response suppression to distracter stimuli determines attention-filtering performance in primate prefrontal neurons. Neuron. 2011;70:141–52.
23. APA. Diagnostic and statistical manual of mental disorders (DSM- III). 3rd ed. Washington: American Psychiatric Association; 1980.
24. Daley D, Jones K, Hutchings J, Thompson M. Attention deficit hyperactivity disorder in pre-school children: current findings, recommended interventions and future directions. Child Care Health Dev. 2009;35:754–66.
25. International Classification of Diseases. 10th ed. Geneva, Switzerland: World Health Organization (WHO); 1992.
26. Schatz AM, Ballantyne AO, Trauner DA. Sensitivity and specificity of a computerized test of attention in the

diagnosis of attention–deficit/hyperactivity disorder. Assessment. 2001;8:357–65.

27. Granet DB, Gomi CF, Ventura R, Miller-Scholte A. The relationship between convergence insufficiency and ADHD. Strabismus. 2005;13:163–8.
28. Rouse M, Borstring E, Mitchell L, Kulp MT, et al. Academic behaviors in children with convergence insufficiency with and without parent-reported ADHD. Optom Vis Sci. 2009;86:1169–77.
29. Gillberg C, Gillberg IC, Rasmussen P, Kadesjö B, et al. Co-existing disorders in ADHD-implications for diagnosis and intervention. Eur Child Adolesc Psychiatry. 2004;13:I/80–92.
30. Goldman LS, Genel M, Bezman RJ, Slanetz PJ, et al. Diagnosis and treatment of attention deficit/hyperactivity disorder in children and adolescents. JAMA. 1998;279:1100–7.
31. Biedermann J. Attention-deficit hyperactivity disorder. Biol Psychiatry. 2005;57:1215–20.
32. Harpold T, Bierderman J, Gignac M, Hammerness P, et al. Is oppositional defiant disorder a meaningful diagnosis in adults? Results from a large sample of adults with ADHD. J Nerv Ment Dis. 2007;195:601–5.
33. Borstring E, Rouse M, Chu R. Measuring ADHD behaviors in children with symptomatic accommodative dysfunction or convergence insufficiency: a preliminary study. Optometry. 2005;76:588–92.
34. Farrar R, Call M, Maples WC. A comparison of the visual symptoms between ADD/ADHD and normal children. Optometry. 2001;72:441–51.
35. Damari DA, Liu J, Smith KB. Visual disorders misdiagnosed as ADHD case series and literature review. J Behav Optom. 2000;11:87–91.
36. Available from: www.drugs.com. Last Accessed June 9, 2011.
37. NIMH Attention Deficit Hyperactivity Disorder (ADHD) Children and Adolescents. Available from: www.nimh.nih.gov/health/publications/attention-deficit-hyperactivity-disorder/complete-index.shtml. Last Accessed May 20, 2011.
38. Pharmacy Times. Top prescription drugs of 2009. Available from: www.pharmacytimes.com/publications/issue/2010/May2010/RxFocusTopDrugs-0510. Last Accessed May 20, 2011.
39. Langworthy-Lam KS, Aman MG, Van Bourgondien ME. Prevalence and patterns of use of psychoactive medicines in individuals with autism in the Autism Society of North Carolina. J Child Adolesc Psychopharmacol. 2002;12: 311–22.
40. Young J, Kavanagh M, Anderson G, Shaywitz B, et al. Clinical neurochemistry of autism and related disorders. J Autism Dev Disord. 1982;12:147–65.
41. National Association of School Psychologists' NASP Delegate Assembly. Position statement on students with attention problems. NASP 2003. Available from: www.nasponline.org. Last Accessed on May 20, 2011.
42. Root RW, Resnick RJ. Professional psychology. Res Pract. 2003;34:34–41.
43. Conners CK, March JS, Wells KC, Ross R. The expert consensus guidelines ®: treatment of attention-deficit/hyperactivity disorder. J Atten Disord 2001;4(suppl1): A1–50.

CHAPTER 10

Kenneth J. Ciuffreda, OD, PhD, FCOVD-A, FAAO
Neera Kapoor, OD, MS, FCOVD-A, FAAO

Acquired Brain Injury

Acquired brain injury (ABI) is an umbrella term that includes traumatic brain injury (TBI) or concussion, cerebral vascular accident (CVA) or stroke, aneurysm, brain tumor, vestibular dysfunction, and/or postsurgical complications resulting in anoxia or hypoxia, to name a few (1). In terms of deficits evident subsequent to ABI, the crux of research has been performed in the areas of TBI and CVA. Neurologic deficits evident following TBI and CVA include altered cognition, affect, and/or sensorimotor abilities (often including vision) (1,2). While the period of natural recovery following ABI varies and is not always complete, using TBI as an example, recovery ranges from a few months to 1 to 2 years following the incident depending upon the nature and severity of the insult (1,2). Therefore, the assessment, rehabilitation/intervention, and monitoring of neurologic and systemic deficits evident following ABI are indicated as deemed appropriate.

Traumatic brain injury refers to an acquired, sudden-onset, nonprogressive and nondegenerative condition, exclusive of birth trauma, affecting neurologic function (1–3). Hospital visit data reported to and compiled by the Centers for Disease Control and Prevention reflect that, in the United States, approximately 1.7 million individuals per year reported having incurred a TBI (3). Since many with mild traumatic brain injury (mTBI) do not report to a hospital immediately following the actual precipitating event, this estimated incidence of TBI is likely an underestimate.

Cerebral vascular accident (stroke) refers to an ischemic (~85% of all strokes) or hemorrhagic vascular event compromising neurologic function (4,5). In the United States, CVA affects approximately 795,000 persons each year, with an estimated 610,000 being new or first strokes (5). Stroke in the United States is the third leading cause of death with 137,000 individuals dying from stroke annually (4). Further, CVA remains the leading cause of serious long-term disability in the United States (5).

Sensorimotor vision symptoms are reported often in those with ABI, specifically TBI and CVA, in frequencies ranging from 30% to 85%. This depends upon the nature of the vision deficit and the criteria used in the clinical research study (1,6–8). Individuals with TBI and CVA manifest a constellation of visually based symptoms (1,6–8), which is not surprising since 7 of the 12 cranial nerves deal directly or indirectly with vision (CN II, III, IV, V, VI, VII, and VIII). This is also not surprising when one considers the pervasiveness and extent of many brain injuries, especially TBI with its underlying multifaceted coup–contrecoup mechanism of damage (1). The visual symptoms may encompass and be derived from one or more of the following areas: oculomotor and accommodative dysfunctions, binocular vision deficits, visual field loss/reduced sensitivity, photosensitivity, visual motion sensitivity, visual memory deficits, visual attentional problems, vestibular impairment, spatial localization errors, perceptual deficits and visual information processing problems, and visuomotor coordination impairment (Table 10.1) (1,6–9).

Fortunately, all of these dysfunctions can be remediated, at least in part, using a range of optical devices and/or therapeutic techniques: nearpoint lenses, vergence prisms, yoked prisms, field-enhancing prisms, binasal occlusion, vestibular therapy, optometric vision therapy, and perceptual/cognitive therapy (9–11). In addition, these individuals have a high frequency of occurrence of corneal, lenticular, vitreal, and/or retinal abnormalities, which produce a wide range of symptoms (e.g., dry eye) (12). These problems often require medical and/or surgical, rather than rehabilitative, intervention.

Individuals with ABI often demonstrate a full range of oculomotor problems that have been found in much higher frequency than in a matched non-ABI

TABLE 10.1 Visual Sequelae of ABI

Category of Vision Problem	Specific Deficit
Eye movement dysfunctions	Deficits of saccades, deficits of pursuit, fixation anomalies, nystagmus
Accommodative dysfunctions	Impairment of accommodative amplitude, facility, and sustainability
Binocular vision deficits	Convergence insufficiency, exophoria, vertical phoria, fusional vergence dysfunction
Visual field loss	Central scotoma, congruous/incongruous homonymous hemianopia, congruous/incongruous quadrantanopia, unilateral visual–spatial inattention (i.e., neglect), altitudinal defects
Visual–vestibular dysfunctions	Vestibular impairment, vertigo, loss of balance, visual motion sensitivity, spatial localization errors, impaired visual motor integration/coordination
Perceptual dysfunctions/visual information processing problems	Contrast sensitivity, color vision, photosensitivity, spatial relationships, body image, agnosias, laterality and directionality, visual memory deficits, visual attentional problems

Modified from Suchoff IB, Ciuffreda KJ, Kapoor N. Visual and vestibular consequences of acquired brain injury. Santa Ana: Optometric Extension Program Foundation; 2001.

population. This is not surprising, as 4 out of the 12 cranial nerves deal with fine oculomotor control (CN III, IV, VI, and VIII). These deficits may encompass the vergence, version, and/or accommodative systems, as well as the pupil and visuomotor postural systems (1,6–11,13).

The incidence of the above oculomotor problems was recently quantified in a retrospective study of comprehensive clinical vision examinations of symptomatic adults with ABI (n = 160 with mTBI and n = 60 patients with CVA) who were referred to and assessed in a specialty vision rehabilitation clinic (7). The results presented in Table 10.2 reveal a considerable commonality in both mTBI and CVA, with convergence insufficiency, CNIII paresis/palsy, and saccadic deficits being most prominent. In addition, accommodative insufficiency and accommodative facility dysfunctions were prevalent in both mTBI and CVA. The oculomotor problems were found with up to 10-fold greater frequency of occurrence in the ABI versus non-ABI populations. Fortunately, with optometric vision therapy, positive outcomes were evident in 90% of the group who were identified, received, and completed therapy (10).

More recently, Ciuffreda et al. (13) have developed a targeted/focused clinical oculomotor diagnostic protocol in this population, in particular those with mTBI (Table 10.3). This diagnostic protocol includes a range of high-yield parameters that can be readily assessed in the clinical optometric practice (e.g., near point of convergence). A targeted protocol facilitates more accurate and complete diagnoses, which in turn should result in rapid and efficient therapeutic interventions to improve sensorimotor vision function.

Sensorimotor vision function deficits are important to assess and treat because they affect the progress of rehabilitation, as well as basic activities of daily living (ADLs). It is important to keep in mind that many aspects of rehabilitation and daily living tasks are vision based. Some reading-related or visual search tasks used in cognitive and occupational rehabilitation may be affected if deficits of saccades, fixation, accommodation, or vergence are evident. In addition, those presenting with visual field defects, blur,

TABLE 10.2 Summary of the Percentage of Individuals in Each Subgroup (Where for TBI n = 160 and for CVA n = 60) within a Given Category of Ocular Motor Dysfunction and the Most Common Anomaly Present

Ocular Motor Dysfunction	TBI (%)	Most Common Anomaly (TBI)	CVA (%)	Most Common Anomaly (CVA)
Accommodation	41.1	Accommodative insufficiency	12.5	Accommodative infacility
Versional	51.3	Deficits of saccades	56.7	Deficits of saccades
Vergence	56.3	Convergence insufficiency	36.7	Convergence insufficiency
Strabismus	25.6	Strabismus at near	36.7	Strabismus at far
CN Palsy	6.9	CN III	10	CN III

Note: For accommodation, the "n" represents the number of persons actually tested for accommodation (TBI n = 51, CVA n = 8), which only included those under the age of 40 years (i.e., prepresbyopic).
Reprinted with permission from Ciuffreda et al. Occurrence of oculomotor dysfunctions in acquired brain injury: a retrospective analysis. Optometry. 2007;78(4):155–61.

TABLE 10.3 Targeted Clinical Oculomotor Parameters

Vergence	• Near point of convergence break (especially with repetition) • Near point of convergence recovery (especially with repetition) • Positive relative vergence break • Positive relative vergence recovery • Vergence facility (prism flipper baseline) • Vergence facility (prism flipper fatigue) • Horizontal near dissociated phoria • AC/A ratio • Fixation disparity at near • Associated phoria at near • Stereoacuity (per its relation to vergence error)
Accommodation	• Accommodative amplitude • Accommodative facility (lens flipper fatigue) • Positive relative accommodation/Negative relative accommodation
Version	• Fixational stability • Saccadic accuracy • Pursuit accuracy • Developmental Eye Movements test

Modified from Ciuffreda et al. Oculomotor diagnostic protocol for the mTBI population. Optometry. 2011;82:61–63.

or diplopia may experience difficulty progressing with their rehabilitation if their vision problems have not been addressed with neuro-optometric intervention. Neuro-optometric rehabilitation options may benefit those with deficits of accommodation, tear film integrity, versional ocular motility, vergence ocular motility, visual–vestibular interaction, light–dark adaptation, and visual field integrity. Therefore, assessment and treatment of persistent, residual sensorimotor vision deficits following TBI and CVA may improve a patient's ability to perform the requisite aspects of rehabilitation, as well as their independent ADLs.

DEFICITS OF ACCOMMODATION

The frequency of occurrence of accommodative anomalies among prepresbyopic individuals with TBI ranges from 10% to 40% (6,7). While fewer data are available on accommodation in stroke, approximately 12.5% of visually symptomatic individuals with stroke presented with an accommodative anomaly in a recent retrospective study (7). Typical symptoms include constant or intermittent blur in conjunction with eyestrain or brow aches (7,9,10). Neuro-optometric rehabilitation treatment options for accommodative deficits are restorative, compensatory, and adaptive.

ANOMALOUS TEAR FILM INTEGRITY

Dry eye syndrome relates to anomalous composition and/or uniformity of volume and flow of the tear film, suggesting two predominant categories of dry eye: aqueous deficiency and evaporative loss. While dry eye has a reported frequency of occurrence of 10% in the general population >65 years of age (14), an incidence ranging from 15% to 22% has been reported in those with ABI (6,12,14). Further, dry eye is also a common ocular side effect of some antidepressant and antihypertensive medications (6,12,14). Since many with ABI are prescribed antidepressant and antihypertensive medications, an elevated occurrence of dry eye in this population is understandable.

With the two types of dry eye coexisting or presenting in isolation, patients may report intermittent distortion of clarity of vision varying with blinking, frequent blinking, and a possible foreign-body sensation (6,12,14). Typical treatment options for managing dry eye are compensatory and, depending upon the severity of the dry eye, range from prescribing artificial tears over the counter to inserting punctal plugs (14).

DEFICITS OF VERSIONAL OCULAR MOTILITY

Versional ocular motility includes fixation, smooth pursuit, and saccades. Anomalies of versional ocular motility have been reported in those with ABI with a study-dependent frequency of occurrence ranging from 40% to 85% (1,6–10). Associated symptoms include reduced reading speed, loss of place when reading, and dizziness or sensation of motion when reading (7,8,10). Neuro-optometric rehabilitation treatment options for managing versional ocular motor deficits are restorative, compensatory, and adaptive.

DEFICITS OF VERGENCE OCULAR MOTILITY

Vergence anomalies have been reported with study-dependent frequencies, ranging from 40% (6) to 56% (7) in those with TBI and up to 37% (10) in those with stroke. The most commonly reported vergence dysfunction in TBI and stroke is convergence insufficiency (6–8,10). A common associated symptom with vergence anomalies is constant or intermittent diplopia, which is temporarily eliminated with monocular occlusion (i.e., the diplopia is not evident under monocular conditions). Additional symptoms of vergence dysfunction include eyestrain when reading, vision-related headaches, avoidance of vision-related tasks, and dizziness or sensation of motion when reading (7,9,10). The neuro-optometric rehabilitation treatment options for anomalies of vergence are restorative, compensatory, and adaptive.

DEFICITS OF VISUAL–VESTIBULAR INTERACTION

The main purpose of the vestibuloocular reflex (VOR) is gaze stabilization or, more specifically, the stabilization of the retinal images while the head is in motion (1,15). Many neural areas contribute to the VOR. However, the simplest is the neural arc for the horizontal VOR, in which the oculomotor nerve communicates with the abducens nerve via the medial longitudinal fasciculus and onward to communicate with the acoustic (also known as the vestibulocochlear) nerve, thereby stabilizing horizontal gaze while the head moves horizontally (1,15,16). The VOR, which is also referred to as "gaze stabilization" by many vestibular therapists, is a valuable component of the vestibular rehabilitative regimen, which requires stable and accurate extraocular motility (1,15).

Many patients with ABI manifest anomalies of visual–vestibular interaction (also referred to as visual vertigo or "supermarket syndrome"), which is accompanied by symptoms such as disequilibrium and increased sensitivity to visual motion in supermarkets, malls, crowds, and other multiply visually stimulating environments (1,16). These same patients may also report difficulty performing "gaze stabilization" tasks in vestibular rehabilitation. For such individuals, neuro-optometric vision therapy for ocular motor anomalies in patients with visual–vestibular disturbances is compensatory, adaptive, and, to a moderate degree, restorative. Neuro-optometric vision therapy addressing anomalies of both versional and vergence ocular motility should occur prior to commencing VOR training in vestibular rehabilitation (1,9).

PHOTOSENSITIVITY

Photosensitivity in the ABI population refers to increased light sensitivity with discomfort in the absence of ocular inflammation (9,17,18), and it may present as increased sensitivity to all lighting or selectively to fluorescent lighting (17,18). Although the precise neurologic substrate responsible for photosensitivity in ABI remains unknown, anomalies of light (i.e., photopic) and dark (i.e., scotopic) adaptation have been hypothesized as being responsible for general photosensitivity (17,18). Those with selective photosensitivity to fluorescent lighting often manifest elevated critical flicker fusion frequency thresholds and may report symptoms of increased sensitivity to visual motion and visual–vestibular disturbances (18).

Reasonable diagnostic testing for photosensitivity includes assessment of scotopic threshold and/or critical frequency fusion threshold values, which may be measured and compared to normative data. Treatment options are compensatory and adaptive, rather than restorative (9,17,18).

ANOMALIES OF VISUAL FIELD INTEGRITY

Visual field anomalies may present as diffuse or lateralized (i.e., a left or right hemianopia or quadrantanopia). Diffuse visual field defects are more common in those with TBI and demyelinating disease. Conversely, homonymous lateralized visual field defects are more common in those with stroke. Visual field integrity assessment usually involves visual field testing under monocular viewing conditions while controlling for visual fixation, such as confrontation testing and perimetry.

The occurrence of visual field defects in those with TBI has been reported with a study-dependent frequency ranging from 35% to 39% (19). A recent retrospective study on a sample of visually symptomatic persons with TBI and stroke reported that visual field defects were evident in approximately 39% and 67% of those with TBI and stroke, respectively (19). That same retrospective study of visually symptomatic persons with TBI and stroke reported that, out of those presenting with visual field defects, homonymous lateralized visual field defects were manifest in approximately 23% and 48% of those with TBI and stroke, respectively (19).

There is a spectrum of four major diagnostic categories of visual field integrity, regarding postchiasmal, homonymous lateralized visual field defects (20): (a) no visual field defect and no unilateral spatial inattention (USI); (b) no visual field defect, but evident USI; (c) a visual field defect with USI; or (d) a visual field defect without USI. To diagnose a lateralized (i.e., left or right hemi- or quadrant-inattention) USI, additional pencil and paper diagnostic tests such as drawing of a daisy/clock/person or cancellation are beneficial (20).

Associated symptoms related to anomalous visual field integrity include bumping into objects on one side of visual space, difficulty with reading-related eye movements due to the field defect, and possible lack of awareness that one's visual field is no longer intact. Since lateralized homonymous visual field defects do not usually resolve completely or spontaneously, treatment options (9,20) remain compensatory and adaptive for the most part, rather than restorative, despite evident case reports of restored visual field integrity for those with postchiasmal lateralized visual field defects (20).

CONCLUSION

In summary, given the pervasiveness of the brain injury, a constellation of visual, sensorimotor, visual perceptual, and related dysfunctions is often present. It is important for the primary eye care provider to make the appropriate diagnoses and then to treat or refer out for treatment to remediate any visual dysfunctions present. Treatment allows immediate and long-term improvement in the patient's life, impacting ADLs. Fortunately, remediation is successful in most cases.

REFERENCES

1. Suchoff IB, Ciuffreda KJ, Kapoor N, editors. Visual and vestibular consequences of acquired brain injury. Santa Ana: Optometric Extension Program Foundation; 2001.
2. McHugh T, Laforce R Jr, Gallagher P, Quinn S, Diggle P, Buchanan L. Natural history of the long-term cognitive, affective, and physical sequelae of mild traumatic brain injury. Brain Cogn. 2006;60:209–11.
3. Faul M, Xu L, Wald MM, Coronado VG. Traumatic brain injury in the United States: emergency department visits, hospitalizations and deaths 2002–2006. Atlanta: Centers for Disease Control and Prevention, National Center for Injury Prevention and Control; 2010.
4. Heron MP, Hoyert DL, Murphy SL, Xu JQ, Kochanek KD, Tejada-Vera B. Deaths: final data for 2006, [PDF–5.3M] National Vital Statistics Reports; 57(14). Hyattsville: National Center for Health Statistics; 2009.
5. Lloyd-Jones D, Adams R, Carnethon M, et al. Heart Disease and Stroke Statistics—2009 Update. A Report from the American Heart Association Statistics Committee and Stroke Statistics Subcommittee. Circulation. 2009;119:e21–181.
6. Suchoff IB, Kapoor N, Waxman R, Ference W. Prevalence of visual and ocular conditions in a non-selected acquired brain-injured patient sample. J Am Optom Assoc. 1999; 70:301–8.
7. Ciuffreda KJ, Kapoor N, Rutner D, Suchoff IB, Han ME, Craig S. Occurrence of oculomotor dysfunctions in acquired brain injury: a retrospective analysis. Optometry, 2007; 78: 155–61.
8. Goodrich GL, Kirby J, Cockerham G, Ingalla S, and Lew Ht alsual function in patients of a polytrauma rehabilitation center: a descriptive study. Journal of Rehabilitation Research and Development, 2007; 44: 929–36.
9. Kapoor N, Ciuffreda KJ. Vision disturbances following traumatic brain injury. Curr Treat Options Neurol. 2002; 4:271–80.
10. Ciuffreda KJ, Rutner D, Kapoor N, Suchoff IB, Craig S, Han ME. Vision therapy for oculomotor dysfunctions in acquired brain injury: a retrospective analysis. Optometry, 2008; 79:18–22.
11. Ciuffreda KJ, Ludlam DP. Conceptual model of optometric vision care in mild traumatic brain injury. J Behav Optom. 2011;22:10–2.
12. Rutner D, Kapoor N, Ciuffreda KJ, et al. Occurrence of ocular disease in traumatic brain injury in a selected sample: a retrospective analysis. Brain Inj. 2006;20:1079–86.
13. Ciuffreda KJ, Ludlam D, Thiagarajan P. Oculomotor diagnostic protocol for the mTBI population. Optometry. 2011;82:61–3.
14. Rutner D, Kapoor N, Ciuffreda KJ, et al. Frequency of occurrence and treatment of ocular disease in symptomatic individuals with acquired brain injury: a clinical management perspective. J Behav Optom. 2007;18:31–6.
15. Leigh RJ, Zee DS. The neurology of eye movements. 4th ed. New York: Oxford University Press; 2006.
16. Bronstein AM. Vision and vertigo: some visual aspects of vestibular disorders. J Neurol. 2004;251:381–7.
17. Du T, Ciuffreda KJ, Kapoor N. Elevated dark adaptation thresholds in traumatic brain injury. Brain Inj. 2005; 19:1125–38.
18. Chang TT, Ciuffreda KJ, Kapoor N. Critical flicker frequency and related symptoms in mild traumatic brain injury. Brain Inj. 2007;21:1055–62.
19. Suchoff IB, Kapoor N, Ciuffreda KJ, Rutner D, Han ME, and Craig S. The frequency of occurrence, types, and characteristics of visual field defects in acquired brain injury: a retrospective analysis. Optometry, 2008; 79: 259–65.
20. Suchoff IB, Ciuffreda KJ. A primer for the optometric management of unilateral spatial inattention. Optometry. 2004;75:305–19.

CHAPTER 11

Garth N. Christenson, OD, MSEd, FCOVD, FAAO
Eric Borsting, OD, MSEd, FAAO, FCOVD

Learning Disabilities

INTRODUCTION

This chapter provides a pragmatic foundation for the clinical aspects of learning disability (LD), and reviews the rich history of optometric involvement in the field. The stage will be set for the clinician to understand the laws, procedures, and practicalities regarding qualification for and provision of LD services in the public schools. The chapter also provides the clinician with the background knowledge necessary to manage the learning-related vision issues for those patients with an LD or who are struggling with learning issues but do not qualify for LD services.

Optometry's involvement in the diagnosis and management of visual problems associated with LD dates back to the mid-1900s. Decades before LDs were formally recognized in the public school system, optometric pioneers such as Gerry Getman were studying and writing about visual development and learning (1). Getman and others, such as Gessel et al. (2), laid the groundwork for the concept of visual developmental skills, which evolve out of sensory motor play and maturational experiences during childhood. Getman noted that "vision develops out of the tutelage of touch." Visual information processing (VIP) skills such as laterality/directionality, visual form perception, visual figure ground, visual–motor integration, and auditory–visual integration were brought to the forefront of inquiry pertinent to optometric research in the area of visual development and learning (3–5). Flax wrote about the difference in visual skills needed when "learning to read" (grades 1–3) and those required for the advanced skill of "reading to learn" (grades 4 and up) (6). Poor VIP skills are more likely to be involved in youngsters who are struggling to learn to read. Meanwhile, visual efficiency skills such as eye alignment/binocularity, eye movements, and accommodation are more likely to cause difficulty in reading to learn. An inefficient visual system will impede information acquisition resulting in less proficient reading ability. Solan et al. elaborated on the positive correlation between VIP skills and learning, especially in the early grades (7).

More recently, formal VIP evaluation batteries for assessing and managing deficiencies of learning-related visual skills in the child with learning problems have been developed by optometric scholars and clinicians (8,9) (see Chapter 21, Diagnosis and Treatment of Vision Information Processing Disorders for more detail on VIP).

This introduction establishes the involvement of optometric clinicians as pioneers in the field of diagnosis and treatment of vision-related learning difficulties. Learning-related vision problems are often closely associated with various LDs. The next section provides the definitions, details, and various important distinctions for the clinician working with patients in the field of LD.

DEFINITION, PREVALENCE, AND ETIOLOGY FOR LEARNING DISABILITY

The term LD denotes a heterogeneous group of learning problems. Affected individuals often show anomalies in neurologic functioning, educational achievement, social/emotional status, and/or attention issues. These lead to difficulties in one or more of the following areas: listening, reading, writing, reasoning, or mathematical skills. Approximately 5% of the population has been classified as learning disabled (10). In 1975, the passage of public law (PL) 94–142 included this definition of learning disabilities:

Specific LD means a disorder in one or more of the basic psychological processes involved in understanding or in using language, spoken or written, which may manifest itself in an imperfect ability to listen, think, read, write, spell, or do mathematical calculations. The term includes such conditions as perceptual handicaps, brain injury, minimal brain dysfunction, dyslexia, and developmental aphasia. The term does not include children who have learning problems that are primarily the result of visual, hearing, or motor handicaps, mental retardation, emotional disturbance, or those at an environmental, cultural, or economic disadvantage.

In 1980, an alternative definition to that written in the PL 94–142 was proposed by the National Joint Committee on Learning Disabilities as follows:

A heterogeneous group of disorders manifested by significant difficulties in the acquisition and use of listening, speaking, reading, writing, reasoning, or mathematical abilities. These disorders are intrinsic to the individual and presumed to be due to central nervous system dysfunction. Even though an LD may occur concomitantly with other handicapping conditions (e.g., sensory impairment, mental retardation, social and emotional disturbance) or environmental influences (e.g., cultural differences, insufficient/inappropriate instruction, psychogenic factors), it is not the direct result of those conditions or influences.

Both definitions include the idea of significant difficulties in learning language, reading, writing, or math. In addition, these difficulties cannot be attributed to another disability or environmental factors.

TYPES OF LEARNING DISABILITY

Various types of LD arise from deficient information processing that adversely affects academic achievement. The areas of deficient processing include input, integration, memory, and output. Input involves sensory processing of visual and auditory stimuli. Examples of deficiencies in this area include poor recognition and ability to consistently identify shapes and sounds, difficulties sequencing information in a proper timeline, and left–right recognition issues. These issues often result in persistent letter reversals, sequential memory problems, and difficulty distinguishing primary auditory sounds from background sounds. Integration problems can lead to difficulties in being able to relate sounds with shapes, as in number and letter recitation. Additionally, there is often a poor ability to motorically reproduce what was seen when drawing or writing. On a more global level, a child may have trouble integrating previous knowledge with new information. Memory or storage problems obviously make learning difficult due to problems retaining new material either through short- or long-term visual or auditory memory. Lastly, output problems involve the areas of motoric production such as drawing, writing, verbal expression, socially appropriate gestures, etc. With these areas of processing deficiency in mind, we can look at some of the recognized types of LD.

Reading disorders are the most prevalent of all the types of LD with estimates as high as 70% to 80% (11). The differentiation of nonspecific reading disability versus specific reading disability is worth mentioning in this regard.

Nonspecific reading disability includes all the potential causes of reading failure such as sociocultural disadvantage, educational deprivation, primary emotional problems, sensory impairment (auditory or visual disability), low intellectual quotient (IQ) issues, etc. In specific reading disability, none of these general exclusionary problems would be the primary cause of the reading failure. The term dyslexia is often used in this arena as synonymous with specific reading disability. Varying definitions of dyslexia have lead to individuals confusing a variety of reading-related difficulties including problems with word recognition, eye tracking, ocular dominance, comprehension, oral fluency, spelling, letter reversals, and letter transpositions within words, and many other factors.

A model of dyslexia should be based on valid constructs, which underlie and define a specific written language problem. It should be based on repeatable behavioral characteristics owing to underlying language-based neurologic functions and validated by genetic principles as well as prevalence issues. Such a model is discussed below and again later in the chapter. Currently, dyslexia is a term that has been de-emphasized in the school system. Rather, educators and members of the multidisciplinary team dealing with LD evaluation and placement look for specific reading-related issues (i.e., perceptual strengths and weakness, verbal intelligence versus performance IQ, word recognition level, reading comprehension, etc.), which comprise the reading problem. These diagnostic revelations ideally become part of the educational plan for the child.

If there were identifiable types of specific reading disability which could be diagnosed reliably based on characteristic reading (decoding) and spelling (encoding) patterns, this would be very helpful when treating LD. Then diagnosis of one of three main types of dyslexia would lead to a remediation protocol which could be consistently applied for that type of case so that the wheel would not have to be reinvented each time an individualized education plan (IEP) was written for the child. It turns out there is such a diagnostic system (12). Although this procedure is currently not widely used in the school system, it offers clarity for improved recognition and management of children with LD. The types of dyslexia recognized in this system include dyseidesia, dysphonesia, and the mixed type dysphoneidesia (Table 11.1). Interestingly, this system of classification for dyslexia has many proponents who agree on the dual model of phonetic and eidetic coding although terminology varies in some cases (13–25). It has construct validity based on neurologic modeling (26) and has led to clarification of the genetics of reading disability. The dyseidesia type has been found to be inherited via an autosomal dominant pattern (27). These issues are the subjects of entire texts that provide detail including a robust neurologic model, advanced diagnostic procedures, and management specifics (28,29).

Math disability is sometimes referred to as dyscalculia. Such a disorder occurs in students who struggle with recalling math facts, grasping concepts of fractional volume and geometric principle, and plain number sense.

Nonverbal LD may involve issues with motor coordination, social awkwardness, poor organizational skills, and problems with math. Children with nonverbal learning disabilities often show deficits in VIP. These difficulties often occur in the presence of excellent abilities in other areas such as verbal expression, vocabulary, and retention skills.

Delayed speech and language development and/or auditory processing disorders can lead to problems performing in the classroom. Examples of these problems include when multiple verbal directions are given rapidly, or when there is a significant amount of background noise in the classroom. Additionally, the affected individual may be a better visual learner versus learning via audition.

CAUSES AND RISK FACTORS

Most cases of LD do not have an identifiable cause but certain factors can increase the risk of a child manifesting LD. Heredity is a factor as some cases run in families. For example, one of the types of dyslexia, dyseidesia, has been found to be caused by an autosomal dominant genetic anomaly (27). This means that if one parent is affected, the theoretical risk for each child born is 50%. (See Chapter 2, Genetics)

Gestational and birth problems such as low birth weight, oxygen deprivation, prematurity, and exposure to toxic substances such as alcohol and drugs can be risk factors. Childhood accidents including head injuries, toxic substance exposure (lead paint, pesticides), and malnutrition are also risk factors. Socioeconomic factors can lead to various issues that put the child at risk for LD: poor preschool development for the child in terms of reading activities, lack of stimulating developmental play activities for motor and visual skill acquisition, and nutritional deficiencies.

UNDERSTANDING LEARNING DISABILITY IN THE SPHERE OF PUBLIC EDUCATION, DIAGNOSIS, AND TREATMENT

Treatment of the child with LD may require proper educational instruction and/or allied health care intervention. In order for parents, professionals and

TABLE 11.1 Types of Dyslexia

Type	Definition	Characteristics
Dyseidesia	Difficulty matching whole words and whole-word sounds, especially nonphonetic words, that is, light may be pronounced l-i-g-t	Slow reader, decodes words phonetically, spells phonetically ("brij" for bridge), genetic type (autosomal dominant)
Dysphonesia	Difficulty dividing words into syllables and matching sounds with symbols	Reads fairly well until comes to an unknown word, semantic substitution (i.e., glove for mitten), spelling errors are nonphonetic ("sak" for ask) may include letter transpositions
Dysphoneidesia	Difficulty with whole word processing and phonetic processing as in both types above	Combined traits of both types above creating great learning and spelling

the school system to work together for the benefit of the child with learning disabilities, all parties need an understanding of the Individuals with Disabilities Education Act (IDEA). This law started with legislation in 1975 as Public Law 94–142.

In essence, IDEA states that students with disabilities are entitled to an IEP that provides free and appropriate instruction in the least restrictive environment. In educational terms, this means the child will be taught in a setting with his nondisabled peers to the greatest extent possible. This first requires that the child qualify for special services through the school's special education department. In order to appreciate how the system works, the practitioner needs to be cognizant of the stages through which most children pass before they can receive LD services in the public school. Table 11.2 details the stages for identification of, need for, and delivery of LD services: (a) referral stage, (b) assessment stage, and (c) instructional stage. (10)

Once the referral is made for evaluation, the school psychologist and the multidisciplinary team convenes to complete testing and determine, based on the state regulated criteria, whether or not the student qualifies for special services. Table 11.3 provides a comprehensive listing of areas to be surveyed in the psychoeducational evaluation. The results of the assessment determine whether the child qualifies as having a disability. The exact criteria for classifying a child as having an LD vary from state to state. As an example, a child would qualify for special education services if there is a 2-year discrepancy between IQ and academic achievement.

The multidisciplinary team is comprised of specialists that often include occupational therapists, speech and language personnel, special education teachers, adaptive physical education personnel, school psychologists, and others as needed. An IEP is developed in conjunction with the parents after it is determined that the child has qualified for special education services. Once approved, the IEP becomes the child's blueprint for his educational experience each day at school. It includes when the child will be in the classroom or pulled out for special services like occupational, speech and language, and multisensory-linguistic therapy. Some specific areas of the IEP form include (a) present level of function for the student (e.g., reading level and knowledge of math facts), (b) annual goals and short-term benchmarks, and (c) related services (i.e., occupational therapy, physical therapy, adaptive physical education, counseling, and speech and language therapy). The school recommends goals for the child's progression through the program. An example of a long-term

TABLE 11.3 Areas of Evaluation for the Psychoeducational Evaluation

History	Medical Social Academic
Cognitive ability	IQ level (verbal and nonverbal) Language ability Attention and concentration Memory Visual processing skills Auditory processing skills Cognitive style Processing speed
Academic achievement	Reading evaluation (word recognition–decoding level and comprehension level) Spelling (encoding ability) Mathematics Written language abilities (i.e., composition, handwriting, grammar)
Emotional–behavioral development	Self-concept Resilience and coping strategies Relationships with others Reality testing

TABLE 11.2 Stages in the Process of Obtaining LD Services in the Public School System

Referral stage	*Screening*—teacher observations, formal or informal assessment of academic, and or behavioral functioning *RTI (Response to Intervention)*—rather than proceeding directly to formal psychoeducational assessment, therapy is instituted to ascertain the response of the child to early intervention
Assessment stage	Formal psychoeducational evaluation to determine (A) If there is a significant discrepancy between cognitive ability and academic achievement in the various areas of instruction (i.e., math and reading, etc.) (B) Adequacy of emotional/behavioral functioning
Instructional stage	If the child qualified for services in the assessment stage: Writing educational goals including instructional techniques and strategies, tailoring special services to the child's needs (occupational therapy, physical therapy, speech and language therapy, counseling, etc.), and implementing the IEP

goal is "reading at a third-grade level by the end of the academic year." This broad goal requires a short-term benchmark that allows for incremental, measurable progress toward the long-term goal. For example, the IEP may state that the child "will be able to successfully decode one syllable words using the vowel consonant e rule, in 4/5 trials by the end of quarter one." The IEP is generally reviewed annually by the parents and the multidisciplinary team. Specific intervention strategies for general consideration in the instructional arena for LD are listed in Table 11.4.

Reading and Learning Disability Reading delay accounts for the vast majority of LD cases. Research conducted over the last two decades points to phonology and rapid naming as potential core deficits associated with problems in decoding words (30,31). One of the critical core processing deficits causing poor decoding is difficulty with phonologic awareness or the ability to analyze and synthesize sounds in the English language (30,32). Phonologic awareness is a strong predictor of reading problems. More importantly, interventions that improve phonologic awareness and phonetic decoding skills have been shown to have a positive impact on reading achievement in children.

There is general agreement that decoding problems can affect both phonologic word-attack strategies and the ability to develop an adequate sight-word vocabulary. Decoding problems in phonetic, word-attack skills, and/or sight-word recognition are often classified, respectively, as either dysphonetic or dyseidetic (11).

This classification system called the PEC (phonetic–eidetic coding) model is based on the work of Griffin and Walton (11). This system borrowed from the work of Boder and Jarrico (12) and shared terminology as to naming the types of dyslexia but differed in terms of the associated characteristics and inferential causes of dyseidesia and dysphonesia (see Table 11.1). Detailed discussion of the PEC model of dyslexia is beyond the scope of this chapter but is reviewed elsewhere (28,29).

Much has been written about tinted lenses (33–35), magnocellular deficit theory (36–38), and rapid naming/dual-deficit hypothesis paradigms (39). To date, these issues have been shown to be of relatively limited clinical relevance. Various reviews of the tinted lens theory showed there was little long-lasting benefit from wearing tinted lens (40,41) and that likely the real problem was attributable to undiagnosed visual disorders such as binocular and accommodative dysfunction (which are usually best treated with optometric vision therapy) (42,43). Another theory discusses the notion that magnocellular processing deficits (attributed to causing timing difficulties in the visual system, i.e., poor saccadic suppression) may actually be an associated finding coexisting with dyseidesia or dysphoneidesia rather than being a causative factor (44).

To distill the information regarding the nature of specific reading disability, the practitioner would be wise to heed the admonition of the clinical professor who instructed his interns regarding arriving at a diagnosis, "When you hear hoof beats look for a horse not a zebra" (i.e., the most likely cause).

TABLE 11.4 Instructional Strategies for Learning Disabilities

General concepts	Student works at his/her own level of mastery, that is, not being promoted just because a certain amount of class time was spent on a particular curricular concept
	Repetition and practice with relevant motivational consideration when appropriate
	Emphasis of fundamental skill acquisition before moving to advanced material
Direct instruction	Highly structured, sequentially based instruction
	Emphasis on small increments of material to be digested with planning for repetition
	Scripted lesson plans
	Upbeat interaction between learners and teacher
	Redirection of negative behaviors to keep child on task
	Correction of mistakes in a positive nonjudgmental manner
	Grouping of students based on similar skill level
	Ability to assess progress to ensure competency building instruction
Classroom modifications	Seating considerations
	Modified assignments when appropriate
	Testing alterations such as allowing spell checking on essays, etc.
	Control setting for reduced distractions
	Possible partnering with classmate or teacher's aide for one-on-one feedback

In the field of LD when evaluating an individual with reading disability, the likely cause is dyseidesia or dysphoneidesia (i.e., PEC model dyslexia) and not magnocellular deficiencies, rapid naming problems, or tinted lens issues. This is further supported by the prevalence issue where PEC model dyslexia accounts for up to 23% of students in a regular classroom and 71% in a resource room for children with reading disability (45).

The PEC model approach leads to the realization that once reading readiness skills are appropriately developed (perhaps with intervention of occupational therapy and/or VIP therapy), the child with dyseidesia or dysphoneidesia will need some kind of direct instruction, that is, multisensory language therapy (MLT). Additionally, it is important to note that many intervention programs assume that the child has normal visual processing skills in areas such as right/left awareness, form perception, and/or visual–auditory integration. Problems in these areas may make it difficult for the child to benefit from the MLT techniques. Optometric vision therapy is often very helpful in such cases (see Chapter 25, Optometric Management of Functional Vision Disorders for more information regarding optometric vision therapy)

All the programs listed in Table 11.5 (46–50) use multisensory procedures combined with phonologic awareness instruction to improve the child's single-word decoding skills and are generally based on the Orton-Gillingham method (46). In this system, letter names and sounds are learned by associating sensory information from the visual, auditory, and kinesthetic modalities. Consonant and vowel sounds are learned first followed by consonant blends, vowel combinations, and phonetic irregularities. Emphasis is placed on learning the rules for exceptional symbol–sound associations. This brings logic to the written language. Finger spelling is a technique that allows the student to process symbol–sound sequences along with knowledge of how to attack phonetically irregular words based on learning the rules. This approach may sound cumbersome to the good reader, who has refined whole-word, symbol–sound decoding abilities, but for the dyslexic student (with dyseidesia or dysphoneidesia), it is very beneficial.

Some practitioners integrate low-level multisensory language techniques into therapy to teach patients with dyseidesia or dysphoneidesia to transfer visual processing skills into language competency, as in symbol–sound association for basic word recognition and spelling. One program, which bridges VIP therapy with MLT techniques, is called the dyslexia program teaching (DPT) (50).

The next step in therapy is fluency of continuous text reading that is necessary for the child to move from learning to read to reading to learn. This is a critical issue since many children with reading disabilities are not evaluated until grade 3. At that point, they have missed so much reading-related activity that they have to read for 8 hours per day for a year to "catch up" to the experience equal to that of a good reader (51). One program that helps with fluency and builds confidence in terms of continuous text reading is called read naturally (52).

TABLE 11.5 Examples of Multisensory, Phonetic, and Language Therapy Programs

Program	Description
Orton-Gillingham (46)	Letter names and sounds are learned by associating sensory information from the visual, auditory, and kinesthetic modalities. Consonant and vowel sounds are learned first followed by consonant blends, vowel combinations, and phonetic irregularities.
Slingerland (47)	Adaptation and extension of Orton-Gillingham
Project Read (48)	Adaptation and extension of Orton-Gillingham
Wilson Reading System (49)	Based on Orton-Gillingham, students learn decoding principles through a 12-step program that takes 1–3 y to complete
Dyslexia Program Teaching (50)	The DPT method utilizes concepts and teach the DPT method utilizes concepts and techniques from three proven methods: 1. Motor planning and laterality therapy to improve fundamental readiness skills such as attention and directional awareness 2. Halapin letter dynamics for development of concrete written language principles through movement, vision, and audition 3. Multisensory language therapy (such as Orton-Gillingham) using finger spelling and language knowledge for irregular phoneme patterns (which are so common in the English language)

Math and Learning Disability Traditional math curricula have been problematic for students with LD. The reasons for this include the reading vocabulary is too difficult, material is poorly sequenced, and students do not possess the requisite skills to understand basic math concepts (53). Remedial math programs often use concrete manipulatives such as blocks and shapes to instill the concepts of spatial relations and numerical values to help the LD child in this area. Two specific programs that are used for LD instruction in cases of math difficulties are project math (54) and connecting math concepts (55). An interesting concept involving consideration of visual processing skills underlying math ability is the concept of subitizing. Subitizing is a visual skill involving how one visually recognizes groups of objects, for example, grouping numbers together for storage and processing and its relationship to math ability (56). This may become a meaningful area to consider for clinical diagnosis and management of visual deficiencies in the LD child with math issues.

The Response to Intervention Concept for Early Intervention in LD An important consideration involves the conventional IQ versus achievement disparity criterion to determine whether or not children qualify for special education. The many problems with this method are pointed out by Bos and Vaughn (57) and include the following:

1. The achievement versus IQ gap is difficult to determine in younger children. As a result, the identification process is often delayed until second grade or beyond.
2. Many younger children in the 5- to 7-year-old category may benefit from early intervention which is effective at preventing a more profound reading dysfunction.

An alternative to the IQ versus achievement disparity special education criterion is a fairly new concept called the response to intervention (RTI) (58). In this paradigm, the child is identified informally as needing extra help. Rather than going through an in-depth psychoeducational evaluation, age-appropriate therapy for the particular deficient skill area is instituted to measure the RTI. With early intervention, it is thought that a more extensive evaluation and remediation services may be avoided.

The RTI framework appears to have great potential for limiting some of the failures that children with mild reading disabilities suffer in the early grades. Those students with marked dyseidesia or dysphoneidesia, who usually end up decoding two or more grade levels below grade placement, would generally benefit from a complete psychoeducational evaluation and IEP. However, some of those students could also be identified using the RTI paradigm since they would likely need more intensive instruction to accomplish the objectives of the RTI. This would be preferable to just waiting for the students to fall 2 years behind in reading before instituting any intervention. Other RTI examples for elementary grades are found in Table 11.6.

Incidentally, an efficient and validated method to measure the ability of kindergarten students to recognize letters, write letters, and sound out letters is the predyslexia letter coding test (63).

By intervening early and instituting the RTI techniques noted, two things are likely to happen: (a) students would gain the skills that otherwise they would be unlikely to achieve, and (b) the students who have marked difficulties would be identified early for possible special education qualification. The interesting point here is that by using the RTI precept, the school would save dollars by intervening early and preventing the need for special education in the later years. Once failure occurs, the reading or learning problem is often compounded by secondary emotional and behavioral problems, which tend to be recalcitrant to therapy and ultimately lead to greater expense for the school system.

TABLE 11.6 Response to Intervention Suggestions for Students with Reading Problems in Elementary School

Kindergarten	Alphabet Story (50) Discrimination Motor Alphabet (50)
1st Grade	Vowel Mat (long and short vowels) (59) Syllable Synthesis (ba, ab, bi, ib etc., on vowel mat) (59)
Other options	**Phonemic Awareness** (phonics, consonants, vowels, diagraphs, diphthongs) Spelling Smart (60) Dyslexia Program Teaching (DPT) (50) Project Read (48) Systematic, Sequential Phonics (61) **Word Meaning and Vocabulary** Read Aloud Handbook (62) **Comprehension** Read Naturally (52) Informal Ask for three main points in story, have student predict end of story, ask for two or three facts from story, etc.

Caveats for Children in the Learning Disability System The enactment of PL 94–142 and its implementation across the country in public schools was obviously a step forward for children with disabilities. There are some potential drawbacks, however. For example, Heward (64) cites some of the misunderstandings that can lead to unsuccessful outcomes for students with disabilities:

- Some educators and administrators are taught that a structured curriculum, including daily lessons to develop specific skills, is not necessary for effective student learning.
- Some educators also believe that student performance cannot be measured.

These kinds of attitudes are counterproductive for the child with LD to be able to achieve success in the academic environment. Students with dyslexia and other disabilities need tasks to be highly structured and broken down into smaller manageable units which can be monitored for individual progress and measurement of proficiency.

Parent Advocacy To wrap up the ideas presented regarding parents advocating for their child in the special education setting, a couple of notions of a general nature would be worth considering.

For parents who are having a child evaluated in the public school system, a positive, cooperative, and conscientious approach is generally preferable to being overly demanding and threatening litigation. Certainly, it is important for parents/guardians to be informed and aware of their rights in the process, but obviously maintaining a good working relationship with the school officials, teachers, and specialists will benefit the student in the long run.

Most school districts do not currently recognize the term dyslexia. They may refer to specific reading disability or LD involving reading and writing, etc. In any event, if the parents understand the characteristics and best teaching methods for their child's specific reading disability, then they will be able to advocate for the most appropriate long-term goals, benchmarks, and instructional methods in the IEP. Parents may need to be educated as to the appropriate instructional methods available for their child's learning difficulty. This is another area where an informed eye care professional specializing in the field of children's vision can be of great assistance. Additionally, along these lines as a parent, it would be appropriate to have the child receive pull-out instruction with other students with similar types of specific reading dysfunction rather than lumping them with other LD students who may have other issues which do not allow instruction to be complimentary and effective (i.e., students with cognitive disabilities, primary emotional behavioral disorders, etc.)

As a practical matter, parents also need to know that not all students with dyslexia will qualify for special education. In other words, the severity of the dyslexic pattern may not be of such a degree that a 2-year gap between IQ and achievement is present, thereby not allowing the child to qualify for an IEP and special placement. Furthermore, many public schools do not currently utilize the RTI approach. As a result, parents may want to seek professional help from outside the school system and/or choose to homeschool the child. In many cases, the outside help is in the form of tutoring or allied professional clinics that specialize in children's learning problems.

CONCLUSION

This review of current practices for identifying learning problems in the public school system, together with the information and theory as to management of LD, both educationally and from an allied health care perspective, should lead to greater understanding for clinicians dealing with patients who are struggling with learning issues. Emphasis has been placed on the PEC model of dyslexia and the importance of parents advocating appropriately for their children. This approach will hopefully lead to utilization of appropriate research-based innovative methods, as well as reforming the qualification process, to help the many students who struggle with learning disabilities such as dyslexia. Additionally, all allied professionals in the educational and health care field are called upon to continue to move toward a shared common knowledge base for recognizing and managing children with general reading dysfunction as well as dyslexia and other learning disabilities.

REFERENCES

1. Getman GN. Techniques and diagnostic criteria for the optometric care of children's vision. Duncan: Optometric Extension Program Foundation, Inc.; 1960.
2. Gesell A, Ilg FL, Bullis GE. Vision: its development in infant and child. New York: Paul Hober, Inc.; 1949.

3. Richman J. Visual developmental profile. Philadelphia: Pennsylvania College of Optometry; 1972.
4. Hoffman LG. An optometric learning disabilities evaluation, (Parts I-III). Optom Mon. 1979;70:118–21, 201–5, 279–83.
5. Solan HA, Groffman S. Understanding and treating developmental and perceptual motor disabilities. In: Solan HA, editor. The treatment and management of children with learning disabilities. Springfield: Charles C Tomas; 1982.
6. Flax N. Problems in relating visual function to reading disorder. Am J Optom. 1970;47:366–72.
7. Solan HA, Mozlin R, Rumpf DA. Selected perceptual norms and their relationship to reading in kindergarten and the primary grades. J Am Optom. 1985;56:458–67.
8. Suchoff IB. Visual spatial development in the child: an optometric theoretical and clinical approach. New York: State University of New York; 1981.
9. Scheiman MM, Rouse MW. Optometric management of learning-related vision problems. St. Louis: Mosby/Elsevier; 2006.
10. Lerner JW. Learning disabilities: theories, diagnosis, and teaching strategies. 9th ed. Boston: Houghton Mifflin; 2003.
11. Griffin JR, Walton HN. The dyslexia determination test (DDT). Los Angeles: Instructional Materials and Equipment Distributors; 1981, 1987, 2003.
12. Boder E, Jarrico S. The Boder test of reading and spelling patterns. New York: Grune and Stratton; 1982.
13. Geshwind N. Specializations of the human brain. Sci Am. 1979;241:180–99.
14. Galaburda AM, Kemper TL. Cytoarchitectonic abnormalities in developmental dyslexia: a case study. Ann Neurol. 1979;6:94–100.
15. Duffy FH, Denkla MD, Bartels PH, et al. Dyslexia: automated diagnosis by computerized classification of brain electrical activity. Ann Neurol. 1980;7:421–28.
16. Fried I, Tnaguay PE, Boder E, et al. Development of dyslexia: electrophysiological evidence of clinical subgroups. Brain Lang 1981;12:14–22.
17. Rosenthal JH. EEG even-related potentials in dyslexia and its subtypes. In: DAB Lindberg, MF, Collen EE, Van Brunt, editors. AMIA Congress on Medical Informatics (1st 1982 San Francisco). New York: Mason Pub;1982.
18. Roeltgen DP, Sevush S, Heilman KM. Phonological agraphia: writing by the semantic route. Neurology (Cleveland). 1983;33:755–65.
19. Hynd GW, Hynd CR. Dyslexia: neuroanatomical/neurolinguistic perspectives. Reading Res Q. 1984;19:482–98.
20. Roeltgen DP, Heilman KM. Lexical agraphia. Brain. 1984; 107:811–27.
21. Flynn JM, Deering WM. Subtypes of dyslexia: investigation of Beder's classification system using quantitative neurophysiology. Dev Med Child Neurol. 1989;31:215–23.
22. Hynd GW, Semrud-Clikeman M. Dyslexia and neurodevelopmental pathology: relationships to cognition, intelligence, and reading skill acquisition. J Learn Disabil. 1989;22:204–16.
23. Ridder WH, Borsting E, Cooper M, et al. Not all dyslexics are created equal. Optom Vis Sci. 1997;74:99–104.
24. Shaywitz SE, Shaywitz BA, Pugh KR, et al. Functional disruption in the organization of the brain for reading in dyslexia. Proc Natl Acad Sci U S A. 1998;95:2636–641.
25. Ridder WH, Borsting E, Banon T. Dyseidetic and dysphonetic dyslexics display an elevated motion coherence threshold. Invest Ophthalmol Vis Sci. 1992;69:148–51.
26. Cardinal DN, Griffin JR, Christenson GN. A neurological-behavioral model of dyslexia. J Behav Optom. 1992;3:35–9.
27. Griffin JR. Genetics of dyseidetic dyslexia. Optom Vis Sci. 1992;69:148–51.
28. Griffin JR, Christenson GN, Wesson M, et al. Optometric management of reading dysfunction. Boston: Butterworth-Heinemann; 1997.
29. Christenson GN, Griffin JR. Helping children overcome dyslexia: a guidebook for parents, educators and other professional specialists. Santa Ana: Optometric Extension Program Foundation; 2011.
30. Torgerson JK, Wagner RK. Alternative diagnostic approaches for specific developmental reading difficulties. Learn Disabil Res Pract. 1998;13:220–32.
31. Wolf M, Bowers P, Biddle K. Naming-speed processes, timing, and reading: a conceptual review. J Learn Disabil. 2000;33:387–407.
32. Rosner J. Phonological awareness skills program. Austin: Pro-ed; 1999.
33. Irlen H. Successful treatment of learning disabilities. Paper presented to the 91st Annual Convention of the American Psychological Association. Anaheim, CA; 1983.
34. Irlen H. Reading by colors: Overcoming dyslexia and other reading disabilities by the Irlen method. New York: Avery; 1991.
35. Williams MC, LeCluyse K, Rock-Faucheux A. Effective interventions for reading disability. J Am Optom Association. 1992;63:411–17.
36. Lovegrove W Martin F, Slaghuis W. A theoretical and experimental case for a visual deficit in specific reading disability. Cogn Neurolophysiol. 1986;3:225–67.
37. Skottun BC. The magnocellular theory of dyslexia: the evidence from contrast sensitivity. Vis Res. 2000;40:111–27.
38. Solan HA, Shelby-Tremblay J, Hansen PC, et al. M-cell deficit and reading disability: a preliminary study of the effects of temporal vision processing therapy. Optometry. 2004;75:640–50.
39. Schatchneider C, Carlson CD, Francis DJ, et al. Relationship of rapid naming and phonological awareness in early reading development: implications for the double deficit hypothesis. J Learn Disabil. 2002;35:245–56.
40. Rosner J, Rosner J. The Irlen lens treatment: a review of the literature. Optician. 1987;194:26–33.
41. Cardinal DN, Griffin JR, Christenson GN. Do tinted lenses really help students with reading disabilities? Interv School Clinic. 1993;28:275–9.
42. Solan HA. An appraisal of the technique of correcting reading disorders using tinted overlays and tinted lenses. J Learn Disabil. 1990;23:621–3.
43. Blaskey P, Scheiman M, Parisi M, et al. The effectiveness of Irlen filters for improving reading performance: a pilot study. J Learn Disabil. 1990;23:604–12.
44. Christenson GN, Griffin JR, Taylor M. Failure of blue tinted lenses to change reading scores of dyslexic individuals. Optometry. 2001;72:627–33.
45. Griffin JR. Prevalence of dyslexia. J Optom Vis Dev. 1992; 23:17–22.

46. Gillingham A, Stillman B. Remedial training for children with specific disability in reading, spelling, and penmanship. Cambridge: Educators Publishing Service; 1970.
47. Slingerland B. A multisensory program for language arts for specific language disability children: a guide for primary teachers. Cambridge: Educators Publishing Service; 1970.
48. Greene VE, Enfield ML. Project Read Curriculum. Language Circle Enterprises, Inc. Available from: www.projectread.com/curriculum-ccon-3.html Last Accessed February 21, 2011.
49. Wilson BA. Wilson reading system. Milbury: Wilson Language Training; 1988.
50. Christenson GN. Dyslexia program teaching (DPT). Hudson: Christenson Vision Care, 2215 Vine Street; 1999.
51. Torgerson JK, Wagner RK, Rashotte CA, et al. Intensive remedial instruction for children with severe reading disabilities. J Learn Disabil. 2001;34:33–58.
52. Ihnot C, Ihnot T. Read Naturally. St. Paul: Read Naturally, Inc; 1991.
53. Blankenship CS. Curriculum and instruction: an examination of models in special and regular education. In: Cawley JE, editor. Developmental teaching of mathematics for the learning disabled. Rockville: Aspen; 1984.
54. Cawley J, Fitamaurice AM, Goodstein H, et al. Project math. Tulsa: Educational Progress Corporation; 1976.
55. Bernadette K, Carnine D, Engelmann S, et al. Connecting math concepts. Chicago: Science Research Associates; 2003.
56. Fischer B, Gebhardt C, Hartnegg K. Subitizing and visual counting in children with problems acquiring basic arithmetic skills. Optom Vis Dev 2008;39:24–9.
57. Bos CS, Vaughn S. Strategies for teaching students with learning disabilities and behavior problems. Boston: Pearson Education; 2006.
58. Vaughn SR, Fuchs LS. Redefining learning disabilities as inadequate response to instruction: the promise and potential problems. Learn Disabil Res Prac. 2003;18:137–46.
59. Halapin R. Vowel mat, syllable synthesis. Trumbul: Halapin Learning Systems, Inc.; 1995.
60. Stowe CM. Spelling smart. San Francisco: Jossey-Bass, a Wiley Imprint; 2002.
61. Cunningham PM. Systematic sequential phonics they use, for beginning readers of any age. Greensboro: Carson-Dellosa Publishing Company, Inc.; 2000.
62. Trelease J. Read aloud handbook. New York: Penguin Group, Inc.; 2006.
63. Wesson MD, Griffin JR, Christenson GN. Pre-dyslexia Letter Coding Test (PLCT). Culver City: Reading and Perception Therapy Center; 1991.
64. Heward WL. Ten faculty notions about teaching and learning that hinder the effectiveness of special education. J Spec Educ. 2003;36:288–300.

CHAPTER 12

Pamela H. Schnell, OD, FAAO
Dominick M. Maino, OD, MEd, FAAO, FCOVD-A
Robert Jespersen, MD

Psychiatric Illness and Associated Oculovisual Anomalies

Individuals with one or more psychiatric illnesses (PIs), as well as those with a dual diagnosis (DD) of mental illness and substance abuse and/or intellectual disability and mental illness, require eye and vision care as much as, if not more than, the general population. These individuals tend to be taking one or more psychiatric medications and are often at greater risk for drug-induced ocular anomalies, frequently suffer ocular trauma, and are less likely to report having any eye or vision problems. This chapter reviews the major PIs frequently encountered in an optometric practice and the oculovisual problems typically seen in this population.

DEPRESSION

Depression is one of the most commonly encountered mental illnesses. It affects 6.7% of the adult population in the United States (1) with approximately one-third of these individuals classified as having severe disease. Up to 50% of adults in the United States will experience a depressive episode at some point in their lives (2,3). Approximately 15% to 20% of adolescents have an episode of depression by age 20 (4). This disorder is also becoming more common in younger populations (5). Depression is a serious mood disorder that is hallmarked by sadness that does not go away and is disruptive to daily functioning and interpersonal relationships. The condition needs to persist for more than 2 weeks in order to be officially diagnosed, and patients must demonstrate at least five symptoms. There is no predilection for any particular race or sex, although females are diagnosed with this disorder more frequently (6,7). This is possibly due to a greater number of females feeling comfortable talking about emotional issues and presenting more often for treatment. Evidence has shown that patients with a first-degree relative with depression are at higher risk for developing the disorder themselves. Certain personality types and those experiencing periods of extreme stress are susceptible to episodes of depression as well (8–10).

Symptoms of depression, also known as major depression, clinical depression, or depressive disorder, are varied. They include sadness, loss, anger, and frustration, as well as agitation, hopelessness, irritability, fatigue, and/or restlessness. In addition, individuals may experience a change in appetite, weight gain/loss, and difficulty concentrating. They also exhibit a lack of energy, unexplained crying spells, and sleep changes. Unexplained physical manifestations are frequently seen including headaches and back pain. In extreme cases, psychotic symptoms such as hallucinations are possible. Patients tend to have negative feelings and thoughts relating to themselves as well, including feelings of worthlessness, self-hate, guilt, and withdrawal. Suicidal thoughts can lead to attempts on their own lives (6).

In both younger and older populations, symptoms may vary somewhat from those of the typical adult patient. In younger children, for example, depression often presents as irritability, moodiness, and worry. In adolescents anger, anxiety, and avoidance of normal social activities are common, and these are often associated with behavioral problems that could be misread as typical teenage rebellion or confused with other disorders such as attention deficit hyperactivity disorder (ADHD) or oppositional-defiant disorder (ODD). In the elderly, symptoms of depression are often overlooked or attributed to other illnesses or diagnoses. These patients may show a general dissatisfaction with life and boredom that do not seem indicative of the larger underlying problem of depression (11,12).

In general, the combination of symptoms seen in the various forms of depression frequently leads to poor communication with health care professionals and the underreporting of ocular symptoms. The hopeless patient may have a strong feeling of "why bother." The worried and anxious patient may be overly focused on worst possible outcomes and may even withhold information or avoid contact, or conversely, exaggerate symptoms to express their patient's worries and deepest fears (for instance, irrational fear of going blind). If health care professionals do not realize that their patient suffers from depression, they may obtain inadequate information or experience the relationship with the patient in a negative way. Awareness of depression and its effect on the patient and the health care professional is essential in order to obtain the best assessment.

There are multiple treatments currently available for depression, and often more than one form of management is necessary for an individual. If a patient's symptoms are serious, ongoing, or disruptive to their functioning, medication may be necessary. There are several types of antidepressant medications classified by their effects on the neurotransmitters that are believed to be associated with major depression. These include selective serotonin reuptake inhibitors (SSRIs—e.g., Prozac, Zoloft, Paxil, Luvox, Celexa, Lexapro), serotonin/norepinephrine reuptake inhibitors (SNRIs—e.g., Pristiq, Effexor, Cymbalta, Remeron), norepinephrine/dopamine reuptake inhibitors (NDRIs—e.g., Wellbutrin), tricyclic antidepressants (e.g., Elavil), and monoamine oxidase inhibitors (MAOIs—e.g., Nardil, Parnate, Marplan). In treatment-resistant cases, or when the depression is complicated with psychotic symptoms, antipsychotic medications, lithium and other mood stabilizers, and/or thyroid medications may be added to the regimen to boost the effectiveness of the antidepressant medication (13,14). Medications may be needed for extended periods of time for best results. Unfortunately, there can be numerous unwanted side effects associated with the medications used for depression (Table 12.1). The tricyclic antidepressants tend to have higher side effects than newer medications for depression and are not as frequently prescribed as in the past. Monoamine oxidase inhibitors can be highly effective, but they have the potential for the most severe side effects due to their common interaction with various food items (e.g., cheese, pickles, wine), and are often used as a last resort (15).

In addition to prescription medications, there are several herbal remedies used for depression. St. John's wort is perhaps the most common of these and is used primarily for mild cases. It is important to note that St. John's wort can interact with other medications (particularly birth control pills) and render them less effective, so patients must be educated about interactions just as they would be with prescription medications (14,15). Other supplemental remedies include *S*-adenosylmethionine (SAMe), available as a prescription in Europe, and omega-3 fatty acids (16).

One of the mainstays of depression treatment is psychotherapy. Various forms are available, including cognitive–behavioral therapy (CBT), one-on-one counseling, and group therapy. Psychotherapy is often

TABLE 12.1 Side Effects of Psychotropic/Neuroleptic Medications

Drug	Ocular Side Effects
Antipsychotics	Decreased vision, visual hallucinations, mydriasis, nonspecific ocular irritation, eyelid or conjunctiva irregularities, decreased accommodation, night blindness, color vision defects, diplopia, oculogyric crises
Antidepressants	Decreased or blurred vision, decreased accommodation, dry eye, visual hallucinations, photophobia, mydriasis, cycloplegia, color vision defects, extraocular muscle irregularities, eyelid or conjunctiva irregularities
Anticonvulsants	Diplopia, nystagmus, oscillopsia, decreased vision, ptosis, visual hallucinations, mydriasis, myopia, photophobia, decreased accommodation, color vision defects, eyelid or conjunctiva irregularities
Antianxiety agents	Risk of narrow-angle glaucoma, decreased or blurred vision, dry eye, conjunctivitis, diplopia, decreased corneal reflex, extraocular muscle irregularities, decreased accommodation, visual field defects, visual hallucinations

From Donati RJ, Maino DM, Bartell H, Kieffer M. Polypharmacy and the lack of oculo-visual complaints from those with mental illness and dual diagnosis. Optometry. 2009;80:249–54, used with permission of the editor.

employed in conjunction with medications for the best prognosis for long-term improvement and prevention of recurrences. The patient's therapist can recommend one or more coping strategies, including journaling, stress and time management techniques, joining community support groups, and finding outside activities in which to participate in order to avoid isolation. Involving the family members or other support team members in the educational and therapeutic process is highly beneficial (16). Alternative therapies such as yoga, acupuncture, massage therapy, and guided imagery are also becoming more widely used (14–16). Additional options for treatment exist and may be used in conjunction with electroconvulsive therapy (ECT) for those with suicidal or psychotic symptoms who are not responding to medical treatment or psychotherapy, transcranial magnetic stimulation (TMS), vagus nerve stimulation, or light therapy.

There are numerous subcategories of depression which the eye care professional may encounter. Among these are atypical depression, postpartum depression, postpartum psychosis, dysthymia, seasonal affective disorder (SAD), psychotic depression, and schizoaffective disorder. A discussion of symptomatology and treatment for these is beyond the scope of this text, and the reader is referred to any number of excellent sources for further and more detailed information.

In general, depressive illnesses can cause major dysfunction to a patient's life, including symptoms that can affect their ability to communicate with caregivers and to follow through with treatment recommendation. The depressed patient may be on multiple treatments, including medications that each have potential side effects relevant to eye care.

BIPOLAR DISORDER

Bipolar disorder (also known as manic depression or bipolar affective disorder) is a mood disorder characterized by large cyclical swings between a hyperaroused (manic) state and depression. Both the elevated mood and the depression are disruptive to normal functioning and may persist for extended periods. Usually, the manic and depressed phases are distinct from one another, but when the two phases of the cycle overlap, the condition is known as a mixed state. Bipolar disorder is classified into several distinct types. Type I, the classic manic depression with which most readers may be familiar, is usually more severe, with more intense symptoms than type II. In type II bipolar disorder, the patient usually presents with a typically depressed pattern, with interspersed periods of mild mania. However, the individual can develop full-blown mania under certain circumstances (usually when the disorder is unrecognized and the seemingly "depressed" patient is treated with antidepressant medications that "switch" the depression into full mania).

Prevalence rates for the two types are similar, ranging from 0.4% to 1.6% for type I and approximately 0.5% for type II (17,18). There is no significant race, ethnicity, or sex predilection for bipolar disorder, although females may show increased lifetime prevalence for type II (19). A third, and still less intense, form of bipolar disorder is cyclothymia, which is highlighted by shallower mood swings and less intense symptomatology than either type I or type II. It has a similar prevalence rate to the other types at 0.4% to 1.0% (19). Risk factors for bipolar disorder include having a first-degree relative with either bipolar or another mood disorder, going through periods of high stress or major life changes (such as recent childbirth or the death of a loved one), or the abuse of drugs or alcohol. In addition to environmental influence, genetic factors appear to play a role in the course of the disorder (19–21). The symptoms in either phase of bipolar disorder, whether manic or depressed, are similar between the subtypes. Symptoms typically appear at some time between the mid-teen years and the patient's early 20s (21) but may present later in life, often with a triggering event. Patients with type II will show fewer symptoms than those with type I, with cyclothymia patients showing the least. Symptoms associated with the manic phase may include agitation, irritation, inflated self-esteem, delusions of grandeur, and little need for sleep. Patients in a manic phase have a noticeably elevated mood, displaying hyperactivity, restlessness, increased energy, racing thoughts, and a lack of self-control. In addition, these patients display poor temper control and often engage in reckless or risky behavior such as spending sprees, binge drinking or eating, recreational drug use, or promiscuity. The behaviors associated with a manic phase can result in poor work or school performance. Individuals with this disorder may be unaware that what they are experiencing is part of a manic cycle (21).

Symptoms encountered when a patient is in a depression phase are similar to what has been previously described for major depression. They may lose interest in activities they once enjoyed, feel overwhelming sadness, fatigue, or listlessness, and have a sense of hopelessness about the future. The patient can feel worthless or guilty and have difficulty concentrating or making decisions. Eating disturbances are common, whether they take the form of loss of appetite and weight loss or overeating and weight gain. Similarly, sleep disturbances often manifest as either insomnia or excessive sleepiness. Thoughts of self-harm or suicide are common, which puts these individuals at risk for self-injurious behaviors.

In children and adolescents, mood swings and other symptoms can be difficult to separate from the normal emotional changes of puberty. Individuals at these ages may be more likely to show constant irritability rather than more clear-cut depression (21) and can show rapid temper tantrums and explosive aggressive behavior. Cycling through the phases may be much more rapid than in adult patients, often with wide swings from one extreme to the other occurring within hours. The diagnosis is also often found in conjunction with (or misdiagnosed as) ADHD or ODD (21) since these symptoms often overlap.

The diagnosis of bipolar disorder varies slightly with each type. In order to have a diagnosis of type I bipolar disorder, the patient must have at least one episode of mania or mixed state, but do not need to have experienced a phase of depression. For type II, at least one major depressive episode (MDE) is required, as well as one or more periods of hypomania, or mania less symptomatic than the true manic phase of type I. The symptoms must cause distress in some aspect of the patient's life to qualify for the diagnosis of type II bipolar disorder. For a diagnosis of cyclothymia, the patient must have experienced repeated episodes of both hypomania and depression, lasting for >2 years (1 year for children or adolescents). These symptoms cannot disappear for longer than 2 months at a time and must cause significant distress in some aspect of the patient's life (21).

The manic and depressive episodes must also follow certain criteria in order to qualify as such for diagnostic purposes. A manic episode is characterized as a distinct period of abnormally and persistently elevated, expansive, or irritable mood lasting at least 1 week, or less if the patient is hospitalized (21). There must be three or more of the symptoms listed above, and the episode should be disruptive enough to significantly interfere with work, school, or other functioning; to require hospitalization or to trigger a psychotic break. In addition, the symptoms cannot be due to some other diagnosis, such as substance abuse. In order to be classified as hypomania, the episode must be different from the patient's nonmanic state and cause a noticeable change in functioning, but not be such that the patient cannot function at work, school, etc. These periods are also not severe enough to cause a psychotic break. To be classified as a MDE, there must be five or more symptoms over a 2-week period which occur nearly every day. The symptoms must not be due to another natural cause, such as grief over the death of a loved one. Mixed episodes meet the criteria for both manic and depressed episodes nearly every day for at least 1 week.

The major goals of treatment for bipolar disorder involve minimizing a patient's cycling and avoiding hospital stays. Treatment aims to improve the patient's functioning between episodes, to reduce the severity and frequency of the episodes, and to prevent self-destructive behavior and suicide. The most frequent treatment modalities used are medications, psychotherapy, and structured support programs. Medication options are varied, with mood stabilizers often employed as a first-line choice. These mood stabilizers include such drugs as carbamazepine, lamotrigine, lithium, and valproate (valproic acid). Other drugs used frequently are antiseizure medications, antipsychotics, antianxiety medications (benzodiazepines), and antidepressants. The latter are used only in conjunction with mood stabilizers as they have been shown to exacerbate manic episodes (21). Psychotherapy, generally used in conjunction with medications, may consist of CBT, family therapy, or group therapy. Alternatives that may be needed for nonresponsive cases include ECT and TMS. Omega-3 fatty acids, which appear to improve brain functioning in periods of depression, have been used for the treatment of bipolar disorder as well. St. John's wort and SAMe, both used for major depression, may be beneficial, but these should be used with caution as they can trigger mania (21). Therapies such as acupuncture, yoga, and massage therapy have been used with varying success. It is important to note, however, that these are not a replacement for medication and psychotherapy.

Several milder subtypes of bipolar disorder exist. These include such entities as SAD in which patients experience depression with the onset of autumn or winter and mania or hypomania in spring or summer. Rarely, patients may reverse this trend and experience their depression in the warmer months. Rapid cycling bipolar disorder is a subset in which the patient experiences four or more cycles within the span of 1 year; some patients may cycle so rapidly that they swing from one extreme to the other within hours. With any type of bipolar disorder, psychosis may occur. This detachment from reality may occur within either a manic or depressed state, and may include either delusions or hallucinations. A psychotic break may be the first sign of bipolar disorder in many cases.

As noted with major depressive disorder, the combination of symptoms seen in depression frequently leads to poor communication with health care professionals and the underreporting of ocular symptoms. The hopeless patient may have a strong feeling of "why bother" while the worried and anxious patient might withhold information or avoid contact. This pattern is seen in bipolar depression as well, but can be interspersed with periods of manic grandiosity and even psychosis. Frequently, manic patients are highly unfocused with poor attention to practical matters. They may be very hard to interview or examine without careful redirection to the task. Awareness of bipolar syndromes and their effect on the patient is essential to obtain the best outcomes. As with major depression, the bipolar patient will likely be on one or more medications with a possibility of side effects disrupting ocular functioning.

SCHIZOPHRENIA

Schizophrenia is a complex group of mental disorders characterized by a patient's abnormal interpretation of reality. Patients have difficulty thinking logically and demonstrate abnormal social behavior and emotional responses. They show a combination of hallucinations, delusions, and disordered thinking. Schizophrenia should not be confused with multiple personality disorder or "split personality," which is a distinct clinical entity (21).

Schizophrenia occurs in approximately 1% of the population worldwide and shows no particular race or sex predilection. It does, however, tend to appear later in women and have a milder presentation than it does in men (22). Childhood-onset schizophrenia, which begins after age 5, is rare and is often confused with autism (23). The cause of schizophrenia is unclear, but research indicates a possible genetic component (23–25). Dopamine and glutamate imbalance may play a role; brain structure and central nervous system differences have been shown with neuroimaging (22). Other risk factors include a family history of schizophrenia; first or second trimester intrauterine exposure to viruses, toxins, or malnutrition; stressful life circumstances; older paternal age; and taking psychoactive drugs during adolescence or young adulthood (22,23).

Signs and symptoms of schizophrenia develop slowly, over months or even years. In men, onset is typically in the teens or 20s; in women it may be as much as 10 years later (22). Symptoms of schizophrenia are categorized into groups: positive or negative, cognitive or affective. Positive symptoms include delusions (the most common), hallucinations (usually hearing voices), disordered thoughts, and disorganized behavior (26). Negative symptoms involve the diminishment or absence of normal functioning. Examples include loss of interest, lack of emotion, reduced planning ability, poor personal hygiene, social withdrawal, and loss of motivation. Those symptoms considered cognitive involve thought processes, such as the ability to make sense of information, attention, and memory. The affective symptoms involve the patient's mood; the patient may show odd or inappropriate behavior or may experience mood swings (27).

There are several types of schizophrenia, and symptoms vary between these. Patients with paranoid schizophrenia are typically anxious, angry, or argumentative. They may falsely believe that others are trying to harm them or a loved one. These individuals tend to have less functional impairment than patients in some of the other categories and have the best prognosis for long-term improvement (22). Patients with the disorganized type of schizophrenia have problems thinking and expressing ideas and may show childlike behavior and minimal emotion. These individuals, unfortunately, carry the worst prognosis for improvement and are generally the most impaired (22). Catatonic schizophrenic patients are either in a constant state of unrest or they may not move at all. They may be rigid, grimace, and have odd facial expressions, or be minimally responsive. Finally, undifferentiated schizophrenia is characterized by a mixture of the above symptoms. This is the largest of the subtypes. For any of the subtypes, once patients are stabilized and no longer in a full-blown crisis, they could be diagnosed with residual schizophrenia, where they demonstrate only some symptoms that are often milder than those noted during the crisis.

Schizophrenic patients with relatively mild illness, or who are in remission, can appear "normal" without the hallmarks of the disease. They may not show delusions, hallucinations, or overt thought disorder. However, they often continue to have ongoing issues with poor thought cohesion, lack of motivation, apathy, or social avoidance.

Definitive diagnosis of schizophrenia is the purview of psychiatry and requires certain criteria. Patients must show at least two of the following: disordered thoughts, speech, or behavior; delusions; hallucinations; or catatonic behavior. They must show negative symptoms for a significant time over the course of 1 month. The diagnosis is generally made based on a thorough interview and observation over time, but laboratory tests, EEG, or brain scan such as computerized tomography (CT) scanning can be used as well to rule out other diagnoses.

Treatment usually involves one or more medications. Antipsychotics are generally the most effective but cause significant side effects, such as sedation, dizziness, weight gain, and an increased chance of diabetes and high cholesterol (28). Less frequently seen side effects include restlessness, gait or movement problems, difficulty with muscle contractions or spasms, and tremors. A serious long-term risk of antipsychotic use is the development of tardive dyskinesia, a neurologic disorder in which the patient makes involuntary, repetitive, purposeless movements. The drug clozapine can be added to the treatment regimen if the patient is unresponsive to antipsychotics, which may have greater effectiveness but also generally causes an increase of unwanted side effects (23). Injections of antipsychotic medications are also possible for individuals who cannot tolerate oral dosing. The use of support groups and psychotherapy, especially psychoeducation involving the patient's family, is also important. Treatment for adolescents is similar to that for adults, although at present, only two antipsychotics are approved for use in patients between 13 and 17 years old (risperidone [Risperdal] and aripiprazole [Abilify]).

As noted with the previously discussed disorders in schizophrenia, the combination of symptoms frequently leads to poor communication with health care professionals and the underreporting of ocular symptoms. The paranoid patient may have a belief that the caregiver is "against" the patient and withhold information or avoid contact. As with the depressed patient, schizophrenic patients can present as flat or avoidant, unmotivated, and noncompliant. Schizophrenic patients can be highly distracted with poor attention to practical matters. They can also have a difficult time processing basic instructions about eye care follow-up.

The patient with schizophrenia can also be very difficult to interview or examine without careful redirection to the task. A patient with bizarre behavior or appearance and psychotic thought can be frightening for the health care professional. For the most part, psychotic thought and behaviors are not dangerous, and an accepting/nonjudgmental approach is best. Many patients with schizophrenia can focus on a task (such as an eye examination), even when they are psychotic, if given thoughtful redirection. In rare but significant cases, however, psychotic patients can be threatening and even aggressive. If the health care professional feels threatened, it is essential to increase the distance you are from the patient and seek assistance from other staff. If the health care provider is aware of a history of psychosis with aggression, it is best to see the patient in a clinic with support staff available. Best outcomes are achieved when the health care professional is aware of the various schizophrenic syndromes and their effects on the patient and themselves.

ANXIETY/PANIC DISORDER

Anxiety and panic disorders are most easily discussed when separated into subcategories and addressed individually. Among the most common of the subtypes include generalized anxiety disorder (GAD), panic disorder, obsessive–compulsive disorder (OCD), and posttraumatic stress disorder (PTSD).

Generalized Anxiety Disorder Generalized anxiety disorder affects approximately 6.8 million American adults, with women affected twice as often as men (29). The onset of symptoms is generally gradual and can occur at any age, although the most common period of onset is between childhood and middle age. It is less common to have GAD onset occur in either young children or the elderly. GAD is often accompanied by other anxiety disorders, depression, or substance abuse. Risk factors for GAD include female sex, childhood adversity, stress, illness, genetic influence, and substance abuse (30). Certain personality types are at higher risk for GAD as well.

Patients with GAD experience excessive, irrational dread of everyday situations. They may have a sense of impending doom or death, anticipate disaster, or be overly concerned about health, finances, or family or work issues. Physical symptoms are frequently seen. Among these symptoms are hyperventilation, sweating, shortness of breath, and dizziness, as well as nausea, headaches, chest pain, and rapid heart rate. Abdominal cramping, faintness, difficulty swallowing, and tightness in the throat are also noted. In addition, individuals may experience fatigue, muscle aches or tension, irritability, and a frequent need to use the bathroom. They can have difficulty either falling asleep or staying asleep, often can't relax, and startle easily (30–32). Symptoms generally begin suddenly and without warning. They usually peak in about 10 minutes and last for approximately half an hour, but may persist for longer periods. In children, symptoms may tend more toward excessive worry—about school or sports performance, about punctuality, or about perfection with tasks. They also exhibit a severe lack of confidence and seem to be always striving for approval and need constant reassurance about their performance (32).

The diagnosis of GAD is made when patients experience excessive worry about a variety of issues for at least 6 months (32). The individual must show difficulty controlling their worry and that worry must have a significant effect on their daily life. Some evidence suggests that chemical differences in the brain are at least partially responsible for the symptoms associated with GAD (33). Treatment, as with the previously discussed conditions, generally involves both medication and some form of psychotherapy. Antidepressants, benzodiazepines, and buspirone (BusPar), as well as alternative remedies such as kava, valerian, and vitamin B/folic acid supplements are utilized.

Panic Disorder In contrast to GAD, panic disorder involves more frank attacks of terror and intense fears that develop for no apparent reason (34). It affects a similar number of adults as does GAD, and women are affected at nearly twice the rate of men (30). The tendency toward panic disorder may be partially inherited (31). Panic attacks often begin in late adolescence or early adulthood and may occur at any time, even during sleep. During an attack, the terror is often accompanied by a pounding heart, sweatiness, weakness, faintness, or dizziness. Patients flush or feel chilled, and they often have nausea, chest pain, or a sense of feeling smothered. Symptoms generally begin suddenly and without warning. They usually peak in about 10 minutes and last for approximately half an hour, but may persist for longer periods. Many individuals often feel exhausted following an attack (35). Risk factors may include significant stress, the death or illness of a loved one, childhood abuse, or other traumatic event. The patient may develop specific phobias or begin to avoid social situations and experience an increase in thoughts of suicide (1). Approximately one-third of individuals end up housebound due to agoraphobia, which occurs when the patient is intensely afraid of being outdoors since they do not feel safe anywhere but at home (30).

An official diagnosis of panic disorder requires four or more attacks and there must be a history of a month or more of intense fear of having another attack. The patient displays a significant change in their behaviors that are directed at preventing another attack. The attacks cannot be attributable to another cause, such as social phobia (36). As with GAD, treatment includes both medication and psychotherapy. Specific medication classes include SSRIs, SNRIs, tricyclic antidepressants, benzodiazepines, and MAOIs. Cognitive–behavioral therapy and alternative therapies such as yoga, massage, aerobic exercise, and meditation are all used to varying degrees and with varying success on a patient-by-patient basis.

Obsessive–compulsive Disorder A third category of anxiety disorder is OCD. In this disorder, unreasonable thoughts and fears (obsessions) give rise to repetitive behaviors (compulsions). Both obsessions and their accompanying compulsions tend to revolve around themes. Some common obsessive themes include the fear of contamination or dirt; the need to have items arranged in an orderly or symmetrical fashion; the inability to throw things away; or the excessive worry concerning possible intruders. Accompanying compulsive themes can include washing and cleaning, extreme orderliness, hoarding, counting and checking, or repeating the same activity over and over (i.e., locking the door). The disorder may have a genetic influence and be affected by serotonin levels (36). Approximately 2.2 million American adults have OCD (30), with men and women equally affected (30,37). The disease course is varied and symptoms may come and go. Approximately one-third of patients develop symptoms as children (30).

Specific diagnostic criteria exist for the diagnosis of OCD. In general, individuals must experience either obsessions or compulsions, they should realize that these are excessive or unreasonable, and these behaviors have to significantly interfere with the patient's daily routine (37). Obsessions are persistent, intrusive thoughts that cause distress, not simply excessive worries that the patient knows are a product of their own mind. Compulsions must be behaviors that the patient feels compelled to perform which are meant to prevent or reduce distress about their obsessions (37). Patients may not realize that their symptomatic thoughts and behaviors are excessive or unreasonable; however, treatment outcomes are usually much better if the patient recognizes that the symptoms are problematic and seeks help. Treatments include medications and various types of psychotherapy, including CBT in the form of exposure and response prevention. Psychiatric hospitalization or residential treatment is also used as needed.

Posttraumatic Stress Disorder Posttraumatic stress disorder has become much more widely discussed in the media of late, primarily due to the large number of soldiers returning from war zones such as Iraq and Afghanistan. Posttraumatic stress disorder is a serious mental health disorder triggered by a terrifying event in which the patient has been directly involved or to which they have been a witness. There could have been actual physical harm, or there may have been only the threat of physical harm, to either the patient or to a loved one. Posttraumatic stress disorder can occur after a mugging, rape, torture, kidnapping, child abuse, car accidents, plane crashes, bombings, or natural disasters, or any event that is perceived as highly threatening (30,38). It can occur in patients of all ages, but currently affects approximately 7.7 million adult Americans. Women experience PTSD more often than men, and the condition is often accompanied by depression, substance abuse, or other anxiety disorders (30). The clinical course varies, with some patients recovering in 6 months and others becoming chronic. Complications of PTSD include substance abuse, depression, eating disorders, and suicidal thoughts or actions. Individuals also have an increased risk of certain physical diagnoses, such as cardiovascular disease, autoimmune disease, chronic pain, and/or musculoskeletal disorders (39).

Patients with PTSD startle easily and become emotionally numb and can lose interest in things they once enjoyed. They often display irritability, aggressiveness, or violence, or become withdrawn and experience loss of affection toward their loved ones (39). Patients often have flashbacks, which can be triggered by sights, sounds, smells, or feelings. The patient may begin to avoid situations that remind them of the event. Anniversaries of the triggering event are often particularly difficult. Symptoms generally begin within 3 months of the event and can persist for years afterward (39). Those affected must have experienced these symptoms for at least 1 month for a definitive diagnosis to be made. As with other anxiety disorders, medications and psychotherapy are commonly recommended treatments. Antipsychotics, antidepressants, and antianxiety medications are the most frequently used. Prazosin, a medication used in the treatment of hypertension and which blocks the brain's response to the neurotransmitter norepinephrine, has been utilized with some success for patients with insomnia and/or recurrent nightmares. Finally, a specialized form of therapy called eye movement desensitization and reprocessing has been applied to alleviate some symptoms of PTSD (39).

The individual with PTSD can be highly avoidant of any situation that increases stress, including entering the examination room. In a general way, just going to see a health care professional could be experienced as highly stressful, or the patient could have specific triggers for the severe symptoms seen in panic attacks or PTSD. For instance, a panic attack could be triggered by a feeling of being "closed in" by the health professional that is starting an examination. Or, for a patient with a history of childhood sexual abuse who suffers from PTSD, being in a darkened room and having eye examination equipment placed "over" their face could trigger a flashback to their childhood abuse.

The health care professional can greatly reduce anxiety by first being aware that their patients may be suffering from extreme anxiety, and then by enacting general and specific measures to reduce the anxiety as much as possible. The examination room should be as calming as is possible. The patient should be greeted and asked how they are doing. The examination process should be reviewed and the patient asked if they are ready to proceed with the examination. If the health care provider is watchful, signs of anxiety can be recognized early and gently acknowledged by asking the patient how they are doing and if they can proceed. If caregivers do not realize that their patients suffer from anxiety disorders, they will often obtain inadequate information or experience the relationship with the patient in a negative manner.

DUAL DIAGNOSIS: PSYCHIATRIC ILLNESS AND SUBSTANCE ABUSE

A patient who has simultaneous diagnoses of both a mental illness and a substance use disorder (SUD) is known as having a dual diagnosis (DD), also called co-occurrence or comorbidity. The mental illnesses involved vary and include such diagnoses as major depression, schizophrenia, and various anxiety disorders. A strong association has been shown between SUD and mental illness (39,40). Patients with mental illness are twice as likely to have a problem with drugs or alcohol, and vice versa. Either disorder can present first, and can be causative for the other (41–44). It is often difficult to determine which disorder came first, since symptoms are often subclinical for many mental illnesses.

There are approximately 2.7 million adults in the United States with co-occurring MDE and alcohol use disorder (45,46). In addition, there has been a significant amount of research conducted on the prevalence of DD in specific populations. Young adults between the ages of 18 and 25 have been shown to be at increased risk for initiating drug or alcohol use if they have had an episode of major depression within the past year (47). Veterans in the same age range are more likely to have serious psychological distress than older veterans (48). In adolescents there is an association between inhalant use and depression. If there has been an episode of major depression within the past year, the individual is up to three times more likely to initiate inhalant use (49,50).

Signs and symptoms of the mental disorders encountered in DD have been described in previous sections. Substance abuse disorders have their own symptoms, including a high tolerance for drugs and alcohol, withdrawal, the use of the substances in dangerous situations, a higher rate of arrest or incarceration, and significant interference with their abilities at work, school, or home (51). Patients often use alcohol or drugs, including cigarettes, as a form of self-medication. Cigarette smoking, for example, has been shown to cause a temporary decrease in symptoms and improved cognition in patients with schizophrenia (42–44). Research has also noted that approximately 40% of cigarettes smoked in the United States are smoked by patients with a psychiatric disorder. This increases both their morbidity and mortality rates (44). Individuals who have a DD encounter more adverse behaviors and consequences than patients with a single diagnosis. Among these are a higher tendency to be violent (52), a greater likelihood to be arrested or jailed (53), decreased compliance with medications, higher failure rates with treatment, and a higher risk of relapse. Those with DD tend to be in poorer overall health with higher rates of psychosis or side effects such as tardive dyskinesia. They are also at higher risk for the social phenomenon of "downward drift." They often find themselves living in more dangerous neighborhoods if they lose a source of income and any social support network they may have had. Those with DD often associate more with other drug or alcohol abusers, which reinforces their own difficulty with or dependence on the substance. Finally, they are at greater risk for becoming homeless, especially if there is limited or no family interaction and support (54). Dual diagnosis patients are also at increased risk for suicidal thoughts or suicide attempts (55,56).

Treatment for those with DD is more difficult than that for either the substance use disorder or psychiatric illness alone. The treatment plan must address both aspects of the DD for best prognosis and the least chance for relapse. Generally, treatment follows a stepwise progression that includes detoxification with rehabilitation of the SUD and treatment for the mental illness following. Patients who can overcome their substance abuse are more likely to have successful treatment for their mental illness. Treatment may often include specialized group therapy, since patients with mental illness may not fit well into established programs such as Alcoholics Anonymous or Narcotics Anonymous (55). It is important to note that denial is common among patients with SUD or DD, so treatment plans should be geared toward building trust between the individual and the doctor, developing adequate support systems, and realizing that recovery is a long-term process.

Comorbidity of Mental Illness with Intellectual and Developmental Disability

There is another form of DD that includes not only the presence of a PI but also varying levels of intellectual and developmental disability (IDD). Intellectual and developmental disability is diagnosed in a patient if intellectual disability (formerly known as mental retardation) is recognized through testing before the age of 18. Intellectual disability is usually divided into mild, moderate, severe, and profound based upon IQ scores. Other forms of developmental disabilities include the autism spectrum disorders such as autism or Asperger syndrome. These are primarily diagnosed by observed deficits in social communication capabilities but can often include mild to profound intellectual deficits.

Most clinicians and researchers believe that patients with IDD have at least the same but most likely higher rates of PI. This could be based on a combination of biologic, psychological, and social factors. Patients with intellectual deficits frequently have genetic abnormalities or have suffered injury to the brain (such as lack of oxygen at birth, head trauma, or severe fever). These cerebral injuries could very well have a biologic effect on the neurotransmitter systems thought to be related to mental illness.

Psychologically, individuals growing up with IDD can have trouble "fitting in," have difficulty maintaining self-esteem, and feel that they cannot "be themselves." On a social level, persons with IDD suffer unusually high rates of abuse and neglect. This abuse ranges from the teasing that many IDD patients endure in classroom situations to high levels of physical and sexual abuse.

The prevalence of mental illness among adults with intellectual disability varies between 10% and 39%. One study noted that the rate of PI among those with developmental disability was similar to that found in the general population (16%). Schizophrenic and phobic disorders, however, were seen in significantly higher numbers than those reported for the general population (0.04% and 1.1%, respectively). As with many disorders, various comorbidities have an additive effect. For instance, it has been reported that the added combination of advanced age and physical disability significantly increase chances of having a PI (57). White et al. (58) evaluated the prevalence of intellectual disability and mental illness in an Australian community sample and found that of those with an intellectual disability 1.3% were psychotic, 8% demonstrated depression, and 14% had an anxiety disorder.

Fletcher (59), a member of the National Association of the Dually Diagnosed (60), wrote in an article published in the *Journal of Intellectual Disability Research* that the estimated prevalence of intellectual disability comorbid with a PI is anywhere from 20% to 60%. He also noted that these individuals are being deinstitutionalized, but without adequate community support. Several programs in the past have been developed to serve the needs of the dually diagnosed including the Illinois-Chicago Mental Health Program based at the University of Illinois Chicago and the Ulster County Comprehensive Community Care System located in Ulster county, New York. More recently, Neumann Family Services (61) in Chicago, IL has developed multiple programs serving the dually diagnosed including bringing health care professionals to the facility to serve clients when they are on campus. These services include routine physicals, primary care medical services, dental examinations, and podiatry services, as well as comprehensive eye and vision examinations, nursing services, psychiatric services, and referrals to various specialists when needed.

The National Down Syndrome Society (NDSS) (62) reports that at least half of those with Down syndrome (DS) will experience a mental health issue. National Down Syndrome Society's web site states that the various psychiatric problems for younger children with DS include but are not limited to

- *Disruptive, impulsive, inattentive, hyperactive, and oppositional behaviors*
- *Anxious, ruminative, inflexible behaviors*
- *Deficits in social relatedness, self-immersed, repetitive stereotypical behaviors*
- *Chronic sleep difficulties, daytime sleepiness, fatigue, and mood-related problems*

Older school-aged DS children and adolescents often experience

- *Depression, social withdrawal, diminished interests, and coping skills*
- *Generalized anxiety*
- *Obsessive–compulsive behaviors*
- *Regression with decline in loss of cognitive and social skills*
- *Chronic sleep difficulties, daytime sleepiness, fatigue, and mood-related problems*

And finally, adults with DS exhibit

- *Generalized anxiety*
- *Depression, social withdrawal, loss of interest, and diminished self-care*
- *Regression with decline in cognitive and social skills*
- *Dementia*

Unlike the NDSS webpage that has a fair amount of information regarding mental health and DS, the United Cerebral Palsy webpage (63) hardly mentions any comorbid mental health conditions at all. The National Fragile X Foundation (64), on the other hand, notes that children with Fragile X often have problems with anxiety and that girls and women with fragile X tend to be shy, socially anxious, and often demonstrate schizotypal behaviors and depression. Bacalman et al. (65), in a paper that evaluated the psychiatric phenotype of males with fragile

X–associated tremor/ataxia syndrome, reported that various mental health problems such as delusions, hallucinations, agitation/aggression, and depression, as well as anxiety, apathy, disinhibition, and irritability were present. Unfortunately, many of those with an intellectual disability are often either misdiagnosed when it comes to a PI or not diagnosed at all.

MEDICAL CONDITIONS, MENTAL ILLNESS, AND VISION PROBLEMS

Individuals with PIs often do not have access to routine medical care. The result is undiagnosed and untreated medical conditions that can also affect the individual's eye health and vision. Those with schizophrenia and bipolar disorders frequently experience a higher incidence of cardiovascular disease, diabetes, various pulmonary problems, stroke, and hypertension. Many of these medical conditions can cause serious visual impairment if not treated in a timely fashion (66).

Oculovisual Problems and Psychiatric Illness Although there have been few studies that have evaluated the oculovisual problems of those with a PI, there seems to be support for a trend toward various eye and vision anomalies being associated with specific forms of mental illness. Depending upon the anomaly being studied, visual acuity, refractive error, and oculomotor issues are areas of concern for this population.

Donati et al. (67) reported that even though those with mental illness and the dually diagnosed were taking up to 10 or more major psychotropic and neuroleptic drugs (many of which have unwanted ocular side effects), almost 50% had no visual complaints. This may mean that when the optometrist reviews the patient's case history, that they should look upon the lack of symptoms and complaints with suspicion.

They also found that the most frequent ocular anomalies encountered were astigmatism (50% PI and 37.84% DD), myopia (60.71% PI and 62.16% DD), presbyopia (35.71% PI and 37.84% DD), and blepharitis (32.14% PI and 32.43% DD). When these individuals did complain, those complaints most frequently noted were blurry vision (17.74% PI and 17.72% DD) and the need for new glasses (11.29% PI and 17.72% DD).

In an article by Maino et al. (68), it was noted that individuals with a PI exhibited uncorrected refractive error, strabismus, and blepharitis, as well as pigmentary retinopathy and cataracts. Those with intellectual disability and mental illness (DD) showed similar findings, with the exception of cataracts. A statistically significant amount of astigmatism was seen in those with a PI.

Depression Although few studies have evaluated the presence of vision problems that are associated with depression, at least one study reports that those with depression appear to have problems with saccadic accuracy (69). However, we do know that individuals with various vision disorders are frequently depressed. For instance, Mathew et al. (70) reported that having age-related macular degeneration led to depressive symptoms both directly and indirectly because of reduced general health and social functioning, while a second study has shown that dry eye syndrome is associated with the development of depression as well (71). In general, any patient who is medically ill has a tendency toward developing signs and symptoms of depression (72).

Schizophrenia Those with schizophrenia often have reduced visual acuity and problems with visual perception and visual memory. It has been noted that impaired visual acuity increases the risk of injuries and falls and can also lead to an increase in social isolation by schizophrenics who already demonstrate problems in this area. It has been recommended by at least one study that those with mental illness be examined every year if 40 years of age or older and every 2 years for those <40. They also stated that any using antipsychotic drugs should be evaluated for vision problems on a routine basis as well (73). Those with schizophrenia exhibit many oculomotor dysfunctions including fewer fixations, longer fixation duration, longer saccade duration and peak velocity, and smaller saccade amplitude compared with healthy controls (74) and also have deficits in smooth pursuit eye movements (75) and visual tracking (76).

CONCLUSION

Those with a PI have at least the same, if not an increased need for eye and vision care. Although current research suggests various areas of oculovisual function and eye health that may be severely affected by and be comorbid with PI, a great deal of additional research in this area is needed. Those with dual diagnosis (mental illness and IDD) not only have all the visual problems associated with a developmental disability, but any that may also be associated with a mental illness. Eye care professionals will need to use adaptive examination techniques, as documented in this book in Chapter 16, Comprehensive Examination Procedures, and be aware of all of the potential ocular side effects of the many major psychotropic drugs these individuals are prescribed to provide the best possible care.

REFERENCES

1. National Institute of Health. Statistics. Available from: www.nimh.nih.gov/statistics/index.shtml. Last Accessed June 20, 2011.
2. Merikangas KR, Ames M, Cui L, Stang PE, et al. The impact of comorbidity of mental and physical conditions on role disability in the US adult household population. Arch Gen Psychiatry. 2007;64:1180–8.
3. Kessler RC, Berglund P, Demler O, Jin R, et al. Lifetime prevalence and age-of-onset distributions of DSM-IV disorders in the National Comorbidity Survey replication. Arch Gen Psychiatry. 2005;62:593–602.
4. Garber J, Horowitz JL. Depression in children. In: Gotlib IH, Hammen CL, editors. Handbook of depression. New York: Guilford Press; 2002.
5. Staley JK, Sanacora G, Tamagnan G, Maciejewski PK, et al. Sex differences in diencephalon serotonin transporter availability in major depression. Biol Psychiatry. 2006;59:40–7.
6. Feldman RS, editor. Psychological disorders. In: Essentials of understanding psychology. 8th ed. New York: McGraw-Hill; 2009.
7. Mayo Clinic. Depression. . Available from: www.mayoclinic.com/health/depression/DS00175. Last Accessed July 11, 2011.
8. Kendler KS, Gatz M, Gardner CO, Pedersen NL. A Swedish national twin study of lifetime major depression. Am J Psychiatry. 2006;163:109–14.
9. Kendler KS, Kessler RC, Walters EE, MacLean C, et al. Stressful life events, genetic liability, and onset of an episode of major depression in women. Am J Psychiatry. 1995; 152:833–42.
10. Kendler KS, Karkowski LM, Prescott CA. Causal relationship between stressful life events and the onset of major depression. Am J Psychiatry. 1999;156:837–41.
11. Seroczynski AD, Jacquez FM, Cole DA. Depression and suicide during adolescence. In: Adams GR, Berzonsky MD, editors. Blackwell handbook of adolescence. Malden: Blackwell Publishers; 2003.
12. Wenar C. Developmental psychopathology: from infancy through adolescence. 3rd ed. New York: McGraw-Hill; 1994.
13. PubMed Health, National Institutes of Health. Depression. Available from: www.ncbi.nlm.nih.gov/pubmedhealth/PMH0001941/. Last Accessed July 11, 2011.
14. Medline Plus, National Institutes of Health. Depression. Available from: www.nlm.nih.gov/medlineplus/ency/article/000945.htm. Last Accessed July 11, 2011.
15. Mayo Clinic. Depression. Available from: www.mayoclinic.com/health/depression/DS00175. Last Accessed July 11, 2011.
16. Corrigan PW, River LP, Lundin RK, Penn DL, et al. Three strategies for changing attributions about severe mental illness. Schizophrenia Bull. 2001;27:187–95.
17. Kelly J. Epidemiology. Bipolar web page. Appalachian State University. Available from: www1.appstate.edu/~hillrw/BipolarWebPage/Epidemiology.html. Last Accessed June 11, 2011.
18. Kelly J. Bipolar index. Bipolar web page. Appalachian State University. Available from: www1.appstate.edu/~hillrw/BipolarWebPage/BipolarIndex.html. Last Accessed June 11, 2011.
19. Craddock N, Jones I. Molecular genetics of bipolar disorder. Brit J Psych. 2001;178:s128–33.
20. PubMed Health, National Institutes of Health disorder. Available from: www.ncbi.nlm.nih.gov/pubmedhealth/PMH0001924/. Last Accessed June 11, 2011.
21. Mayo Clinic. Bipolar disorder. Accessed May-June 2011. Available from: www.mayoclinic.com/health/bipolar-disorder/DS00356. Last Accessed June 11, 2011.
22. PubMed Health, National Institutes of Health. Schizophrenia. Available from: www.ncbi.nlm.nih.gov/pubmedhealth/PMH0001925/. Last Accessed June 11, 2011.
23. Sullivan PF, Kendler KS, Neale MC, et al. Schizophrenia as a complex trait: evidence from a meta-analysis of twin studies. Arch Gen Psychiatry. 2003;60:1187–92.
24. Kato T. Molecular genetics of bipolar disorder and depression. Psychiatry Clin Neurosci. 2007;61:3–19.
25. Ben-Shachar S, Lanpher B, German JR, Qasaymeh M, et al. Microdeletion 15q13.3: a locus with incomplete penetrance for autism, mental retardation, and psychiatric disorders. J Med Genet. 2009;46:382–8.
26. Coltheart M, Langdon R, McKay R. Schizophrenia and monothematic delusions. Schizophrenia Bull. 2007;33:642–7.
27. Buchanan RW, Javitt DC, Marder SR, Schooler NR, et al. The Cognitive and Negative Symptoms in Schizophrenia Trial (CONSIST): the efficacy of glutamatergic agents for negative symptoms and cognitive impairments. Am J Psychiatry. 2007;164:1593–602.
28. Remington G. Understanding antipsychotic 'atypicality:' a clinical and pharmacological moving target. J Psychiatry Neurosci. 2003;28:275–84.
29. National Institutes of Health. Anxiety disorders. Available from: www.nimh.nih.gov/health/publications/anxiety-disorders/complete-index.shtml. Last Accessed June 11, 2011.
30. Hettema JM, Neale MC, Kendler KS. A review and meta-analysis of the genetic epidemiology of anxiety disorders. Am J Psychiatry. 2001;158:1568–78.
31. Mayo Clinic. Generalized anxiety disorder. Available from: http://www.mayoclinic.com/health/generalized-anxiety-disorder/DS00502. Last Accessed June 11, 2011.
32. Starcevic V, et al. Pathological worry, anxiety disorders and the impact of co-occurrence with depressive and other anxiety disorders. J Anxiety Dis. 2007;21:1016–27.

33. Holmes A, et al. Mice lacking the serotonin transporter exhibit 5-HT-sub(1A) receptor-mediated abnormalities in tests for anxiety-like behavior. Neuropsychopharmacology. 2003;28:2077–88.
34. Rachman S, deSilva P. Panic disorders: the facts. Oxford: Oxford University Press; 2004.
35. Mayo Clinic. Panic attacks. Available from: www.mayoclinic.com/health/panic-attacks/DS00338. Last Accessed June 11, 2011.
36. Mayo Clinic. Obsessive-compulsive disorder. Available from: www.mayoclinic.com/health/obsessive-compulsive-disorder/DS00189. Last Accessed June 11, 2011.
37. Welkowitz LA, et al. Obsessive-compulsive disorder and comorbid anxiety problems in a national anxiety screening sample. J Anxiety Dis. 2000;14:471–82.
38. Mayo Clinic. Post-traumatic stress disorder. Available from: www.mayoclinic.com/health/post-traumatic-stress-disorder/DS00246. Last Accessed June 11, 2011.
39. Jane-Llopis E, Matytsina I. Mental health and alcohol, drugs and tobacco: a review of the comorbidity between mental disorders and the use of alcohol, tobacco and illicit drugs. Drug Alcohol Rev. 2006;25:515–36.
40. Regier DA, Farmer ME, Rae DS, Locke BZ, et al. Comorbidity of mental disorders with alcohol and other drug abuse. Results from the Epidemiologic Catchment Area (ECA) Study. JAMA. 1990;264:2511–8.
41. Medline Plus, National Institutes of Health. Dual diagnosis. Available from: www.nlm.nih.gov/medlineplus/dualdiagnosis.html. Last Accessed June 11, 2011.
42. DBS Alliance. Dual diagnosis. Available from: www.dbsalliance.org/pdfs/dualdiag.pdf. Last Accessed June 11, 2011.
43. Research Report Series—comorbidity: addiction and other mental illnesses. Available from: www.drugabuse.gov/researchreports/comorbidity/index.html. Last Accessed June 11, 2011.
44. Sinha R, Rounsaville BJ. Sex differences in depressed substance abusers. J Clin Psychiatry. 2002;63:616–27.
45. Hasin DS, Nunes E. Comorbidity of alcohol, drug and psychiatric disorders: epidemiology. In: Kranzler HR, Rounsaville B, editors. Dual diagnosis and treatment: substance abuse and comorbid mental and psychiatric disorders. New York: Marcel Dekker Inc.; 1997.
46. Substance Abuse and Mental Health Services Administration, Office of Applied Studies. The NSDUH Report: co-occurring major depressive episode (MDE) and alcohol use disorder among adults. Rockville, MD, February 16, 2007.
47. Substance Abuse and Mental Health Services Administration, Office of Applied Studies. The NSDUH Report: depression and the initiation of cigarette, alcohol, and other drug use among young adults. Rockville, MD, November 15, 2007.
48. Kubik MY, Lytle LA, Birnbaum AS, Murray DM, et al. Prevalence and correlates of depressive symptoms in young adolescents. Am J Health Behav. 2003;27:546–53.
49. Sakai JT, Hall SK, Mikulich-Gilbertson SK, Crowley TJ, et al. Inhalant use, abuse, and dependence among adolescent patients: commonly comorbid problems. J Am Acad Child Adolesc Psychol. 2004;43:1080–8.
50. Wu LT, Pilowsky D, Schlenger WE, Galvin DM. Misuse of methamphetamine and prescription stimulants among youths and young adults in the community. Drug Alcohol Depend. 2007;89:195–205.
51. Farooque R, Ernst F. Filicide: a review of eight years of clinical experience. J Natl Med Assoc. 2003;95:90–4.
52. Blake PY, Pincus JH, Buckner C. Neurologic abnormalities in murderers. Neurology. 1995;45:1641–7.
53. National Alliance on Mental Illness. Comorbidity. Available from: www.nami.org/Template.cfm?Section=By_Illness&Template=/TaggedPage/TaggedPageDisplay.cfm&TPLID=54&ContentID=23049. Last Accessed June 11, 2011.
54. Substance Abuse and Mental Health Services Administration, Office of Applied Studies. The OAS Report: suicidal thoughts, suicide attempts, major depressive episode, and substance use among adults. Rockville, MD, Issue 34, 2006.
55. Moscicki EK. Epidemiology of completed and attempted suicide: toward a framework for prevention. Clin Neurosci Res. 2001;1:310–23.
56. Deb S, Thoma M, Bright C. Mental disorder in adults with intellectual disability: prevalence of functional psychiatric illness among a community-based population aged between 16 and 64 years. J Intellect Disabil Res. 2001;45:495–505.
57. White P, Chant D, Edwards C, Waghorn G. Prevalence of intellectual disability and comorbid mental illness in an Australian community sample. Aust N Z J Psychiatry. 2005;39:395–400.
58. Fletcher RJ. Mental illness-mental retardation in the United States: policy and treatment challenges. J Intellect Disabil Res. 1993;37:25–33.
59. National Association of the Dually Diagnosed. Available from: www.thenadd.org/. Last Assessed July 11, 2011.
60. Neumann Family Services. Available from: www.neumannfamilyservices.org/. Last Accessed July 11, 2011.
61. National Down Syndrome Society. Mental health issues and Down syndrome. Available from: www.ndss.org/index.php?option=com_content&view=article&id=171%3Amental-health-issues&catid=60%3Aassociated-conditions&Itemid=88&showall=1. Last Accessed July 11, 2011.
62. United Cerebral Palsy. Available from: www.ucp.org/resources/health-and-wellness. Last Accessed July 11, 2011.
63. National Fragile X Foundation. Available from: www.nfxf.org/html/anxiety.html. Last Accessed July 11, 2011.
64. Bacalman S, Farzin F, Bourgeois JA, Cogswell J, et al. Psychiatric phenotype of the fragile X-associated tremor/ataxia syndrome (FXTAS) in males: newly described fronto-subcortical dementia. J Clin Psychiatry. 2006;67:87–94.
65. Kilbourne AM, McCarthy JF, Welsh D, Blow F. Recognition of co-occurring medical conditions among patients with serious mental illness. J Nerv Mental Dis. 2006;194;598–602.
66. Donati RJ, Maino DM, Bartell H, Kieffer M. Polypharmacy and the lack of oculo-visual complaints from those with mental illness and dual diagnosis. Optometry. 2009;80:249–54.
67. Maino DM, Rado ME, Pizzi WJ. Ocular anomalies of individuals with mental illness and dual diagnosis. J Am Optom Assoc. 1996;67:740–8.
68. Jergelova M, Jagla F. Central and peripheral correlates of eye movements in selected mood disorders. Neuro Endocrinol Lett. 2010;31:731–7.
69. Mathew RS, Delbaere K, Lord SR, Beaumont P, et al. Depressive symptoms and quality of life in people with age related macular degeneration. Ophthalmic Physiol Opt. 2011;31:375–80.

70. Li M, Gong L, Sun X, Chapin WJ. Anxiety and depression in patients with dry eye syndrome. Curr Eye Res. 2011;36:1–7.
71. Stewart DE. Physical symptoms of depression: unmet needs in special populations. J Clin Psychiatry. 2003;64:12–6.
72. Viertio S, Laitinen A, Perla J, Saarni S, et al. Visual impairment in persons with psychotic disorder. Soc Psychiatry Psychiatr Epidemiol. 2007;42:902–8.
73. Bestelmeyer PE, Tatler BW, Phillips LH, Fraser G, et al. Global visual scanning abnormalities in schizophrenia and bipolar disorder. Schizophr Res. 2006;87:212–22.
74. Kathmann N, Hochrein A, Uwer R, Bondy B. Deficits in gain of smooth pursuit eye movements in schizophrenia and affective disorder patients and their unaffected relatives. Am J Psychiatry. 2003;160:696–702.
75. Levy DL, Sereno AB, Gooding DC, O'Driscoll GA. Eye tracking dysfunction in schizophrenia: characterization and pathophysiology. Curr Top Behav Neurosci. 2010;4:311–47.

CHAPTER 13

Denise A. Valenti, OD, FAAO

The Visual System in Neurodegenerative Disease

INTRODUCTION

Even though the mechanisms of diseases that damage neuroprocessing are poorly understood, these conditions impact the visual system in very concrete ways. Though, there is limited knowledge of how the visual system is involved in the degenerative processes. This chapter discusses three diseases and how the pathology affects the visual system: Alzheimer disease (AD), Parkinson disease (PD), and Huntington disease (HD).

ALZHEIMER DISEASE

It is estimated that over 5.1 million Americans have AD (1–3). It is the most common form of dementia among the aged (3). Alzheimer disease is irreversible and progressive, and it affects memory processing in the early stages. There are some indications that visual integration processing, such as contrast and motion, is affected even before memory. The definitive diagnosis for AD is generally made at autopsy and is characterized by deposits of plaques containing amyloid structures and tau tangles in the brain (4,5). There are strategies to develop biomarkers utilizing positron emission tomography (PET) imaging of the brain and amyloid in cerebral spinal fluid (6). An additional finding is the loss of the connective nerve fibers between cells. The clinical diagnosis currently is made based on observation, history, and neuropsychological testing. Alzheimer disease–related pathology of the visual system, even in those not clinically diagnosed with AD, has been identified in elderly brain donors. In a study of 41 donors in the Framingham Heart Study, McKee et al. (7) found that 52% of those donors who had been considered cognitively intact had dense neurofibrillary tangles, neuropil threads, and tau-immunoreactive neurites surrounding neuritic plaques and amyloid beta angiopathy in the visual association area, Brodmann 19. All the donors that had been diagnosed with cognitive impairment showed such findings. The visual association area processes signals from the magnocellular visual pathway, which is sensitive to contrast and motion.

Even though there is a rare hereditary version affecting those younger than 60, the majority of people affected have late-onset AD. Genetic factors related to different types of apolipoprotein E (APOE) have been identified in late-onset AD. One of them, APOE4, increases a person's risk of getting the disease. While 40% of all people who develop late-onset AD have APOE4, having this form of the gene does not always result in the development of the disease. In addition to the APOE genes, there are now 15 additional genes identified as possibly contributing to the development of late-onset AD (8).

Methods of assessment that can be used when symptoms occur include a comprehensive medical history, cognitive screening, neuropsychological evaluation, and testing of blood, urine, and spinal fluids and imaging of brain structures and functions. Cholinesterase inhibitors (ChEI) such as Donepezil (Aricept), Rivastigmine (Exelon), and Galantamine (Razadyne) and a single neuroprotective drug, Memantine (Namenda), are used to treat symptoms, but do not slow the progression of the disease. These medications regulate neurotransmitters and may help with some of the presenting behavioral symptoms. These drugs do not alter the disease process and lose their effectiveness over time (9).

Alzheimer disease impacts visual function early in the course of the disease and correlates with cognitive loss. Visual function loss in AD has many aspects in common with the identified losses in other neurodegenerative processes affecting the eye, such as age-related macular degeneration (AMD), and glaucoma. Contrast sensitivity deficits in the lower spatial frequencies, motion perception deficiency, and visual field defects are found in patients with AD (10,11). Deficits specific to blue wavelengths have been reported (12); however, groups with protocols accounting for the presence or absence of an intact lens with cataracts did not find color deficits specific to any wavelengths (13). Glaucoma also affects lower spatial frequencies in contrast sensitivity, produces visual field defects (14), causes deficits in the blue (short) wavelength color range (15), and reduces motion perception (16). Age-related macular degeneration causes changes to all frequencies in contrast sensitivity (17), color deficits across all wavelengths (18), and foveal detection of motion (19).

Glaucoma When patients with AD also have glaucoma, the course of vision loss related to glaucoma has been described as being rapidly progressive and severe (20). Studies demonstrate a higher rate of glaucoma among AD patients compared to the normal population (21,22). If there are two neurodegenerative processes, such as glaucoma and AD, affecting one of the major relay centers for visual function, it is easy to appreciate that the loss in function can be substantial. Cholinesterase inhibitors have been found to lower intraocular pressure (IOP). This is a positive side effect of pharmaceutical interventions for AD and may be protective for glaucoma. Cholinesterase inhibitors have been approved for the treatment of AD and are generally the first-line approach. Estermann et al. (23) showed an 8.8% reduction of IOP in 63 eyes of those newly diagnosed with AD when placed on Donepezil, a selective form of ChEI. It was also shown to have a neuroprotective effect in retinal ganglion cells exposed to glutamate toxicity in rats, both in vivo and in vitro with an orally administered dose (24). Topical Rivastigmine, which is a selective carbamate-type ChEI, was demonstrated to have a dose-dependent lowering of IOP in rabbits. This selectivity inhibits the isoform of the enzyme that is almost exclusively found in the central nervous system. One topical administration of Rivastigmine lowered IOP 23% with a 5% concentration, 20% with a 2% concentration, and 15% with a 1% concentration. The effect was maintained upon measurement at 5 hours (25).

Both AD and glaucoma affect the same visual pathways but in different regions. Glaucoma causes loss in the magnocellular layers of the lateral geniculate nucleus (LGN) (26,27). There is shrinkage and change in the LGN neurons early on in the glaucoma disease process which can be observed even before nerve fiber loss in the optic nerve (28,29). Deficits specific to the magnocellular pathway have also been identified in individuals with AD even in brain areas devoid of plaques and neurofibrillary tangles. The magnocellular pathway shows signs of significant cell loss in the primary visual cortex of AD individuals (30). Amyloid plaques and neurofibrillary tangles have been identified in the cuneal and lingual gyri of participants with AD, which correlates with the incidence of functional visual field loss (10). Magnocellular layers in the LGN have been shown to have plaques associated with AD (31).

Age-related Macular Degeneration A report from the Age-Related Eye Disease Study group indicates that there is a relationship between the severity of AMD and cognitive dysfunction in older patients (32). Studies suggest that AD and AMD may have pathologic processes in common. The deposits in the brain with AD and deposits of drusen (the precursor of AMD) in the retina both contain amyloid beta (33–35). In comparing nine retinas from individuals with AMD versus a control group, it was found that four of nine AMD retinas but none of the control group retinas had amyloid beta proteins (31). None of the individuals in either group had a diagnosis of AD at death, and studies of brain tissue were not performed so that we cannot conclusively relate the two diseases. Immunotherapy treatment targeting amyloid beta has been shown to reduce the volume of drusen and improve visual function in a mouse model of AMD (36). There was an association of APOE polymorphism in both AMD and AD in a study involving 49 participants with AMD, 32 participants with AD, and 27 control participants in a study undertaken in Hungary (37). The study showed a higher rate of APOE2 among those with AMD and a higher rate of APOE4 in those with AD. There was an 8% rate of AMD found in those with AD. In the meta-analysis literature review, there was a differential effect of the APOE2 and APOE4 alleles where the APOE2 was associated with a 20% risk for AMD and APOE4 was associated with a protective rate of 40% (38). The relationship of APOE factors to glaucoma is less clear.

Anterior Segment Individuals with AD appear to have lens opacities that may be specific to AD. Goldstein et al. (39) identified amyloid beta proteins in the cytoplasm of lens fiber cells in four lenses of those with AD. Upon autopsy, supranuclear equatorial opacities were identified in nine of those with AD, but not in the eight eyes from control donors. Growth factor receptors are functional only in the equatorial peripheral cells of human lenses (40) making this area more vulnerable to cell proliferation that can induce opacities. Drugs that work on cholinergic receptors can cause miotic activity and protein transport into the lens, creating cataracts. The drug treatments for glaucoma using echothiophate iodide (Phospholine), Humorsol, and Florpyryl also caused lens miotic activity and protein transport into the lens creating cataracts (41,42). Donepezil has a similar mechanism of action and may be contributory to cataract development as well.

Multiple reports describe an exaggerated mydriatic response to dilute tropicamide in those with AD (43–48). This excessive reaction is related to the cholinergic system. Recent work using a prospective longitudinal design, which followed participants over a period of 2 to 4 years, found that an exaggerated pupil response to mydriatics predicted a threefold risk for developing significant cognitive impairment. When there was an associated APOE4 allele, the risk increased to four (49). Donepezil was shown to constrict the pupil with an average change from 3.9 to 3.6 mm (50). There are losses of neuronal structures in the Edinger-Westphal nucleus, which is one of the primary neural structures involved in pupillary response (51). The Edinger-Westphal nucleus shows signs of AD pathology in the form of tau-tangle deposits (52). The Edinger-Westphal nucleus controls ocular accommodation through the ciliary muscle. The ciliary muscle contraction is mediated by muscarinic receptors, and the ciliary muscle contraction is what facilitates outflow of aqueous and the subsequent lowering of IOP (53). The ChEI affects the ciliary muscle, lowering IOP.

Optic Nerve Fiber Imaging Parisi et al. (54) used the Stratus OCT to assess the optic nerve fiber layer thickness in 34 subjects (17 individuals with AD, 14 age-matched control individuals). A significant reduction in nerve fiber thickness in the AD individuals was reported. Iseri et al. (55) looked at macular volume and found that in 28 eyes of those with AD, there was significant thinning of the macula compared to 30 eyes tested from a control group. Further, they found thinning of the retinal nerve fiber layer in those with AD. The macular and the nerve fiber layer thinning showed correlations with the severity of dementia and cognitive function. Valenti (56) reported reductions in nerve fiber layers using the Stratus OCT. Berisha et al. (57) in a study comparing those with either glaucoma or AD and age-matched controls found reductions in the superior quadrant in the AD group and reduced disc ratios only in the glaucoma group. This study demonstrated that the reductions identified with Stratus OCT are unique to AD and are not undiagnosed ocular pathology such as glaucoma. A study undertaken by Paquet et al. (58) looked at 14 participants with mild AD, 12 participants with moderate AD, and 15 noncognitively impaired age-matched participants. They also included 23 participants with mild cognitive impairment, which is considered clinically to be the precursor to AD. The results showed the nerve fiber layer to be thinned in those with mild cognitive impairment, and both mild and moderate to severe AD. The study did not find any significant difference between those with mild AD and mild cognitive impairment.

Frequency-doublingTechnology Frequency-doubling technology (FDT) is hypothesized to isolate the magnocellular pathway. It uses low-spatial frequency sinusoidal gratings (<1 cycle/degree) that undergo a high-temporal frequency counterphase flicker at 25 Hz or greater. Preliminary reports indicate reductions in regions of the FDT that correlate with the superior nerve fiber layer deficits (59). The temporal flicker component of FDT has been shown to be reduced in those with AD. A study of ten subjects with AD compared to subjects with no dementia (60) found significant reductions in the response of the magnocellular pathway when measured using PET. The stimulus was a grid pattern with increasing temporal frequency. With lower temporal frequencies, there were minimal differences but as the frequencies approached 15 Hz, the reduction in neural response in those with AD became greater compared to age-matched controls. Using the critical flicker fusion test, there was a loss of detection in the descending component of the test in those with AD compared to both normal controls and subjects with vascular dementia (61).

Down Syndrome Down syndrome (DS) is caused by a complete or partial additional, extra chromosome 21 and is expressed in approximately 1/800 live births (62). Those born with DS are now surviving into adulthood and advanced age. In 1929, the life expectancy for a child with DS was 9 years and now it is 50 or greater (62) (see Chapter 4, Down Syndrome for further information) According to some reports, AD occurs in nearly 100% of those with DS over the age of 40 (63,64). Rates of AD-type symptoms in those with DS are reported to be zero under the age 30, 33% between 30 and 39, and 55% between ages of 40 and 52.

Adults with DS experience a dementia that resembles AD and it is not related to existing atherosclerotic complications (65). In a group of 225 adults with DS who at initial evaluation had not shown any signs of dementia or cognitive decline, it was found that blood plasma levels of AB42 and AB40 had changed upon reevaluation 14 to 20 months later. The adults also had cognitive and functional ability testing demonstrating decline in function. The study indicated that in DS, a decrease in levels of plasma AB42, a decline in the AB42/AB40 ratio, or an increase in levels of AB40 may be sensitive indicators of conversion to AD (66). In a study of 187 adults with DS, with and without a diagnosis of AD, 28 genes were evaluated. The most strongly associated gene was the APOE4 (67).

PARKINSON DISEASE

Parkinson disease is a group of neurodegenerative diseases that occurs secondary to the loss of dopamine-producing brain cells. Symptoms of PD include trembling, tremor of the hands, arms legs, jaw, and face. There is a slowing of movement known as bradykinesia. Other changes include rigidity or stiffness in limbs and the trunk, problems with balance and coordination, and postural instability (68). There is no laboratory or blood test to diagnose PD; the diagnosis is made based on neurologic exam and symptoms. PD generally affects those over the age of 50 and is more prevalent among men than women. There are 50,000 to 60,000 newly diagnosed cases of PD in the United States each year with over one million Americans now living with PD (69). There is a subtype of PD that involves deposits both in the retina (70) and neural tissue (71).

Individuals with PD show deficits in color perception (72), contrast sensitivity (73), motion (72), visual field, and eye movement. Dry eye is frequently reported as well (74,75). Motor deficits frequently include abnormal saccades, poor convergence, blink abnormalities, and gaze deficits. Retinal deficits may contribute to circadian abnormalities, and deficits in the autonomic system can contribute to reflex tear production and quality. Conventional eye examinations may not readily identify the subtle loss in the visual system that is common in PD.

Retina Retinal structures are affected by dopamine depletion (72) and changes in the photoreceptors (70). The optic nerve fiber layer shows loss of structure (76) and there is evidence of dopamine depletion impacting neuroprocessing regions further along the visual pathway (77,78). Changes in dopamine levels may cause retinal ganglion cell functional and structural deficits. Dopaminergic innervation around the fovea is reduced in those with PD (79), while autopsy findings in patients who were unmedicated at death showed decreased retinal dopamine concentrations (80). Pale inclusion deposit pathology containing synuclein has been identified in the retinas upon autopsy of those who had PD syndromes with symptoms of hallucinations (70). Visual hallucinations are present in 30% to 60% of PD patients receiving treatment (81–83). In a study looking at visual hallucinations in AD, it was found that the hallucinations were associated with a higher likelihood of Lewy body disease (84) indicating a mixed pathology. Visual hallucinations often occur in the presence of retinal disease, but with the absence of cognitive impairments (85,86), explaining the probability of those with PD and retinal pathology having a greater and more frequent manifestation of visual hallucinations.

Neural Pathways and Glaucoma Dopaminergic innervation also exists at the level of the LGN (87). Dopamine receptor agonists have been found to influence the function of the LGN in detection of contrast in animal models. This led researchers to conclude that visual contrast deficits in PD do not all originate in the retina but occur in higher neural pathways as well (77). Different diseases alter the magnocellular and parvocellular pathways leading up to the LGN and may play a role in the quality of deficits in contrast sensitivity discrimination (88). Glaucoma, like PD, impacts the LGN. There are losses in the M (25,26), P (26), and K layers (89) of the LGN in glaucoma. There is shrinkage and change in the LGN neurons early on in the glaucoma disease process, which can be observed even before nerve fiber loss in the optic nerve (27,28). Studies have found a higher rate of glaucoma among PD patients compared to non-PD patients (75,90).

Eye Movements It has been found that poor saccades, asthenopia, upgaze deficiency, and convergence insufficiency are more common in individuals with PD compared to age-matched controls. Saccades, both reflexive and complex, are also abnormal (91).

Nerve Fiber Layer Imaging Reductions in axonal retinal nerve fiber layer in participants with PD have been reported (76,92–94). Yavas et al. (95) not only found reductions in the nerve fiber layer but also that treatment with levodopa had less of a reduction in nerve fiber layer thickness compared to those being treated with dopamine agonists. Moschos et al. (96) found reductions in the nerve fiber layer temporally and nasally with these individuals having visual acuities of 20/20 or better, normal visual fields and normal color vision.

Frequency-doubling Technology Reduced contrast is found in those with PD (73). When responding to a questionnaire, 27% of participants with PD reported difficulties attributed to probable contrast sensitivity deficits (97). Silva et al. (98), using a target similar to the FDT (variable contrast stimuli at a high-frequency testing), found that those with PD had reductions in the magnocellular pathway. This correlated with the stage of the disease. Preliminary studies with FDT have identified deficits in those with PD compared to age-matched control participants (99–101).

Vision, Mobility, and Laterality A study of mobility in PD found significant laterality effects (102). Those with predominantly right hemisphere disease had symptoms primarily on their left side. These same subjects demonstrated greater problems with spatial orientation when walking (103). The right posterior parietal lobe is dominant for a variety of spatial functions (102). It is not unusual for patients with PD to have an initial-onset presentation of unilateral brain deficits. This asymmetry is maintained long after the disease has progressed to become bilateral (104,105). The asymmetry of physical presentation is due to pronounced changes in dopamine metabolism in the contralateral regions of the brain (104,106,107). A result of asymmetric neural involvement is poor navigation and subsequent collisions with objects and door frames in the visual space that is ipsilateral to the predominant lesion. Mobility problems are associated with self-reports of visual and spatial disorders. Those with PD use sensory cues, including visual input, as a means of initiating movement (108) making optimum visual input critical for safe movement.

A study undertaken by Hely et al. (109) found that older PD patients deteriorated more rapidly and were significantly more likely to develop problems with balance and dementia. Visual functions that impair mobility such as contrast sensitivity and visual field (110) decline in all patients as they age, but those with PD have greater deficits in these visual functions. This places them at an even greater risk for falls secondary to balance and mobility problems. Lee et al. (111) tested eight PD subjects with left unilateral disease expression, eight with right expression, and 8 age-matched controls on a vertical line bisection task. Results found probable altitudinal neglect in those with left unilateral PD. This supports the hypothesis of dopaminergic involvement in the encoding of visual space in the superior visual field. There may be brain laterality and retinal region specificity for detecting and processing contrast. This has implications for PD with and without glaucoma as it frequently has distinct laterality as its initial presentation.

HUNTINGTON DISEASE

Huntington disease is caused by an increased number of triplet (CAG) repeats in the Huntington gene (112). It manifests at a rate of between 7 and 10 persons per 100,000 (113). The disease is expressed by the degeneration of neurons in certain areas of the brain. The process causes uncontrolled movements, loss of cognitive functions, and emotional disturbances. Huntington disease is an autosomal dominant inherited disorder. The age of onset and rate of progression varies from person to person. In 1% to 3% of those diagnosed with HD, there is no previous history in the family (114).

Retina Huntington disease causes degeneration of several different transmitter systems in the brain and retina affecting visual function. Retinal degeneration that is readily apparent has yet to be structurally documented. However, the expression of the disease may be subtle so as not to produce deficits when measured by conventional eye examination procedures.

In a study of 19 participants with HD, there was significantly reduced functioning of the cone triad in the outer plexiform layer of the retina (115). The threshold detection was significantly reduced in HD compared to age-matched controls. A single study of brain tissue from transgenic HD mice found that there was significant immunoreactivity in the LGN (116). No such studies are reported in the literature for humans, however. A single reported histology study of human retina found atrophy of the caudate nucleus, the putamen and cortical areas, as well as abundant inclusions or aggregates in the cingular gyrus with staining specific to HD pathology. No inclusions or aggregates were found in the retina. Abnormal staining in the nerve fiber layer, not specific to HD, was also documented. The study was reported to be hampered by the detachment of the pigment epithelium during sectioning (117).

Animal models have shown pronounced retinal degeneration. Studies in mice have mutant huntingtin (the protein encoded by the HD gene) in the retina, which leads to substantial vision deficits and retinal dystrophy. Neuronal intranuclear inclusions appear in all three layers, but histologic abnormalities affect the inner retina, inner nuclear layer, and the ganglion cell layer. The aggregates accumulate progressively and are prevalent in animals that exhibit a strong neurologic phenotype. As animals age, the photoreceptor cell layer becomes irregular and disorganized. Dysfunction in photoreceptors and neurons, specifically the rod bipolar cells with postsynaptic transmission to photoreceptors and cone function (118,119), is found to be impaired when tested with an electroretinogram.

Binocular Function and Motility The most frequently reported ocular dysfunctions are related to saccades and pursuits. What is conspicuously absent is the reporting of diplopia with the saccadic or pursuit dysfunction. However, diplopia is often reported even in early stages in spinocerebellar ataxia type 3 (SCA3) (120). Spinocerebellar ataxia and other genetic diseases that have loss of neurons resulting in movement dysfunction have many attributes in common with HD. The diplopia in SCA3 is hypothesized to be associated with vergence (yoked eye movement) deficiencies (120). The most dramatic symptom of poor yoked visual function is amblyopia or strabismus. In general population studies, the rate for strabismus is 3% to 4% (121,122); however, in those with HD, the prevalence is three times the average rate. A dysfunction in vergence has been reported in 33% of HD patients (123). Retinal degeneration resulting in legal blindness is present in a subset of patients with SCA who survive beyond middle age (124). One hypothesis is that those with HD may have retinal dysfunction, possibly neurodegenerative, but do not survive long enough to show structural changes that are evident in a conventional eye exam.

Functional Vision In a study of 13 subjects with HD using the visual evoked potential (VEP), reduced amplitude compared to controls was documented. The same study found that in four of nine offspring of those with HD, VEP amplitude was also reduced (125). In a 13-year study of five participants at risk for HD, but clinically free of symptoms, serial visual electrodiagnostic testing, a neuropsychological assessment, physical exam, and brain imaging using CT were performed. Of the original five, three became symptomatic. Visual electrodiagnostic testing predicted the diagnosis preclinically (126). Another investigation using the VEP found that when using two criteria to indicate the presence of disease (diminution of amplitudes and either distortion of amplification or alterations in the VEP waveforms) in 36 participants with HD, 24 (67%) could be considered abnormal (127). However, this differed from yet another study that looked at a total of 12 participants with HD using a variety of electropotentials including pattern-reversal visual (PRVEPs), brain stem auditory (BAEPs), and somatosensory evoked potentials (SSEPs). The cortical SSEP amplitude was decreased compared with that of age-matched controls. The SSEP latency, PRVEPs, and BAEPs were normal (128).

O'Donnell et al. (129) studied a large group of participants in four categories: (a) 32 prediagnostic gene carriers with minimal neurologic abnormalities, (b) 20 prediagnostic gene carriers with moderate neurologic abnormalities, (c) 36 gene carriers diagnosed with HD, (d) 201 nongene carriers. They evaluated participants using contrast sensitivity for stationary and moving sinusoidal gratings and motion discrimination. The participants diagnosed with HD demonstrated deficits in contrast sensitivity for moving gratings. The prediagnostic gene carriers that showed moderate neurologic findings also demonstrated deficits compared to the nongene carriers. The group concluded that those with HD show dysfunction in the magnocellular pathway occurs early in the neurodegenerative process. Deficits have also been identified using FDT in clinical patients with HD (99).

Visual Pathways Structural imaging using MRI in those with HD showed significant cerebral white matter loss. Occipital white matter was more affected than other cerebral white matter (130). A second study also found occipital white matter loss, but found it to be lateralized to the right occipital lobe (131). At autopsy, 19 HD brains were studied along with 10 age-matched control brains using staining specific to HD pathology. Huntington disease pathology was found in the LGN of those with HD that was significantly more pronounced than the controls (132).

CONCLUSION

Visual pathways and visual function is impacted by neurodegenerative disease. Despite limited knowledge, it is clear that visual deficits can impact function and quality of life. Combined with motor dysfunction or cognitive decline, visual deficits can create even greater concerns for falls and injury. A thorough assessment of the visual system, optical, functional, and structural, is important for patients with a probable or definitive diagnosis of neurodegenerative disease.

REFERENCES

1. Valenti DA. Alzheimer's disease: visual system review. Optometry. 2010;81(1):12–21.
2. Valenti D. The anterior visual system and circadian function with reference to Alzheimer's disease. In: Cronin-Golomb A, Hof PR, editors. Vision in Alzheimer's disease. Interdiscipl top gerontol. Basel: Karger; 2004;34:1–29
3. US National Institutes of Health. Alzheimer's disease Fact Sheet. National Institute on Aging. Available from: http://www.nia.nih.gov/Alzheimers/Publications/adfact.htm. Last Accessed February 9th, 2011.
4. Jalbert JJ, Daiello LA, Lapane KL. Dementia of the Alzheimer type. Epidemiol Rev. 2008;30:15–34.
5. Hof PR, Cox K, Morrison JH. Quantitative analysis of a vulnerable subset of pyramidal neurons in Alzheimer's disease: I. Superior frontal and inferior temporal cortex. J Comp Neurol. 1990;30:44–5.
6. Anoop A, Singh PK, Jacob RS, et al. CSF biomarkers for Alzheimer's disease diagnosis. Int J Alzheimer Dis. 2010; doi:10.4061/2010/606802.
7. McKee AC, Au R, Cabral HJ, et al. Visual association pathology in preclinical Alzheimer disease. J Neuropathol Exp Neurol. 2006;65:621–30.
8. Belbin O, Carrasquillo MM, Crump M, et al. Investigation of 15 of the top candidate genes for late-onset Alzheimer's disease. Hum Genet. 2010;129:273–82.
9. Wollen KA. Alzheimer's disease: the pros and cons of pharmaceutical, nutritional, botanical, and stimulatory therapies, with a discussion of treatment strategies from the perspective of patients and practitioners. Altern Med Rev. 2010;15:223–44.
10. Armstrong RA. Visual field defects in Alzheimer's disease patients may reflect differential pathology in the primary visual cortex. Optom Vis Sci. 1996;73:677–82.
11. Trick GL, Trick LR, Morris P, et al. Visual field loss in senile dementia of the Alzheimer's type. Neurology. 1995;45:68–74.
12. Cronin-Golomb A, Sugiura R, Corkin S, et al. Incomplete achromatopsia in Alzheimer's disease. Neurobiol Aging. 1993;14:471–7.
13. Pache M, Smeets CH, Gasio PF, et al. Colour vision deficiencies in Alzheimer's disease. Age Ageing. 2003;32:422–6.
14. Quigley HA, Addicks EM, Green R. Optic nerve damage in human glaucoma III: quantitative correlation of nerve fiber loss and visual field defect in glaucoma, ischemic optic neuropathy, papilledema and toxic optic neuropathy. Arch Ophthalmol. 1982;100:135–46.
15. Pacheco-Cutillas M, Edgar DF, Sahriae A. Acquired colour vision defects in glaucoma-their detection and clinical significance. Br J Ophthalmol. 1999;83:1396–402.
16. Shabana N, Cornilleau PV, Carkeet A, et al. Motion perception in glaucoma patients: a review. Surv Ophthalmol. 2003;48:92–106.
17. Mei M, Leat SJ. Suprathreshold contrast matching in maculopathy. Invest Ophthalmol Vis Sci. 2007;48:3419–24.
18. Feigl B, Brown B, Lovie-Kitchin J, et al. Monitoring retinal function in early age-related maculopathy: visual performance after one year. Eye. 2005;19:1169–77.
19. Ruppertsberg AI, Wuerger SM, Bertamini M. When S-cones contribute to chromatic global motion processing. Vis Neurosci. 2007;24:1–8.
20. Bayer AU, Ferrari F. Severe progression of glaucomatous optic neuropathy in patients with Alzheimer's disease. Eye. 2002;16:209–12.
21. Bayer A, Ferrari F. Severe progression of glaucomatous optic neuropathy in patients with Alzheimer's disease. Eye. 2002;16:209–12.
22. Bayer AU, Ferrari F, Erb C. High occurrence rate of glaucoma among patients with Alzheimer's disease. Eur Neurol. 2002;47:165–8.
23. Estermann S, Daepp G, Cattapan-Ludewig K, et al. Effect of oral donepezil on intraocular pressure in normotensive Alzheimer patients. J Ocul Pharmacol Ther. 2006;22:62–7.
24. Miki A. Protective effect of donepezil on retinal ganglion cells in vitro and in vivo. Curr Eye Res. 2006;31:69–77.
25. Goldblum D, Garweg JG, Bohnke M. Topical rivastigmine, a selective acetylcholinesterase inhibitor, lowers intraocular pressure in rabbits. J Ocul Pharmacol Ther. 2000;1:29–35.
26. Chaturvedi N, Hedley-Whyte T, Dreyer EB. Lateral geniculate nucleus in glaucoma. Am J Ophthalmol. 1993;116:182–8.
27. Yucel YH, Zhang Q, Qupta N, Kaufman PL, et al. Loss of neurons in magnocellular and parvocellular layers of the lateral geniculate nucleus in glaucoma. Arch Ophthalmol. 2000;118:378–84.

28. Weber AJ, Chen H, Hubbard WC, et al. Experimental glaucoma and cell size, density and number in primate lateral geniculate nucleus. Invest Ophthalmol Vis Sci. 2000;41:1370–9.
29. Yucel YH, Zhang Q, Weinreb RN, et al. Atrophy of relay neurons in mango-and parvocellular layers in the lateral geniculate nucleus in experimental glaucoma. Invest Ophthalmol Vis Sci. 2001;42:3216–22.
30. Hof PR, Morrison JH. Quantitative analysis of a vulnerable subset of pyramidal neurons in Alzheimer's disease: II. Primary and secondary visual cortex. J Comp Neurol. 1990;301:55–64.
31. Leuba G, Saini K. Pathology of subcortical visual centres in relation to cortical degeneration in Alzheimer's disease. Neuropathol Appl Neurobiol. 1995;21:410–22.
32. AREDS. Cognitive impairment in the age related eye disease study. Arch Ophthalmol. 2006;124:537–43.
33. Anderson D, Talaga K, Rivest A, et al. Characterization of beta amyloid assemblies in drusen: the deposits associated with aging and age-related macular degeneration. Exp Eye Res. 2004;78:243–56.
34. Yoshida T, Ohno-Matsui K, Ichinose S, et al. The potential role of amyloid beta in the pathogenesis of age-related macular degeneration. J Clin Invest. 2005;115:2793–800.
35. Dentchev T, Milan A, Lee V, et al. Amyloid-beta is found in drusen from some age-related macular degeneration retinas, but not in drusen from normal retinas. Mol Vis. 2003;9: 184–90.
36. Ding JD, Lin J, Mace B, et al. Targeting age-related macular degeneration with Alzheimer's disease based immunotherapies: anti-amyloid beta antibody attenuates pathologies in an age-related macular degeneration mouse model. Vis Res. 2008;48:339–45.
37. Kovacs KA, Pamer Z, Kovacs A, et al. Association of apolipoprotein E polymorphism with age-related macular degeneration and Alzheimer's disease in south-western Hungary. Ideggyogy Sz. 2007;60:169–72.
38. Thakkinstian A, Bowe S, McEvoy M, et al. Association between apolipoprotein E polymorphisms and age-related macular degeneration: a HuGE review and meta-analysis. Am J Epidemiol. 2006;164:813–22.
39. Goldstein L, Muffat J, Cherny R, et al. Cytosolic beta-amyloid deposition and supranuclear cataracts in lenses from people with Alzheimer's disease. Lancet. 2003;361:1258–65.
40. Collinson DJ, Duncan G. Regional differences in functional receptor distribution and calcium mobilization in the intact human lens. Invest Ophthalmol Vis Sci. 2001;42:2355–63.
41. Shaffer RN, Hetherington J. Anticholinesterase drugs and cataracts. Am J Ophthalmol. 1966;62:613–8.
42. Deroetth A. Lenticular opacities in glaucoma patients receiving echothiophate iodide therapy. JAMA. 1966;195:152–4.
43. Scinto LFM, Rentz D, Potter H, et al. Pupil assay and Alzheimer's disease: a critical analysis. Neurology. 1999;52:673–7.
44. Reitner A, Baumgartner I, Thuile C, et al. The mydriatic effect of tropicamide and its diagnostic use in Alzheimer's disease. Vis Res. 1997;37:165–8.
45. Hanyu H, Hirao K, Shimizu S, et al. Phenylephrine and pilocarpine eye drop test for dementia with Lewy Bodies and Alzheimer's disease. Neurosci Lett. 2007;414:174–7.
46. Grunberger J, Linzmayer L, Walter H, et al. Receptor test (pupillary dilation after application of 0.01% tropicamide solution) and determination of central nervous activation (Fourier analysis of papillary oscillations) in patients with Alzheimer's disease. Neuropsychobiology. 1999;40:40–6.
47. Granholm E, Morris S, Galasko D, et al. Tropicomide effects on pupil size and pupillary light reflexes in Alzheimer's disease and Parkinson's disease. Int J Psychophysiol. 2003;47:95–115.
48. Gomez-Tortosa E, Jimenz-Alfaro DBA. Pupil response to tropicamide in Alzheimer's disease and other neurodegenerative disorders. Acta Neurol Scand. 1996;94:104–9.
49. Scinto LRM. Pupillary hypersensitivity predicts cognitive decline in community dwelling elders. Neurobiol Aging. 2008;29:222–30.
50. Estermann S, Daepp GC, Cattapan-Ludewig K, et al. Effect of oral donepezil on intraocular pressure in normotensive Alzheimer patients. J Ocul Pharmacol Ther. 2006;22:62–7.
51. Scinto LF, Wu M, Daffner CK, et al. Selective cell loss in Edinger-Westphal in asymptomatic elders and Alzheimer's patients. Neurobiol Aging. 2001;22:729–36.
52. Scinto LF. ApoE allelic variability influences pupil response to cholinergic challenge and cognitive impairment. Genes Brain Behav. 2007;6:209–15.
53. Kaufman P. Enhancing trabecular outflow by disrupting the actin cytoskeleton, increasing uveoscleral outflow with prostaglandins, and understanding the pathophysiology of presbyopia. Exp Eye Res. 2008;86:3–17.
54. Parisi V, Restuccia R, Fattapposta F, et al. Morphological and functional retinal impairment in Alzheimer's disease patients. Clin Neurophysiol. 2001;112:1860–7.
55. Iseri P, Altinas O, Today T, et al. Relationship between cognitive impairment and retinal morphological and visual functional abnormalities in Alzheimer's disease. J Neuro-Ophthalmol. 2006;26:18–24.
56. Valenti D. Neuroimaging of retinal nerve fiber layer in AD using optical coherence tomography. Neurology. 2007;69:1060.
57. Berisha F, Feke GT, Trempe CL, et al. Retinal abnormalities in early Alzheimer's disease. Invest Ophthalmol Vis Sci. 2007;48:2285–9.
58. Paquet C, Boissonnot M, Roger F, et al. Abnormal retinal thickness in patients with mild cognitive impairment and Alzheimer's disease. Neurosci Lett. 2007;420:97–9.
59. Valenti DA, Laudate T, Cronin-Golomb A. Vision screening of Alzheimer's disease with frequency doubling technology (FDT). Invest Ophthalmol Vis Sci. 2004;45(E-Abstract 231):231-B04.
60. Mentis MJ, Horwitz B, Grady CL, et al. Visual cortical dysfunction in Alzheimer's disease evaluated with temporarily graded stress test during PET. Am J Psychiatry. 1996;153:32–40.
61. Curran S, Wilson S, Musa S, et al. Critical Flicker Fusion Threshold in patients with Alzheimer's disease and vascular dementia. Int J Geriatr Psychiatry. 2004;19:575–81.
62. US National Institutes of Health. Facts About Down Syndrome. Eunice Kennedy Shriver National Institutes of Children's Health and Human Development. Available from: http://www.nichd.nih.gov/publications/pubs/downsyndrome.cfm. Last Accessed February 9th, 2011.

63. Burger PC, Vogel FS. The development of the pathologic changes of Alzheimer's disease and senile dementia in patients with Down's syndrome. Am J Pathol. 1973;73:457–76.
64. Cork LC. Neuropathology of Down syndrome and Alzheimer disease. Am J Med Genet Suppl. 1990;7:282–6.
65. Lott IT, Dierssen M. Cognitive deficits and associated neurological complications in individuals with Down's syndrome. Lancet Neurol. 2010;9:623–33.
66. Schupf N, Zigman WB, Tang MX, et al. Change in plasma A{beta} peptides and onset of dementia in adults with Down syndrome. Neurology. 2010;75:1639–44.
67. Patel A, Rees SD, Kelly MA, et al. Association of variants within APOE, SORL1, RUNX1, BACE1 and ALDH18A1 with dementia in Alzheimer's disease in subjects with Down syndrome. Neurosci Lett. 2011;487:144–8.
68. US National Institutes of Health. Parkinson's disease information. National Institute of Neurological Disorders and Stroke. Available from: http://www.ninds.nih.gov/disorders/parkinsons_disease/parkinsons_disease.htm. Last Accessed February 9th, 2011.
69. National Parkinson's Foundation. Parkinson's disease review. 2010; Available from: http://www.parkinson.org/parkinson-s-disease.aspx. Last Accessed February 9th, 2011.
70. Maurage CA. Retinal involvement in dementia with Lewy bodies: a clue to hallucinations? Ann Neurol. 2003;54: 542–7.
71. Jelllinger KA. A critical reappraisal of current staging of Lewy-related pathology in human brain. Acta Neuropathol. 2008;116:1–16.
72. Pieri V, Diederich NJ, Raman R, et al. Decreased color discrimination and contrast sensitivity in Parkinson's disease. J Neurol Sci. 2000;172:7–11.
73. Uc EY, Rizzo M, Anderson SW, et al. Visual dysfunction in Parkinson disease without dementia. Neurology. 2005;65:1907–13.
74. Tamer C, Melek IM, Duman T, et al. Tear film tests in Parkinson's disease patients. Ophthalmology. 2005;112:1795.
75. Nowacka B, Lubiński W, Karczewicz D. Ophthalmological and electrophysiological features of Parkinson's disease [abstract only]. Klin Oczna. 2010;112:247–52.
76. Inzelberg R, Ramirez JA, Nisipeanu P, Ophir A. Retinal nerve fiber layer thinning in Parkinson disease. Vis Res. 2004;44:2793–7.
77. Zhao WQ, Latinwo L, Liu XX, et al. L-dopa upregulates the expression and activities of methionine adenosyl transferase and catechol-O-methyltransferase. Exp Neurol. 2001;171:127–38.
78. Braak H, Ghebremedhin E, Rüb U, et al. Stages in the development of Parkinson's disease-related pathology. Cell Tissue Res. 2004;318:121–34.
79. Nguyen-Legros J. Functional neuroarchitecture of the retina: hypothesis on the dysfunction of retinal dopaminergic circuitry in PD. Surg Radiol Anat. 1988;10:137–44.
80. Harnois C. Decreased dopamine in the retinas of PD. Invest Ophthalmol Vis Sci. 1990;31:2473–5.
81. De Maindreville AD. Hallucinations in PD. Mov Disord. 2005;20:212–7.
82. Crevits L. Abnormal psychophysical visual perception in PD patients. Acta Neurol Belg. 2003;103:83–7.
83. Diederich NJ. Repeated visual hallucinations in PD. Mov Disord. 2005;20:130–40.
84. Terao T. Visual hallucinations in Alzheimer's disease: possible involvement of low visual acuity and dementia with Lewy bodies. J Neuropsychol Clin Neurosci. 2000;12:516–7.
85. Menon GJ, Rahman I, Menon SJ, et al. Complex visual hallucinations in the visually impaired: the Charles Bonnet Syndrome. Surv Ophthalmol. 2003;48:58–72.
86. Scott IU. Visual hallucinations in patients with retinal disease. Am J Ophthalmol. 2001;131:590–8.
87. Papadopoulos GC, Parnavelas JG. Distribution and synaptic organization of dopaminergic axons in the lateral geniculate nucleus of the rat. J Comp Neurol. 1990;29:356–61.
88. Tebartz van Elst L, Greenlee MW, Foley JM, et al. Contrast detection, discrimination and adaptation in patients with Parkinson's disease and multiple system atrophy. Brain. 1997;120:2219–28.
89. Gupta N, Ang LC, Noel deTilly L, et al. Human glaucoma and neural degeneration in intracranial optic nerve, lateral geniculate nucleus and visual cortex. Br J Ophthalmol. 2006;90:674–8.
90. Bayer AU, Keller ON, Ferrari F, et al. Association of glaucoma with neurodegenerative diseases with apoptotic cell death: Alzheimer's disease and Parkinson's disease. Am J Ophthalmol. 2002;133:135–7.
91. Mosimann UP, Müri RM, Burn DJ, et al. Saccadic eye movement changes in Parkinson's disease dementia and dementia with Lewy bodies. Brain. 2005;128:1267–76.
92. Altintas O, Iseri P, Ozkan B, et al. Correlation between retinal morphological and functional findings and clinical severity in Parkinson's disease. Doc Ophthalmol. 2008;116:137–46.
93. Valenti D. Vision Assessment in Neurodegenerative disease. American Public Health Association National Conference. Philadelphia, PA, 2005.
94. Valenti DA. Neuroimaging of retinal nerve fiber layer in Alzheimer's disease and Parkinson's disease using optical coherence tomography. Alzheimer's Association 2006 (Abstract National Meeting).
95. Yavas GF, Yilmaz O, Kusbeci T, et al. The effect of levodopa and dopamine agonists on optic nerve head in Parkinson's disease. Eur J Ophthalmol. 2007;5:812–6.
96. Moschos MM, Tagaris G, Markopoulos I, et al. Morphologic changes and functional retinal impairment in patients with Parkinson disease without visual loss. Eur J Ophthalmol. 2011;21:24–9.
97. Lee A, Harris J. Problems with perception of space in Parkinson's disease: a questionnaire study. Neuroophthalmology. 1999;22:1–15.
98. Silva MF, Faria P, Regateiro FS, et al. Independent patterns of damage within magno, parvo and koniocellular pathways in Parkinson's disease. Brain. 2005;128:2260–71.
99. Valenti DA, Auerbach S. Movement disorders: deficits in visual processing as measured by frequency doubling technology. Invest Ophthalmol Vis Sci. 2009;50(E-Abstract 210):2010-D785.
100. Valenti DA. Neurologic disease: use of frequency doubling technology. Invest Ophthalmol Vis Sci. 2010;51(E-Abstract 2334):2334-A584.
101. Valenti DA. Functional Losses in Parkinson's disease: frequency doubling technology. Invest Ophthalmol Vis Sci. 2005;46(E-Abstract 626):626-B00.

102. Previc FH. The neuropsychology of 3-D space. Psychol Bull. 1998;124(2):123–64.
103. Bowen FP, Hoehn MM, Yahr MD. Parkinsonism: alterations in spatial orientation as determined by a route-walking test. Neuropsychologia. 1972;10(3):355–61.
104. Antonini A, Leenders KL, Vontobel P, et al. Complementary PET studies of striatal neuronal function in the differential diagnosis between multiple system atrophy and Parkinson's disease. Brain. 1997;120:2187–95.
105. Laulumaa V, Kuikka JT, Soininen H, et al. Imaging of D2 dopamine receptors of patients with Parkinson's disease using single photon emission computed tomography and iodobenzamide I 123. Arch Neurol. 1993;50:509–12.
106. Innis RB, Seibyl JP, Scanley BE, et al. Single photon emission computed tomographic imaging demonstrates loss of striatal dopamine transporters in Parkinson disease. Proc Natl Acad Sci U S A. 1993;90:11965–9.
107. Marek KL, Seibyl JP, Zoghbi SS, et al. [123I] beta-CIT/SPECT imaging demonstrates bilateral loss of dopamine transporters in hemi-Parkinson's disease. Neurology. 1996;46:231–7.
108. Slatt B, Loeffler JD, Hoyt WF. Ocular motor disturbances in Parkinson's disease electromyographic observations. Can J Ophthalmol. 1966;4:267–73.
109. Hely MA, Morris JG, Reid WG, et al. Age at onset: the major determinant of outcome in Parkinson's disease. Acta Neurol Scand. 1995;92:455–63.
110. Luciani F, Cappello E, Tollot L, et al. Normal values for fundus perimetry with the microperimeter MP1. Ophthalmology. 2010;117:1571–6.
111. Lee AC, Harris JP, Atkinson EA, et al. Dopamine and the representation of the upper visual field: evidence from vertical bisection errors in unilateral Parkinson's disease. Neuropsychologia. 2002;40:2023–9.
112. The Huntington's Disease Collaborative Research Group. A novel gene containing a trinucleotide repeat that is expanded and unstable on Huntington's disease chromosomes. The Huntington's Disease Collaborative Research Group. Cell. 1993;72:971–83.
113. Spinney S. Uncovering the true prevalence of Huntington's disease. Lancet Neurol. 2010;9:760–1.
114. US National Institutes of Health. Huntington's Disease Information Page. National Institute of Neurological Disorders and Stroke. Available from: http://www.ninds.nih.gov/disorders/huntington/huntington.htm. Last Accessed February 10th, 2011.
115. Paulus W, Schwarz G, Werner A, et al. Impairment of retinal increment thresholds in Huntington's disease. Ann Neurol. 1993;34:574–8.
116. Petrasch-Parwez E, Nguyen HP, Lobbecke-Schumacher M, et al. Cellular and subcellular localization of Huntington aggregates in the brain of a rat transgenic for Huntington Disease. J Comp Neurol. 2007;501:716–30.
117. Petrasch-Parwez E, Saft C, Schlichting A, et al. Is the retina affected in Huntington disease? Acta Neuropathol. 2005;110:523–5.
118. Petrasch-Parwez E, Habbes HW, Weickert S, et al. Fine-structural analysis and connexin expression in the retina of a transgenic model of Huntington's disease. J Comp Neurol. 2004;470:181–197.
119. Helmlinger D, Yvert G, Picaud S, et al. Progressive retinal degeneration and dysfunction in R6 Huntington's disease mice. Hum Mol Genet. 2002;11:3351–9
120. Ohyage Y, Ymada T, Okayama A, et al. Vergence disorders in patients with spinocerebellar ataxia 3/Machado-Joseph disease: a synoptophore study. J Neurol Sci. 2000;173:120–3.
121. Robinson B, Bobier WR, Martin E, et al. Measurement of the validity of a preschool vision screening program. Am J Public Health. 1998;89:193–8.
122. Donnelly UM, Stewart NM, Hollinger M. Prevalence and outcomes of childhood visual disorders. Ophthalmic Epidemiol. 2005;12:243–50.
123. Leigh RJ, Newman SA, Folstein SE, et al. Abnormal ocular motor control in Huntington's disease. Neurol. 1983;33:1268–75.
124. Gouw LG, Kaplan CD, Haines JH, et al. Retinal degeneration characterizes a spinocerebellar ataxia mapping to chromosome 3p. Nat Genet. 1995;10:89–93.
125. Oepen G, Doerr M, Thoden U. Huntington's disease: alterations of visual and somatosensory cortical evoked potentials in patients and offspring. Adv Neurol. 1982;32:141–7.
126. Cala LA, Black JL, Collins DW, et al. Thirteen years longitudinal study of computed tomography, visual electrophysiology and neuropsychological changes in Huntington's chorea patients and 50% at-risk asymptomatic subjects. Clin Exp Neurol. 1990;27:43–63.
127. Hennerici M, Hömberg V, Lange HW. Evoked potentials in patients with Huntington's disease and their offspring. II. Visual evoked potentials. Electroencephalogr Clin Neurophysiol. 1985;62:167–76.
128. Ehle AL, Stewart RM, Lellelid NA, et al. Evoked potentials in Huntington's disease. A comparative and longitudinal study. Arch Neurol. 1984;41:379–82.
129. O'Donnell BF, Blekher TM, Weaver M, et al. Visual perception in prediagnostic and early stage Huntington's disease. J Int Neuropsychol Soc. 2008;14:446–53.
130. Fennema-Notestine C, Archibald SL, Jacobson MW, et al. In vivo evidence of cerebellar atrophy and cerebral white matter loss in Huntington disease. Neurology. 2004;63:989–95.
131. Henley SM, Wild EJ, Hobbs NZ, et al. Relationship between CAG repeat length and brain volume in premanifest and early Huntington's disease. J Neurol. 2009;256:203–12.
132. Herndon ES, Hladik CL, Shang P, et al. Neuroanatomic profile of polyglutamine immunoreactivity in Huntington disease brains. J Neuropathol Exp Neurol. 2009;68:250–61.

CHAPTER 14

Barry S. Kran, OD, FAAO
D. Luisa Mayer, PhD

Vision Impairment and Brain Damage

Brain-related visual impairment is called *cortical* or *cerebral* visual impairment (CVI). For the purposes of this review, CVI denotes a significant deficit in visual acuity, with possible visual field loss, and other impaired visual behaviors that cannot be explained by ocular, ocular motor, or refractive anomalies. These latter conditions may and do coexist with CVI. The causes of vision impairment in children due to brain damage* are numerous. Brain damage is the leading cause of pediatric vision impairment in high-income countries (1–4). Clinically, the extent of vision impairment generally correlates with the extent of brain damage. The types and ranges of visual function, however, can be variously and differentially affected in any specific causal condition.

Cognitive and motor disabilities that accompany brain damage in children increase the challenges in determining various facets of vision impairment. Despite this, it is essential to identify impaired visual functions and affected behaviors in order to generate a management plan that best fits the needs of the patient. This chapter provides a model to help diagnose brain-related vision impairment in children who may also present with cognitive, neuromotor, and/or hearing deficits. (See Chapters 2, Genetics; 3, Cerebral Palsy; 6, Intellectual Disabilities of Unknown Etiology; 13, Neurodegenerative Diseases; and 23, Special Assessment Procedures and to a lesser extent Chapters 4, Down Syndrome; 5 Fragile X syndrome; and 8, Autism, which discuss many of the affected populations.)

***Brain damage* is preferred when referring to central nervous system (CNS) insult before the brain and its pathways are fully developed, while *brain injury* is more appropriate for insult to fully mature CNS.

CAUSES OF CVI IN CHILDREN

The causes of CVI in children include hypoxic ischemia in the preterm and term brain, brain malformations, focal brain lesions (e.g., stroke), central nervous system infections, neonatal hypoglycemia, metabolic disorders, chromosomal disorders, traumatic brain injury, and intractable epilepsy (1,2,5). Damage to the brain of the preterm infant, now called encephalopathy of prematurity, includes white matter loss or periventricular leukomalacia (PVL) and germinal matrix hemorrhage (6). Numerous biochemical pathways lead to white and gray matter destruction depending on the cause (e.g., hypoxic ischemia) and the timing of insult on the developing brain. Volpe et al. have elucidated these destructive processes in the premature brain (6,7).

Imaging and histopathologic studies reveal differences in areas and structures damaged in the preterm versus term brain. From 24 to 34 weeks gestation, damage to immature periventricular white matter is more likely than in the older gestation brain (1,2,8). Loss of cerebral blood flow causes variable and more diffuse injuries of white and gray matter, and of subcortical basal ganglia, thalamus, and brainstem (1,2,8). It has been postulated that the appearance of optic nerve head may indicate the preterm gestational age of brain damage. For example, small optic nerves, secondary to retrograde transsynaptic degeneration, may occur in the infant with evidence of brain damage between gestational age 24 to 34 weeks (9,10). A large optic disc cup with a normal optic nerve head size is associated with brain damage between gestational age 28 and 34 weeks (9,10). While optic disc appearance may not be an absolute marker for the timing of brain damage nor a predictor of visual function, it is important to consider retrograde transsynaptic degeneration in the differential diagnosis in an infant with large optic disc cups (10,11).

Over the past decade, it has become apparent in adult and in pediatric populations that malformed or injured cerebellar structures can have significant impact beyond the well-described motor and speech functions. Nonmotor behaviors that may be impaired include visual–spatial, executive control, and social–emotional (12). Although rarely seen or underappreciated in clinical practice, children with cerebellar abnormalities may have visual–spatial problems typically associated with dorsal stream dysfunction, such as optic ataxia, which may confound a differential diagnosis as to cause (12,13). Damage or maldevelopment of the cerebellum in children born very prematurely also complicates interpretation of the complex visual difficulties typically attributed to white matter loss of immaturity (PVL) (7,13). Attention deficits such as regulation of shifts in attention, social/affective disturbances such as extreme mood changes, and autistic behaviors have in recent studies been correlated with damage to the cerebellum (12–14). Thus, the role of the cerebellum in conditions such as attention deficit hyperactivity disorder and autism must now be considered, especially in former preterm infants (12,13). This newly described potential role for the cerebellum in visual processing is fascinating and deserves to be considered in the differential of the loci of visual impairment.

Etiologies causing vision impairment can be separately identified by damage or dysfunction to visual pathways from anterior to posterior structures as follows: *ocular* (ocular media, retina, optic nerve, anterior chiasm), *ocular motor* (brain stem, basal ganglia, thalamus, and cerebellum), *cortical* (postchiasm, optic tract and radiations, occipital cortex), and *cerebral* (occipital cortex connections with parietal and temporal lobes, i.e., vision association areas of dorsal and ventral streams). As noted in the previous paragraph, the role of the cerebellum as a locus of sensory vision impairment must now be included in this scheme of differential diagnosis. It is the examiner's responsibility to investigate the extent to which damage or dysfunction of these structures contributes to the child's visual impairment. Important considerations in the differential diagnosis of cortical/cerebral vision impairment include significant refractive error, nystagmus, oculomotor apraxia (saccadic initiation failure), abnormal retinal development, optic nerve hypoplasia, and generalized cerebral damage (8).

CLASSIFICATION OF CVI

Vision impairment secondary to brain damage in children has been reported since the mid-1980s (5,8,15–20). Initially called cortical vision impairment because of abnormal striate (occipital) images on CT brain scans, later investigations have highlighted extrastriate cortical and subcortical structures as potential causes of childhood visual impairment (5,8). Some characteristics of childhood visual impairment correspond closely to visual problems observed in soldiers with war-related brain injuries reported early in the 20th century (5,8,20–22). These visual disorders caused by cortical and noncortical visual structures have led to the more encompassing term for brain-based vision disorders, "cerebral visual impairment" (8,25). Cortical/cerebral visual impairment is now the leading cause of pediatric visual impairment in developed countries (3,4,17,18,23). This chapter highlights the key points regarding the identification and evaluation of individuals with CVI. There are two texts on this topic which explore critical aspects of CVI with implications for habilitation in greater detail than is possible here (24, 25). After summarizing key concepts and an approach to collaborative assessment, two cases will be presented to highlight the diversity of presentation of individuals with vision impairment secondary to brain damage.

Cortical Visual Impairment Characteristics that are generally accepted as indicating *cortical* visual impairment include light gazing or avoidance of lights, better visual attention for moving versus static objects and for familiar versus novel objects, better visual responses to simple versus complex displays, difficulty integrating gaze with reach, difficulty integrating looking with listening, poor social gaze, delayed responses to visual stimulation, and variability in functional vision (26–30).

Cerebral (Complex) Visual Impairment Conceptually, higher-level cerebral vision functions are separated into dorsal and ventral streams. Though they are considered parallel and separate processing streams, they necessarily connect and interact. The dorsal stream has been described as the "vision for action" system ("where" and "how") (31,32). Input from occipital cortex to parietal cortex integrated with other sensory input, and with reciprocal connections to the frontal cortex, control head/eye movements that are driven by visual attentive processes, and ultimately control visual guidance of movement. Dysfunctions associated with dorsal stream include an inability to see objects in complex environments (simultanagnosia), inability to direct one's gaze to objects, and impaired visual guidance of limbs (optic ataxia) (31–34).

The ventral steam is considered the "vision for recognition" ("what") pathway and codes the brain's visual "library" (31,32,35). Specific modules in the anterior temporal lobes encode input from occipital cortex that process faces, colors, complex symbols (e.g., letters), shapes, and routes. For example, damage to a relatively localized area in the ventral stream can result in an inability to recognize people by sight (prosopagnosia), and damage to another ventral area results in the inability to identify landmarks (topographic disorientation) (35). Isolated ventral stream dysfunctions in children are rare (36,37). Much more frequent are children with dorsal stream dysfunction, although some children also exhibit behaviors suggesting ventral stream dysfunction (38). However, ventral stream dysfunction may be underdiagnosed in younger children who have not developed the cognitive abilities or communication skills necessary to assess recognition vision.

OVERVIEW OF THE CLINICAL ASSESSMENT OF THE CHILD WITH CVI

Approach to the Clinical Evaluation The evaluation of children with brain damage by eye care providers should include a summary of findings of information from other health professionals. Reports from specialists in neurology, metabolism, genetics, and others who have diagnosed and are managing the child's medical care as well as reports of neuroimaging studies should be reviewed prior to examining the child. Neuropsychological evaluations are often helpful. This information should aid in formulating a differential diagnosis for the possible cause(s) of visual impairment and suggest interpretation of visual behaviors, as well as lead to developing a management approach.

Concerns and observations by the parents, therapists, teachers, and vision service providers are critical for a thorough understanding of the child. The teacher of students with vision impairment (TVI), the orientation and mobility (O&M) specialist, as well as the deaf–blind educator and early intervention professional with a background in vision should provide reports of their community-based evaluations and their rationale for services. Review of the Individualized Family Service Program (for birth to age 3 years), or the Individualized Educational Plan (for age 3 to 22 years), with supporting documentation of the psychological–educational evaluation, enables a better understanding of the child's developmental status, educational needs and goals, and provision for therapeutic interventions in relation to functional vision concerns.

Our approach to clinical evaluation is based upon the need to determine how the individual uses and sustains vision from the time we meet them in the waiting area until they leave the exam room. In our view, a patient is neither uncooperative nor untestable. It is the responsibility of the provider to create an environment where the patient can both feel comfortable and utilize their vision. Information is gained by observing the child's functional visual behaviors during the particular test of visual function as well as how we need to modify the test procedures to obtain reliable responses. Visual functions assessed must relate to the child's functional vision in daily life, at home, and at school. Appropriate tests to assess visual functions, examination of ocular health and refractive error, comprise the assessment. Chapters 16, Comprehensive Examination Procedures and 23, Special Assessment Procedures provide a comprehensive review of clinical assessment, while this section highlights our approach vis-à-vis selected crucial visual functions.

Many young patients are apprehensive about being touched or tested, so it is important to determine how to approach a patient prior to attempting any formal testing of acuity or other visual functions. Caregivers and teachers can be helpful in that regard. It may be necessary to "play" with the child before obtaining acuity. Getting on the floor to play catch while rolling a ball or approaching the child with a colorful toy or object of interest and gaining a sense of when he is aware of it, how it is tracked (i.e., with head and/or eye movements), and how long it is fixated. Whether the child reaches for the ball, observing for the presence of nystagmus or null point, and how well visual attention is sustained enable the establishment of a rapport with the patient while collecting standard information in a nonconventional manner and order. We have seen patients with brain damage who were engaged visually only when the visual space was very simplified (dark room) and a lighted toy with an auditory output was used. Patients who can perform the acuity task quickly and in a normally illuminated environment are very different from individuals who need a quiet room, simplified presentation, frequent breaks, and 20 to 30 minutes to ensure that threshold was obtained.

Visual Acuity To measure visual acuity, we test the child with both eyes open before testing each eye separately. This allows the child to become familiar with the task without being stressed about something on his face and allows us to assess fixation preference, the integrity of conjugate eye movements, and gross eye alignment. Visual acuity with both eyes viewing also represents the child's best visual acuity and is more relevant to functional vision than monocular acuity (39). Testing acuity first with both eyes open is especially important when measuring grating acuity with a preferential looking technique (PLT), which is the only way behavioral acuity can be measured in young and developmentally delayed children. Preferential looking technique acuity testing often requires a modified presentation for the child's ocular motor disorder (e.g., vertical card presentation for the child with hemifield loss, or in large angle esotropia, or horizontal nystagmus), and to accommodate a neuromotor disability (e.g., placing the card at angle appropriate to child's head–eyes in wheelchair).

Teller Acuity Cards (TAC) is a semiobjective PLT used to obtain grating acuity. Acuity is interpreted in relation to binocular and monocular TAC age norms (40), and in relation to treatment (e.g., for amblyopia or after spectacle correction). Of equal importance to these interpretations of visual acuity are observations made of the child's "functional" visual and other responses when being presented with the TACs. These responses include time needed for the child to respond to the gratings, ease of gaze shifts to the gratings, side biases, head–eye positions, and reaching, touching, or pointing to the grating. Children with CVI may look away from the cards, possibly because of the novelty of the stimulus. Fixations may be very brief and fleeting or the child may stare at suprathreshold gratings. They may be unable to attend to the stimuli if the examiner talks or makes noises. Lighting conditions may need to be changed (e.g., light directed onto the card for improved attention; decrease in overhead lighting because of light gazing). Thus, although visual acuity is the quantitative outcome of TAC testing, the child's visual responses during the test provide information on their visual fixation abilities, visual attention capabilities, visual motor behaviors, possible visual field loss, responses under competing sensory input, and the effects of other environmental conditions. A study of TAC II (second generation of TAC) acuity in children designated deaf–blind found larger test–retest differences than expected for children developing typically (41). This finding substantiates observations in daily life as well as in clinical practice of greater variability in visual behaviors in atypically developing children compared with typically developing children.

Visual evoked potential (VEP) methods, which take advantage of the large macular projection in the occipital cortex, have great appeal for testing visual acuity in young and disabled children. Unlike PLT, neither the child's voluntary behavioral response nor subjective judgment of patient's response is required. However, several factors mitigate against routine use of VEP acuity measurement in pediatric low-vision clinical settings. Visual evoked potential technology to measure acuity requires considerable experience and expertise with the equipment, test parameters and methodologies, as well as efficient test procedures with infants and disabled children. Norms for VEP acuities need to be obtained by each clinical setting as well (42). Our experience using TACs mirrors the results of longitudinal studies of PLT and VEP grating acuities in children with CVI (42,43). PLT and VEP grating acuities improve somewhat with age in most children with CVI; however, rarely do acuities reach normal values.

Recognition Acuity With children who have adequate cognitive, language, and motor skills (as well as awareness of a world "out there"), recognition acuity for letters or other optotypes at both distance and near can be obtained. Matching paradigms with single optotypes (i.e., Patti Pics, Lea Symbols, HOTV) can be used if the child is unable to name them. The impact of the complexity of the visual array on visual function can be obtained by comparing, for example, full chart or line acuity with single optotype presentation. Young and delayed children, however, typically can only be tested with single optotypes. Information about the child's visual–perceptual abilities can be derived by observing performance difficulties on optotype naming or matching tests.

Visual Field The functional consequences of major field loss in children, especially those with other visual impairments, and cognitive and motor deficits, should not be minimized. Clinical observations and anecdotal reports by parents and therapists provide evidence that visual field loss in children impairs visually guided behaviors, including mobility and fine motor skills, and may delay motor milestones. Despite a lack of formal studies in this area, a presumption of the effects of visual field loss on visual development provides strong motivation to assess the visual field carefully and thoroughly in any child with CVI.

Visual field in most children with severe CVI can be tested using modified confrontation techniques with appropriate stimuli. Lighted stimuli presented in dim room illumination are necessary for children with global and severe CVI. Children with less severe CVI can be tested with small toys or lighted stimuli. A wand containing a light at its end that flickers to elicit orienting and with variable intensity enables assessing the spectrum of visual loss. More extended lighted devices, such as a small light box, or a cell phone or iPad-like digital display can provide useful, but rough, information on visual field status.

Goldmann manual kinetic perimetry (GMKP) is possible with typical children age 4 years and older (44). It is also useful in assessing field loss in children with CVI who are not severely developmentally delayed. Children who can play computer games may be testable by GMKP. Automated perimetry is not feasible for most children with CVI even using new automated kinetic perimeters because of the demands for visual attention and vigilance.

Children with CVI are at risk of lower visual field impairment (20,45). The superior optic radiations, damage to which causes inferior field loss, course along the lateral ventricles and thus are extremely vulnerable to hypoxic ischemic injury and encephalopathy of prematurity. Spastic diplegia (neuromuscular weakness of lower limbs), the most common form of cerebral palsy, is a frequent outcome of encephalopathy of prematurity due to damage to the upper motor neuron downstream pathway that also courses through periventricular white matter (20,45). Thus, inferior field loss is strongly associated with spastic diplegia.

With experience, confrontation testing using light wands and small toys can reveal inferior field losses. However, it is important NOT to present targets along the horizon as is typical in clinical practice, because an inferior field loss will be missed. Targets should be presented in each quadrant along the major oblique meridia and on other trials moved perpendicular to the horizontal meridian at some eccentricity from fixation. The child with inferior field loss will detect the target at or near the horizontal meridian.

Inferior field defects may be more difficult to detect if they are relative rather than dense and complete. Relative inferior field loss would present as constriction of the inferior field, which, in Goldmann perimetry, requires testing of several isopters (45). However, it may be difficult in confrontation testing to differentiate field constriction from impaired attention. An interesting central fixation target, such as the examiner's face, may cause suppression of normal orienting to a salient peripheral target. Children with CVI are often more attracted to environmental sounds and to the examiner's voice than to any nonnoisy visual target.

Other Visual Functions Other visual functions that may be important to assess in the child with CVI include color vision and contrast sensitivity. Children with good visual acuity and dorsal and/or ventral stream dysfunction should be assessed for color vision. Formal color vision testing is possible at a developmental age of 4 to 5 years when the child is capable of shape matching or naming or sorting. Naming or matching colors of objects can suggest intact color identification at earlier ages. Contrast sensitivity tests appropriate for young, visually impaired children have significant limitations and commercially available test results do not contribute significantly to understanding the child's CVI visual impairment. Visual acuity testing using high-contrast grating stimuli, done in a conscientious and careful manner with results related to age norms, arguably is the most useful behavioral measure of spatial vision possible in clinical settings for children with CVI.

Functional Visual Behaviors Additional visual behaviors that contribute to understanding of the child's visual impairment are broadly defined as "functional vision." These include informal observations of the child's visual and visual motor skills, for example, visual behaviors while reaching for objects, stringing beads, matching and fitting puzzle pieces, and drawing and copying. Observing how the child attends and scans pictures in books, whether and how accurate the child points to images in pictures, how they attend to their own and others' images in a mirror, and whether they make eye contact with examiners and others provides important information about visual attention and visual–perceptual abilities. Observing the child moving around in the examining room and in the hallway provides clues to visually guided mobility. These observations are augmented by neurologic examinations, neuropsychological evaluations, Roman-Lantzy CVI assessments, Dutton CVI inventory responses, discussed below, and evaluations by the child's TVI and O&M specialist (26,46).

CASE EXAMPLES

The following two cases are emblematic of the extremes which constitute the range of patients with CVI. The first case is of a child with low cognitive and motor abilities and very limited use of vision. The second case is a highly functional individual whose career goals and independence are threatened by her previously undocumented complex visual dysfunctions.

CASE 1:

The child, age 5.5 years when assessed, had a history of neonatal sepsis and infantile spasms. His brain MRI showed severe cerebral atrophy. Walking was delayed; language and other cognitive abilities were limited. Ocular status included a variable angle exotropia, wandering gaze, and significant hyperopia. Retinae and optic nerves were normal. Spectacles were well tolerated. His family and educators wondered how useful his vision was for instruction and activities of daily living.

Significant Clinical Findings With correction and both eyes open, grating visual acuity with TACII was 1.7 cycles per degree (20/360). A quiet, visually simplified environment was necessary to test his visual acuity; the acuity card was moved until he stopped his extraneous movements and attended to (without looking directly at) the grating location. His visual field, tested by confrontation using lights of different size and brightness, was severely constricted. When shown salient objects without sound and with sufficient time to respond, he rarely oriented or attended to the object. If the object made a sound or was tapped by the examiner, the child might orient toward the object, then turn away from it, and then reach for it. Usually, he would reach for or grope for the object without looking clearly on the basis of the direction of sound or where he expected the object to be. The child would then explore the object tactually and if allowed, orally. These observations indicated that vision was not a reliable source of information regarding the location (or type and nature) of objects. He used auditory and tactual cues to apprehend objects.

Notably, this child's grating acuity improved up to age 18 months and then remained unchanged. His acuity is outside the normal limits of grating acuity beyond age 6 months (40). Remarkably, he has always worn his glasses despite no measurable improvement in grating acuity or observable changes in visual function. He may benefit from the reduced need for accommodation or appreciate the magnification sufficiently to continue to wear them.

Impression Given the health of this child's eyes, as well as the severity of cerebral atrophy and severity of visual impairment despite correction for significant hyperopic refractive error, CVI is the best explanation for his visual impairment. This child is appropriate for assessment and intervention by a vision educator using the Roman-Lantzy's approach (26). The assessment component of this approach is summarized immediately after the discussion of this case.

Comments This child's ability to sustain use of vision, even in a significantly modified environment, was limited. Yet, as eye care providers, we do not have the training to determine the most appropriate sensory modalities for developing life skills, educational instruction, and the possibility of literacy. To assess these issues, a comprehensive evaluation by a qualified teacher of the visually impaired is needed that includes a learning media assessment (LMA) with emphasis on the sensory channels component (47). The LMA is a formalized approach to determining the most effective literacy media for an individual with vision impairment. The vision teacher notes how a child approaches a variety of tasks. Does the child use visual, auditory, or tactual information in different activities and in which activities does he use them? With this assessment, the TVI determines the child's preferred modality (or modalities), the synergy between modalities during the child's interactions with objects and people, and how the child can most efficiently acquire information. The outcome of this evaluation, the report of our clinical assessment, and consultation with the educational team and the child's parents will enable the best approaches for reaching life skills and educational goals.

In advocating for the child's need for vision services, the doctor can cite the evidence from the assessment to support using a modified environment when presenting visual materials. Parents and therapists are encouraged to give the child opportunities to match or name optotypes for future testing of acuity. Optimal distance for viewing visual materials can be suggested. Reporting only the child's acuity without the conditions under which it was obtained would not accurately portray how the child was using their vision. Emphasizing that the child's PLT or single optotype acuity represents significant vision impairment, although possibly not at legal blindness level, may be required to ensure that the school system provides appropriate vision services. However, the exact nature and intensity of vision services must be determined by the child's vision educators.

Roman-Lantzy Assessment and Intervention Approach Assessment and habilitation of *cortical* visual impairment have been advanced by the work of Christine Roman-Lantzy (26). Roman-Lantzy developed an instrument intended for TVIs to assess children with cortical visual impairment; this assessment tool is linked with a methodology for intervention/habilitation (26). It provides the TVI with a semiquantitative means of monitoring changes in behaviors and an intervention method intended to effect positive changes in these behaviors. The CVI evaluation is administered in the child's environment by a trained TVI. The child's visual behaviors are scored in two ways. In each of ten domains of concern (color preferences, object movement, visual latency, visual field preference, visual complexity, purposeful gaze, distance viewing, visual reflexes, visual novelty, and visually guided reach), the patient is scored from 0 to 1, in increments of 0.25. These 10 individual scores are summed and defined in discrete ranges that represent overall visual functioning. This scoring paradigm is termed the "within CVI characteristics assessment method."

A separate "across CVI characteristics assessment" is performed by grading behaviors across grouped domains outlined in a recording form. Ranges of visual function are scored from 1 to 2 which indicates "student functions with minimal visual response" to a score of 9 to 10 which means "Student spontaneously uses vision for most functional activities." This two-level scoring system allows for nonuniform domains of visual difficulties within similar CVI ranges. Roman-Lantzy's overall model of assessment is still being refined; however, it is the only quantitative and programmatic approach to intervention for children with CVI. It is currently being used by many TVIs in the United States. Roman-Lantzy's approach aids in understanding the visual behaviors of children with classically defined CVI, rather than for individuals with more complex and discrete visual–perceptual difficulties associated with post-striate brain damage, discussed below. The latter children may not have significant visual acuity deficits and may be without visual field loss and will score close to typical high levels in the Roman-Lantzy assessment. Thus, the nature and extent of their visual–perceptual dysfunctions may not be identified by the Roman-Lantzy instrument. Case 2 is an example of such a child.

CASE 2:

An 18-year-old high school senior who plans to attend college had concerns about her ability to use and sustain her vision. She reported her eyes tire easily with demanding near work, and she had difficulty walking on uneven terrains. She wondered if she could drive.

She was born at 26 weeks gestation. There was bilateral germinal matrix hemorrhage, MRI evidence of occipital and parietal volume loss (i.e., white matter loss), and evidence for encephalopathy of prematurity (6). She had hypotonia of the trunk and extremities.

Ocular history included retinopathy of prematurity (treated with laser), right eye worse than left, very high myopia and anisometropia (right eye worse), staphylomas in both eyes, right esotropia, and amblyopia (refractive and strabismic). Goldmann visual fields were constricted overall to the largest light target with the nasal field more constricted than the temporal field.

Neuropsychological evaluation found her IQ to be normal. A comprehensive driving evaluation reported that she could not relate how to handle a hypothetical event such as a tire blowout. In a driving simulator, she had great difficulty determining what to do in complex situations. The evaluator noted that "she does not have the life skills necessary to cross a street or manage her self independently at home or in the community."

Clinical Findings Corrected distance acuity with full-letter chart was right eye 20/150 and left eye 20/60. The isolated letter acuity for the left eye was 20/40 – 2. The acuity testing took 15 minutes. As testing proceeded, her skin color became pale, her voice softer, and her body position went from erect and straight to bent and twisted. A break was needed before continuing the examination. Assessment of refractive error, ocular alignment, and ocular health were consistent with the records of her long-standing ophthalmologist.

Impression This patient has several visual function deficits due to known ocular causes. Importantly, this patient would not be classified visually impaired based upon her full chart or single-letter acuity. However, given her behavior during acuity testing, the MRI findings of white matter loss and the driving evaluation, CVI was strongly suspected. To explore this possibility further, the Dutton Cerebral Visual Impairment Inventory of visual behaviors was given separately to the patient and her mother (46).

Dutton CVI Inventory This 51-item inventory is broken into seven sections, each with a different number of items. The first 13 items explore evidence of visual field impairment or impaired visual attention on one side. The next five items seek evidence of impaired perception of movement. Nine items then ask about potential visual difficulties in complex environments. Another nine items question impairment of visually guided movement of the body and further evidence of visual field impairment. Four items seek evidence of impaired visual attention. Another four items seek evidence of behavioral difficulties associated with crowded environments. The final seven items evaluate the ability to recognize what is being looked at and to navigate. These latter seven items appear to assess the ventral stream, while the previous 44 items assess dorsal stream behaviors. Each behavior is scored as *never, rarely, sometimes, often, always*, or *not applicable.*

The mother and patient in the case described above, responded as either *often* or *always* on 26 of the 44 dorsal stream items. This is an extraordinary level of agreement for significant dorsal stream problems with this inventory. Examples of agreement include issues with impaired perception of movement (3/5 items), difficulty with complex visual scenes (6/9 items), difficulty in crowded environments (3/4 items), and impaired visual attention (3/4 items). However, they completely disagreed regarding ventral stream items with the patient indicating significant concerns and her mother none or minor concerns. For example, the patient noted that identifying known people was always a problem, yet her mother reported the opposite.

For years, the patient and her mother were told by eye doctors and educators that her mildly reduced acuity was not impeding academic pursuits and was not contributing to symptomatology. However, she clearly had complex visual difficulties which now can be classified as CVI—dorsal plus ventral dysfunction. Considering her difficulties, we advocated for a community-based functional vision assessment by a qualified TVI in addition to an LMA (47). Further, we strongly recommended she has an assessment by an O&M instructor to assess her ability to travel in familiar and unfamiliar environments of varying complexity. As a result, this patient is receiving some services and accommodations that enable her to succeed in a local community college. A driver's license is not being pursued at the current time.

CONCLUSION

Cortical or cerebral visual impairment is the most common type of vision impairment in the developed world (3,4). It is present in children with other disabling conditions and can coexist with other causes of visual impairment (i.e., ocular and ocular motor). Varying levels of cognitive and motor factors as well as other sensory problems can make the determination of CVI even more difficult. Flexibility during the evaluation is critical. The data collected, the methods of testing, and the patient's responses are important to state in the report. These observations can aid the child's educational team and therapists in understanding how the child is best able to use vision, and how long vision can be sustained under optimal conditions. Aside from using results obtained from other professionals, the report often uses evidence from the evaluation to recommend additional assessments or to provide input regarding visual considerations for educational placement. This type of collaborative care is necessary for assuring proper diagnosis and for the development of an integrated treatment plan.

Spectacles are an important consideration. However, a poor fit or tactile defensiveness could cause rejection of spectacles. Proper frame selection and/or desensitization training may be necessary before deciding on the functional impact of spectacles. Plus for near as well as prisms for visual field expansion should be considered. Inferior field defects are a contraindication for bifocals. Maximizing of visual function is aided by treating ocular and ocular motor disorders, if possible, as well as by providing compensatory strategies. Vision therapy for habilitation of dorsal and or ventral dysfunction has not been well established and is an area of opportunity. Some elements of Chapters 24, Neuroplasticity and 25 Optometric Management of Functional Vision Disorders may be appropriate for consideration with patients with CVI.

Except for Dr. Roman-Lantzy's CVI approach which follows definite protocols, intervention, generally speaking, is presently geared toward compensatory strategies (26,34,48–52). Examples include a child who has difficulty finding a toy in a toy box might have an easier time if toys were stored linearly and neatly on shelves rather than in a crowded box. An individual who gets lost easily in crowded places may benefit from training to preview the space so that landmarks can be identified for future encounters. A child who cannot identify people by sight may benefit from a person verbally self-identifying, or the child could be taught to identify the person by specific features that are vocalized in singsong ("She's the lady with white hair who wears pink glasses!").

This brief overview of visual impairment secondary to brain damage is intended to provide the reader with the range of issues surrounding the identification and evaluation of children with visual and other impairments. Parents and caregivers of children with complex medical, sensory, and motor problems who also have poorly understood visual impairments benefit from the information on probable causes of visual impairment. Once these issues are identified and described by the eye practitioner, caregivers are given appropriate recommendations for the child's educational and therapeutic team which optimally lead to the best educational practices and maximal habilitation.

ACKNOWLEDGMENT *Darick W. Wright, M.Ed., COMS, CLVT, is a key member of our evaluative team and, though not an author, is a vital contributor to our understanding of our patients.*

REFERENCES

1. Soul J, Matsuba C. Causes of damage to the visual brain: common aetiologies of cerebral vision impairment. In: Dutton GN, Bax M, editors. Clinics in developmental medicine no. 186: visual impairment in children due to damage to the brain. London: Mac Keith Press; 2010. p. 20–6.
2. Flodmark O, Jacobson L. Pathogenesis and imaging of disorders affecting the visual brain. In: Dutton GN, Bax M, editors. Clinics in developmental medicine no. 186: visual impairment in children due to damage to the brain. London: Mac Keith Press; 2010. p. 50–66.
3. Gogate P, Gilbert C. Blindness in children: a worldwide perspective. Community Eye Health. 2007;20:32–3.
4. World Health Organization. Childhood blindness. Available from: www.who.int/blindness/causes/priority/en/index4.html. Last Accessed March 11, 2011.
5. Hoyt CS. Visual function in the brain-damaged child. Eye. 2003;17:369–84.
6. Volpe JJ. Brain injury in premature infants: a complex amalgam of destructive and developmental disturbances. Lancet Neurol. 2009;8:110–24.
7. Khwaja O, Volpe JJ. Pathogenesis of cerebral white matter injury of prematurity. Arch Dis Child Fetal Neonatal Ed. 2008;93:F153–61.
8. Dutton G, Jacobson L. Cerebral visual impairment in children. Semin Neonatol. 2001;6:477–85.
9. Jacobson L, Hellstrom A, Flodmark O. Large cups in normal-sized optic discs: a variant of optic nerve hypoplasia in children with periventricular leukomalacia. Arch Ophthalmol. 1997;115:1263–9.

10. Jacobson L, Hard AL, Svensson E, et al. Optic disc morphology may reveal timing of insult in children with periventricular leukomalacia and/or periventricular haemorrhage. Br J Ophthalmol. 2003;87:1345–9.
11. Brodsky MC. Periventricular leukomalacia and intracranial cause of pseudoglaucomatous cupping. Arch Ophthalmol. 2001;119:626–7.
12. Schmahmann JD. Disorders of the cerebellum: ataxia, dysmetria of thought, and the cerebellar cognitive affective syndrome. J Neuropsychiatry Clin Neurosci. 2004;16:367–78.
13. Volpe JJ. Cerebellum of the premature infant: rapidly developing, vulnerable, clinically important. J Child Neurol. 2009;24:1085–104.
14. Schmahmann JD, Sherman JC. The cerebellar cognitive affective syndrome. Brain. 1998;121:561–79.
15. Whiting S, Jan JE, Wong PK, et al. Permanent cortical visual impairment in children. Dev Med Child Neurol. 1985;27:730–39.
16. Lambert SR, Hoyt CS, Jan JE, et al. Visual recovery from hypoxic cortical blindness during childhood. Computed tomographic and magnetic resonance imaging predictors. Arch Ophthalmol. 1987;105:1371–7.
17. Huo R, Burden S, Hoyt CS, et al. Chronic cortical visual impairment in children: etiology, prognosis, and associated deficits. Br J Ophthalmol. 1999;83:670–5.
18. Good WV, Jan JE, deSa L, et al. Cortical visual impairment in children: a major review. Surv Ophthalmol. 1994;38:351–64.
19. Cioni G, Fazzi B, Coluccini M, et al. Cerebral visual impairment in preterm infants with periventricular leukomalacia. Pediatr Neurol. 1997;17:331–8.
20. Dutton GN, Saaed A, Fahad B, et al. Association of binocular lower field VF impairment, impaired simultaneous perception, disordered visually guided motion and inaccurate saccades in children with cerebral visual dysfunction: a retrospective study. Eye. 2004;18:27–34.
21. Gillen JA, Dutton GN. Balint's syndrome in a 10 year old male. Dev Med Child Neurol 2003;45:349–52.
22. MacDonald I. Gordon Holmes lecture: Gordon Holmes and the neurological heritage. Brain. 2007;130:288–98.
23. Hatton DD, Schwietz E, Boyer B, et al. Babies Count: the national registry for children with visual impairments, birth to 3 years. JAAPOS. 2007;11:351–5.
24. Dennison E, Hall-Lueck A, editors. Proceedings of the summit on cerebral/cortical visual impairment: educational, family and medical perspectives, April 30, 2005. New York, NY: AFB Press; 2006.
25. Dutton GN, Bax M, editors. Clinics in developmental medicine no. 186: visual impairment in children due to damage to the brain. London: Mac Keith Press; 2010.
26. Roman-Lanzky C. Cortical visual impairment: an approach to assessment and intervention. New York, NY: AFB Press; 2007.
27. Jan JE, Groenveld M. Visual behaviors and adaptations associated with cortical and ocular impairment in children. J Vis Imp Blind. 1993;87:101–5.
28. Jan JE, Groenveld M, Sykanda AM. Light gazing by visually impaired children. Dev Med child Neurol. 1990;32:755–9.
29. Jan JE, Wong PEKH. The child with cortical visual impairment. Semin Ophthalmol. 1991;6:194–200.
30. Matsuba C, Soul J. Clinical manifestations of cerebral visual impairment. In: Dutton GN, Bax M, editors. Clinics in developmental medicine no. 186: visual impairment in children due to damage to the brain. London: Mac Keith Press; 2010. p. 41–9.
31. Goodale MA, Milner AD. Sight unseen: an exploration of conscious and unconscious vision. Oxford: Oxford University Press; 2004.
32. Dutton GN. Cognitive vision, its disorders and differential diagnosis in adults and children; knowing where and what things are. Eye. 2003;17:289–304.
33. Holmes G. Disturbances of visual orientation. Br J Ophthalmol. 1918;2:449–68, 506–16.
34. McKillop E, Dutton GN. Impairment in children due to damage in the brain: a practical approach. Br Ir Orthopt J. 2008;5:8–14.
35. Farah MJ. Visual agnosia. 2nd ed. Cambridge: MIT Press; 2004.
36. Dutton GN. Email communication. January 23, 2011.
37. Lam FC, Lovett F, Dutton GN. Cerebral visual impairment in children: a longitudinal case study. Outcomes beyond the visual acuities. J Vis Imp Blind. 2010;104:625–35.
38. Dutton GN. "Dorsal stream dysfunction" and "dorsal stream dysfunction plus" a potential classification for perceptual vision impairment in the context of cerebral vision impairment? Dev Med Child Neurol. 2009;51:170–2.
39. Colenbrander G. Towards the development of a classification of vision-related functioning—a potential framework. In: Dutton GN, Bax M, editors. Clinics in developmental medicine no. 186: visual impairment in children due to damage to the brain. London: Mac Keith Press; 2010. p. 282–94.
40. Teller DY, Dobson V, Mayer DL. Teller acuity cards II handbook. Chicago: Stereo Optical Company, Inc.; 2005.
41. Johnson C, Kran BS, Deng L, Mayer DL. Teller II and Cardiff Acuity testing in school-age deafblind population. Optom Vis Sci. 2009;86:188–95.
42. Fulton AB, Hansen RM, Moskowitz A. Assessment of vision in infants and young children. In: Celesia CG, editor. Disorders of visual processing handbook of clinical neurophysiology. vol. 5. New York: Elsevier BV; 2005. p. 203–30.
43. Good WV, Fulton AB. Impairments of central visual function and its measurement. In: Dutton GN, Bax M, editors. Clinics in developmental medicine no. 186: visual impairment in children due to damage to the brain. London: Mac Keith Press; 2010. p. 77–84.
44. Mayer DL, Fulton AB. Visual fields. In: Hoyt C, Taylor D, editors. Pediatric ophthalmology and strabismus. London: Elsevier Science Ltd.; 2004.
45. Jacobson L, Flodmark O, Martin L. Visual field defects in prematurely born patients with white matter damage of immaturity: a multiple-case study, Acta Ophthalmol Scand. 2006;84:357–62.
46. Dutton GN, Calvert J, Ibrahim H, et al. Impairment of cognitive vision: its detection and measurement: structured clinical history-taking for cognitive and visual perceptual dysfunction and for profound visual disabilities due to damage to the brain in children. In: Dutton GN, Bax M, editors. Clinics in developmental medicine no. 186: visual impairment in children due to damage to the brain. London: Mac Keith Press; 2010.

47. Koenig AJ, Holbrook MC. Learning Media Assessment of students with visual impairments. A resource guide for teachers. 2nd ed. Austin: Texas School for the Blind and Visually Impaired; 1995.
48. Dutton GN, Cockburn D, McDaid G, et al. Practical approaches for the management of visual problems due to cerebral visual impairment. In: Dutton GN, Bax M, editors. Clinics in developmental medicine no. 186: visual impairment in children due to damage to the brain. London: Mac Keith Press; 2010. p. 217–26.
49. Buultjens M, Hyvärinen L, Walthes R, et al. Strategies to support the development and learning of children with cerebral visual impairment at home and at school: communication, orientation and mobility. In: Dutton GN, Bax M, editors. Clinics in developmental medicine no. 186: visual impairment in children due to damage to the brain. London: Mac Keith Press; 2010. p. 227–336.
50. Buultjens M, Hyvärinen L, Walthes R. Approaches to the management in schools of visual problems due to cerebral visual impairment. In: Dutton GN, Bax M, editors. Clinics in developmental medicine no. 186: visual impairment in children due to damage to the brain. London: Mac Keith Press; 2010. p. 236–44.
51. Aitken S. Strategies to help children who have both visual and hearing impairments. In: Dutton GN, Bax M, editors. Clinics in developmental medicine no. 186: visual impairment in children due to damage to the brain. London: Mac Keith Press; 2010. p. 245–56.
52. Campbell M, Buultjens M. Setting up integrated services for children with cerebral visual impairment. In: Dutton GN, Bax M, editors. Clinics in developmental medicine no. 186: visual impairment in children due to damage to the brain. London: Mac Keith Press; 2010. p. 257–64.

CHAPTER 15

Mary Bartuccio, OD, FAAO, FCOVD
Nadine Girgis, OD, FAAO

Vision Screening

INTRODUCTION

As public awareness increases regarding eye and vision care, the need for a quick, effective, and inexpensive method to detect visual problems is mounting. Vision problems in children without special needs are frequently encountered. It has been found that 25% of school-aged children and 11.5% of teenagers have undetected or untreated vision problems (1–3). Furthermore, children aged 5 to 14 have a high prevalence of refractive error, which, if left untreated, can develop into a visual problem that affects their quality of life and school performance (4,5). In Indiana, "students who failed the vision screening in 1st grade were found to be more at risk for poorer academic performance on standardized testing in grade 3" (6). Further research indicates that there is a high prevalence of vision disorders in patients with intellectual disability (ID) as compared to the normal population (7). These disorders include strabismus, amblyopia, high refractive error, accommodative dysfunction, ocular health anomalies, visual–perceptual deficiencies, and ocular motor dysfunctions (5,8–24).

Vision screenings were created to help address this public health issue. Screenings provide an opportunity for children to be evaluated who otherwise do not have access to vision care. Nonetheless, recent research shows that it is difficult to determine if vision screenings are effective in detecting critical vision problems in children (25,26). In a recent review of the literature, Beauchamp et al. (25) found that having good vision is valuable and that vision screenings are not effective in detecting amblyopia. They noted that vision screenings are not appropriate as the sole method of detecting vision problems in children and patients with special needs.

Legislative policies regarding vision screenings are inconsistent from state to state. A vision screening can vary from simply checking visual acuity to a requirement of 11 tests including evaluation of accommodation and visual tracking (27). This lack of uniformity, in itself, can lead to undiagnosed visual problems in children.

The Special Olympics – Lions Clubs International Opening Eyes is one of the few programs that facilitates vision screenings for athletes with ID. (This topic is discussed in more detail later in this chapter.) Since patients with special needs have a high risk for developing severe visual problems, a comprehensive eye examination is essential to properly diagnose and successfully treat these conditions (7).

Inconsistencies exist within the medical community with regard to the best method for the detection of vision problems in children. Various organizations state different recommendations. According to the American Academy of Pediatrics, "Examination of the eyes should be performed beginning in the newborn period and at all well-child visits" (28). These would occur at the annual physical examination. The American Academy of Ophthalmology states, "Examination of the eyes should be performed beginning in the newborn period, and then as an infant, preschooler and school-age" (29). The American Optometric Association recommends that "Vision screening programs that are well-designed and properly administered in public or private schools should be utilized to assist in the identification of children in need of care who have not had access to comprehensive examination services" (30).

VISION SCREENING AND COMPREHENSIVE EYE EXAMINATIONS: NOT THE SAME

The purpose of a vision screening program is to "help identify children or adults who may have undetected vision problems and refer them for further evaluation" (30). More specifically, Blum defines a school screening by its principal objective: "to detect children who have vision problems or potential vision problems that affect physiologic or perceptual processes of vision and to find those who have vision problems that interfere with performance in school" (31). Due to monetary constraints, lay personnel often conduct the vision screening instead of a well-trained eye care professional. In addition, the environment is usually not well controlled and the lighting or other aspects of the setting may not be appropriate. Furthermore, a vision screening is not diagnostic; only part of the visual system is being assessed and conclusions cannot be derived from that minimal data.

It should be recognized that the public perceives that passing a vision screening guarantees that the child has no visual problems. Parents also falsely assume that the screening is a complete eye examination (32). This lack of public awareness of the problems associated with vision screenings results in even more children who are not being appropriately diagnosed and treated (33).

Vision screenings do not typically occur in children under three years of age. Only 66% of children 3 to 5 years of age are screened (usually using some type of visual acuity measurement) at the pediatrician's office (34). The AOA created the InfantSEE program providing free comprehensive eye examinations for any infant 6 to 12 months of age to address this glaring need in the community (30).

There are specific guidelines to follow when establishing a vision screening (Table 15.1). It is important to keep in mind that there are numerous screening batteries that can conform to these guidelines. However, a screening test should be simple, rapid, inexpensive, safe, and acceptable (35).

The greatest concern when conducting a vision screening is low sensitivity. This results in undiagnosed vision problems and underreferrals. Failure to identify children who need further attention jeopardizes the effectiveness and credibility of any screening endeavor and will result in hidden costs to the community. During a vision screening, patients with special needs may not respond well or may not understand the instructions of the test, making it very difficult to assess their visual status. Therefore, a comprehensive eye examination conducted by a well-trained eye care professional is essential in evaluating and treating the visual needs of these high-risk patients (7).

TABLE 15.1 Guidelines for a Vision Screening

The condition sought should be an important health problem.

1. There should be an accepted treatment for patients with recognized disease.
2. Facilities for diagnosis and treatment should be available.
3. There should be a recognizable latent or early symptomatic stage.
4. There should be a suitable test or examination.
5. The test should be acceptable to the population.
6. The natural history of the condition, including development from latent to declared disease, should be adequately understood.
7. There should be an agreed policy on whom to treat as patients.
8. The cost of case finding (including diagnosis and treatment of patients diagnosed) should be economically balanced in relation to possible expenditures on medical care as a whole.
9. Case finding should be continuing process and not a "once-and-for-all" project.

Wilson JMG, Jungner F. Principle in practice of screening for disease. In: Public Health papers, no.34. Geneva: World Health Organization; 1968.

Vision Screening Batteries

The Orinda Study In the 1950s, this multidisciplinary vision screening battery was designed to minimize overreferral by creating "the least expensive, least technical and most efficient screening program for finding essentially all elementary-school children with vision problems" (36). This study involved the administration of six different screening batteries followed by a comprehensive eye examination on children that failed the screening. Through comparison of the data of 3,889 children screened, the modified clinical technique (MCT), consisting of distance visual acuity, near cover test, retinoscopy, and ocular health assessment (Table 15.2), effectively identified 96% of children with visual problems and 98% of those without (32). This study also determined that less than half the children with vision problems were detected using only Snellen visual acuity testing (37). The high direct cost of this screening resulted from the salaries of optometrists; however, the lower indirect cost to the community was offset as fewer underreferrals were guaranteed (32). Today, the high direct cost of the MCT is the main reason for underutilization of this technique (31).

The New York State Optometric Association Battery In the 1980s, the New York State Optometric Association (NYSOA) investigated the relationship between vision problems and learning (38). The testing battery used assessed visual skills in

TABLE 15.2 Clinical Procedures and Referral Criteria for MCT

Testing Procedure	Characteristic Measured	Criteria of Referral
Snellen distance visual acuity	Visual acuity	20/40 or less, either eye
Retinoscopy with lens rack neutralization	Refractive error:	
	Hyperopia	+1.50 DS or more
	Myopia	−0.50 DS or more
	Astigmatism	± 1.00 DC or more
	Anisometropia	± 1.00 D or more
Distance cover test	Coordination at distance:	
	Tropia	Any tropia
	Esophoria	5^ or more
	Exophoria	5^ or more
	Hyperphoria	2^ or more
Nearpoint cover test	Coordination at distance:	
	Tropia	Any tropia
	Esophoria	6^ or more
	Exophoria	10^ or more
	Hyperphoria	2^ or more
Observation and direct ophthalmoscopy	Organic	Any verified pathology or medical anomaly of the eye and/or adnexa

Adapted from Blum H, Peters HB, Betterman JW. Vision screening for elementary schools: the Orinda study. Berkeley: University of California Press; 1959.

relation to school performance, whereas the Orinda study did not. However, the NYSOA battery was time consuming. After receiving 2 to 3 hours of training, parent volunteers administered the nine clinical techniques described in Table 15.3 (39). A referral criterion can also be found in this table (38). The vision screening battery's specificity (ability to detect children with vision problems) was 72%, much lower than the Orinda study, as was the specificity (65%) (40).

The Vision in Preschoolers Battery The vision in preschoolers (VIP) study is an ongoing multiphase, multicenter, multidiscipline, clinical investigation to evaluate the accuracy of screening tests used to identify preschool-aged children in need of further evaluation for vision disorders (41–43). The primary goal of the VIP study is to determine whether there are tests or combinations of tests, which can be used effectively to determine which preschoolers would benefit from a comprehensive eye examination to detect amblyopia, strabismus, significant refractive errors, and other associated risk factors (41–43). The study compared 11 screening tests and used laypersons, pediatric nurses, pediatric optometrists, and pediatric ophthalmologists. During the three phases of the study, it was found that nurses and laypeople have the same reliability when administering the screening tests (43). Also, of the 11 screening tests, the 4 most sensitive tests (with 90% specificity) were noncycloplegic retinoscopy, Lea symbols for visual acuity testing, Welch Allyn Suresight Vision Screener, and Retinomax autorefractor (41,42). Vision in preschoolers found that a vision screening, administered by an eye care professional, must include a unilateral cover test and autorefraction in order to maintain high sensitivity and specificity for strabismus. However, if a layperson is performing a strabismic sensitive screening, the Stereosmile II and the Suresight tests must be performed together. Other combinations of tests will not increase the sensitivity and specificity for strabismus (41–43). This study has not been completed and will further enhance this area of research in the future.

VISION REGULATIONS AND LEGISLATIVE POLICIES IN THE UNITED STATES

Universal comprehensive eye examinations would help more children succeed in school through the early detection of visual problems (6). As of 2011, only three states (Missouri, Kentucky, and Illinois) mandate comprehensive eye evaluations for children, 27 require vision screenings only and five require vision screening and follow-up. Unfortunately, 10 states do not mandate any form of vision assessment (Fig. 15-1) (44,45). With recent studies indicating a high incidence of vision problems (4–6), more states should be mandating vision care requirements for all children, especially those with physical, mental, and intellectual disabilities.

Some states have begun to develop improved guidelines for children in special education programs. Iowa and Delaware both require that children in special education programs undergo a vision screening. In addition, Ohio has regulations that require children with disabilities to have an examination with an optometrist or fully trained physician (45). Due to the constantly changing state regulations regarding vision requirements, every eye care professional should make a point to review the guidelines in the states in which they have licensure.

TABLE 15.3 Clinical Procedures and Referral Criteria for the NYSOA Screening Battery

Test	Condition Screened	Criteria for Referral
Snellen chart—20 ft.	Myopia, high astigmatism, amblyopia, high hyperopia	20/40 or worse in either eye or more than 2 line difference between the eyes.
Reduced Snellen chart—13 ft.	High refractive error, focus dysfunction	Same as above
+1.50 sphere VA test—20 ft.	Mild hyperopia	Less than 2 line blur of the best distance acuity
+/-2.00 flippers—13 ft.	Accommodative facility, focus ability	Less than 3 cycles in 30 s.
Bell push up	Convergence ability	4 ft. or greater
Keystone skills		
(a) vertical imbalance	Suppression, fusion ability, muscle balance	Line through any figure other than ball
		2 or 4 balls
(b) 4 ball fusion—distance		2 or 4 balls
(c) 4 ball fusion—near		
Titmus stereo tests	Stereopsis perception, binocularity	7 or less
NYSOA K-D	Eye tracking skills	Greater than 1 standard deviation above age norms in the NYSOA manual
Winterhaven copy forms	Eye–hand coordination, visual motor coordination, visual organization, form reproduction	Less than age norms in the NYSOA manual
Keystone color card	Color deficiency	Failure to read numbers

From Cohen AH, Lieberman S, Stolzberg, et al. The NYSOA vision screening battery: a total approach. J Am Optom Assoc. 1983;54:981. Copyright 1983 by the American Optometric Association, reprinted with permission.

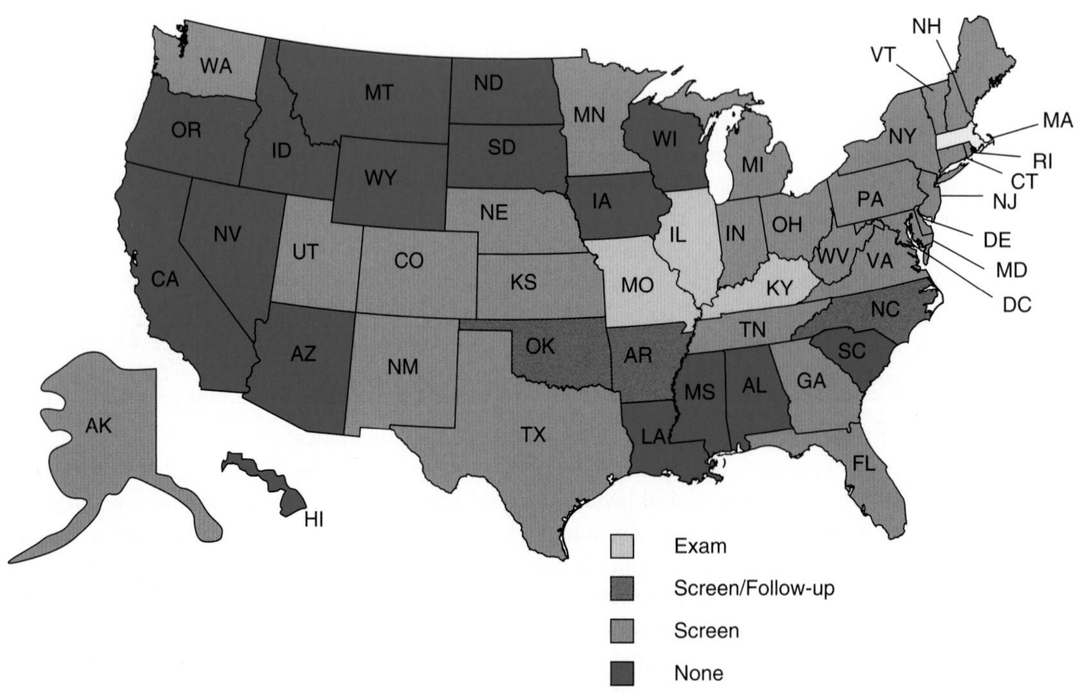

FIGURE 15-1. State preventive vision care requirements for children, United States, 2007 (See also Color Section). (Reprinted from Abt Associates. Building a comprehensive child vision care system: a Report of the National Commission on Vision and Health. Alexandria, VA, June 2009.)

The United States Preventative Services Task Force (USPSTF) is a major authority on clinical recommendations that strongly influence policy makers and insurance company payers. The USPSTF recently reported that it "recommends vision screening for all children at least once between the ages three and five years, to detect the presence of amblyopia or its risk factors" (46). In addition, it also "concludes that current evidence is insufficient to assess the balance of benefits and harms of vision screening for children" (46). However, no recommendation was made for children less than 3 years of age. According to the AOA, this was "based on the misguided belief that infants and young children cannot be examined due to 'the child's inability to cooperate.' The USPSTF's action will cause harm to the efforts of eye doctors nationwide to reverse the high rate of preventable vision loss in children from the first year of life through age 5, a widely recognized public health emergency" (47).

SPECIAL OLYMPICS

In 1962, Eunice Kennedy Shriver began the first summer camp for children and adults with ID at her home in Maryland. Her vision was to create an international organization that would provide these special athletes a place to play sports, "regardless of whatever different abilities they may have" (48). In the summer of 1968, the first Special Olympic Games were held at Soldier Field in Chicago, IL. Included in these games were 1,000 athletes from the United States and Canada that competed in various track, field, and swimming events. In 1986, Special Olympics was declared an international organization by the United Nations. Over the years, the leaders of this organization realized the lack of care that existed for people with ID. They found that these athletes had a 40% greater risk for developing health problems (7). Healthy athletes became an official Special Olympics initiative, providing health care services to athletes worldwide. These services included free vision, dental and hearing screenings, injury prevention clinics, and nutrition education. Through a partnership of the Lions Club International (2001), Essilor International (2002), the Safilo group (2003), and Liberty Sport (providing education about sport-related eye injuries), the Healthy Athletes Opening Eyes program continues to grow (47). In a limited review of the data for the year 2009, 16.2% of 11,023 athletes screened had an eye health problem. These included, but were not limited to, blepharitis, conjunctivitis, corneal anomalies, pinguecula, glaucoma suspect, cataracts, pterygium, and optic nerve anomalies. It was also found that approximately 18% of examined athletes had strabismus. During a period from 1995 to 2009, over 169,265 athletes were screened and 75,126 glasses were dispensed.* This number will certainly increase as Special Olympics continues to help a greater number of these athletes.

CONCLUSION

In general, uncorrected vision problems that are not diagnosed and treated appropriately can lead to poor school performance and increased overall personal and community cost. There is a high prevalence of visual problems in patients with special needs which can affect their overall quality of life. With the exception of statistics provided by Special Olympics, there is little to no clinical research conducted to determine the benefits of vision screenings in this population. Early detection and treatment of these conditions can help prevent poor visual development, produce better outcomes, and improve quality of life. With this in mind, a system to help detect these conditions early in life is strongly advocated, especially in patients with special needs.

REFERENCES

1. Roberts J. Eye examination findings among youth aged, 12–17 years, United States. Vital and Health Statistics, Series 11, No. 155, DHEW Publication (HRA) 76-1637, Rockville, MD. November 1975.
2. Peters HB. Vision care of children in comprehensive health program. J Am Optom Assoc. 1966;37:113–s8.
3. Bloom B. Use of selective preventive care procedures United States, 1982. Vital and Health Statistics, Series 10 No.157, DHHS publication (PHS) 86-1585, Hyattville, MD. September 1986.
4. Kleinstein RN, Jones LA, Hullett S, et al. Refractive error and ethnicity in children. Arch Ophthalmol. 2003;121:1141–7.
5. Woodruff ME, Cleary TE, Bader D. The prevalence of refractive and ocular anomalies among 1942 institutionalized mentally retarded person. Am J Optom Physiol Opt. 1980; 57:70–84.

*Data provided by Sandra S. Block, Global Clinical Advisor, Special Olympics Lions Club International Opening Eyes. Dec 1, 2010.

6. Marshall EC, Meetz M, Harmon LL. Through our children's eyes—the Public health impact of the vision screening requirements for Indiana school children. Optometry. 2010;81: 71–82.
7. Woodhouse JM, Adler P, Duignan A. Vision in athletes with intellectual disabilities: the need for improved eye care. J Intellect Disabil Res. 2004;48:736–s45.
8. Maino DM. The mentally handicapped patient: a perspective. J Am Optom Assoc. 1987;58:14–7.
9. Zwaan J. Ophthalmological disorders. In: Rubin IL, Crocker AC, editors. Developmental disabilities: delivery of medical care for children and adults. Philadelphia: Lea & Febiger; 1989. p. 240–50.
10. Levy B. Incidence of oculo-visual anomalies in an adult population of mentally retarded persons. Am J Optom Physiol Opt. 1984;61:324–6.
11. Amos C. Refractive error distribution in a profoundly retarded population. Am J Optom Physiol Opt. 1976;54:234–8.
12. Green M, Courtney G. Stereoacuity in mentally retarded and intellectually normal adolescents. Am J Optom Physiol Opt. 1977;54:821–5.
13. Courtney G. Refractive errors in institutionalized mentally retarded and emotionally disturbed children. Am J Optom Physiol Opt. 1971;48:492–7.
14. Woods G. Visual problems in the handicapped child. Child Care Health Dev. 1979;5:303–22.
15. Bradley B. Differential responses in perceptual ability among mentally retarded brain-injured children. Optom Wkly. 1964;55:31–3.
16. Smith W. Visual and perceptual performances of mental retardates—preliminary report. Opt J Rev Optom. 1966;103:39–42.
17. Edwards W, Price W, Weisskopf B. Ocular findings in developmentally handicapped child. J Pediatr Ophthalmol. 1972;9:162–7.
18. Manley J, Schuldt W. The refractive state of the eye and mental retardation. Am J Optom Arch Am Acad Optom. 1970;47:236–9.
19. Tuppurainen K. Ocular findings among mentally retarded children in Finland. Acta Ophthalmol. 1983;61:634–44.
20. Mackay D, Bankhead I. Fine motor performance in subjects of subnormal, normal and superior intelligence. Aust N Z J Dev Disabil. 1985;11:143–50.
21. Crozier G. Genetic ocular disorders. Rev Optom. 1979; 116:49–53.
22. Crozier G. Genetic counseling and single gene disorders. Rev Optom. 1979;116:45–51.
23. Murphee A. Ophthalmologic signs in genetic disease. Hosp Prac. 1984;19:85–92.
24. Duckman R. Visual problems. In: Mcdonald E, editor. Treating cerebral palsy for clinicians by clinicians. Austin: Pro-Ed Inc.; 1987. p. 105–31.
25. Beauchamp GR, Ellepola C, Beauchamp C. Evidence-based medicine: the value of vision screening. Am Orthop J. 2010;60:23–7.
26. Schmucker C, Grosselfinger R, Riemsma R, et al. Effectiveness of screening preschool children for amblyopia: a systemic review. BMC Ophthalmol. 2009;9:3. Available from: http://www.biomedcentral.com/1471-2415/9/3. Last Accessed on February 20, 2011.
27. Ciner EB, Dobson V, Schmidt PP, et al. A survey of vision screening policy of preschool children in the United States. Surv Ophthalmol. 1999;43:445–57.
28. American Academy of Pediatrics. Available from: www.AAP.org. Last Accessed on October 12, 2010.
29. American Academy of Ophthalmology. Available from: www.AAO.org. Last Accessed on October 12, 2010.
30. American Optometric Association. Available from: www.AOA.org. Last Accessed on October 12, 2010.
31. Peters HB, Blum HB, Beltman JW, et al. The Orinda vision study. Am J Optom Arch Am Acad Optom. 1959; 36:455–69.
32. Mozlin R. Epidemiology of school vision screenings. J Behav Optom 2002;13:59–64.
33. Zaba J, Mozlin R, Reynolds W. Insights on the efficacy of vision examinations and vision screening for children first entering school. J Behav Optom. 2003;14:123–6.
34. Wasserman RC, Croft CA, Brotherton SE. Preschool vision screening in pediatric practice: a study from the pediatric research in office settings (PROS) network. Pediatrics. 1992;89:834–8.
35. Wilson JMG, Jungner F. Principle in practice of screening for disease. In: Public Health papers, no.34. Geneva: World Health Organization; 1968.
36. Blum HL, Peters HB, Bettman JW. Vision screening for elementary schools: the Orinda study. Berkeley: University of California Press; 1959.
37. Peters H. Vision screening with a Snellen chart. J Optom Arch Am Acad Optom. 1961;38:487–505.
38. Cohen AH, Liberman S, Stolzberg M, et al. The NYSOA vision screening battery—a total approach. J Am Optom Assoc. 1993;54:979–84.
39. Bodack MI, Chung I, Krumholtz I. An analysis of vision screening data from New York City public schools. Optometry. 2010;81:476–84.
40. Lieberman S, Cohen AH, Stolzberg M, et al. Validation study of the New York state Optometric Association (NYSOA) vision screening battery. Am J Optom Physiol Opt. 1985;62: 165–8.
41. Vision in Preschoolers (VIP). Threshold visual acuity testing using the crowded HOTV and Lea symbols acuity tests. J Pediatr Ophthalmol Strabismus. 2003;7:396–9.
42. Vision in Preschoolers (VIP). Does assessing eye alignment along with refractive error or visual acuity increase sensitivity for detection of strabismus in preschool vision screening. Invest Ophthalmol Vis Sci. 2007;48:3115–25.
43. Vision in Preschoolers (VIP). Preschool vision screening tests administered by nurse screeners compared with lay screeners in the vision in preschooler study. Invest Ophthalmol Vis Sci. 2005;46:2639–48.
44. Abt associates. Building a comprehensive child vision care system: a Report of the National Commission on Vision and Health, Alexandria, VA, June 2009.
45. Prevent blindness America: State mandated school eye exam and vision screening laws. Available from: http://www.

preventblindness.org/advocacy/StateVisionScreeningLaws 11907.pdf. Last accessed on October 2, 2010.

46. Chou R, Dana T, Bougatsos C. Screening for visual impairment in children ages 1–5 years: update for the USPSTF. Pediatrics. 2011;127:e442–79.

47. AOA response to USPSTF recommendation on children vision screening. Available from: www.aoa.org. Last accessed on March 9, 2011.

48. Special olympics. Available from: http://www.specialolympics.org/. Last accessed on October 21, 2010.

CHAPTER 16

Marc B. Taub, OD, MS, FAAO, FCOVD

Comprehensive Examination Procedures

The examination of a patient with a physical, mental, psychological, or behavioral disorder is often one of the greatest challenges any health care provider can face. As with nonhandicapped patients, every clinician has methods of obtaining the information necessary to make a proper diagnosis. A clinician must creatively alter his or her examination techniques in order to improve diagnostic and therapeutic outcomes.

Those involved in health care should not assume that the patient with special needs cannot participate in the examination sequence. Speaking directly with the patient's parent, guardian, or caretaker prior to the start of the examination will often provide useful information and a starting point for your approach to the care of your patient. Instead of relying heavily on subjective testing, you should consider using objective testing to get the best assessment of ocular health and vision function possible.

HISTORY

A clinician's preparation for a special needs patient examination ideally should begin before the patient enters the practice. Intake forms and questionnaires on the patient's social, educational, medical, and ocular history should be sent out before the appointment so that time is not spent completing this task in the office (see Chapter 30, The Optometric Practice for more detail). The information gathered in these documents not only provides insight into the patient's needs and level of functioning but also enables an efficient check-in process. The longer a patient, especially one with special needs, waits to be seen, the more nervous, agitated, and/or scared he or she might become.

An appropriate questionnaire that is both broad and specific at the same time is the College of Optometrists in Vision Development Quality of Life (COVD-QOL) questionnaire (1). Developed in 1995, it is available in a long (30 questions) or short (19 questions) form (2). The questionnaire has several benefits: (a) it has excellent test–retest reliability (3), (b) it identifies visual symptoms that are correlated with academic performance (4), (c) it is an accurate means of documenting post optometric vision therapy outcomes (5), and (d) it is effective in measuring the quality-of-life changes patients experience after vision therapy (6).

The COVD-QOL's questions cover a broad range of topics, including somatic sensation (headaches, asthenopia, pain, diplopia, dizziness, nausea, and blurry vision), physical–occupational (mobility, job, school, self-care, and ability to manage life without assistance), social interaction (personal relationships with friends, family, peers, and community), and psychological well-being (overall satisfaction with life, anxiety, memory, and self-image) (Appendix 1). In completing the COVD-QOL, the patient or his or her caregiver answers questions on a 0 to 4 scale: "always" = 4 points, "frequently" = 3 points, "occasionally" = 2 points, "seldom" = 1 point, and "never" = 0 points. The total score is obtained by summing the scores for each question. A score of >20 is indicative of a visual efficiency or vision information processing disorder (1,2).

One of the difficulties in trying to determine the level of symptoms in special needs patients is that they often do not report the symptoms. A recent study highlights the lack of visual complaints in a population ($n = 202$) with a dual diagnosis of mental illness and intellectual disability (7). These patients had a greater incidence of having an oculovisual

APPENDIX 1

COLLEGE OF OPTOMETRISTS IN VISION DEVELOPMENT QUALITY-OF-LIFE CHECKLIST QUESTIONNAIRE COVD-QOL

	NEVER	ONCE IN A LONG WHILE	SOMETIMES	A LOT	ALWAYS
1. Headaches with near work					
2. Words run together reading					
3. Burn, itch, watery eyes					
4. Skips/repeats lines reading					
5. Head tilt/close one eye when reading					
6. Difficulty copying from chalkboard					
7. Avoids near work/reading					
8. Omits small words when reading					
9. Writes up/down hill					
10. Misaligns digits/columns numbers					
11. Reading comprehension down					
12. Holds reading too close					
13. Trouble keeping attention on reading					
14. Difficulty completing assignments on time					
15. Always says "I can't" before trying					
16. Clumsy, knocks things over					
17. Does not use his/her time well					
18. Loses belongings/things					
19. Forgetful/poor memory					

X1 ______ X2 ______ X3 ______ X4 ______
TOTAL SCORE ____________

anomaly (8–14) and were using medications, including antipsychotics, antidepressants, anticonvulsants, and major tranquilizers/anxiolytics. These have been shown to produce a significant number of visually related side effects (15–17). Only 50% of patients in the study who should have complained of visual symptoms actually did so. Some explanations for this phenomenon include lack of verbal communication between the patient (7) and caregiver and perhaps a greater tolerance to pain (15). With or without an indication of visual symptoms from the patient, a clinician must rely on subjective (either the patient's or caretaker's observations) and objective examination data to determine the proper treatment.

Prior to the examination, you should acquire information from the patient's other medical, educational, rehabilitative, and eye care specialists. The patient's physician can provide information concerning systemic anomalies and any functional limitations, while occupational, physical, speech, and language therapists provide information about the individual's developmental, perceptual, speech/oral and gross/fine motor capabilities. Other rehabilitation/educational specialists can provide insights into the presence of any unusual head tilts/turns, unusual body postures, illumination requirements, and educational issues.

When assessing medical history, note any ocular or systemic medications and the length of time they have been taken. Being familiar with commonly used medications and their side effects is important due to the secondary visual side effects that can occur. Antiseizure medications, such as divalproex sodium (Depakote), have been reported to cause visual hallucinations, nystagmus, and subconjunctival or retinal hemorrhages. Some central nervous system (CNS) agents used to treat anxiety, such as alprazolam (Xanax), have been reported to cause blurred vision and color vision defects. Antipsychotic and antiseizure agents, when taken over a long period of time, can produce significant ocular side effects including stellate cataracts, paralysis of extraocular muscles, pigmentary deposits on the cornea, and glaucoma (18). Despite the prevalence of ocular symptoms, it is important to remember that patients with special needs are less likely to report visually related symptoms secondary to these potent medications (7).

VISUAL ACUITY ASSESSMENT

Although in many ways visual acuity may be the least important finding from a comprehensive eye and vision examination, it is the one item all parents, teachers, and other professionals will immediately want to know. Determining visual acuity in a patient with multiple disabilities can prove to be a daunting task. The optotype that will be used to assess the patient's acuity depends on the developmental age and ability to respond verbally and physically. The clinician should choose the appropriate test based on the patient's history (19). The clinician should also realize when assessment methodologies are not providing the information being sought and then be able to switch to an alternative procedure in order to maintain the patient's cooperation.

In a traditional examination, visual acuity is performed immediately following the history. When working with patients with special needs, a clinician should consider performing visual acuity testing during the middle of the examination because of the potentially excessive amount of time it may take to complete. If performed immediately at the beginning of the examination, the patient may lose focus or become tired or anxious, which could affect his or her ability to complete the examination.

In attempting to determine a patient's visual acuity, a clinician should keep in mind that a measure of visual acuity is nothing more than a certain sized object seen at a particular distance. If the size of the object and the distance between the patient and the object are known, then the clinician can measure a visual angle in minutes of arc and convert it to visual acuity or adapt an existing visual acuity tool to the situation. Clinicians should feel free to alter the testing parameters if the patient performs at a higher level when te testing procedure is altered. It is always important, however, to note the changed testing parameters in the record.

Snellen Acuity Test Snellen acuity is an identification visual acuity task and is based on a minimum angle of resolution. The typical Snellen optotype has a particular, simple geometry in which the thickness of the lines equals the thickness of the white spaces between lines and the thickness of the gap in the letter (Fig. 16-1). For example, with the Landolt C, the width and gap of the "C" are identical; the height of the "C" is five times this amount. Snellen acuity can be successfully administered to patients with a developmental age of at least 5 or 6 years. It should not be performed at an earlier age as it is difficult to gauge whether patients can't see it or that they simply do not know their letters. The advantage of Snellen acuity testing with special needs patients is that practitioners are comfortable using the test. In addition, Snellen acuity tests are generally accessible and well standardized. Besides letter recognition issues, one other major disadvantage is that special needs patients may not comprehend looking into a mirror (if the examination room is <20 ft long).

HOTV Test The HOTV test (20) is appropriate for patients with developmental ages of about 2½ to 5 years of age. Four letters (H, O, T, and V) are used in the chart (Fig. 16-2). The test is performed at 10 ft and is administered similarly to Snellen acuity. It comes with a near card, so patients can match the letters at distance by pointing to the corresponding letter on the near card. By using only four optotypes and allowing the patient to point at a matching shape, letter recognition issues are eliminated. The letters chosen are symmetrical around the vertical axis, which avoids left–right confusion. Unfortunately, the symbols do not blur equally, so it may be possible for patients to identify even blurred letters correctly, allowing them to guess. The HOTV test has been shown to have testability rates comparable to the Tumbling E (21) and Lea symbol tests (22,23). The Tumbling E test, however, has been shown to have better test–retest reliability and validity than the HOTV (22). Several studies with subjects aged 3 to 5 years also noted that testability increased as the subject's age increased (22,23).

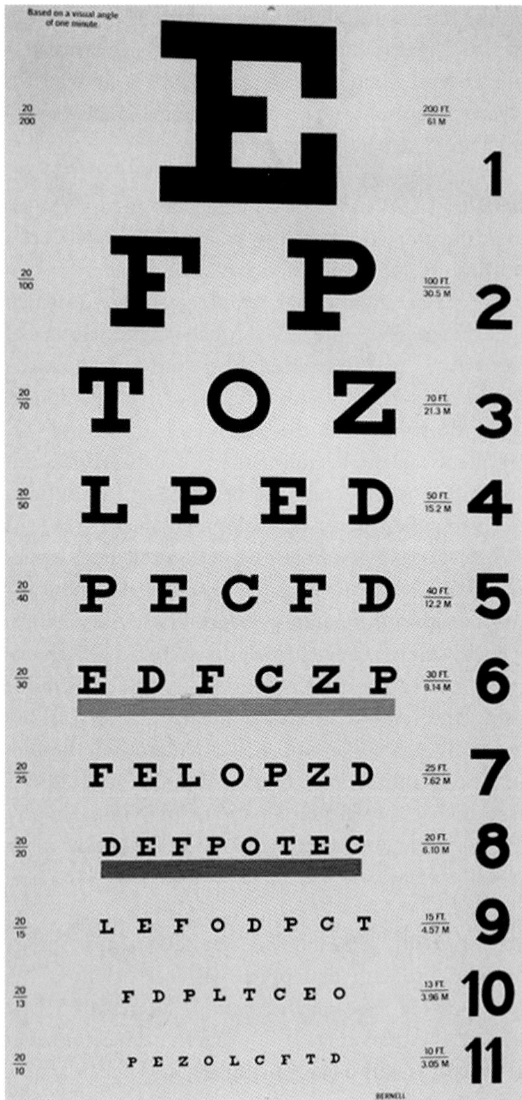

A

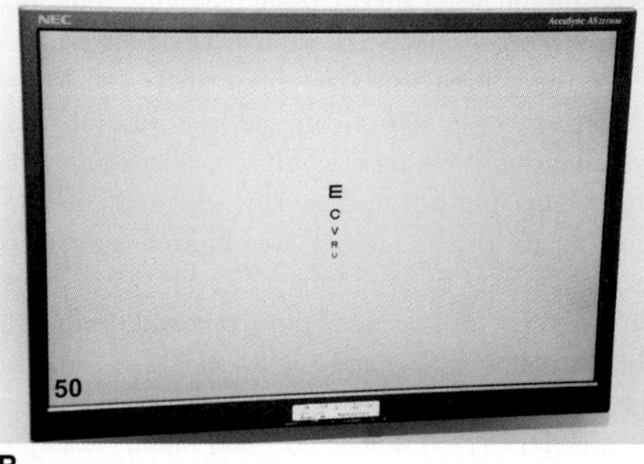

B

FIGURE 16-1. **A:** A traditional Snellen acuity chart. **B:** Electronic acuity systems are becoming increasingly prevalent in the offices of vision care providers.

Lea Symbols Test The Lea symbols (24) test can be used for children between the developmental ages of 2 and 5 years and is extremely useful for nonverbal patients. Performed at 10 ft, the test contains four symbols (circle, square, house, and apple) (Fig. 16-3). Several adaptations can be made rather than having the child call out the shape that he or she sees. The child can match each symbol at a distance to a three-dimensional companion puzzle or two-dimensional picture representations at near. While many other optotypes on various charts can be guessed due to blur or shape interpretation, with Lea symbols, as the patient reaches his or her visual acuity threshold, all the symbols blur out evenly (24). This reduces the likelihood of the patient guessing each symbol correctly. The Lea symbols test is also available as a near visual acuity test.

Broken Wheel Test This test (25) is useful for children between the developmental ages of 3 and 6 years (26). It uses a picture of a car and replaces the wheels of the car with the Landolt C symbol, which is the international standard of visual acuity measurement (27). The test is performed by placing two pictures side by side, although for some children placement of the test plates vertically, one above the other, appears to make it easy to do. One picture has complete wheels, while the other has the Landolt C symbol as the wheels that have a section missing. The child is asked to point to the car with the "broken wheels" and identify the direction of the break. The child must identify three out of four presentations to receive credit for that acuity level. The test is highly sensitive and can detect subtle differences between the two eyes (28,29).

Allen Picture Chart Test The Allen picture chart, which has enjoyed unfortunate worldwide recognition and popularity, can be found in most pediatricians' offices. This chart contains line drawings of objects such as a birthday cake, hand, bird, house, rotary telephone, and army jeep (Fig. 16-4). The symbols have been criticized as archaic and abstract (28). For example, rotary phones and army jeeps are not commonly used or seen today so a patient may have trouble identifying it. Visual closure skills, which may or may not be present, are required as the gap widths are inconsistent and highly variable. This means that the visual acuity measures are inaccurate. The symbols also do not

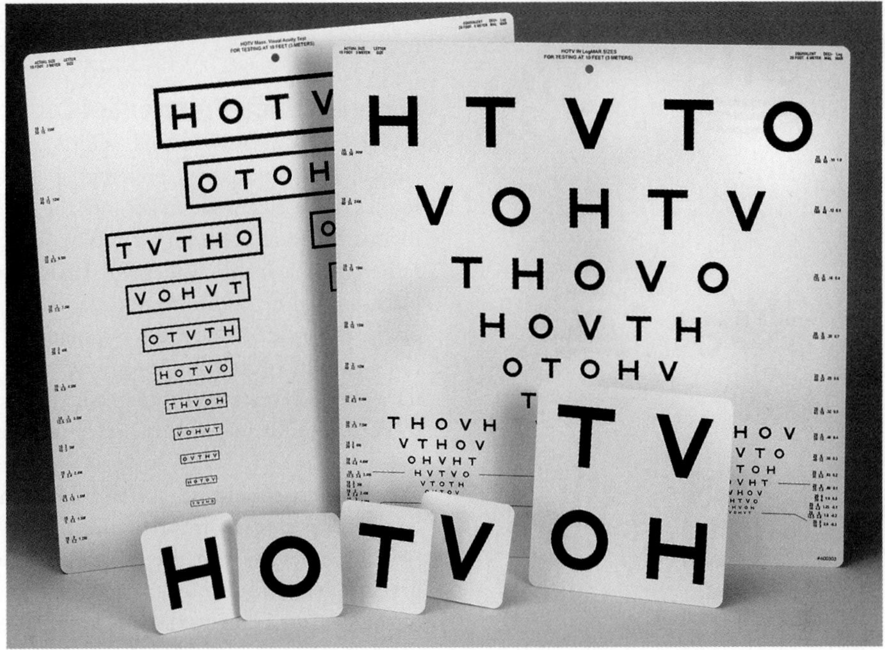

FIGURE 16-2. The HOTV test of visual acuity. (Courtesy of Good-Lite Company.)

blur out equally so patients can guess some symbols correctly (30). Another limitation of the test is that the lowest visual acuity available is 20/30. Therefore, there is no way truly to know if the patient can or cannot see 20/20.

Tumbling E Test With the Tumbling E test, the child must tell the orientation of the legs of the letter "E" (up, down, left, right) (Fig. 16-5). This test is very helpful for nonverbal children because they can point which way the "E" is oriented. However,

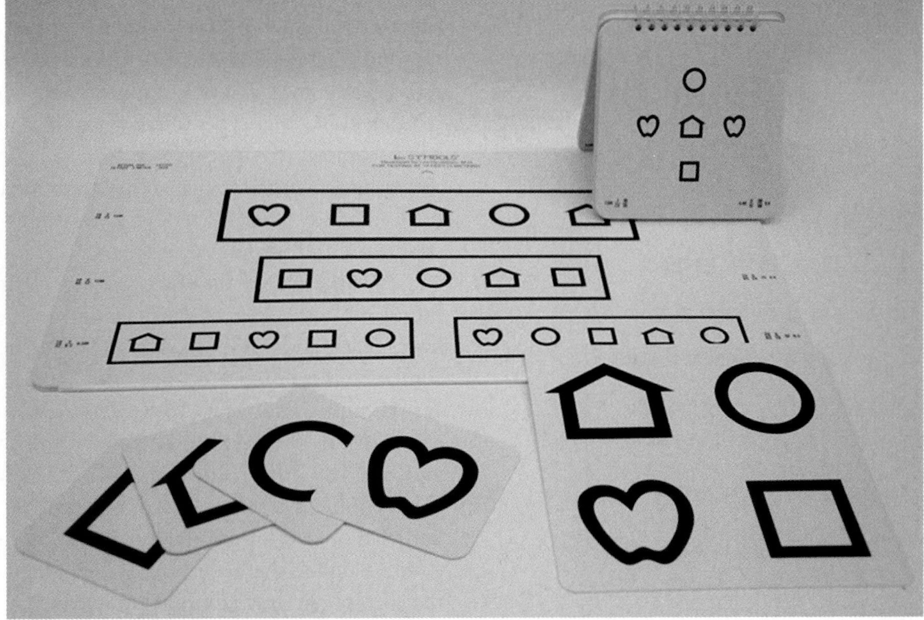

FIGURE 16-3. The Lea symbols test of visual acuity.

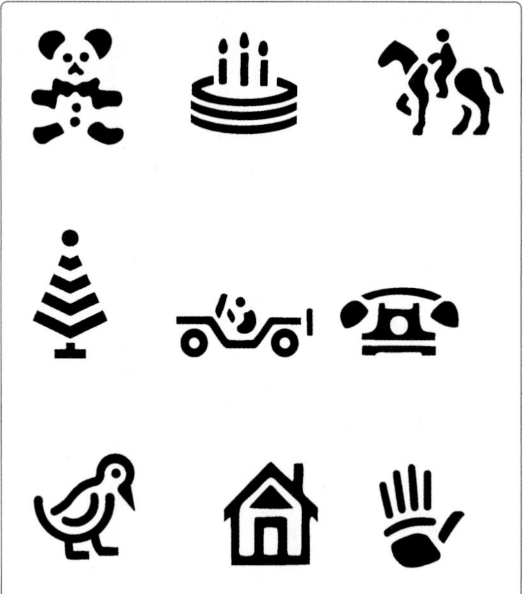

FIGURE 16-4. The Allen picture test of visual acuity. (Courtesy of Good-Lite Company.)

this may pose a problem to children who have issues with laterality and directionality (31). One proposed alteration in the procedure is to have the child point in the direction of left or right (32). The Tumbling E

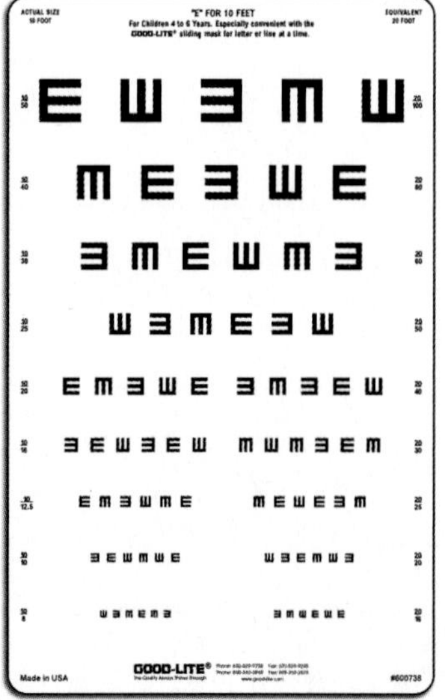

FIGURE 16-5. The Tumbling E test of visual acuity. (Courtesy of Good-Lite Company.)

is useful for children with a developmental age of 4 to 5 years (26).

Forced-choice Preferential Looking Teller acuity cards measure visual acuity using a forced choice, two-alternative preferential looking technique. This technique relies on the preference of infants to fixate bold, high-contrast stripes (grating) rather than a blank field (33). Each card contains black-and-white stripes on one side and a blank field on the other side at the mean luminance of the stripes (Fig. 16-6). This test is appropriate for developmental ages of 2 years and under and has been shown to be successful in patients under the age of 1 year (34–36).

The test should be started by holding a lower-level acuity card in front of the patient at 55 cm (which coincides with the length of the card). The practitioner looks through a small hole in the middle of the card to evaluate the direction of the patient's fixation toward one side of the card versus the other (Fig. 16-7). Pointing toward the side of the card that has the stripes is also considered a correct response. To prevent bias, the practitioner should not know the position of the stripes before it is presented to the patient. Each Teller card is presented to the patient four times with random stripe positioning. The patient receives credit for a particular acuity level only if he or she correctly identifies the correct side in three out of four presentations. To determine the patient's threshold acuity, the cards should be presented until the patient can no longer correctly respond to three out of four presentations. Keep in mind that grating acuity is not necessarily equivalent to Snellen or other types of recognition acuity. It has been reported that testing with preferential looking yields better visual acuity versus traditional identification acuity tests (37). This is especially true for strabismic amblyopes.

A variation of the Teller acuity cards can be found with the Lea or Patty Paddles. These tools have black-and-white stripes of different widths similar to the Teller cards, but have handles to allow easy administration (Fig. 16-8). The paddles are held equally from the midline in front of the child, one gray and the other with stripes. If the child is able to recognize the stripes, he or she will turn his or her head or eyes toward the movement of the striped paddle. Unlike the Teller cards, the patients can see the face of the test administrator and may become easily distracted.

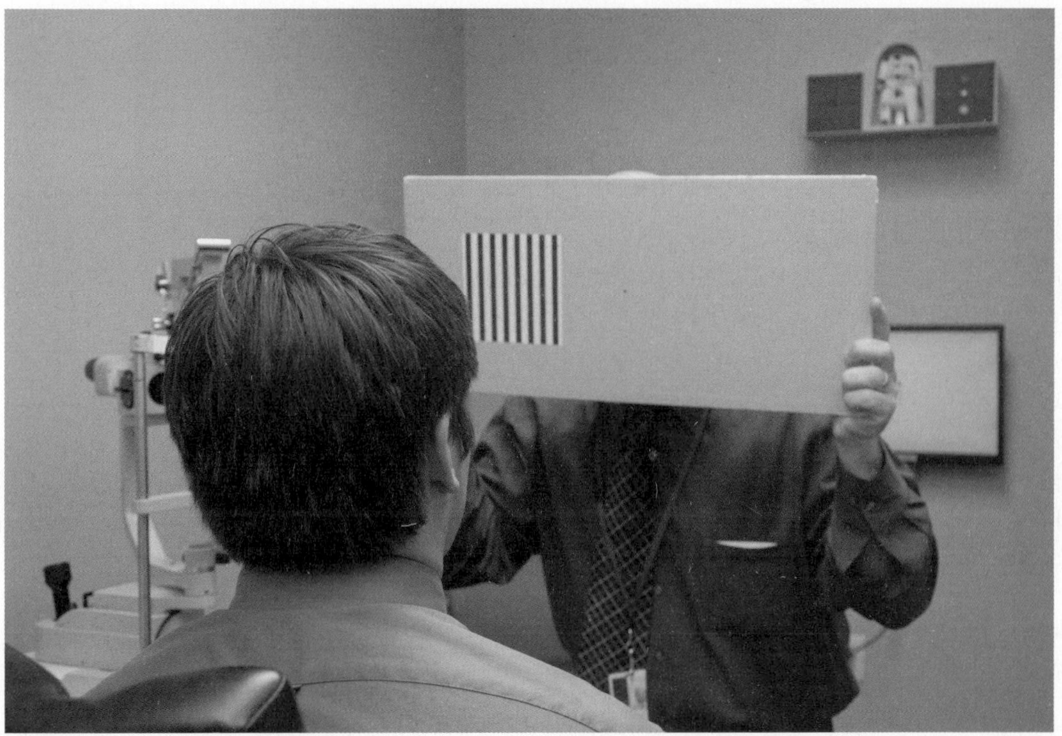

FIGURE 16-6. In the preferential looking technique using the Teller acuity cards, if the patient can see the grating pattern, he or she will look in that direction instead of the solid gray.

Cardiff Acuity Cards Cardiff acuity cards, like the Teller acuity cards, is a preferential looking test, but it uses the principle of vanishing optotypes (38,39) (Fig. 16-9). This means that the targets disappear at the patient's resolution limit. Each card contains a picture of a house, car, fish, train, dog, or duck. The pictures are in an up/down rather than a right/left separation. This makes direction of fixation easier to distinguish in cases of congenital nystagmus (29). The test also does not use a peek-hole as with Teller acuity cards, which may make fixation easier to discriminate. Similar to the Teller cards, the practitioner should not know the position of the target picture so as to be unbiased. The test is continued until the patient can no longer

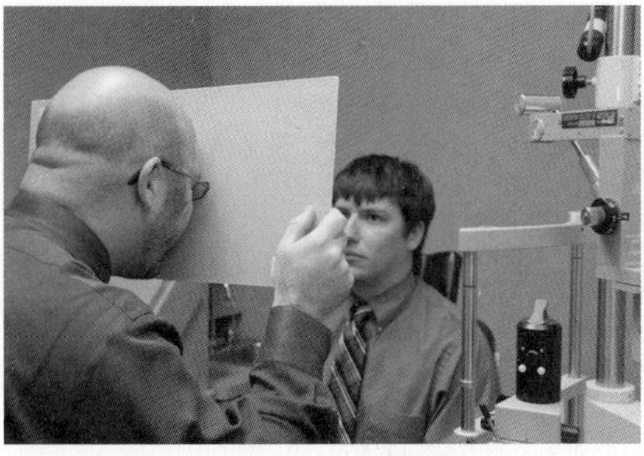

FIGURE 16-7. In the preferential looking technique using the Teller acuity cards, the tester looks through a small hole in the center of the card and determines the direction of the patient's eye movement. The tester should not know the direction of the target prior to testing.

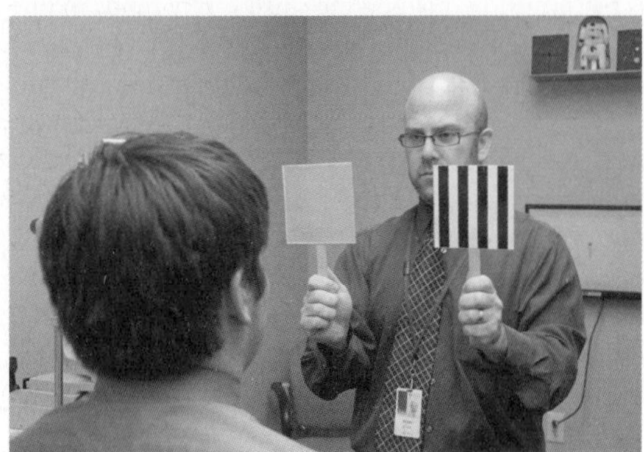

FIGURE 16-8. In the preferential looking technique using grating paddles, the patient may be distracted by the tester.

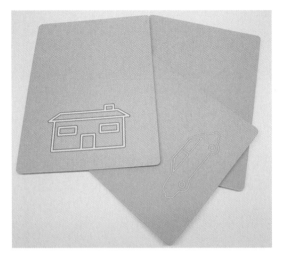

FIGURE 16-9. The Cardiff cards test visual acuity using an increased or decreased contrast optotype.

identify the location of the target on two out of three presentations (38).

Bailey-Hall Cereal Test The Bailey-Hall Cereal (40) Test is a forced-choice test in which the child has to identify which card has the picture of the cereal. It can be used for patients with developmental ages between 18 months and 3 years. The patient is given two cards at a particular acuity level, one with a picture of a piece of cereal and the other with a picture of a square. Giving the child a piece of cereal for all correct responses can be used as a way to keep him or her motivated (41).

Bock Candy Bead Acuity Test The Bock candy bead acuity test grossly estimates near visual acuity by using candy beads (cake decorations). The test is performed by holding the small candy beads in one hand, while leaving the other hand empty. The examiner asks the child if he or she would like some candy. As any parent can attest, if the child can see the candy, he or she will attempt to pick it up instinctually and usually very quickly. If vision is poor, the child may not pay attention to either hand. While this is a test of gross ability, beads or candy of different size can be used to further differentiate between the two eyes (28). Of course, do not use candy if the patient has swallowing or texture issues or dietary restrictions.

Optokinetic Nystagmus (OKN) Optokinetic nystagmus (OKN) testing can be used to verify if the patient possesses a cortical or subcortical visual response. Optokinetic nystagmus testing is appropriate for developmental ages between 18 months and 7 years and requires little to no effort by the patient (Fig. 16-10). The OKN drum contains black stripes that should be oriented vertically in front of the patient. The drum is spun *slowly* and the examiner observes the patient's eye movements as he or she follows the rotating drum. The patient should exhibit a slow pursuit-like motion (slow phase) and then a fast refixation (fast phase) nystagmoid-like movement, which is noted as his or her eyes jump back and forth while looking at the striped pattern (29). By changing the test distance, the minimal stripe visual angle to elicit nystagmus is noted. An alternative to the drum is the use of striped cloth that is pulled across in front of the patient. The visual angle is converted to Snellen acuity. One min arc stripe width is equivalent to 20/20.

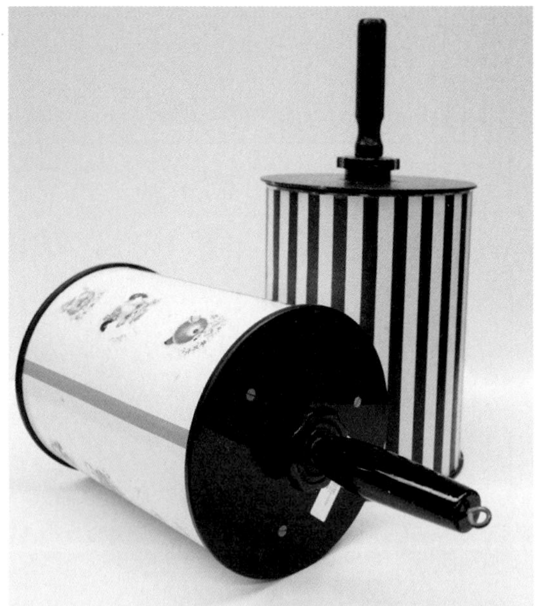

FIGURE 16-10. The traditional (black-and-white grating) and pediatric OKN drums.

Visual Evoked Potential Occasionally, the developmental level and the cooperation of the patient make it very difficult to use traditional methods to assess visual function. Electrodiagnostic testing is a very precise way to quantify the patient's potential visual acuity. The visual evoked potential is a bioelectrical signal that is generated in the visual cortex of the brain in response to a visual stimulation. Scalp electrodes are used to record electrical signals while the patient views a stimulus such as a grating or checkerboard pattern. Several measurements are recorded with various stimulus sizes to determine the minimal visual acuity (42). While this may not be the best choice for many patients, as poor cooperation may make testing difficult, it remains an option if everything else fails. For further information regarding this topic, please refer to Chapter 23, Special Assessment Procedures.

COLOR VISION TESTING

Color vision testing can offer important diagnostic information about a child's ocular health and capabilities. Color deficiency may be either congenital or acquired. Congenital color deficiency is bilateral and stable over the life of the patient. It is more common in males than females as it is an X-linked condition. Approximately 8% of males and 0.5% of females are color deficient. Congenital color deficiency is typically red-green in nature (43).

Acquired color defects are typically monocular or asymmetric and found equally in males and females. They can progress or regress and involve a loss of blue sensitivity, leading to blue-green and yellow-violet discrimination loss with an accompanying vision decrease (43).

There are various commercially available tests that allow the measurement of color vision. They can be grouped into four categories: (a) pseudoisochromatic plate tests, (b) arrangement or panel tests, (c) matching tests, and (d) naming tests (44). The tests that practitioners are most familiar with fall into the first two categories, but based upon a patient's abilities, creativity may be needed to obtain the desired information.

Ishihara Plate Test This test was first published in 1906 and is the most used color vision test worldwide. Its efficiency has been studied extensively. It was considered the gold standard for rapid identification of red-green deficiencies (45–56), but the Hardy-Rand-Rittler (HRR) test, discussed next, is now considered to be superior. The patient is asked to identify numbers that are seen on colored plates (Fig. 16-11). There are 38- and 24-plate editions available (44). Even though this test requires a patient response, it can also be performed using a cotton-tipped applicator or a paintbrush if the patient is nonverbal. The test is limited by the lack of tritan plates to test blue-yellow deficiencies, and it does not allow for an assessment of the severity of the color vision deficiency. Also, patients with poor visual discrimination or visual figure ground may have a hard time understanding the test, not because they have a color vision deficiency but due to a perceptual deficit.

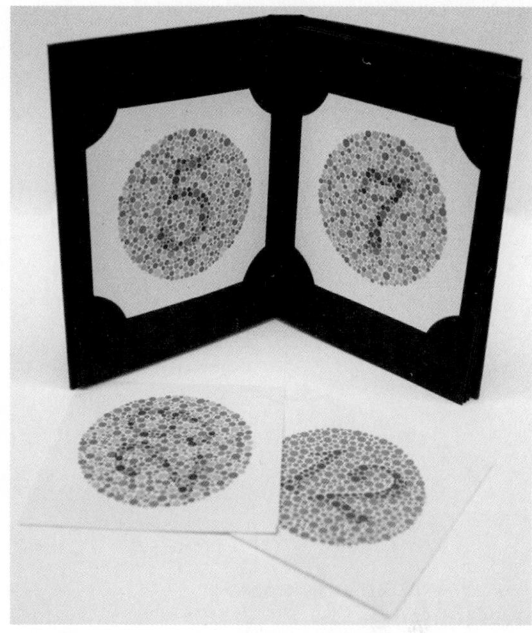

FIGURE 16-11. The Ishihara color vision test (See also Color Section).

Hardy-Rand-Rittler Test The HRR pseudoisochromatic test, first published by the American Optical Company in 1955 (50), can differentiate better than the Ishihara test between protan and deutan deficiencies. It can also assess the severity of the deficiency and test for tritan defects. This test was not available for many years until it was reproduced by Richmond products in 2002 (57). Colorimetric analyses of the new version indicate that it should actually outperform the previous version in differentiating protans and deutans and in grading severity (58,59).

The test comprises 24 plates, each displaying either one or two pictures including a cross, circle, or triangle (Fig. 16-12). There are four demonstration plates to confirm test understanding on the part of the patient. These plates can be seen by all observers. There are six screening plates: four for protan/deutan deficiencies and two for tritan deficiencies. These are followed by 14 plates designed to differentiate the three types of defects. The colors of the symbols

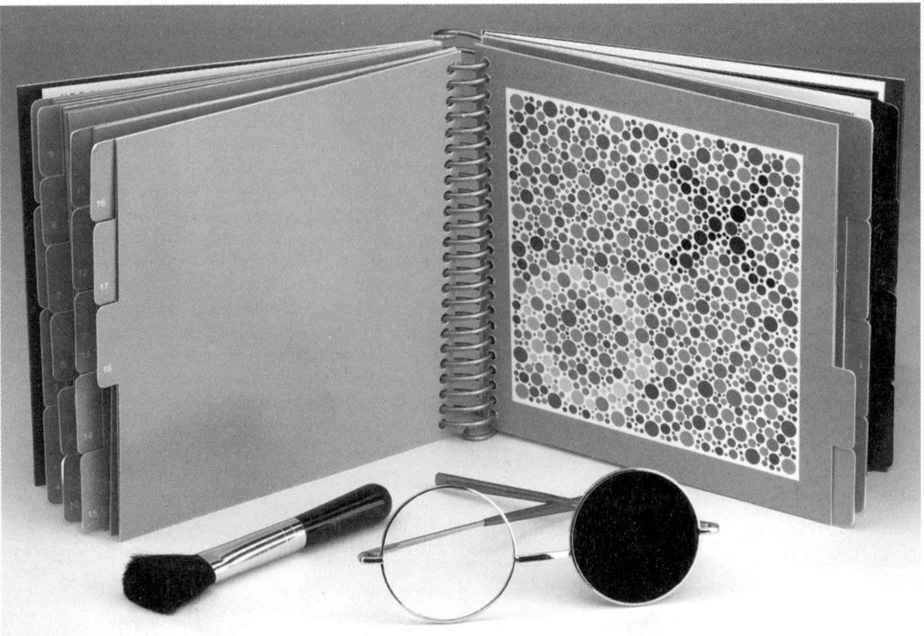

FIGURE 16-12. The Hardy-Rand-Ritter (HRR) test of color vision. (See also Color Section.) (Courtesy of Good-Lite Company.)

become increasingly saturated as the patient progresses through the test. The greater the saturation, the more likely the target will be identified. Grading is mild, medium, or severe, depending on the number of plates missed (57). As with the Ishihara, a paintbrush can be used for patients who are not able to name the symbol or with those who are nonverbal.

Color Vision Testing Made Easy Color vision testing made easy (CVTME) is an alternative method of testing color vision in patients who do not know their numbers. It consists of 9 to 14 pseudoisochromatic plates with simple symbols such as a star, circle, and square on earlier plates and complex forms such as a balloon, sailboat, and dog on later plates (Fig. 16-13).

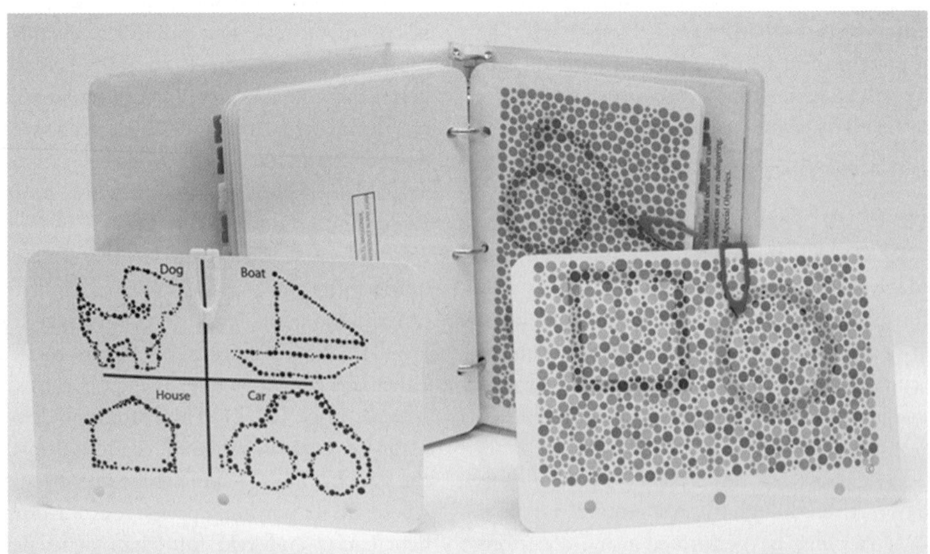

FIGURE 16-13. The color vision made easy color vision test. (See also Color Section.)

The patient is asked to name or point to the shape. In a patient with special needs, asking them to point to a specific shape will often produce better results than simply asking the name of the shape. Similar to the Ishihara test, drawbacks of CVTME include the lack of tritan plates and the inability to assess severity of the color vision losses (44).

Farnsworth-Munsell Dichotomous D-15

This arrangement or panel test is sensitive at detecting and assessing the type and severity of the color vision deficit, although it cannot distinguish between moderate and severe deficiencies. It consists of a set of 16 different colored chips or caps that are arranged in order starting with a fixed color (Fig. 16-14). While this test can take longer than a traditional Ishihara, it does in fact give greater detail concerning the patient's visual deficiency. Tritan defects can be assessed as well (44,60). A version of this test that is magnetic is made by Bernell. This test is sealed and can be presented as a game to the patients. When a complete loss of red, green, or blue color vision is present, a "neutral point" exists in which colors are confused with white. The inclusion of a grayish-white cap can detect this. When testing is completed, the results are charted onto a recording sheet, allowing the practitioner to assess the type of defect and severity.

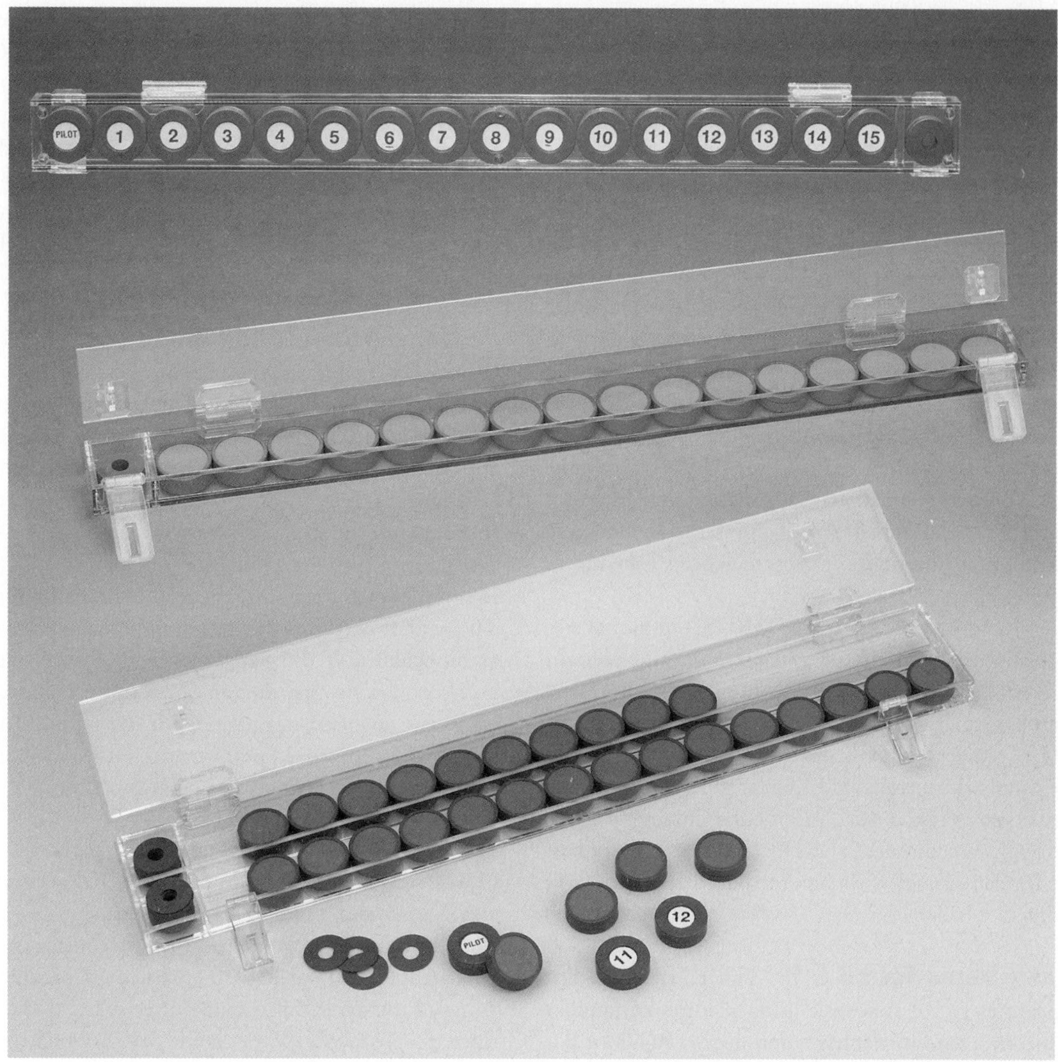

FIGURE 16-14. The Farnsworth D-15 Dichotomous color vision test. (See also Color Section.) (Courtesy of Good-Lite Company.)

Wool/Yarn Test This procedure is akin to a matching test. It can be performed in various fashions, but the most common method involves asking the patient to match colored pieces of yarn to standard pieces of yarn. The practitioner should be able to determine if the patient's chromatic challenges based on the colors of yarn the patient has trouble matching (61).

TESTING THE BINOCULAR VISION SYSTEM

Stereo Vision Testing The most basic characteristic of binocular vision is stereoscopic vision, in which the disparity of two images in each eye is used to determine the relative depth of objects (43). Abnormal visual development, like strabismus or amblyopia, can prevent this process. As these two conditions are found in greater incidence in patients with Down syndrome and other genetic abnormalities, stereo vision testing can be a crucial aspect of the examination.

Two types of stereoscopic stimuli are used in many commercially available tests. Contour stereoscopic targets or local stereopsis have monocular edges or boundaries separated on a background to produce disparity. However, the displacement of the targets in one eye relative to the other can be detected without stereoscopic vision, allowing cheating on the test. As fusion is not required for stereopsis, the targets can be presented centrally or peripherally. Also, targets can be aimed at obtaining the stereoacuity (minimum threshold) or gross stereopsis (maximum appreciation) (62).

Random dot stereograms (RDSs) or global stereopsis are often computer generated and contain a lateral shift in the central core of dots, lines, patterns, or pictures that create the stereoscopic form. RDS requires bifoveal fusion, so a patient with a constant strabismus will not be able to appreciate this type of target (23). Monocular cues are present though, as commercial RDS tests use Polaroid or red/green glasses with superimposed left and right targets.

Lang Stereo Tests I & II The Lang stereo test measures global stereopsis using pictures of familiar objects (a cat, an elephant, and a car). Random dot stereogram images are imprinted on a grating of fine parallel cylindrical strips (63). The images vary in disparity, ranging from 1,200 to 550 seconds of arc on Test I to 600 to 200 seconds of arc on Test II. Test II has the additional feature of having a picture of a star that is visible monocularly, but to observers with binocular vision provides a stereoscopic effect. This also helps to attract and maintain the interest of the patient. The major advantage of the Lang stereo test is that polarized spectacles are not needed. This is helpful for patients who have extreme aversion to placing objects on or near their face. Nonverbal patients simply have to reach for the target to acknowledge that stereopsis is present. This test should not be used in patients that rock or cannot keep their head still as this can produce monocular cues (62).

Frisby Stereo Test This test consists of three plates of Plexiglas of varying thickness (6, 3, and 1.5 mm), each containing four squares of dot patterns. On each plate, one of the four squares contains a central stereoscopic circle printed on the opposite surface. Depending upon the plate used and the testing distance, stereoacuity ranging from 600 to 7 seconds of arc can be assessed. As with the Lang test, monocular cues can be a confounding factor if the patient has difficulty with head and/or body control (43,64).

Pointer and Straw This test provides the practitioner with an idea of the patient's gross depth perception. A regular household straw and a pickup stick are required. The doctor holds the straw vertically approximately 40 cm from the patient. The patient attempts to put the stick in the open end of the straw. If successful, the straw is moved to another location. The patient must use a fluid motion, making sure not to slow down as the pointer nears the straw's opening. The patient performs this action monocularly as well as binocularly. If the performance is similar under both conditions, the doctor can assume that stereopsis was not used to judge depth during binocular testing (61). Improved performance under binocular conditions suggests good binocular function.

Titmus Fly Test This test has three parts: the fly (3,000 seconds of arc), animals (400–100 seconds), and Wirt circles (800–40 seconds) (64) (Fig. 16-15). The fly is used to measure gross stereopsis. Using polarized filters, the patient is asked to pinch the wings of the fly. If this occurs in free space, it is considered a positive response. If the patient touches the page, it is either considered a negative response or simply that the patient did not understand the test. The

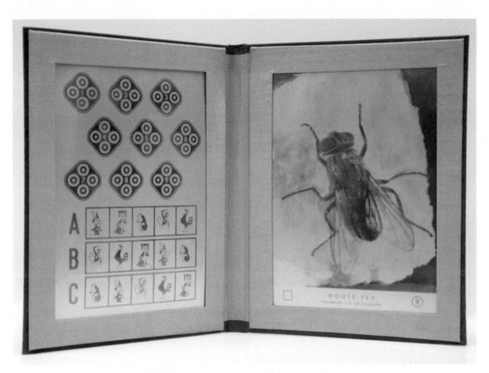

FIGURE 16-15. The "Stereo Fly" test of stereopsis.

practitioner must consider that some patients may be frightened by this picture since it is an enlarged fly.

The animal portion of the test contains five animated animals in each of three rows. The doctor asks the patient to identify the character having crossed disparity. The patient is questioned as to which character is "jumping out at him or her," "popping off of the page," or looks funny or different. The Wirt circles are similar in that the patient must identify which of the four circles is "jumping out at him or her." Whereas the lower-level stereo Wirt targets can be seen using monocular cues, this is not the case with the animal targets.

Randot Stereo Test As with the Titmus Fly, this test also consists of three parts. The "forms" section consists of two groups of four squares, three of which contain a geometric shape seen in stereo. The shapes, including a circle, square, and star should be familiar to young children as well as patients with special needs (Fig. 16-16). The stereo threshold is 500 and 250 seconds of arc depending on the group of squares. The animals and Wirt circle sections are similar to those found on the Titmus test, with the exception that the stereoacuity measured with the circles ranges from 600 to 20 seconds of arc.

Random Dot E Test The Random Dot E test also measures global stereopsis. This stereo test uses two targets and polarized spectacles. A raised model "E" card should be shown to the patient as an example of the target (Fig. 16-17). The patient should be allowed to feel the card so that he or she knows what to expect throughout the test. Two test targets (one that is

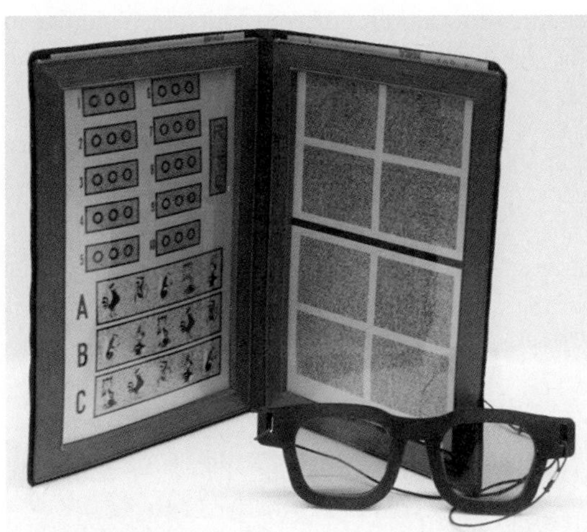

FIGURE 16-16. The Randot test of stereopsis.

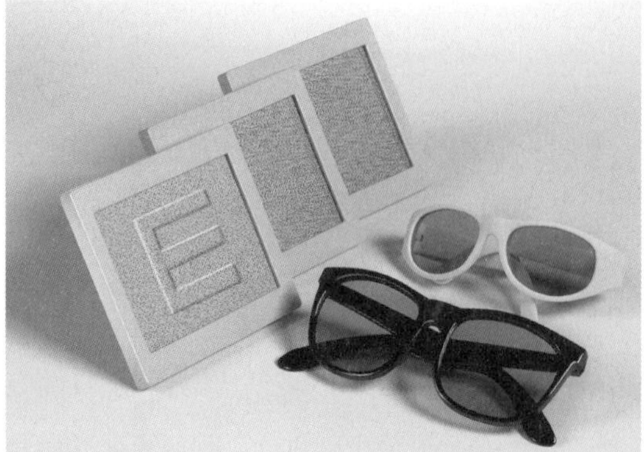

FIGURE 16-17. The Random Dot Stereo "E's" can be used at varying distances. (Courtesy of Good-Lite Company.)

blank and the other containing the stereoscopic "E") are then shown. The patient must identify which target has the letter "E" on it (61,62). The patient must correctly choose three out of four targets to pass this test (62).

This procedure can be performed at different distances in order to evaluate different disparities. For example, if the patient is able to correctly identify the target at 50 cm, this corresponds to a disparity of 504 arc seconds, whereas a distance of about 5 m corresponds to a disparity of 52 arc seconds. This test is very useful for nonverbal patients, because they can simply point to the card with the floating "E." The disadvantage is that it requires the use of polarized spectacles (61).

Stereo Smile Based on a preferential looking format, the Stereo Smile test can be used in very young children successfully (65,66). This test is similar to the Teller acuity cards, in that on the presentation card there is a target on only either the right or left side of the card. The child will look at the side of the card in which he or she sees the stereo target, a smiley face (Fig. 16-18). A demonstration card is available to show the target to the patient prior to testing. The procedure is normed for two test distances, 0.55 and 1.1 m, so that a total of four levels of stereopsis (640, 240, 120, and 60 seconds of arc) can be tested (67). Leat showed that 73% of 6-month- to 2-year-olds could cooperate with this test (65). In a comparison between the Stereo Smile, Random Dot E, and Randot Preschool stereoacuity tests in children age 3 years through 3 years 6 months, it was shown that the testability with the Stereo Smile (77%) was greater than both the Random Dot E (74%) and Randot Preschool (56%) tests (66). The disadvantage of this test, similar to other stereopsis evaluations, is the need for polarized lenses. It can also be challenging to assess eye movements behind the darkened lenses, making a proper determination difficult (67).

VISUAL FIELD TESTING

The goal of visual field testing in special needs patients is to uncover gross peripheral defects and areas of constriction or neglect. A visual field defect may be compensated for by a head turn or a shift in posture that parents and caregivers might ignore as usual behavior for the child. To assess the patient's visual field, the practitioner should sit in front of the child to observe his or her visual response and hold a target (puppet or noise-making toy). The practitioner will need an assistant to stand behind the child and slowly present another toy (one that does not make noise) in the horizontal and vertical meridians

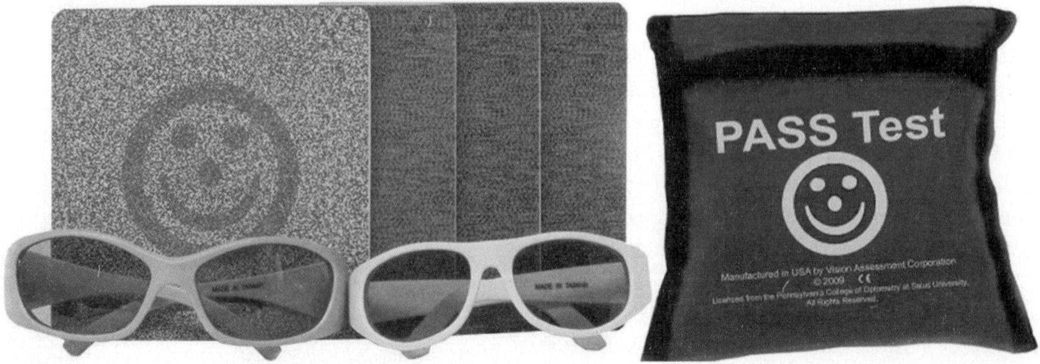

FIGURE 16-18. The Stereo Smile test is similar to the preferential looking technique, as the patient will be drawn to the stereo picture instead of the blank card. (Courtesy of Good-Lite Company.)

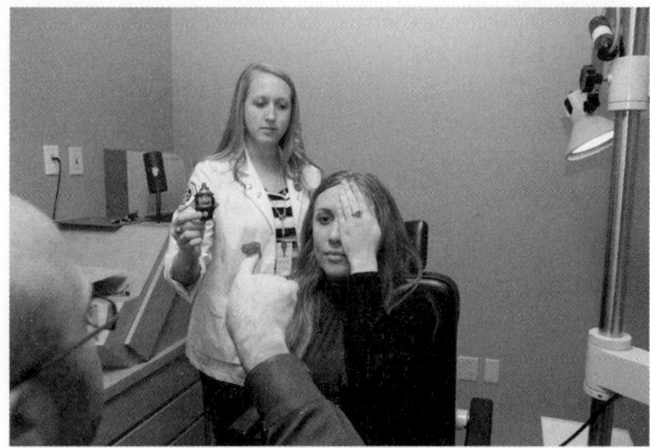

A

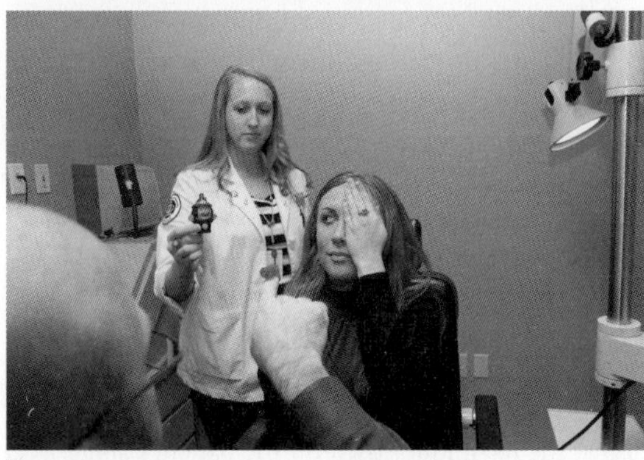

B

FIGURE 16-19. **A** and **B:** Visual field testing involves bringing a target from the side while the patient fixates on a central target. When the patient's eyes move to pick up the peripheral target, it is considered a positive response.

(Fig. 6-19A). The assistant must be careful not to make any noise as it will not be possible to ascertain if the child hears or sees the target as it comes into view. The position where the patient first detects the stimulus should be noted (61) (Fig. 16-19B).

An alternative procedure involves the Lea flicker wand for a quick estimate to determine whether major field losses exist (Fig. 16-20). As with the use of the puppet, the findings are approximate. A diode at the end of the flexible wand can be used either as a flickering or nonflickering illuminated stimulus. The intensity of the stimulus can be changed from 4 cd/m^2 as the weakest luminance to 40 and 400 cd/m^2 when measured at the side of the diode. The wand can be used as the stimulus on an arc perimeter, which results in more exact measurements (68) (a video on how to use the Lea Flicker Wand is available at http://www.lea-test.fi/en/vistests/instruct/flickerw/flickerw.html).

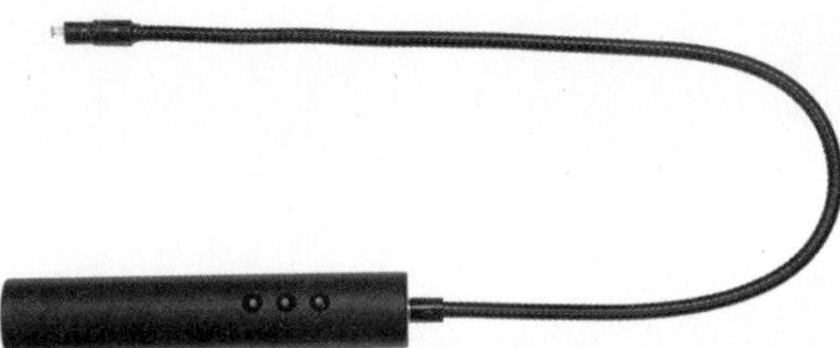

FIGURE 16-20. The Lea Flicker Wand can be used to perform visual field testing as an alternative to a toy or finger puppet. (Courtesy of Good-Lite Company.)

ACCOMMODATIVE ASSESSMENT

Accommodative testing should be considered as many patients with special needs have reduced accommodative function (69,70). Medications frequently prescribed for individuals with disability often interfere with accommodative function (71).

Monocular Estimation Method Retinoscopy Monocular estimation method (MEM) retinoscopy, a form of dynamic retinoscopy, is an objective method to evaluate the accuracy of the accommodative response (72). It is used to diagnose an accommodative or binocular deficiency as well as the need for any near-point therapeutic lenses. This is performed at the Harmon distance (distance from the patient's elbow to the middle knuckle of the middle finger) using an age and educationally appropriate card with words or pictures on it. It should be held directly under the retinoscope light. Most retinoscopes have a method of attaching the MEM card to their heads. If the card is either too difficult or easy, a false response will be found as the accommodative response can be tied to the level of stress put on the visual system (73) (Fig. 16-21).

Retinoscopy should be performed along both the horizontal and vertical axes, in order to detect astigmatism (Fig. 16-22). The amount of plus or minus needed to neutralize the motion of the reflex should be estimated and then confirmed using a trial lens (43,72,74,75). The key to this test is the speed at which the lens is inserted and removed in front of the eye. The lens must not be left in place for more than two seconds (73). With motion indicates an accommodative lag, and against motion indicates a lead. When performing this test, it is important to use normal room illumination. The expected value for MEM retinoscopy is +0.25 D to +0.50 D with a standard deviation of ±0.25 D (75).

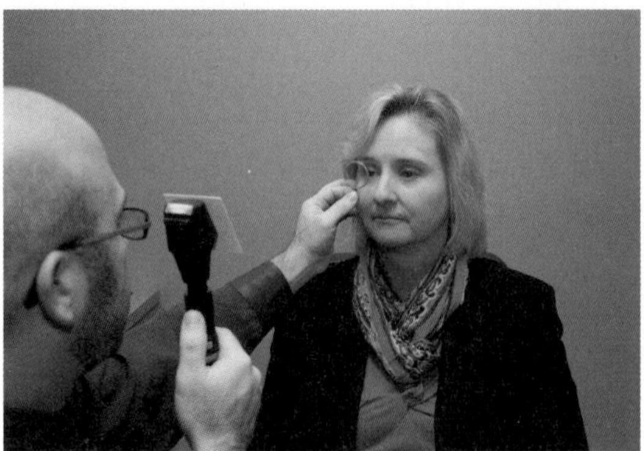

FIGURE 16-21. When performing the MEM technique, it is important to test at the appropriate distance from the patient and move the lens in and out of the patient's view at the correct speed.

Accommodative Amplitude Pull-away Method Traditionally, accommodative amplitude is performed via the push-up method; however, the pull-away variation may prove more successful with special needs patients. The two variations have been found to produce equal results (76). Instead of moving the target (a 20/30 letter/figure) closer to the patient and requesting that the patient indicate the first blur, the target is started close to the patient's eye and brought away until he or she can call out the shape or letter. It is best to have a single target versus a row of letters to minimize patient confusion.

It can be a challenge with any patient to manipulate a card or stick on which the target is imprinted (Fig. 16-23). The use of an accommodation rule (Bernell) can assist in proper measurement. It has a clip and slide mechanism that allow for smooth, controlled movement of the target. The average expected amplitude of accommodation can be derived from the following formula put forth by Hofstetter: AA = 18.5–1/3(Age) (77).

EYE MOVEMENT ASSESSMENT

Evaluating ocular motilities in the special needs patient is crucial due to the high incidence of ocular motor abnormalities in the population. In order to completely assess eye movement skills, the clinician should assess motilities, pursuits, saccades, and near point of convergence (NPC). The Developmental Eye Movement (DEM) test and the King-Devick (K-D) can be used to assess reading eye movements.

To assess ocular motilities, the practitioner should stand at least 50 cm away from the patient and should instruct the patient to follow a fixation target with only his or her eyes. If this is difficult for the patient, place a hand on top of the patient's head to prevent head movement. The target can be any object that gets and maintains the patient's attention, like a finger puppet, penlight, or a novelty item that makes sound and light. While a double H pattern should typically be slowly traced with the fixation target, the practitioner should adjust the technique based on the patient's ability and attention. The patient should be able to keep the target single and follow it in all fields of gaze. An overaction or limitation in movement should be noted.

Pursuit and Saccadic Testing The Northeastern State College of Optometry (NSUCO) method can be performed to evaluate the patient's pursuits and saccades. It has been shown to have good reliability between and within clinicians (78), good test–retest reliability (79,80), and good validity (81–83). The NSUCO method, performed both

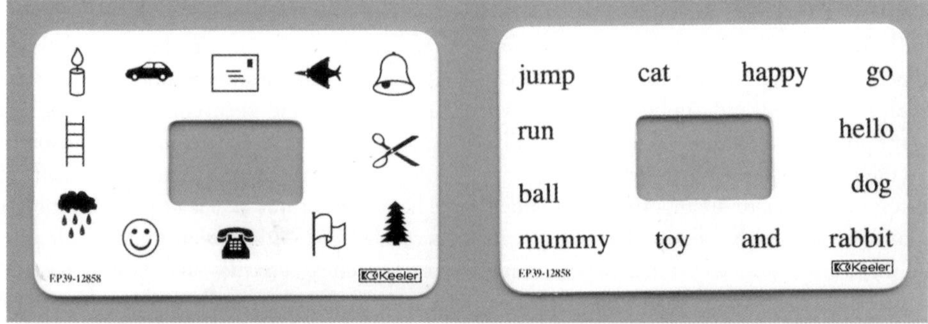

FIGURE 16-22. The MEM cards come in various cognitive levels. Choosing the correct level for the patient is crucial as the results may vary depending on the cognitive load.

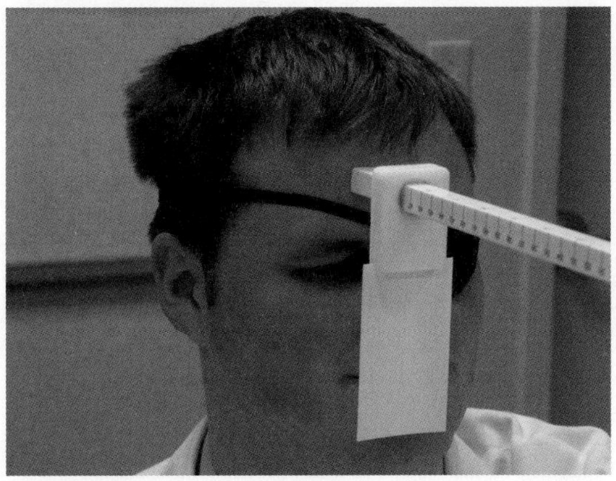

FIGURE 16-23. The pull-away technique for measuring accommodative amplitude. The patient calls out the letter when he or she can first make it out.

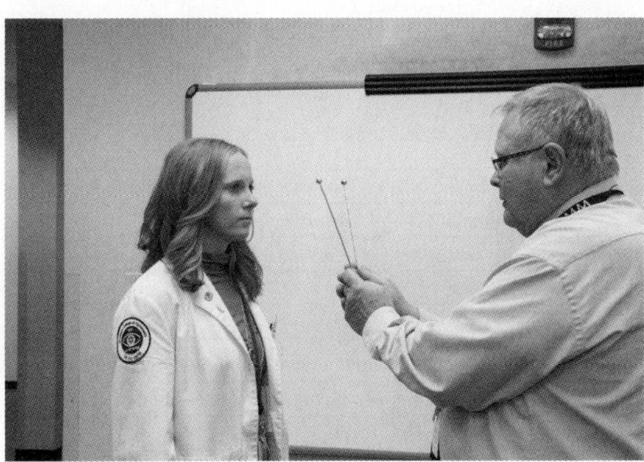

FIGURE 16-25. The NSUCO test of saccades is performed with two Wolff wands. The patient is asked to make five round trips.

monocularly and binocularly, requires the patient to stand. This can be difficult for patients who use a wheelchair or those with poor balance. The NSUCO pursuit method uses a single target that is moved both clockwise and counterclockwise each for two rotations (Fig. 16-24). The circumference of the rotation should be slightly larger than the size of the patient's head, which is about 20 cm. Grading is based on four categories: the patient's ability to complete the test, his or her accuracy, the presence of head movement during the test, and the presence of body movement during the test (84).

The NSUCO procedure for evaluating saccades involves two targets that are held 20 to 25 cm apart (Fig. 16-25). The patient alternates between the two targets upon command and makes five round trips back and forth. Grading is again based on four categories (84) (Appendix 2).

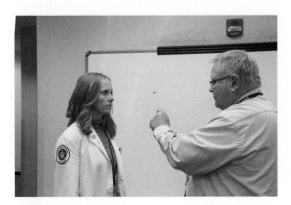

FIGURE 16-24. The NSUCO test of pursuits is performed with one Wolff wand that is moved smoothly in a clockwise and counterclockwise manner.

Near Point of Convergence The NPC evaluates the patient's maximum convergence ability including tonic, proximal, accommodative, and disparity convergence. Testing the patient's NPC is one of the quickest and easiest tests to perform. Near point of convergence can be measured objectively or subjectively (43,75). The target used can be an interesting picture to help keep the patient's attention, or a letter, number, or penlight. The target, which is initially held about 2 ft away on the patient's midline, is slowly brought toward the patient's nose. The NPC break occurs either when the examiner notices one eye turning out or the patient reports diplopia. The target is then pulled away from the patient until fusion (either subjectively or objectively) is regained. This point is known as the recovery (Fig. 16-26).

Repeating this procedure several times can increase its sensitivity and reveal fatiguing of convergence. Scheiman et al. (85) found a recession of the NPC after repetition in both normal patients and those with convergence insufficiency (CI), though the amount of recession was four times greater after ten repetitions in the CI group. While ten repetitions may be difficult and time-consuming, Wick (86) and Mohindra and Molinari (87) recommend only four to five repetitions, which may be easier to accomplish with a special needs patient. The results of the NPC are recorded as break and recovery in centimeters. The expected values for NPC are 6 cm and 10 cm for break and recovery, respectively (75).

APPENDIX 2

NSUCO scoring criteria: direct observation of pursuits

Ability

1	Cannot complete 1/2 rotation in either clockwise or counterclockwise direction
2	Completes 1/2 rotation in either direction
3	Completes one rotation in either direction but not two rotations
4	Completes two rotations in one direction but less than two rotations in the other direction
5	Completes two rotations in each direction

Accuracy (Can the patient accurately and consistently fixate so that no noticeable refixation is needed?)

1	No attempt to follow the target or requires greater than ten refixations
2	Refixations 5 to 10 times
3	Refixations 3 to 4 times
4	Refixations 2 times or less
5	No refixations

Head Movement (Can the patient accomplish the pursuit without moving his or her head?)

1	Large movement of the head or body at any time
2	Moderate movement of the head or body at any time
3	Slight movement of the head or body (> 50% of time)
4	Slight movement of the head or body (<50% of time)
5	No movement of head or body

Body Movement (Can the patient accomplish the pursuit without moving his or her body?)

1	Large movement of the head or body at any time
2	Moderate movement of the head or body at any time
3	Slight movement of the head or body (> 50% of time)
4	Slight movement of the head or body (<50% of time)
5	No movement of head or body

NSUCO scoring criteria: direct observation of saccades

Ability

1	Completes less than two roundtrips
2	Completes two roundtrips
3	Completes three roundtrips
4	Completes four roundtrips
5	Completes five roundtrips

Accuracy (Can the patient accurately and consistently fixate so that no noticeable correction is needed?)

1	Large over- or undershooting is noted 1 or more times
2	Moderate over- or undershooting noted 1 or more times
3	Constant slight over- or undershooting noted (> 50% of time)
4	Intermittent slight over- or undershooting noted (<50% of time)
5	No over or undershooting noted

Head Movement (Can the patient accomplish the saccade without moving his or her head?)

1	Large movement of the head or body at any time
2	Moderate movement of the head or body at any time
3	Slight movement of the head or body (>50% of time)
4	Slight movement of the head or body (<50% of time)
5	No movement of head or body

Body Movement (Can the patient accomplish the saccade without moving his or her body?)

1	Large movement of the head or body at any time
2	Moderate movement of the head or body at any time
3	Slight movement of the head or body (>50% of time)
4	Slight movement of the head or body (<50% of time)
5	No movement of head or body

__________ Total Points Date __________ Name ____________________

PED-136 (02-09)

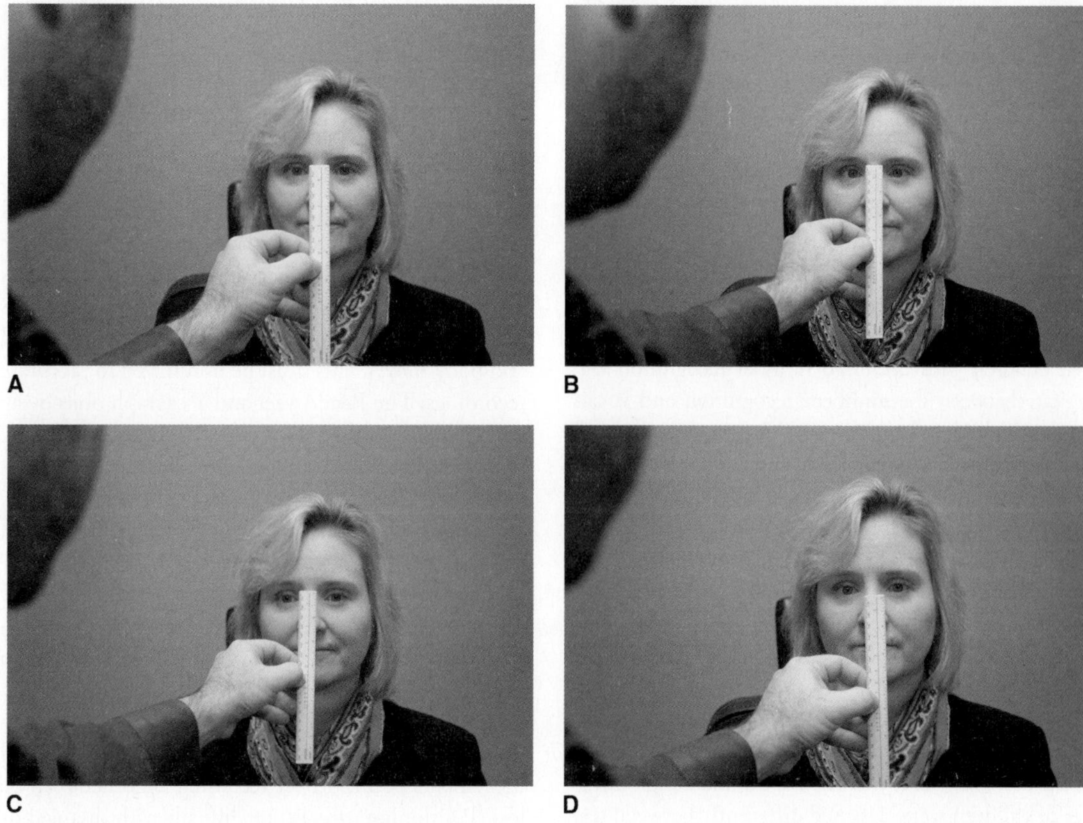

FIGURE 16-26. This sequence demonstrates the three steps in the NPC technique. **A:** The target is brought closer to the patient until he or she indicates that it is blurry. **B:** The target is brought closer until the patient reports two images or the clinician sees the eyes break fixation. **C:** The target is brought closer to confirm loss of fixation. **D:** The target is then brought away from the patient until he or she reports one image or the clinician sees refixation.

The NPC test may also be done with a red lens placed over one eye. The patient will report a "pink" light until fusion is broken. The lightness or darkness of the pink depends upon which eye is dominant. At the "breaking point," the patient should report diplopia with one red and one white light being seen. The use of the red lens makes it easier for the patient to identify when the "break" occurs and has been found to be more sensitive (88).

King Devick The clinician should not assume that simply because patients have special needs that reading is not a part of their life. The K-D (89,90) and DEM (91,92), which are easily administered and have acceptable norms, are two objective tests that can be administered to assess reading eye movements. Kulp and Schmidt (93) showed that while the DEM took longer than the K-D to complete, the relative performance was not significantly different in kindergartners and first graders.

Unfortunately, the tests are loaded with cognitive factors that may skew the results. These tests are difficult to administer in younger children and patients with intellectual disability (94). In the study by Kulp and Schmidt (93), of the 44 kindergartners who were tested with the DEM, 10 (22.7%) were unable to complete the test. Both the K-D and DEM have been shown to be useful in screening for impaired saccadic eye movement following a traumatic brain injury (95–97).

The K-D test contains eight lines of five single-digit numbers. The test becomes progressively more difficult as there are three separate test plates. In the first, the numbers have large spaces between each line and have a black line connecting each number to the next in the line. The second plate also contains large spaces between each of the lines of numbers but the black lines connecting the targets are no longer present. The third and final plate has smaller spacing between each of the lines of numbers, increasing the crowding effect. The numbers also become more randomly staggered as the patient progresses through the three charts. The patient is asked to read aloud each page of numbers as quickly as possible. A score is calculated based on the time needed to complete each chart and the total number of errors made. The calculations are compared to the mean and standard deviation of the test's developmental norms (98). A criticism of the K-D test is that children with decreased number recognition will hesitate between the numbers' recognition and vocalization. If children have decreased information retrieval skills or decreased visual–verbal integration skills, they will display decreased performance on the K-D test even though their saccadic skills may be normal (91,99).

Another criticism is that there is a learning effect with repeated administrations. While the reliability of the K-D has been questioned in 7- to 12-year-olds, reliability was found to be moderately high for kindergartners, first graders, and the group as a whole by Kulp and Schmidt in a study of 79 children. A significant trend toward improved performance was found in the first graders. It was also found that a high number of children were classified differently between test administrations. The percentage ranged from 25% to 35% in kindergartners and 12% to 18.5% in first graders (100).

Developmental Eye Movement Test The DEM evaluates saccadic eye movements by assessing the speed and accuracy in which a series of single-digit numbers are seen, recognized, and verbalized (99). This test compensates for the automaticity component of the K-D test since it compares differences in time scores between vertical and horizontal responses. In this test, the child is first timed while reading two test plates, each composed of two separated vertical columns of numbers; the vertical time score is the sum of these two times. Next, the child reads the same quantity of numbers presented in a randomly spaced, horizontal array (16 rows of 5 randomly spaced single-digit numbers) (92). The time for this section is adjusted if lines or digits are reread or skipped. Scoring is based on a ratio of the time taken to read the horizontal plate versus the time taken to read the two vertical plates. The vertical time score indicates the automaticity of a child's number calling without saccadic eye movements, while the horizontal time score reflects both automaticity of number calling and saccadic eye movement skill. Each score is compared to developmental norms and standard scores developed for the test (98). Concerns have been voiced about reliability and the need to do repeated testing to attain better results (101).

ReadAlyzer/Visagraph The Visagraph and ReadAlyzer are computerized instruments that monitor the subject's eye movements using infrared photocells while a passage of age-appropriate print is read. Subjects must be properly aligned in the instruments, and head and body movements must be minimized for accurate recordings. The ReadAlyzer and Visagraph objectively analyze the recordings, so subjective interpretation by the practitioner is minimal. These programs also calculate eye tracking components including fixations, regressions, directional attack (left to right tendency), average span of recognition, average duration of fixation, reading rate, grade equivalency, and relative eye movement efficiency. The actual eye movement recordings can be printed, analyzed, and demonstrated to the patient and parents. Limitations are that children (grade 3 and younger) can be difficult to test and that once the child is aligned in the instrument, if head movements occur, proper recording alignment can be lost. Positioning can also be difficult with disabled or hyperactive children (98).

EVALUATING BINOCULAR POSTURE

Due to the high incidence of strabismus in special needs patients, the binocular vision assessment is without a doubt an element of the examination that needs to be assessed as thoroughly as possible.

Direct Observation When the patient enters the examination room, the practitioner should examine his or her gait, head and body posture, and eye movements. By watching the patient, the practitioner can detect the presence or absence of strabismus. Direct observation can confirm nystagmus, abnormal lid action, ptosis, epicanthal folds, or facial asymmetry (102).

Brückner Test This red reflex comparison test is useful in the detection and diagnosis of significant refractive error, strabismus, and amblyopia (102,103). Requiring minimal patient cooperation, this test is invaluable when working with special needs patients. While it should not be used as a stand-alone screening technique, the Brückner test does serve as an excellent adjunct to two tests, the Hirschberg test and the cover test, which will be discussed later in this chapter (104).

With the practitioner standing approximately 1 m away from the patient, both eyes are simultaneously illuminated with the ophthalmoscope. The patient's red reflexes are compared for differences in brightness, color, and shape. If one eye has a brighter reflex, it is more likely to be strabismic or amblyopic (102,103).

The brightness differences seen in this procedure have been explained by Roe and Guyton (105) using the principle of conjugacy between the light course and the retina. They indicated that the fundus reflex will appear brighter if the eye is deviated, as the off-axis optical aberrations decrease conjugacy. Therefore, the pupil area will appear brighter and whiter. The darker eye will appear so because the retina is conjugate with the light source.

Hirschberg Test This test allows for an objective examination of binocular alignment as the practitioner is able to make a gross estimate of the magnitude of the deviation. Even though minimal patient cooperation is needed, the patient must be able to attend to the target long enough for the practitioner to make the estimate.

To perform the test, a penlight or transilluminator is directed toward the patient's nose at a 50-cm test distance while the doctor looks over the barrel of the penlight/transiluminator. The patient fixates on the penlight, and the relative placement of the corneal reflexes in relationship to the center of the pupils is evaluated. If the relative positions of the reflexes are symmetric and centered, it is assumed that no strabismus is present (102,103) (Fig. 16-27).

Most patients have symmetrical corneal reflexes with approximately +0.5 mm of nasal displacement. A temporal reflex in one eye indicates esotropia, while a nasal reflex suggests exotropia. A displacement nasally is indicated with a "+" sign, while temporal displacement is signified with a "−" sign. An upward reflex suggests hypotropia of that eye, whereas a downward reflex suggests hypertropia of that eye. If the reflexes are asymmetric, the angle of deviation can be estimated. A 1 mm difference between the reflexes equals approximately 22 prism diopters of deviation (102,103). You can also estimate the deviation present by noting that if the Hirschberg reflex is at the border of the pupil, it is approximately a 30 prism diopter turn. If the reflex is seen between the border of the pupil and the limbus, 60 prism diopters, and at the limbus, approximately 90 prism diopters. (A Hirschberg simulator can be found at http://eyeontechs.com/new/?p=218.)

Krimsky Test When the practitioner is uncertain about the estimate of the displacement in millimeters, the Krimsky test can be performed. This test is performed directly following the Hirschberg test. A prism bar is placed in front of the fixating eye (Fig. 16-28). The practitioner should attempt to find the amount of prism that causes the corneal light reflexes to appear symmetrical. The magnitude and direction of the prism used to estimate the size of the deviation should be recorded (102,103).

There is a caveat to all tests that require using the pupil as a measuring guide. If there is anisocoria (unequal pupil size) or a misshaped, misplaced, or displaced pupil present, the practitioner might

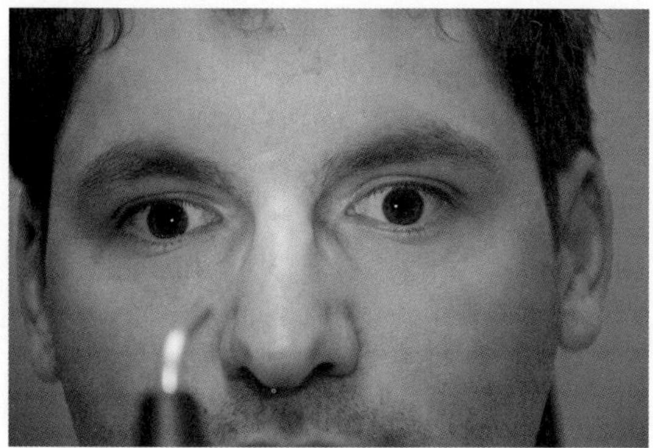

FIGURE 16-27. The Hirschberg test gives a gross estimation of alignment. Notice the white dots on the inner aspects of each iris. This is a normal result. (See also Color Section.)

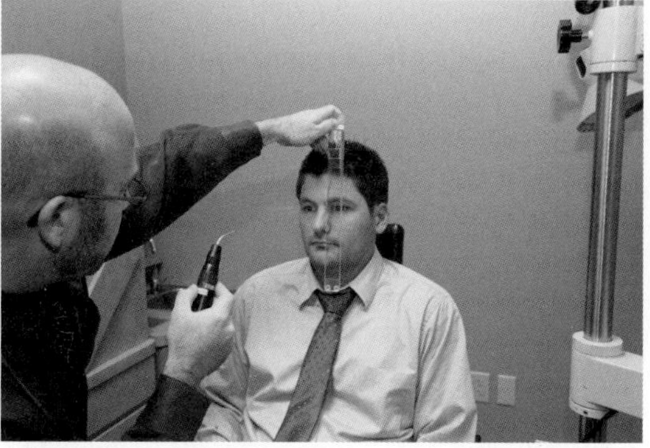

FIGURE 16-28. The Krimsky test is performed if there is an abnormal finding on the Hirschberg test. Prism is introduced to align the reflexes so that they are symmetrical.

not be able to conduct the Hirschberg, Krimsky, and Brückner tests. If the patient has a dark iris and a black pupil, these tests might not be accurate as it would be difficult to obtain a proper measurement.

Cover Test The cover test is the gold standard procedure for determining the type of deviation present, as well as the direction, frequency, laterality, and magnitude of the deviation. Even though it is an objective test, good patient cooperation is vital because poor fixation can cause improper measurement and doctor frustration. This test can be performed at both distance and near with the patient sitting or standing, depending upon physical limitations. The unilateral cover test (UCT) and alternating cover test (ACT) are used in tandem. The UCT is used first to determine whether the patient has a phoria or a tropia, and the ACT is used second to determine magnitude. It is helpful to use an interesting target or a sticker on the nose of the clinician while performing the cover test for special needs patients.

The UCT is performed by occluding one eye while observing the nonoccluded eye for movement. For example, an outward movement of the right eye when the left eye is covered indicates a right esotropia. An inward movement indicates exotropia, an upward eye movement indicates hypotropia, and a downward eye movement indicates hypertropia. This procedure should be repeated for each eye three or four times to allow for an estimate of the frequency of the deviation. A common mistake in administering the UCT, even by the most experienced clinicians, is not giving the patient ample time to refixate and allowing the patient time to fuse the target upon covering and uncovering. Performing this procedure incorrectly will provide the clinician with confusing and often inaccurate results.

If no movement is seen on the UCT, or the magnitude of a heterotropia requires determination, the ACT is used. The occluder is shifted from one eye to the other and back again. The movement of the uncovered eye is observed as the occluder is removed. An outward movement of the eyes indicates esophoria (esotropia), an inward movement indicates exophoria (exotropia), an upward movement indicates a hypophoria (hypotropia), a downward movement indicates a hyperphoria (hypertropia), and no movement indicates orthophoria. The ACT should be repeated several times to identify the direction and magnitude of any movement. Increasing amounts of prism, with the base of the prism bar placed in the direction of the movement, should be continually added until the movement is neutralized and reversal (opposite movement) is noted (102).

The expected value for the distance cover test is one prism diopter of exophoria with a standard deviation of ±1 prism diopter. The expected value for the near cover test is three prism diopters of exophoria with a standard deviation of ±3 prism diopters. Any deviation found on the UCT is considered abnormal (75).

Worth 4 Dot Test The Worth 4 Dot Test is commonly used to determine if suppression exists. The test measures second-degree fusion, which is otherwise known as sensory or flat fusion. With this test, the examiner can also determine the size of the suppression scotoma as well as the depth (102,106).

To perform this test, the patient wears red/green lenses over his or her correction. Older children can view a light with four dots. A pediatric flashlight uses an elephant, a girl, and a ball as targets (Fig. 16-29). Traditionally, the red lens is worn over the right eye, which allows the patient to see the red lights, while the green filter, worn over the left eye allows viewing of the green lights. To improve response results, you might suggest to patients that they "push the buttons" on your flashlight. If they do not see the red "buttons," they will only push the green ones noting that suppression is present.

The test is performed at 40 cm and 6 m. When the test is performed at 40 cm, peripheral fusion is being evaluated. When the test is performed at distance, central fusion is being assessed due to the smaller angular subtense of the target. A patient with normal binocular vision will see one red dot, two green dots, and will perceive the white dot as a mixture of red and green due to retinal rivalry. A response of five dots indicates that the patient is diplopic, while a response of either two red (right eye) or three green

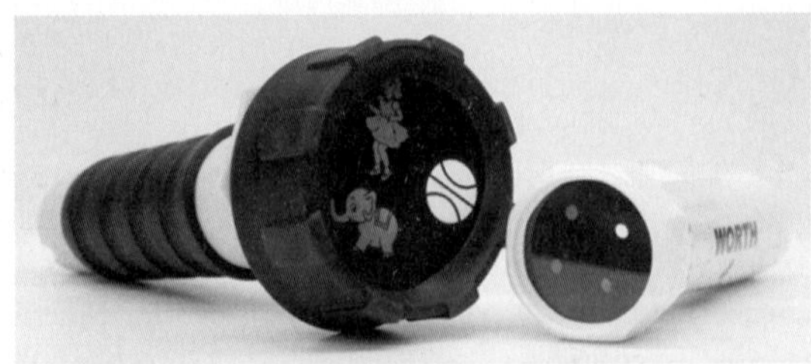

FIGURE 16-29. Adult and pediatric Worth 4 dot tests. (See also Color Section.)

dots (left eye) indicates that the patient is suppressing the image from one eye. The test should be performed first in normal illumination and then in dim illumination to evaluate the depth of suppression. If suppression occurs only with full illumination, it is considered to be shallow. If suppression occurs in both light and dark illumination, the suppression is deemed to be deep. The test distance, room illumination, and patient response should be recorded.

A disadvantage of this test is that the intuitive patient can memorize the number and color of the lights. In order to prevent this, the test can be repeated with the pediatric version which has a three-dot pattern or pictures (102).

REFRACTIVE ERROR ASSESSMENT

When measuring the refractive error of a special needs patient, the clinician might have to rely on purely objective measurements to determine the final prescription. Many of these patients will not be able to participate in a manifest refraction due to either an inability to comprehend the procedure, a lack of ability to verbalize what they see, or any other number of reasons. Commonly, they might not be able to sit still behind the phoropter. The use of retinoscopy racks or skiascopic bars is usually the best option in these situations.

Static Retinoscopy Static retinoscopy is the traditional objective technique used to quantify the patient's refractive error. As previously mentioned, in many cases the doctor must adapt the procedure to the patient. Using retinoscopy racks along with plus spectacles (+1.50 D to +2.00 D depending upon the clinician's working distance) to fog the patient is a quick and simple way to assure a quality result (Fig. 16-30). Since the phoropter is not being used, the practitioner can directly view the patient's fixation and has a better chance of holding the patient's attention. Getting the patient to fixate in the distance might be difficult, so the use of musical toys, bubbles, and video players with cartoons might be useful. Many new electronic acuity systems have videos built in for this very reason. Another hint is to ask the patient's parent or caregiver to bring a favorite object or food that can be used to garner better fixation and attention. The use of a member of the office staff or even the parent could be to help in some capacity.

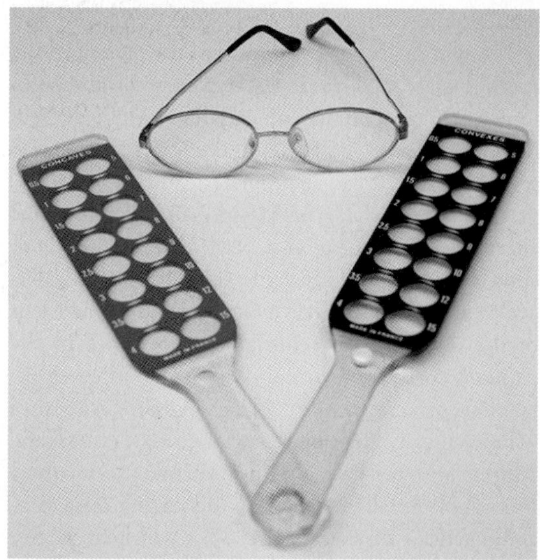

FIGURE 16-30. Retinoscopy racks and bars can help the clinician determine the refractive error when patients cannot use more advanced methods. They come in minus and plus powers. Some clinicians use a pair of reading glasses to neutralize working distance.

Mohindra Near Retinoscopy Method

Mohindra dynamic retinoscopy is an objective, near retinoscopy that is used as an additional refractive method when cycloplegia is contraindicated or unwarranted. Mohindra retinoscopy is performed by having the patient to fixate on the retinoscope light monocularly at 50 cm. Although it is recommended that this test be conducted in complete darkness and with the patient occluded, at times this may not be possible. The refractive error is then determined by algebraically adding −1.25 D to the gross sphere power obtained if the child is 18 months or older. If the child is younger than 18 months, then −0.75 D should be added to the gross sphere power (103).

Keratometry This test is useful to confirm the amount and axis of the corneal astigmatism. Irregular distortions of the mires can give an indication as to the overall health of the cornea. Central corneal distortion or disruption in the integrity of the tear film secondary to disease can easily be seen in the quality of the mires. Proper fixation is required that may prove to be difficult for many patients with special needs. Another difficulty in performing this procedure is that some patients are physically unable to place their chin in the proper position due to an underlying condition.

There are several solutions to this problem. With the advent of handheld equipment that can measure refraction including keratometry, the technology can be brought to the patient instead of the patient to the technology. These handheld autorefractor/autokeratometers are easy to use and very lightweight but still require the patient to fixate on the internal target for several seconds to get an accurate reading.

The keratoscope or Placido disc is a low-cost alternative. It consists of a black disc marked with concentric white and black rings, similar to a bull's-eye target. The examiner looks through a small lens in the center at the reflection of the rings in the patient's cornea. A normal cornea will reflect regular concentric images of the rings. A spherical cornea will produce circular images of the rings. Astigmatic corneas will produce an elliptical image. A cornea that is abnormally curved due to scarring or keratoconus reflects distorted rings. This will help to give a rough estimate of the curvature of the cornea if all else fails.

Cycloplegic Retinoscopy This procedure is very useful in patients with fluctuations in their accommodative system. Cyclopentolate hydrochloride is the drug that is most commonly used for cycloplegic refractions; however, tropicamide can also be used. Studies have shown that tropicamide, which both acts quicker and whose effect lasts a shorter duration than cyclopentolate, is as effective for the measurement of refractive error in numerous populations including healthy, nonstrabismic infants (107), school-aged children with low to moderate hyperopia (108), and myopic adult refractive surgery patients (109). Topical anesthetics should be instilled prior to the cycloplegic agent, followed by two drops of cyclopentolate (0.5% for children from birth to 1 year and 1% for older children), 5 minutes apart (110). Spray administration of the drug appears to be a viable alternative to the use of conventional eye drops for routine cycloplegic retinoscopy in the pediatric population (111–113). A single application can achieve both cycloplegia and pupillary dilation when a mixture of 0.5% cyclopentolate, 0.5% tropicamide, and 2.5% phenylephrine is used (114). Make sure not to give them or the caregiver a tissue until after the spray or drop has been installed as this will stop absorption. Retinoscopy should be performed 20 to 30 minutes after installation (111).

Cyclopentolate produces mydriasis within 30 minutes and maximum cycloplegia in 30 to 45 minutes. The mydriasis and cycloplegia can last up to 24 hours. The onset of the mydriasis and cycloplegia for tropicamide is within 20 to 40 minutes, but lasts for approximately 4 to 6 hours.

Caution must be taken when you use diagnosticc drugs with any individual who has a history to cardiac and/or respriatory problems. These are common problems in patients with Down syndrome, cerebral palsy, and other CNS disorders. Be aware of biologic variations such as low weight which may require a modified dosage (114). Tropicamide 1% may be used in the place of cyclopentolate if dosage is a concern (114–116). Punctal occlusion for several minutes after installation should be considered with all patients to reduce the systemic effects of all diagnostic pharmaceutical agents.

MEASURING INTRAOCULAR PRESSURE

Measuring intraocular pressure (IOP) in special needs patients can be a challenge due to mental and physical constraints. If a patient presents with glaucoma-related signs and the IOP measurements cannot be taken by standard tests, the patient may require tonometry while under sedation (117).

Goldmann Applanation Tonometry Even though this test is considered the standard for determining IOPs, it has several disadvantages for use in a special needs patient. The patient must hold proper fixation and posture, while the practitioner must instill anesthesia prior to use, get very close to the patient, and touch the patient's cornea with the Goldman probe tip to obtain measurements (Fig. 16-31). This may scare some patients, especially those with decreased mental capacity to comprehend the directions and testing (117).

Tono-Pen The Tono-Pen (Medtronics) is a small, handheld device that measures IOP. It is very useful in that multiple, quick measurements of IOP can be obtained. Since the instrument is handheld, it is very useful for patients in wheelchairs (117). Similar to Goldmann tonometry, the probe must touch the cornea (Fig. 16-32). This can be frightening for some patients with special needs. Making matters worse, anesthesia must be instilled prior to measurement. This tends to cause more eyes being clamped shut than being wide open for easy measurement, but the device also provides an indication of the quality of the measurement to reduce abnormal findings.

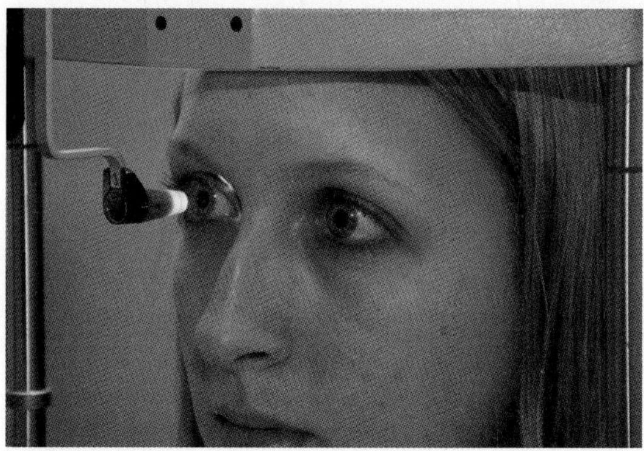

FIGURE 16-31. Goldmann Applanation Tonometry is the gold standard for assessing intraocular pressure, but patients with special needs may not appreciate the need for anesthetic or that the probe touches the eye.

Noncontact Tonometry Noncontact tonometry (NCT) is useful for patients who are uncomfortable with drop instillation and having their eyes touched. Physical constraints may be an issue with this procedure, because the patient must maintain steady fixation. One solution is the Keeler Pulsair tonometer, a handheld NCT. It is valuable when measuring IOPs because the measuring apparatus can be used in almost any situation or location. This makes it useful for patients who use wheelchairs. Prior to taking a reading, the practitioner should demonstrate the puff of air on the patient's hand. This will lessen the chance that the practitioner will only get readings from one eye because of patient apprehension following the first attempt. Patient anxiety about the device and the puff of air can be reduced by saying a phrase such as, "It's going to give you a kiss."

iCare Tonometer Rebound tonometry, which is also known as impact or dynamic tonometry, was first introduced more than 75 years ago but was recently modified and made commercially available in 2003 (118). The method is based on the use of a moving probe that touches the cornea. The motion parameters of the probe are monitored and allow calculation of the IOP. The iCare tonometer uses lightweight, disposable, sterile probes that touch the cornea for such a small amount of time that anesthesia is not required (119).

Favorable comparison of the iCare with Goldmann Applanation Tonometry (GAT) and NCT methods has been found (120,121). Comparing the iCare to the Pulsair 3000, an NCT, it was found that the two tonometers were within ±1 mm Hg in 52.5% of the measurements and within ±2 mm Hg in 71.7% (120). Comparing the iCare to GAT, it was found that 55% of the readings were between ±2 mm Hg and 75% were between ±3 mm Hg from the mean of the Goldmann readings (121).

Digital Tension Estimation When IOPs cannot be obtained using the above methods, digital tension estimation can be used. This method has been found to be a reliable means of obtaining IOP in children, particularly in the range of 6 to 22 mm Hg (122). To perform this test, the patient should close his or her eyes and look down. One index finger should be used to keep the eye in position, and the other index finger should be used to apply pressure above the tarsal plate (Fig. 16-33). The pressure

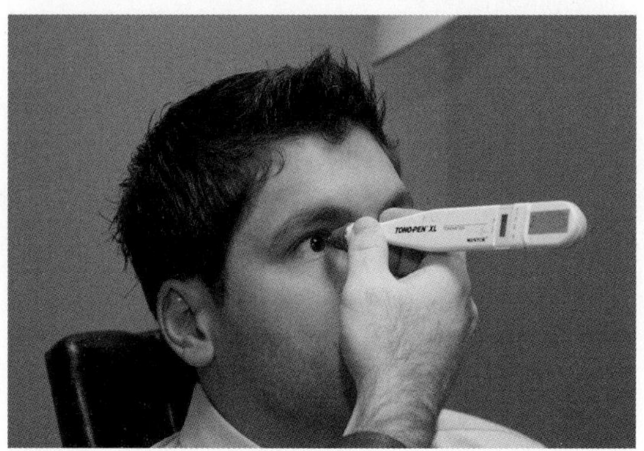

FIGURE 16-32. The Tono-Pen is an alternative to the Goldmann technique.

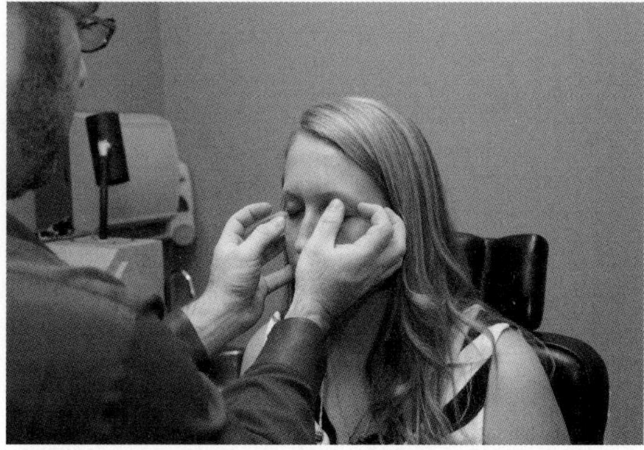

FIGURE 16-33. Digital palpation may be the only assessment of intraocular pressure possible on a patient with special needs.

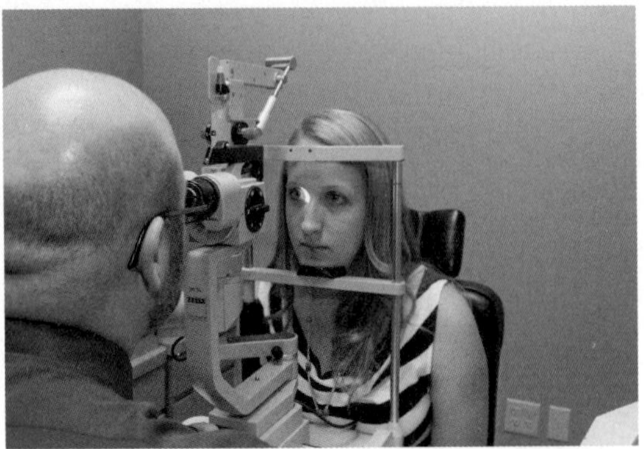

FIGURE 16-34. A slit lamp examination assesses the anterior segment as well as the health of the lids and lashes.

estimation is obtained by the pressing finger force felt by the stationary index finger. Pressures should be recorded as "soft to touch," "medium to touch," or "hard to touch" (122).

ANTERIOR SEGMENT EVALUATION

Gross inspection of the anterior segment should be performed with a high plus lens (20 D lens with a penlight or BIO light) or a handheld or stationary slit lamp (Fig. 16-34). The health of the conjunctiva, lids, lashes, and cornea can be assessed with this method. The depth of the anterior chamber can be evaluated by using a transilluminator and checking for limbal glow. The transilluminator should be placed to the temporal side of the patient's face. The practitioner should note the amount of glow that is transmitted throughout the chamber angle and the amount that is visible on the nasal side of the globe. A shadow may suggest a bowed iris, while a uniform glow suggests a flat iris (117).

POSTERIOR SEGMENT EVALUATION

Evaluation of the vitreous, lens, optic nerve, and retina should be done through dilated pupils using a direct, binocular indirect, or monocular indirect ophthalmoscope. The young patient may lie on the floor or in a parent's lap while the older patient usually remains seated for the practitioner to perform this part of the examination. Photosensitivity is common in patients with special needs because of the medications they are taking or any anatomical/physiological anomalies present. Using low illumination or a red-free filter (green light) may enhance patient cooperation. If the patient is unable to sit for these tests, fundus photography or performing these procedures under general anesthesia may be required (117).

CONCLUSION

Being prepared is the key for any efficient evaluation of a patient. This is especially true when evaluating those with special needs. Having all tools readily available and within easy reach will decrease the time needed for the evaluation and increase the likelihood of the patient being cooperative and capable of giving results that are reliable. Practitioners should consider assembling a kit with equipment for some of the tests/procedures discussed. This will help set the stage for everyone involved and lead to a great examination.

ACKNOWLEDGMENT *I would like to thank Erin Jaffe at Southern College of Optometry for her assistance in taking many of the pictures in this chapter.*

REFERENCES

1. Mozlin R. Quality-of-life outcomes assessment. J Optom Vis Dev 1995;26:194–9.
2. Maples WC. Test-retest reliability of the College of Optometrists in Vision Development Quality of Life Outcomes Assessment short form. J Optom Vis Dev 2002;33:126–34.
3. Maples WC. Test-retest reliability of the College of Optometrists in Vision Development Quality of Life Outcomes Assessment. Optometry 2000;71(9):579–85.
4. Maples WC, Bither M. Efficacy of vision therapy as assessed by the COVD quality of life checklist. Optometry 2002;73(8):492–8.
5. Vaughn W, Maples WC, Hoenes R. The association between vision quality of life and academics as measured by the College of Optometrists in Vision Development Quality of Life questionnaire. Optometry 2006;77:116–23.
6. Daugherty KM, Frantz KA, Allison CL, et al. Evaluating changes in quality of life after vision therapy using the COVD quality of life outcomes assessment. J Optom Vis Dev 2007;38:75–81.
7. Donati RJ, Maino DM, Bartell H, et al. Polypharmacy and the lack of oculo-visual complaints from those with mental illness and dual diagnosis. Optometry 2009;80:249–54.
8. Isralowitz R, Madar M, Lifshitz T, et al. Visual problems among people with mental retardation. Int J Rehabil Res 2003;26:149–52.
9. Maino DM, Maino JH, Maino SA. Mental retardation syndromes with associated ocular defects. J Am Optom Assoc 1990;61:707–16.

10. Maino DM, Rado ME, Pizzi WJ. Ocular anomalies of individuals with mental illness and dual diagnosis. J Am Optom Assoc. 1996;67:740–8.
11. Van SJ, Stilma JS, Bernsen RM, et al. Prevalence of ocular diagnoses found on screening 1539 adults with intellectual disabilities. Opthalmology. 2004;111:1457–63.
12. Viertio S, Laitinen A, Perala J, et al. Visual impairment in persons with psychotic disorder. Soc Psychiatry Pshychiatr Epidemiol. 2007;42:902–8.
13. Warburg M. Visual impairment in adult people with intellectual disability: literature review. J Intellect Disabil Res. 2001;45:424–38.
14. Scheiman M. Assessment and management of the exceptional child. In: Rosenbloom A, Morgan M, editors. Principles and practice of pediatric optometry. Grand Rapids: J. B. Lippincott Co.; 1990. p. 387–419.
15. Fraunfelder FT, Fraunfelder FW. Agents affecting the central nervous system. Drug-induced ocular side effects. 5th ed. Media: Butterworth-Heinmann; 2001. p. 114–58.
16. Fraunfelder FW, Fraunfelder FT. Adverse ocular drug reactions recently identified by the National Registry of Drug-Induced Ocular Side Effects. Ophthalmology. 2004;111:1275–9.
17. Patel M. Ocular side effects of drugs Part 7a: drugs for the nervous system. Optom Today. 2003;43:37–47.
18. Fraunfelder FT, Fraunfelder FW. Drug-induced ocular side effects. 5th ed. Boston: Butterworth-Heinemann; 2001.
19. Maino D. The mentally handicapped patient: a perspective. J Am Optom Assoc. 1987;58:14–7.
20. Sheridan MD, Gardiner PA. Sheridan-Gardiner test for visual acuity. Br Med J. 1970;2:108–9.
21. Friendly DS. Preschool visual acuity screening tests. Trans Am Ophthalmol Soc. 1980;76:383–480.
22. Hered RW, Murphy S, Clancy M. Comparison of the HOTV and Lea symbols charts for preschool vision screening. J Pediatr Ophthalmol Strab. 1997;34:24–8.
23. Vision in Preschoolers Study Group. Preschool visual acuity screening with HOTV and Lea symbols: testability and between-test agreement. Optom Vis Sci. 2004;8:678–83.
24. Hyvarinen L, Nasanen R, Laurinen P. New visual acuity test in preschool children. Acta Ophthalmol. 1980;58:507–11.
25. Richman JE, Petitio GT, Cron M. Broken wheel acuity test: a new and valid test for preschool and exceptional children. J Am Optom Assoc. 1984;55:561–5.
26. Scheiman M. Pediatric visual acuity. In: Eskridge JB, Amos JF, Bartlett JD, editors. Clinical procedures in optometry. Philadelphia: JB Lippincott Co.; 1991. p. 641–50.
27. National Academy of Sciences-National Research Council Committee on Vision. Recommended standard procedures for the clinical measurement and specification of visual acuity. Adv Ophthalmol. 1980;41:103–48.
28. Press LJ. Examination of the preschool child. In: Press LJ, Moore BD, editors. Clinical pediatric optometry. Boston: Butterworth-Heinmann; 1993:47–62.
29. Rowe S, Taub MB, Bartuccio M. Examining special populations: part 4 more examination techniques. Optom Today. 2006:41–4.
30. Mocan MC, Najera-Covarrubias M, Wright KW. Comparison of visual acuity levels on the pediatric patients with amblyopia using Wright figures, Allen optotypes and Snellen letters. J AAPOS. 2005;9:48–52.
31. Lipmann O. Vision screening of young children. Am J Public Health. 1971;61:1586–601.
32. Simons K. Visual acuity norms in young children. Surv Ophthalmol. 1983;28:84–92.
33. Clifford CE, Breann M, Dobson V. Are norms based on the original Teller acuity cards appropriate for use with the new Teller acuity cards II. J AAPOS. 2005;9475–9.
34. McDonald M, Dobson V, Sebris SL, et al. The acuity card procedure: a rapid test of infant acuity. Invest Ophthalmol Vis Sci. 1985;26:1158–62.
35. Dobson V, McDonald M, Kohl P, et al. Visual acuity screening of infants and young children with the acuity card procedure. Am Optom Assoc. 1986;57:285–9.
36. Kohl P, Rolen RD, Bedford AK, et al. Refractive error and preferential looking visual acuity in human infants: a pilot study. J Am Optom Assoc. 1986;57:290–6.
37. Milot J, Navaratil J, Barsoum-Homsy M, et al. Visual acuity in mentally retarded children measured with the forced-preferential looking procedure and the scolatest. Am Orth J. 1988;38:135–41.
38. Woodhouse JM, Adoh TO, Oduwaiye KA, et al. New acuity test for toddlers. Ophthalmic Physiol Opt. 1992;12:249–51.
39. Adoh TO, Woodhouse M. The Cardiff acuity test used for measuring visual acuity development in toddlers. Vision Res. 1994;34:555–60.
40. Bailey IL, Hall AP. New visual acuity tests for children. Am J Optom Physiol Opt. 1984;61:962–5.
41. Haegerstrom-Portnoy G. New procedures for evaluating vision functions of special populations. Optom Vis Sci. 1993;70:306–14.
42. Mackie RT, McCulloch DL. Assessment of visual acuity in multiply handicapped children. Br J Ophthalmol. 1995;79:290–6.
43. Elliot DB. Primary eye care. 2nd ed. Boston: Butterworth-Heinemann; 2003.
44. Dain SJ. Clinical colour vision tests. Clin Exp Optom. 2004;87:276–93.
45. Pickford RW. Tests for colour blindness. Br Med Bull. 1953; 9:82.
46. Cowan A, Tiffin J, Kuhn HS. Color discrimination in industry. Arch Ophthalmol. 1942;28:851–9.
47. Cole BL. Misuse of the Ishihara test for colour blindness. Br J Physiol Opt. 1963;20:113–8.
48. Johnson DD. The Ishihara test: on prevention of job discrimination. J Am Optom Assoc. 1992;63:352–60.
49. Walls GL. How good is the HRR test for color blindness? Am J Optom Physiol Opt. 1959;36:169–93.
50. Hardy LH, Rand G, Rittler MC. The H-R-R Polychromatic plates. J Opt Soc Am. 1954;44:509–23.
51. Rand G, Rittler MC. An evaluation of the AO HRR pseudo-isochromatic plates. Arch Ophthalmol. 1956;56:736–42.
52. Hogan MJ. Evaluation of vision screening methods in industry. AMA Arch Ind Health. 1957;16:93.
53. McCulloch C, Turner NC, Smiley JR. A field study of the H-R-R color vision plate test. Am J Ophthalmol. 1959;48:124–9.
54. Cole BL. Comments on some color vision tests and their use for selection. Aust J Optom. 1964;47:56–64.

55. Paulson H. Colour vision testing. In: Pierce JR, Levene JR, eds. Visual science. Bloomington: Indiana University Press; 1971. p. 164–76.
56. Aroichane M, Pieramici DJ, Miller NR, et al. A comparative study of Hardy-Rand-Rittler and Ishihara colour plates for the diagnosis of non-glaucomatous optic neuropathy. Can J Ophthalmol. 1996;31:350–5.
57. Cole BL, Lian KY, Lakkis C. The new Richmond HRR pesudoisochomatic test for colour vision is better than the Ishihara test. Clin Exp Opt. 2006;89:73–80.
58. Dain SJ. Colorimetric analysis of four editions of the Hardy-Rand-Rittler pseudoisochromatic test. Vis Neurosci. 2004;21:437–43.
59. Bailey JE, Neitz M, Tait DM, et al. Evaluation of the updated HRR color vision test. Vis Neurosci. 2004;21:431–6.
60. Bailey JE. Color vision. In: Eskridge JB, Amos JF, Bartlett JD, editors. Clinical procedures in optometry. Philadelphia: JB Lippincott Co.; 1991. p. 99–120.
61. Taub MB, Rowe S, Bartuccio M. Examining special populations: part 3 examination techniques. Optom Today. 2006;46:49–52.
62. Cooper J. Stereopsis. In: Eskridge JB, Amos JF, Bartlett JD, eds. Clinical procedures in optometry. Philadelphia: JB Lippincott Co.; 1991. p. 121–34.
63. Lang J. A new stereo test. J Pediatr Ophthalmol Strab. 1983;20:72–4.
64. Ohlsson J, Villarreal G, Abrahamsson M, et al. Screening merits of the Lang II, Frisby, Randot, Titmus and TNO stereo tests. J AAPOS. 2001;5:316–21.
65. Leat SJ, Pierre JS, Hassan-Abadi S, et al. The moving dynamic random dot stereosize test: development, age norms, and comparison with the Frisby, Randot, and stereo smile tests. J Pediatr Ophthalmol Strab. 2001;38:284–94.
66. The Vision in Preschoolers Study Group. Testability of preschoolers on stereo tests used to screen vision disorders. Optom Vis Sci. 2003;80:753–7.
67. Leat SJ. Paediatric assessment. In: Rosenfeld M, Logan N, eds. Optometry: science, techniques and clinical management. 2nd ed. Boston: Elsevier; 2009. p. 439–60.
68. Available from: www.lea-test.fil/en/vistests/instruct/flickwew/flickerw.html-Last Accessed February 12th, 2010.
69. Woodhouse JM, Meades JS, Leat SJ, et al. Reduced accommodation in children with Down syndrome. Invest Ophthal Vis Sci. 1993;42:2382–7.
70. Leat SJ. Reduced accommodation in children with cerebral palsy. Ophthalmic Physiol Opt. 1996;16:385–90.
71. Rosenfield M. Accommodation. In: Zadnik K, editor. The ocular examination: measurements and findings. Philadelphia: W.B. Saunders.
72. Daum K. Near point of convergence. In: Eskridge JB, Amos JF, Bartlett JD, eds. Clinical procedures in optometry. Philadelphia: JB Lippincott Co.; 1991. p. 66–8.
73. Valenti CA. The full scope of retinoscopy. 2nd ed. Santa Anna: Optometric Extension Program; 1990.
74. Carlson NB, Kurtz D. Clinical procedures for ocular examination. 3rd ed. Chicago: McGraw-Hill; 1996.
75. Scheiman M, Wick B. Clinical management of binocular vision: heterophoric, accommodative, and eye movement disorders. 2nd ed. Philadelphia: Lippincott Williams & Wilkins; 2002.
76. Woehrle MB, Peters RJ, Frantz KA. Accommodative amplitude determination: can we substitute the pull-away for the push-up method? J Optom Vis Dev. 1997;28:246–9.
77. Hofstetter HW. Useful age-amplitude formula. Optom World. 1950;38:42–5.
78. Maples WC, Atchley J, Ficklin T. Northeastern State University College of optometry's oculomotor norms. J Behav Optom. 1992;3:143–50.
79. Maples WC, Vaughan S, Ficklin T. Verification of the reliability of the King-Devick saccade test. In: Goss D, editor. Proceedings of the NSU symposium on theoretical and clinical optometry. Tahlequah: Northeastern State University; 1988. p. 33–43.
80. Maples WC, Ficklin T. Test-retest reliability of the King-Devick saccade test and NSUCO oculamotor tests. J Behav Optom (Australia). 1991;3:209–14.
81. Maples WC, Ficklin T. A preliminary study of oculomotor skills of learning-disabled, gifted and normal children. J Optom Vis Dev. 1989;20:9–14.
82. Maples WC, Ficklin T. Comparison of eye movement skills between above and below average readers. J Behav Optom. 1990;1:87–91.
83. Solan HA, Ficarra AP. A study of perceptual and verbal skills of disabled readers in grades 4, 5 and 6. J Am Optom Assoc. 1990;61:628–34.
84. Maples WC. Oculomotor dysfunctions: classification of saccades and pursuit deficiencies. In: Press LJ, ed. Applied concepts in vision therapy. St. Louis: Mosby; 1997. p. 120–36.
85. Scheiman M, Gallaway M, Frantz K, et al. The effect of stimulus variables on the near point of convergence. Am Acad Optom (Los Angeles). 1991.
86. Wick BC. Horizontal deviations. In: Amos JF, ed. Diagnosis and management in vision care. Boston: Butterworth, 1987. p. 473.
87. Mohindra I, Molinari J. Convergence insufficiency: its diagnosis and management part I. Optom Monthly. 1980; 71:38–43.
88. Pang Y, Gabriel H, Frantz KA, et al. A prospective study of different test targets for the near point of convergence. Ophthalmic Physiol Opt. 2010;30:298–303.
89. King AT, Devick S. The proposed King and Devick test and its relation to the Pierce saccade test and reading levels. Available from the Carol E. Shepard Memorial Library. Illinois College of Optometry; 1976.
90. Lieberman S, Cohen AH, Rubin J. NYSOA KD test. J Am Optom Assoc. 1983;54:631–7.
91. Garzia R, Richman JE, Nicholson SB, et al. A new visual verbal saccade test: the Developmental Eye Movement test (DEM). J Am Optom Assoc. 1990;61:124–35.
92. Garzia R, Richman JE, Nicholson SB. A new clinical eye movement test compensating for automaticity of number calling. Am J Optom Physiol Opt. 1987;64:54–65.
93. Kulp MT, Schmidt PP. Relationship between visual skills and performance testing on saccadic eye movement testing. Optom Vis Sci. 1998;75:284–7.
94. Maples WC. Oculomotor dysfunctions: classification of saccadic and pursuit deficiencies. In: Press L, editor. Applied concepts in vision therapy. Santa Ana: Optometric Extension Program; 2008. p. 120–36.

95. Galleta KM, Barrett J, Allen M, et al. The King-Devick test as a determinant of head trauma and concussion in boxers and MMA fighters. Neurology. 2011;76:1456–62.
96. Han Y, Cuiffreda KJ, Kapoor N. Reading-related oculomotor testing and training protocols for acquired brain injury in humans. Brain Res Brain Res Protoc. 2004;12:1–12.
97. Suchoff IB, Kapoor N, Waxman R, et al. The occurrence of ocular and visual dysfunctions in an acquired brain-injured patient sample. J Am Optom Assoc. 1999;70:301–8.
98. Vogel G. Saccadic eye movements: theory, testing, and therapy. J Behav Optom. 1995;6:3–12.
99. Richman J, Walker A, Garzia R. The impact of automatic digit naming ability on a clinical test of eye movement functioning. J Am Optom Assoc. 1983;54:617–22.
100. Kulp MT, Schmidt PP. Reliability of the NYSOA King-Devick saccadic eye movement test in kindergartners and first graders. J Am Optom Assoc. 1997;68:589–94.
101. Rouse MW, Nestor EM, Parot CJ, et al. A reevaluation of the Developmental Eye Movement (DEM) test's repeatability. Optom Vis Sci. 2004;81:934–8.
102. Caloroso EE, Rouse MW. Clinical management of strabismus. Boston: Butterworth-Heinemann; 1993.
103. Scheiman M. Hirschberg, Krimsky and Bruckner tests. In: Eskridge JB, Amos JF, Bartlett JD, eds. Clinical procedures in optometry. Philadelphia: JB Lippincott Co.; 1991. p. 651–4.
104. Griffen JR, Cotter SA. The Bruckner test: evaluation of the clinical usefulness. Am J Optom Physiol Opt. 1986; 63:957–61.
105. Roe LD, Guyton DL. The light that leaks: Bruckner and the red reflex. Surv Ophthalmol. 1984;28:665–70.
106. Wick B. Suppression. In: Eskridge JB, Amos JF, Bartlett JD, eds. Clinical procedures in optometry. Philadelphia: JB Lippincott Co.; 1991. p. 698–707.
107. Twelker JD, Mutti DO. Retinoscopy in infants using a near noncycloplegic technique, cycloplegia with tropicamide 1%, and cycloplegia with cyclopentolate 1%. Optom Vis Sci. 2001;78:215–22.
108. Egashira SM, Kish LL, Twelker JD, Mutti DO, Zadnick K, Adams AJ. Comparison of cyclopentolate versus tropicamide cycloplegia in children. Optom Vis Sci. 1993;70:1019–26.
109. Hofmeister EM, Kaupp SE, Schallhorn SC. Comparison of tropicamide and cyclopentolate for cycloplegic refractions in myopic adult refractive surgery patients. J Cataract Refract Surg. 2005;31:694–700.
110. Amos JF. Cycloplegic refraction. In: Bartlett JD, Jaanus SD, editors. Clinical ocular pharmacology. 4th ed. Boston: Butterworth-Heinemann; 2001. p. 425–32.
111. Bartlett JD, Wesson MD, Swiatocha J, et al. Efficacy of a pediatric cycloplegic administered as a spray. J Am Optom Assoc. 1993;64:617–21.
112. Ismail EE, Rouse MW, De Land PN. A comparison of drop instillation and spray application of 1% cyclopentolate hydrochloride. Optom Vis Sci. 1994;71:235–41.
113. Hug T, Cibis GW, Lynd J. The use of spray topical drug delivery system for cycloplegic medications in children. Binocular Vis Strabismus Q. 1997;12:191–4.
114. American Optometric Association. Pediatric eye and vision examination. 2nd ed. St Louis: American Optometric Association; 2002.
115. Gray L. Avoiding adverse effects of cycloplegics in infants and children. J Am Optom Assoc. 1979;50:465–70.
116. Kennerdell JS, Wucher FP. Cyclopentolate associated with two cases of grand mal seizure. Arch Ophthalmol. 1972;87:634–5.
117. Maino DM. Diagnosis and management of special populations. St. Louis: Mosby Year Book; 1995.
118. Kontiola A, Puska P. Measuring intraocular pressure with the Pulsair 3000 and rebound tonometers in elderly patients without an anaesthetic. Graefes Arch Clin Exp Ophthalmol. 2004;242:3–7.
119. Roberts DEC. Comparison of iCARE tonometer with pulsair and tono-Pen in domiciliary work. Optom Prac. 2005;6:33–9.
120. Brusini P, Salvetat L, Zeppieri M, Tosoni C, et al. Comparison of the iCare tonometer with Goldman Applanation Tonometer in glaucoma patients. Glaucoma. 2006;15:213–7.
121. Stampler RL, Lieberman MF, Drake MV. Becker-Schaffer's diagnosis and therapy of the glaucomas. 8th ed. Philadelphia: Mosby Elsevier; 2009. p. 47–67.
122. Ficarra AP, Sorkin R, Morrison C. Assessment of intraocular pressure in children by digital tension. Optometry. 1995;73:499–506.

CHAPTER 17

James M. Newman, MS, OD, FAAO

Diagnosis and Management of Refractive Error

INTRODUCTION

The human refractive state contributes to the clarity and comfort of vision. The individual's adaptation or maladaptation to vision aberrations can affect a person's quality of life (1). These adjustments vary over a lifetime as the vision system undergoes change. Therefore, early intervention and management of refractive errors provide for positive patient outcomes.

Emmetropization is discussed as being a process, both dynamic and passive, where the coordination of the anatomical ocular components of the human eye produces a resultant refractive condition (2). This refractive condition changes from birth throughout the life of the patient, in that there is a general decrease in hyperopia or an increase in myopia till around age 20. The refraction remains relatively stable till around age 40, with a general increase in hyperopia or decrease in myopia until senile cataract formation occurs in the older population (3).

Each of the major refractive ametropias will be discussed with incidence, patient management options and outcomes, and considerations with the special needs populations. Special needs patients present with a prevalence of reduced acuity and possibly undiagnosed refractive conditions that need to be addressed for optimum visual function (4). Since this text is meant for both the optometrist and non–eye care professionals, I will discuss the various aspects of refractive error in such a way so that therapists, special educators, and others involved in the care of patients with special needs will have a better understanding of the topic.

EMMETROPIA

Emmetropia is an ocular condition, where parallel light, with a zero dioptric stimulus, focuses on a patient's retina with no accommodation involved. Patients manifesting emmetropia usually have no complaints because visual acuities are standard at far and near. Emmetropes comprise about 25% of the adult population's refractive status. The classic characteristic of the emmetrope is that they accommodate relatively equal to the distance stimulus. When refracting clinically, patients are made artificially emmetropic by compensatory lenses early in the exam routine to provide a basis of comparison of the subsequent refractive tests. Any refractive condition that differs from emmetropia is termed ametropia, of which there are three major classifications: myopia, hyperopia, and astigmia.

Myopia Myopia is an ocular condition, where parallel light comes to focus in front of the retina without the influence of accommodation (1). The optical elements of the eye are shaped in such a way that the light is focused in front of the retina. The main patient complaint would be distance blur. Minus spherical lenses are used for correcting myopia. Because the main problem for the patient is that distance vision is blurry, the lay term "nearsighted" has evolved, indicating that the patient can see clearly at close ranges, and not at distance. However, in cases of higher-magnitude myopia (>4.00D), patients can also complain of a near blur, that is compensated by holding reading material closer. This allows the light to focus properly on the retina. In this instance, as the uncorrected myope brings reading material closer, the focus of light moves closer to the retina until the light is focused on the retina.

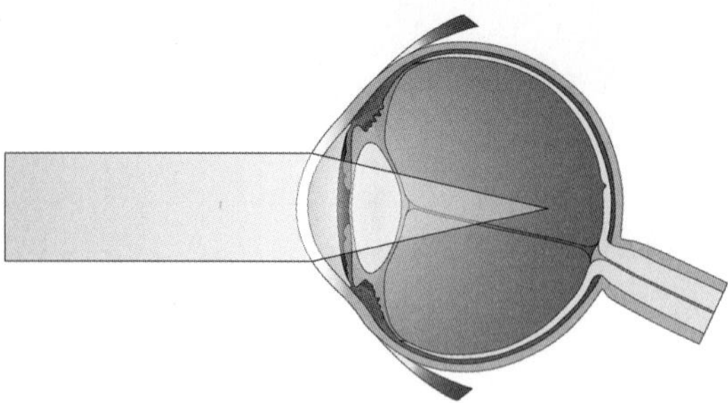

FIGURE 17-1. For an uncompensated myope, parallel light comes to focus in front of the retina, resulting in a vision complaint of blurred vision by the patient.

Figure 17-1 indicates how entering light focuses in the uncorrected myopic eye. Figure 17-2 indicates how the uncorrected myope is made to see clearly by the addition of minus lenses. When the parallel light is focused on the retina with the eye not accommodating, the patient's corrected condition simulates emmetropia. So with the uncorrected myope wearing minus lenses and seeing clearly, this patient has been made an artificial emmetrope.

The incidence of primary myopia in the general population ranges from 25% to 30%, but can vary significantly based on racial ethnicity (1). Because this condition greatly impacts distance clarity and quality of life, the clinical population may be much higher. In the United States, the amount of myopia typically ranges from 0.50D to 4.00D (5). The distribution of high-degree myopia can be directly correlated with the longer than normal axial length of the human eye. For lower magnitudes of myopia, axial length, corneal curvature, or other etiologies may be equally responsible, but with high magnitudes the long axial length is the primary cause.

Selected special needs populations can present with varying magnitudes of myopia, which needs to be addressed for quality-of-life benefits for the individuals affected. Patients with Down syndrome manifest a greater tendency for larger-magnitude myopia (6) (see Chapter 4, Down Syndrome). Premature infants have a tendency to manifest large magnitudes of degenerative myopia, due to the excessive axial length and the accompanying retinal degenerative problems (7). Patients with cerebral palsy do not have a specific predisposition for myopia at a greater incidence than the general population (8) (see Chapter 3, Cerebral Palsy). Traumatic brain injury patients may manifest a transient myopia due to ciliary spasms, so compensation should be delayed, pending resolution of the accommodation problems (9,10).

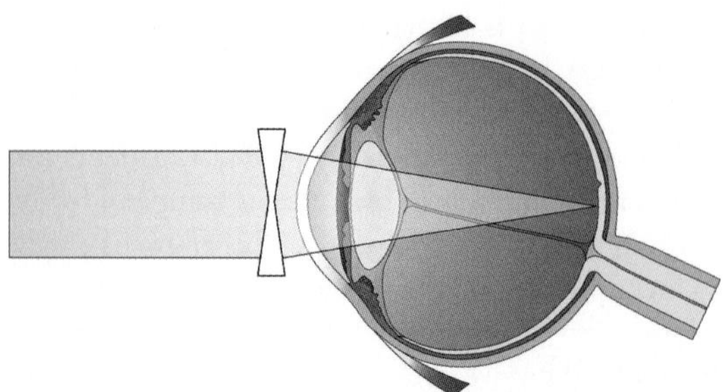

FIGURE 17-2. An uncorrected myopic patient is made artificially emmetropic by the addition of minus lenses, with parallel light now focusing on the retina.

Myopia has been the refractive error most researched. Causation theories that include genetics (11), nutrition (12), accommodation (13) and convergence (14) have been considered. Recently, peripheral retinal blur has been postulated (15). The management options for the myopias are dependent on the etiology determined, so there may be disagreements as to the appropriate management choice. If the patient complains of a distance blur that is constant throughout the day that does not change, the myopia would be considered primary and lens compensation, either with spectacles or contact lenses would be an option.

The retardation of myopia progression in the adolescent population has been a clinical concern for a number of years. Recent studies have affirmed that bifocal additions and bifocal additions with base in prism can reduce the rate of myopic progression in certain patients (16). Topical muscarinic antagonists, such as atropine and pirenzepine, have also shown to delay the progression of myopia (17). Orthokeratology, or corneal reshaping, with conventional gas permeable contact lenses has proven effective in myopia reduction (18). New studies show the potential of overnight contact lens wear having the same effect as conventional daily wear rigid lenses (19).

In the past 20 years, surgical options have been used to compensate for the patient's myopia, most often by surgically altering the shape of the cornea or surgically inserting lenses into the patient's eye. Laser-assisted in situ keratomileusis (LASIK) and photorefractive keratectomy (PRK) are currently the two most popular methods of surgically managing myopia. Both procedures employ lasers to alter the corneal stroma, though LASIK necessitates the creation of a corneal flap, while PRK does not (20).

If distance vision clarity changes throughout the day, the myopia can be thought of as being secondary and the reason for the fluctuation would need to be explored before prescribing lenses. Accommodative dysfunction, divergence excess, convergence insufficiency, fluctuating blood sugar in diabetes, corneal metabolic problems, oral medication side effects, and abuse are a partial list of etiologies that can lead to myopic-like complaints (1).

Because uncorrected myopes accommodate less when viewing a near stimulus, these patients often present with poor accommodative ability during their eye examination. The amplitude of accommodation may be reduced, and a low-positive relative accommodation and high lag of accommodation can be noted. Unaided near phorias should show an exophoric tendency due to the underaccommodation; however, when initially corrected, the near phoria may show less exophoria or even an esophoric tendency. This is due to the fact the patient has been habitually using positive fusional vergence movements to maintain fusion in the absence of available positive accommodative vergence. Now, through lens compensation, the patient has to accommodate more like an emmetrope. The patient is now beginning to use available positive accommodative vergence, along with the habitual positive fusional vergence for fusion, to mimic a convergence excess-type response. This initial response will change as the patient wears the glasses and accommodation approaches normal levels (1).

A general treatment principle is to be careful not to overprescribe minus power for the myopic patient (Table 17.1). If too much minus is given, then parallel light is focused behind the retina, and the patient, if young enough, can accommodate to bring the light to focus on the retina. The patient can still see clearly, yet must overfocus to do so. The patient can habituate to this extra effort and can complain of "blurred" vision if less minus is ever prescribed to them.

TABLE 17.1 Myopic Patient Clinical Pearls

- If distance subjective blur is constant, lens compensation or refractive surgical intervention is acceptable.
- If distance subjective blur varies during the day, secondary causes of the blur should be explored before lens compensation.
- Do not "overminus" or "underminus" myopic patients.
- Be careful in reducing the amount of minus power on an asymptomatic myopic patient.
- Counsel patients concerning lens adaptation, especially when reading.
- Prescribe minimum amount of minus power that answers the patient's blur complaints.
- Because minus lenses minify, large-magnitude myopes may require bifocal additions for magnification, to increase reading clarity.

On initial compensation for myopic patients, there may be some accommodative or focusing adjustment when reading through the new lenses. This is due to the patient habitually accommodating less because of the uncorrected myopia. The patient will now accommodate relatively equal to the stimulus, similar to an emmetrope, yet more than they were used to. The patient should be warned that adaptation to the prescription will take place over days to weeks, but symptoms such as blurred vision while reading and frontal headaches may occur. These near symptoms will abate as the individual adapts to increasing accommodation (1). Encouraging the patient to wear the lenses full time will build up the patient's accommodative ability, increasing the measurable amplitude of accommodation. A bifocal addition for reading may be necessary due to impaired accommodation or if the level of correction is extremely high to improve the near visual acuity.

In patients with special needs, an objective measure of the refractive condition is critical. Keratometry and retinoscopy are of primary importance in obtaining refractive data. The phoropter may need to be ignored in favor of trial frame or loose lens refracting methodology. If fixation or patient attention is a problem, cycloplegic refraction may be indicated. Further information regarding the examination of the special needs patient can be found in Chapter 16, Comprehensive Examination Procedures.

Hyperopia Another variation from emmetropia is hyperopia. Hyperopia is an ocular refractive condition, where parallel light comes to focus behind the retina without the influence of accommodation (1). Unlike myopia, the human eye can respond to light focusing behind the retina by increasing the accommodative effort of the crystalline lens to bring the light to focus on the retina, thus allowing the patient to appreciate clear vision. Hyperopic patients are corrected by means of plus spherical lenses. Whereas emmetropes have clear distance vision with no accommodative effort, uncorrected hyperopes have clear distance vision with accommodative effort. The uncorrected hyperope has the ability to maintain clear vision by overaccommodating for any given stimulus provided the accommodative ability of the eye is adequate.

Figure 17-3 indicates how entering light focuses in the uncorrected hyperopic eye, with the patient not accommodating to parallel light. In the normal human eye, the patient would bring the light focusing behind the retina onto the retina by accommodating to achieve clear distance vision. Figure 17-4 shows the addition of compensatory plus lenses equal to the amount of the uncorrected hyperopia, eliminating the need for the patient's accommodation to bring light into focus on the retina, creating an artificial emmetrope. With the patient accommodating zero to parallel light, the corrected hyperope will simulate an emmetrope, accommodating relatively equal to an accommodative stimulus. In both instances, the patient will have clear distance vision, but in one situation, the eye is accommodating to the zero stimulus of parallel light, but in the other is not accommodating to parallel light with the plus lenses worn. Again, in both instances, the patient would report clear distance vision. Plus lens compensation thus does not necessarily provide clearer vision, but will provide the patient relief from having to accommodate excessively, with more comfortable vision as a positive patient outcome of compensatory lenses.

The ability of the eye to focus light is dependent of the patient's total accommodative ability or the amplitude of accommodation. The amplitude of accommodation decreases with age, most noticeably around age 40. Because younger individuals have greater accommodative ability, these uncorrected hyperopic patients can achieve clarity of vision easily. Due to the reduced focusing ability as the eye ages, older uncorrected hyperopic patients can complain of distance blur directly related to the uncorrected hyperopia.

Most uncorrected hyperopes can see clearly in the distance because the focusing needs are not as great as they are when reading. The closer an object is to the eye, the greater accommodative stimulus of the incident vergence of light and the more dioptric accommodative effort is required (1). Complaints such as blurred vision or difficulty with focus, if present, are usually related to near activities. Thus, the laymen's term "farsighted" is in use because most of the uncorrected hyperopes will have greater problems with reading clarity than distance blur. However, distance blur can result from uncorrected hyperopia when the magnitude comes close to the patient's amplitude of accommodation. As mentioned earlier, this usually occurs in older patients who do not have enough accommodation.

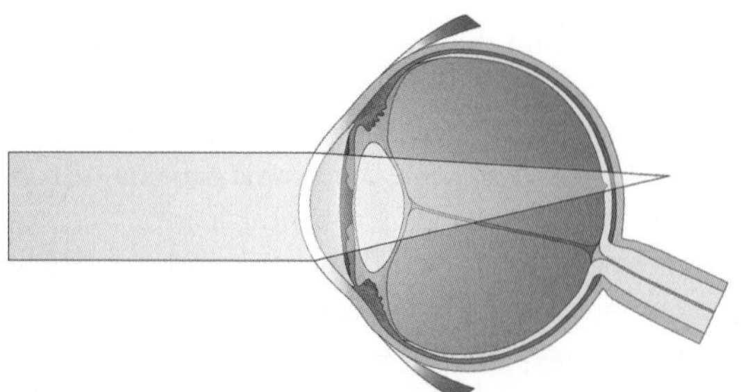

FIGURE 17-3. For an uncompensated hyperope, parallel light comes to focus behind the retina with no accommodation. Accommodation will bring the light to the retina resulting in clear vision.

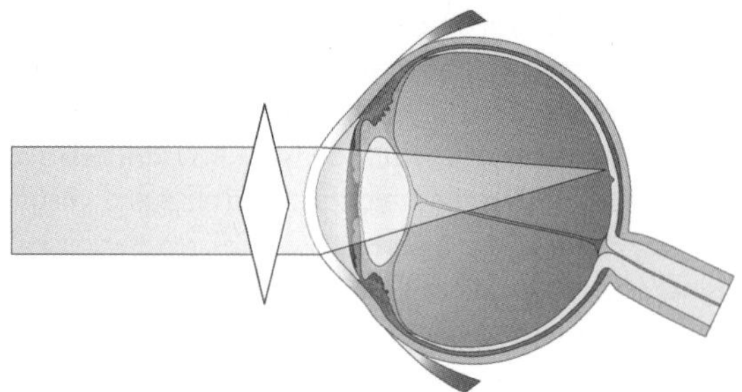

FIGURE 17-4. An uncorrected hyperopic patient is made artificially emmetropic by the addition of plus lenses, with parallel light now focusing on the retina.

The incidence of hyperopia in the general adult population is about 50% to 60% making it the most common refractive condition (1). If all the ocular media and refractive structures coordinate normally as the eye develops, a normal adult refractive error of +0.50D to +0.75D results. If the level of hyperopia is larger, then the axial length of the eye is usually shorter than anatomical human norms (1).

Because small amounts of uncorrected hyperopia is normal in the general population and low-magnitude hyperopia rarely causes patient symptomatology, caution should be used in prescribing plus lenses to asymptomatic uncorrected hyperopes. If all accommodation and convergence relationships are within normal ranges, the low uncorrected hyperopic patient is adequately managed with no lens compensation. Plus lens management would not be necessary unless the patient's reading demands increase with resulting near discomfort. Reading glasses to compensate for the low hyperopia would be considered at that time.

In special needs populations, certain incidences of hyperopia predisposition do occur. Patients manifesting cerebral palsy exhibit some increase in the incidence of hyperopia, but usually <4.00D (8). Patients with Down syndrome tend to show some degree of hyperopia in varying amounts at all ages (21). They also exhibit poor accommodative ability (22), which can exacerbate uncorrected hyperopia, yielding more acuity and reading problems. Current research notes that providing a multifocal prescription (bifocal) for those with Down syndrome and cerebral palsy, no matter their age, should almost always be considered a viable treatment option. Generally, high hyperopia occurs at a higher rate in special needs populations, especially if these individuals have associated learning disabilities (4).

Children, either special needs or otherwise, can present with strabismus as a chief complaint or by parent observation. This may result from the patient manifesting large amounts of uncorrected hyperopia. Strabismus secondary to the uncorrected hyperopia, known as accommodative esotropia, is due to the neurologic connection between accommodation and convergence (23). As the eye accommodates, the two eyes consensually turn in, aiding in reading. However, if the patient is accommodating excessively due to uncorrected hyperopia, one or both of the eyes may turn inward as a result of the extra focusing demands. As a general clinical guideline, a pediatric patient presenting with an esotropia should be considered an uncorrected hyperope until proven otherwise.

Most uncorrected hyperopic patients, if symptomatic, will present with uncomfortable near vision, directly proportional to the amount of reading required, the near-task demands, or the amount of accommodative ability of the patient. The clarity of the vision is usually secondary to the reading fatigue and is accompanied with frontal headaches due to the accommodative difficulty.

Because visual acuity may not be the entire reason for prescribing plus lenses for hyperopes, clinical judgment should be used in counseling patients when and how much to wear the spectacles. Convergence excess, ill-sustained accommodation, and accommodative dysfunction are among the more common refractive reasons for prescribing plus lenses, other than to aid in the uncorrected hyperopia. Since a low amount of hyperopia is the normal refractive condition in the adult population, as a general principle, no lens compensation is made unless the patient has symptoms. The demand for contact lens or surgical refractive management is not as great for hyperopes due to the fact that clarity of vision is not as paramount. However, if clarity of distance vision or cosmetic appearance is important, options other than spectacles can be offered.

Refraction may be difficult either from the inability of the patient's accommodation to relax by routine refractive means or from fluctuations in clarity of vision due to accommodative ciliary muscle spasm. If the patient responses are too problematic, cycloplegic refraction with either tropicamide or cyclopentolate can be considered, allowing a stable refraction to be obtained. The results should be considered in light of the symptoms, visual acuities, and noncycloplegic refractive measurement for final lens management.

Patients presenting with what appears to be a divergence insufficiency or a high-tonic esophoria would need special considerations to insure that all hyperopia or latent hyperopia is manifested. Plus gradient distance phorias would aid in this determination. If the patient's distance phoria does not change with the addition of plus over the manifest refraction, then the patient's esophoria can be considered accurate, and not affected by the uncorrected hyperopia. But if the patient's distance phoria decreases with a repeated phoria through more plus power, then the entire amount of the patient's hyperopia is not revealed, and a delayed subjective or cycloplegic examination would be indicated.

Patients approaching presbyopia (loss of accommodation due to age) that have been previously uncorrected low hyperopes can exhibit "presbyopic-like" symptoms, which can be alleviated by the addition of plus lenses for reading. The amount of plus for reading should not exceed the manifest refraction measurement; this will minimize spectacle adaptation for the patient. Also, the patient will be relieved that bifocal management can be delayed for a few years.

Patients that have Down syndrome show a tendency for underaccommodation with presbyopic-like symptoms occurring at an earlier age than the general population (22). Bifocal management options should be considered to aid in the reading problems occurring with near-point demands, especially when the patients are uncorrected hyperopes. Like all bifocal candidates, considerations should be made for the amount of reading desired by the special needs patient, and the stature of the patient, with more plus needed for individuals with shorter arms. There is more of an art in managing uncorrected hyperopes than uncorrected myopes (Table 17.2). Careful case history and pinpointing the exact nature or absence of complaints is critical. The patient needs to understand fully that management with the plus lenses will not necessarily benefit visual acuity, but will greatly enhance visual comfort. Exhaustive patient education may well be the greatest deterrence to patient maladaptation to plus lens management.

TABLE 17.2 Hyperopic Clinical Pearls

- Uncorrected hyperopes can see clearly at far and near, depending on the magnitude of the amplitude of accommodation.
- Usually, uncorrected hyperopic symptomatology relates to uncomfortable near vision, not blurred vision.
- Children who are manifesting esotropia should be assumed to be uncorrected hyperopes until proven otherwise.
- If a hyperopic patient is symptomatic, prescribe the amount of plus lens compensation that answers the patient's main vision complaint.
- Hyperopic patients should be instructed to wear plus lens correction as directed and counseled heavily concerning adaptation.

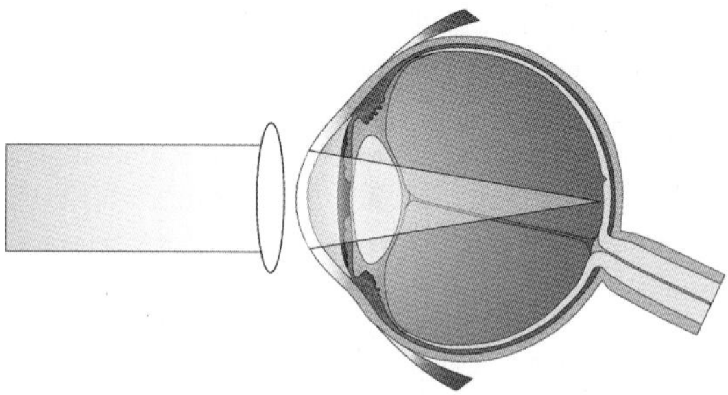

FIGURE 17-6. An uncorrected astigmatic patient is made artificially emmetropic by the addition of sphero-cylinder lenses, with parallel light now focusing both line foci as a point focus on the retina.

Astigmatism Unlike emmetropia, myopia, and hyperopia, in which the focal image is a point of light, astigmia results in line foci. Astigmia is parallel light focusing as two line images, usually perpendicular to each other (1). The perpendicular orientation of the line foci is naturally occurring, or regular astigmatism, and is corrected by spherocylindrical lenses. Line foci that occur in a nonperpendicular fashion are referred to as irregular astigmatism. Irregular astigmatism is usually caused by a disease or traumatic process on the cornea, resulting in corneal abnormalities, producing irregular astigmatism (1).

Figure 17-5 is a representation of how parallel light comes to focus as two line images for regular astigmatism. The figure may be a bit misleading, because the orientation of the two line foci may be in any orientation, and the two line foci are made up of a myriad of light focusing to create the line images. Figure 17-6 illustrates compensatory lenses, termed spherocylinder lenses, causing the two line foci to focus as a point focus on the retina.

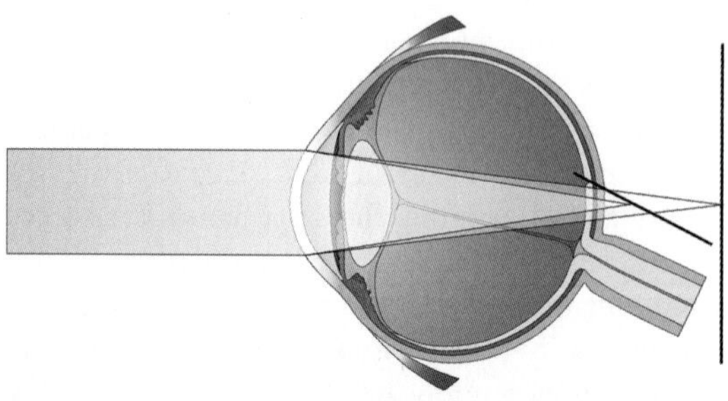

FIGURE 17-5. For an uncompensated astigmat, parallel light comes to focus as two line foci, usually perpendicular to each other.

Astigmatism can be classified by the orientation of the two principle meridians of the line foci. Because of normal lid tension, the cornea has a tendency to have more corneal curvature in the vertical meridian than the horizontal meridian, which is referred to as "with the rule." This anatomical norm occurs more often in the clinical population, and is corrected with minus cylinder axis around 180, or plus cylinder axis around 090.

"Against-the-rule cylinder," which is less common in the general population, goes against the anatomical norms, in that the corneal curvature is greater in the horizontal meridian than the vertical meridian. The minus cylinder correction is located around axis 090, or plus cylinder around axis 180.

Oblique corneas result in oblique astigmatism, which means the orientation of the two line foci fall somewhere between with the rule and against the rule. This is the rarest form and usually occurs in low amounts. The orientation of the line foci images lie between 030 and 060 and 120 and 150.

Astigmatic correction in spherocylinder lenses is one of the most commonly occurring spectacle lens compensation. High amounts of cylinder more often occurs with large-magnitude hyperopia than either myopia or emmetropia and are directly proportional to the corneal curvature. Low amounts of astigmatism can result either from the cornea or the physiologic orientation of the crystalline lens in the eye. In the general population, the distribution of astigmia would be directly proportional to the shape of the cornea, but as patients age, the cornea becomes more spherical, leading to a manifestation of less with-the-rule astigmatism and a greater amount of against-the-rule astigmatism (1). Astigmatism can occur with emmetropia, hyperopia, and myopia. The following classifications are illustrated in Table 17.3.

TABLE 17.3 Types of Astigmia

Type of Astigmia	Definition
Simple myopic astigmia	Parallel light focuses one line image on the retina and the other line image in front of the retina.
Compound myopic astigmia	Parallel light focuses both line images in front of the retina.
Simple hyperopic astigmia	Parallel light focuses one line image on the retina and the other line image behind the retina.
Compound hyperopia astigmia	Parallel light focuses both line images behind the retina.
Mixed astigmia	Parallel light focuses one line image in front of the retina and the other line image behind the retina.

Special needs populations have varying incidences of marked astigmia that is clinically significant. Cerebral palsy patients show a predisposition for larger magnitudes of astigmatism than the general population, especially when severe intellectual impairment exists (24). The prevalence of significant oblique astigmatism has been noted in patients with Down syndrome, with the magnitude of the required cylinder compensation increasing with age (21).

The main etiology of astigmia is the corneal refracting surface. Most large amounts of astigmatism, that is, >1.00D, are the result of the corneal surface being toric, resulting in the need for cylinder correction. In small amounts of astigmatism, the cornea and the crystalline lens cylinder combine to give the resultant cylinder compensation needed. If the cornea is spherical, then all of the naturally occurring toricity of the crystalline lens manifests itself in the resultant refraction.

Vision complaints and the unaided visual acuity vary with the amount of astigmatism correction needed, though a direct relationship between levels of complaints or visual acuity and the amount of astigmatism has not been demonstrated. Asthenopic complaints would be more pronounced when reading, with little complaints of near-reading blur. Compensation for low cylinder is a judgment based on the symptomatology and the patient's criticality in blur interpretation.

The affect of low uncorrected astigmatism does not have a profound impact on the accommodative–convergence system. If the patient manifests asthenopic complaints, then a low accommodative lag or even a lead may be measured due to the patient's accommodative effort to resolve clarity of the blur. This accommodative effort is in vain, because altering the focus does not enable the two line foci to be combined into one point focus. This accommodative fatigue minimally affects accommodation without affecting convergence.

Large amounts of uncorrected astigmatism usually results in reduced vision at far and near, with the patient complaining of blurry vision at both distances. Measurement of visual acuities can be very challenging due to the patient's desire to squint to minimize the blur. The large amounts of uncorrected cylinder directly correlates with the amount of the patient's corneal astigmatism, so keratometry plays a large role in the consideration of management options, including both spectacles and contact lenses. Refractive surgery management can be daunting, due to the shape of the cornea and the criticality of the orientation of the needed astigmatism compensation.

Large amounts of uncorrected astigmia presents some interesting measurements during the refractive routine. Because of the large dioptric amount of the difference between the two line foci, accommodation is greatly affected with lowered positive and negative relative accommodation values, as well as altered lag of accommodation. Vergence ranges also are reduced in both positive and negative directions, with the absolute values being reduced. The expansion of the accommodative and convergence ranges will be accomplished with the patient wearing the indicated amount of astigmatic correction full time, relieving the out-of-focus problem for the eyes (1).

Refracting patients with large amounts of uncorrected astigmatism can be problematic. Because of the patient's habituation to distorted images, patient preferences may gravitate to the uncorrected or habitual spectacle state, even to the point of lowered acuities. Therefore, primary considerations should be given to the objective measures of refraction and to keratometry, regardless of the patient preference. Consequently, great care should be given to patients regarding adaptation to initial correction or correction changes. Clarity of vision may be enhanced when reading, but a general unease may be reported by the patient due to visual distortion noted with full astigmatic correction. Wearing the glasses full time for a period of 1 to 2 weeks will enhance the patients' orientation to this change in image perception (1).

TABLE 17.4 Astigmatic Patient Clinical Pearls

- Most naturally occurring astigmia has both principle meridians perpendicular and can be corrected by conventional spherocylinder lenses.
- The cornea is the main ocular refracting media to be considered for managing astigmatism, so rely heavily on the keratometry when managing astigmatism compensation.
- Prescribing for low astigmia should be considered if the patient symptomatology is mainly reading asthenopia.
- Large amounts of uncorrected astigmatism causes the patient to have trouble making subjective decisions in refraction, therefore rely heavily on objective data when prescribing.
- Be hesitant in changing cylinder axis and power in asymptomatic patients unless this cylinder change markedly increases visual acuity.

If after an adaptive period of full-time wear the patient is still not comfortable wearing the full astigmatic correction, some modifications will need to be made in the spectacle prescription. This maladaptation is usually due to a perceived distortion of what is seen, with the brain not making an adequate adjustment to a nondistorted image. Therefore, the cylinder power may need to be decreased, sacrificing visual acuity. Subsequent prescriptions can gradually increase cylinder power until fully compensated.

Additional caution should be made in changing the orientation of the astigmatic axis and/or powers in the absence of subjective complaints or a decrease in visual acuity. Patients do not adapt well to changes without noticing some benefit in either the clarity or comfort in vision. If the patient is content and visual acuity does not improve, be cautious in changing astigmatic correction from what is being habitually worn (Table 17.4).

PRESBYOPIA

Presbyopia is defined as loss of accommodation or focusing ability due to age (1). Most patients in the United States begin to experience near blurry vision especially when reading around age 40, due to the reduction in accommodation. The classic complaint of "my arms are not long enough" can be heard often from patients that have been relatively asymptomatic, but who now have near-vision problems. The progress of presbyopia continues until around age 65, at which the patient's accommodative ability is essentially nonexistent. The incidence of some amounts of presbyopia in the population over age 40 is 100%, regardless of patient classification (1).

Presbyopic patient symptoms are managed with additional plus lens power over the patient's distance lens correction. This additional plus power takes the place of the patient's accommodation that is problematic, with increased reading clarity. Conventional lined bifocals, blended bifocals, progressive bifocals, and contact lenses afford the patient numerous management options. Refractive surgery management options are usually limited to post–cataract extraction situations, where new multifocal or focusing implants are premium management options. It is important to remember that cosmesis is an important consideration in managing the aging patient, especially in this youth-oriented culture.

Considerations for determining the patient's reading power or bifocal plus power addition include the age of the patient, the patient's desired reading distance, habitual reading prescription, desired near reading ranges through proposed reading prescription, and subsequent refractive measurements. Trial frame refraction for special needs individuals may be more appropriate in determining the bifocal add. All of these criteria need to be evaluated if the patient is to be adequately pleased.

Because presbyopia is an age-related loss of accommodation, then age of the patient can be helpful in determining a starting point for the bifocal addition prescription. As there is a proportional loss of accommodation with aging, bifocal age tables have become a useful tool. Table 17.5 gives prescribing guidelines for the most common reading distances. Additional factors may necessitate modifying the age-based add, as will be discussed later.

TABLE 17.5 Age Table Bifocal Addition Power

Patient Age	Bifocal Addition for 50 cm	Bifocal Addition for 40 cm	Bifocal Addition for 33 cm
40–45	+0.50	+1.00	+1.50
45–50	+1.00	+1.50	+2.00
50–55	+1.25	+1.75	+2.25
55–60	+1.50	+2.00	+2.50
60–65	+1.75	+2.25	+2.75
65–70	+2.00	+2.50	+3.00
Over 70	+2.50	+3.00	+3.50

TABLE 17.6 Presbyopic Clinical Pearls

- Patients that are over 40 should be considered to be presbyopes and questioned about reading difficulties
- Age-based bifocal addition power is a good methodology in special needs populations and a good starting point for the general population.
- The total reading power for an asymptomatic presbyope should not be reduced.
- Presbyopic patients should be given various management options to minimize the social stigma they may perceive.
- All reading distances for which a presbyopic patient needs to read should be within the near reading ranges.

As the patient's focusing ability decreases, the distance at which the patient desires to read is a prime consideration for choosing the bifocal addition. The closer the patient reads, the more power would be required. The converse is also true. As indicated in the age-based table, the practitioner has to assure that the patient's desired working distance is being addressed in the spectacle prescription. There may be more than one working distance needed by the patient, so trifocals, progressive lenses, or multiple pairs of glasses would be prescribing options. Keep in mind that these options are more difficult to use making adaptation an issue for patients with intellectual disability or physical limitations.

To assure that the most appropriate near prescription is issued, the subjective range of clear vision should be measured. If the ranges are too close, the amount of bifocal addition is decreased. If the ranges are too far from patient, then the amount of bifocal addition is increased. Table 17.6 lists several clinical pearls to keep in mind when prescribing glasses for presbyopic patients.

CONCLUSION

When a special needs patient presents for a vision evaluation, compensating for the refractive condition can have an immediate impact on how this patient functions in their environment. Even though the vision examination may have to be altered to obtain sufficient data to make a prescribing judgment, the end results are impactful. Due to the high incidence of refractive problems in the patient with special needs, early intervention cannot be emphasized enough. Having clear and comfortable vision can enhance learning (25), interaction, behavior, and quality of life.

REFERENCES

1. Newman JM. Analysis, interpretation, and prescription for the ametropias and heterophorias. In: Benjamin WJ. editor. Borish's clinical refraction. 2nd ed. St. Louis: Butterworth Heinemann Elsevier Publishers; 2006. p. 963–1024.
2. Mutti DO. To emmetropize or not to emmetropize? The question of hyperopic development. Optom Vis Sci. 2007; 84:97–102.
3. Grosvenor T. Prim eye care. 5th ed. St. Louis: Butterworth-Heinemann Elsevier Publishers; 2007. p. 28–33.
4. Das M, Spowart K, Crossley S, et al. Evidence that children with special needs all require visual assessment. Arch Dis Child. 2010;95:888–92.
5. Vitale S, Sperduto RD, Ferris FL. Increased prevalence of Myopia in the United States between 1971–1972 and 1999–2004. Arch Ophthalmol. 2009;127:1632–9.
6. Bromham NR, Woodhouse JM, Cregg, M, et al. Heart defects and ocular anomalies in children with Down's syndrome. Br J Ophthalmol. 2002;86:1367–8.
7. Gross DA. Development of the ametropias. In: Benjamin WJ. editor. Borish's clinical refraction 2nd ed. St. Louis: Butterworth Heinemann Elsevier Publishers; 2006. p. 55–91.
8. Katoch S, Devi A, Kulkarni P. Ocular defects in cerebral palsy. Indian J Ophthalmol. 2007;55:154–6.
9. London R, Wick B, Kirschen D, Post-traumatic pseudomyopia. Optometry. 2003;74:111–20.
10. Leslie, S. Myopia and accommodative insufficiency associated with moderate head trauma. Optom Vis Dev. 2009;40:25–31.
11. Pacella R, McLellan J, Grice K, et al. Role of genetic factors in the etiology of juvenile-onset myopia based on a longitudinal study of refractive error. Optom Vis Sci. 1999;76:381–6.
12. Lim LS, Gazzard G, Yen-Ling Low, et al. Dietary factors, myopia, and axial dimensions in children. Ophthalmology. 2010;117:993–7.
13. Saw SM, Gazzard G, Au Eong K-G, et al. Myopia: attempts to arrest progression. Br J Ophthalmol. 2002;86:1306–11.
14. Fukushima T, Torii M, Ukai K, et al. The relationship between CA/A ratio and individual differences in dynamic accommodative responses while viewing stereoscopic images. J Vis. 2009;9:21:1–13.
15. Mathur A, Atchison DA, Charman WN. Myopia and peripheral ocular aberrations. J Vis. 2009;9:15:1–12.
16. Cheng D, Scmid K, Woo G, et al. Randomized trial of effects of bifocal and prismatic bifocal spectacles on myopia progression. Arch Ophthalmol. 2010;128(1):12–9.
17. Pang Y, Maino DM, Zhang G, et al. Myopia: can its progression be controlled? Optom Vis Dev. 2006;37(2):7579.
18. Lee TT, Cho P, Discontinuation of orthokeratology and myopic progression. Optom Vis Sci. 2010;87:1053–6.
19. Rah MJ, Jackson JM, Jones L, et al. Overnight orthokeratology: preliminary results of the lenses and overnight orthokeratology (LOOK) study. Optom Vis Sci. 2002;79:598–605.
20. Short AJ, Allan BDS. Photorefractive keratometry (PRK) versus laser-assisted in-situ keratomileusis (LASIK) for myopia. Cochrane Database Syst Rev. 2006;(2):CD005135, DOI:10.1002/14651858.CD005135.pub.2.

21. Al-Bagadady M, Murphy PJ, Woodhouse JM, et al. Development and distribution of refractive error in children with Down's Syndrome. Br J Optom. 2010. Doi:10.1136/bjo.2010.185827.
22. Cregg, M Woodhouse JM, Pakeman VH, et al. Accommodation and refractive error in children with Down Syndrome: cross-sectional and longitudinal studies. Invest Ophthalmol Vis Sci. 2001;42:55–63.
23. Wormald, R, Smeeth, L, Henshaw, K, et al. Evidence based ophthalmology. Bodmin, Cornwall: BMJ Publishing Group; 2004:91.
24. Saunders KJ, Little JA, McClelland JF, et al. Profile of refractive errors in Cerebral Palsy: impact of severity of motor impairment (GMFCS) and CP subtype of refractive outcome. Invest Ophthalmol Vis Sci. 2010;5:2885–90.
25. Nandakumar K, Evans MA, Briand K, Leat SJ. Bifocals in Down syndrome study (BiDS): analysis of video recorded sessions of literacy and visual perceptual skills. Clin Experimen Optom. 2011;94:575–585.

CHAPTER 18

Paul Harris, OD, FCOVD, FACBO, FAAO

Diagnosis and Treatment of Oculomotor Dysfunction

The diagnosis and treatment of the oculomotor system occupies a significant place in optometric care and comes to the fore in patients with special needs. Fixation, the ability to lock onto an object, is a fundamental visual ability from which many characteristics of human behavior emerge. Once fixation has developed, infants begin to follow objects as they move through space (pursuits) and then to jump from one object to another in space (saccades). Dysfunctions in any of these skills can have profound effects in a child's performance in school, at play, and eventually in life. This chapter approaches the subject from a clinical viewpoint to facilitate an understanding of how to assess the fixation, pursuit, and saccadic skills of a patient. Following this, an outline of the therapy available for each of these areas is presented.

ASSESSING FIXATION

In the general population, a clinician does not assess fixation directly. While greeting a patient or performing a case history, a clinician notices a patient's ability to make eye contact or to look at specific objects in the office. A patient might comment about those objects, which clearly indicates that they can and do fixate. Then, a patient reads the eye chart while the clinician performs visual acuity testing, demonstrating appropriate central fixation. In contrast to the general population, it might be necessary to directly assess the degree of fixation ability in many patients with special needs, to understand that patient's visual processing abilities.

A clinician who assesses a child's visual abilities should be cognizant of vision development. Children generally acquire visual abilities according to well-known developmental sequences. Testing should proceed up the developmental ladder moving from what the child can do to what is developmentally beyond their abilities. A clinician can then use the gathered information to determine if the patient responds appropriately.

Fixation is best assessed while a child is alert and, if an infant, during feeding. The most effective target to assess fixation during the first few days of life is a human face or a representation of a face held at about 20 cm from the child. Once the child looks at the face, small horizontal movements of the face should elicit corresponding eye movements in the child. The child's eye movements may not be smooth, but they will tend to move in the direction of the face. With special needs patients, a clinician may need to begin to assess fixation at this fundamental level. If fixation is not obtained on a face or face-like target, then the clinician should not expect fixation on other targets or at other distances.

As children develop, they acquire the ability to fixate on targets that are not as visually attractive as a face. A number of related factors will determine the degree of salience and thus, the degree of fixation affinity of various targets. Some factors involved include, but are not limited to, size, contrast, brightness, intermittency, movement, and spatial frequency of the target (Table 18.1).

A clinician should have available an assortment of fixation targets that match various developmental levels and are likely to be relevant to children. A target that resembles something that a child knows is a more useful target than one with which they have no experience, dislike, or find aversive in some way.

Fixation should not be considered an all-or-none phenomenon. For example, in one case, we may find

TABLE 18.1 Characteristics of the Target and How to Shift toward Greater or Lesser Degrees of Salience

Characteristic	Viewed Preferentially	Reduced View
Size	Bigger	Smaller
Contrast edges	Square wave–like	Sine wave–like
Luminance	Brighter	Dimmer
Spatial frequency	Higher (narrow detail)	Lower (wide detail)
Periodicity (blink, movement, etc.)	Greater amount	Lesser amount

that a child fixates a face nearly 100% of the time, a blinking penlight about 50% of the time, a steady penlight (not blinking) about 20% of the time, and a Wolff wand 1% of the time. It may be important to record all of this to be able to judge changes accurately at a future date. Several months later, the same patient might show an insignificant increase in Wolff wand fixation from 1% to 2% of the time but nearly 100% fixation on the face, blinking light and non-blinking light.

ASSESSING PURSUIT EYE MOVEMENTS

Assuming that a target has been identified that the patient will fixate on at least 50% of the time, a clinician may proceed to assess basic tracking movements. The 50% number is the lower limit time threshold that it takes the clinician to reliably rate the quality of a person's ocular motility. If they are on the target 50% of the time or more, a fairly accurate judgment can be made of what factors cause a decrease in that fixation percentage. This would allow manipulation of various aspects of the target over time and assess loss of fixation from the prior baseline lock on time. In patients with special needs, expecting near 100% central fixation is unrealistic and must be taken into consideration.

As with fixation, a clinician should proceed up the developmental sequence when assessing visual tracking or pursuits. Visual tracking proceeds along a fairly predictable developmental sequence. Development starts with horizontal tracking and moves to tracking vertically and then diagonally. It continues with tracking targets that move in unpredictable paths at varying speeds with stops and starts and that shift through different distances (1).

The target a clinician chooses will affect the assessment of tracking skills. The easier the target is to lock onto with fixation, the better the tracking will look. Once a clinician finds a target on which the patient will fixate, they should first move the target in the horizontal meridian. At first, the target should be moved slowly. As the testing progresses, a clinician should vary as many qualities of the movements as both time and the patients' attention warrant. These qualities include the direction and speed (acceleration and deceleration) of the movement, the distance the target is from the patient, and the use of movement that is both predictable and unpredictable. This provides insight into what factors affect fixation and visual attention in your patient far more sensitively than standard eye muscle or motility testing.

Just as with fixation, multiple factors will determine if a patient can and will track a chosen target. These factors include, but are not limited to, varying qualities such as (a) the direction of movement (simple movements from primary gaze and back in the plane of the horopter would be easier than those that do not remain in the horopter or which never return to primary gaze); (b) the speed of the target (targets moved at a fixed rates of speed are easier to track than targets with varying and unpredictable velocities); and (c) the degree that stops and starts and reversals of movement are interjected into the movement pattern (abrupt stops with quick retrograde movements followed immediately by the same when moving across the midline on a diagonal are examples of this kind of movement). It may be helpful to consider tracking as a manifestation of a patient's ability to fixate. By assessing a patient's ability to track a target, a clinician is asking the patient, "Now that you can fixate on this target, at what point along the movement hierarchies does fixation cease to occur?"

HEAD VERSUS EYE MOVEMENT

Another aspect of fixation and tracking that a clinician should observe is the relative amounts of head and eye movement made when following a target. At lower levels of vision development, an individual maintains fixation on an object only with the resources of the entire body. For example, when testing a 1-week-old infant lying on its back, as the clinician's face moves side to side relative to the infant's face, the infant's entire head will move as the child fixates on the face. If the clinician moves

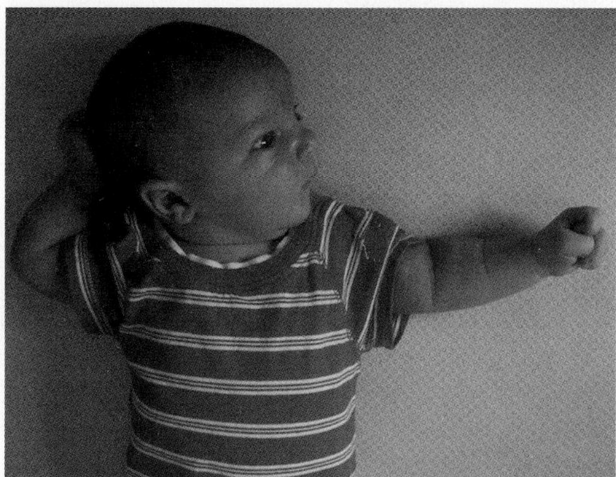

FIGURE 18-1. Child in ATNR elicited by following the face of his mother from primary gaze to his left.

far enough, the infant's asymmetric tonic neck reflex (ATNR) should reveal itself. Asymmetric tonic neck reflex presents with the infant's hand extended on the side of the head turn and the other hand folded up next to the back of the head (Figs. 18-1 and 18-2).

While many eye care professionals have their patients hold steady during an exam, such an instruction might distort how the patient would typically fixate and track. Instead, to maximize the opportunity to observe typical results during the examination, a clinician should simply ask the patient to follow the target.

The amount of head and upper body movement that occurs when testing eye movements should be recorded. The trend in moving toward electronic health records (EHRs) favors the use of a numerical recording system. The Northeastern State University College of Optometry (NSUCO) Oculomotor Test, described in greater detail in Chapter 16, Comprehensive Examination Procedures, assesses four areas, including ability, accuracy, and head and body movement. Each category is given a score ranging from 1 to 5 on which a performance number is produced based on observations made during the testing (2,3).

ASSESSING SACCADIC EYE MOVEMENTS

In most testing protocols for assessing eye movements, pursuit and saccadic eye movements are assessed separately. The seasoned clinician recognizes that life rarely involves activities where only one or the other type of eye movement is needed. When testing pursuits, as soon as any one of the salient factors, discussed above, becomes too hard for a patient to remain locked onto, the clinician will observe the eye movements will fall behind the target. Most patients will compensate with a saccadic eye movement to get back to the target fairly quickly, enabling the keen observer a chance to assess saccadic eye movements indirectly. Thus, a clinician may see both types of eye movements in a more real-world situation.

For most clinicians, however, particularly those with less clinical experience, saccadic eye movements should be assessed separately. Separate assessment of saccadic eye movements requires the introduction of a second target. Selection of the fixation target(s) should follow the same guidelines mentioned above regarding pursuit.

When performing saccadic testing, a clinician must tell the patient when to change fixation between the two targets. Because the instruction to change targets requires, in most cases, a verbal command, a patient's language problems, particularly problems with receptive language, may make the assessment of saccadic eye movements nearly impossible.

How a clinician gives the instruction to change fixation targets can affect both the accuracy of the saccadic eye movement and the amount of head movement relative to the amount of eye movement. If the commands are barked out similar to a drill sergeant yelling out commands to his plebes, a clinician can expect to see more head movement. This result occurs in most patients, not just those with special needs.

Because saccadic eye movements follow the same developmental sequence as pursuit eye movements, saccades in the horizontal direction should mature prior to vertical saccades; horizontal and vertical saccades should emerge before diagonal saccades and so forth, along the expected developmental hierarchies. In many cases where there is no observable supportive head movement with the pursuits, head movement will become a component of the saccadic eye movement. Generally, the further apart the two targets, the higher the probability that head movement will be noted when the patient fixates each target and, in fact, is expected.

Lastly, a clinician should record the degree of accuracy of the movements generated when observing saccadic eye movements. The terms undershoot and overshoot are used to describe inaccuracies. An undershoot is a movement that is hypometric, or smaller than needed to get all the way to the new target in one movement. An overshoot is hypermetric, or larger than needed. When either an under- or

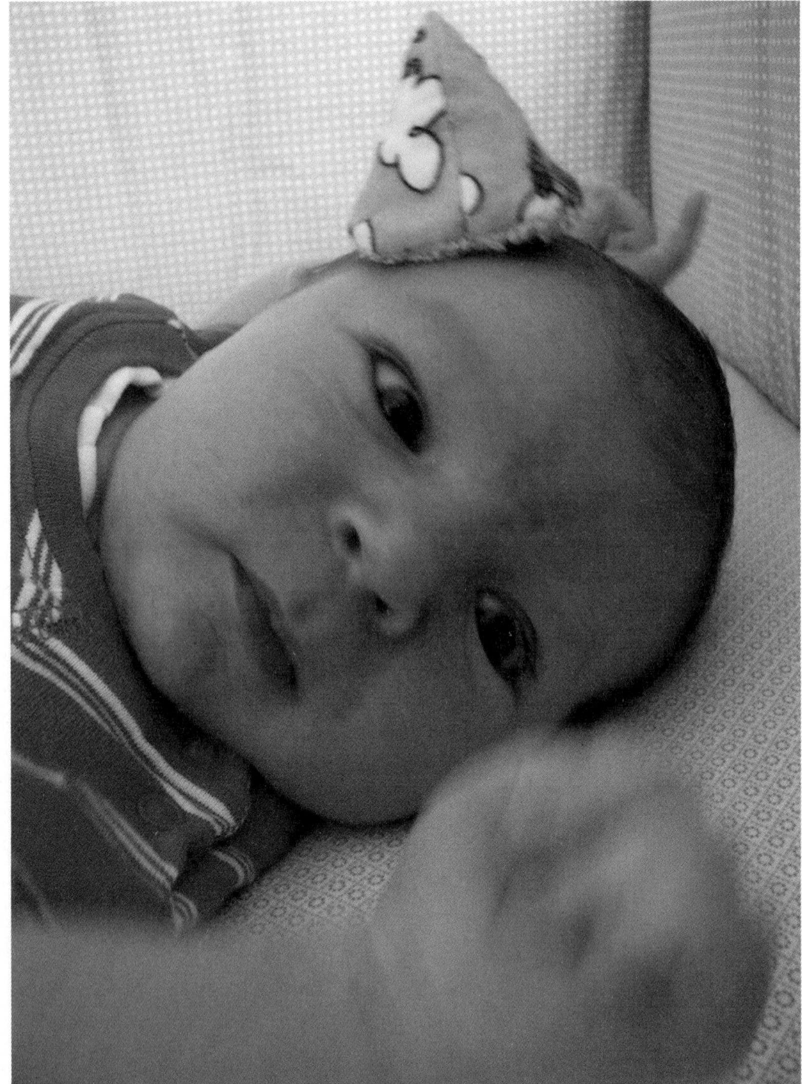

FIGURE 18-2. Once gaze was followed to the extreme, he took up fixation on his extended left hand.

overshoot is observed, a clinician should note how long it takes for corrections to be made and how many attempts it takes for the patient to get back to the target. The dynamic interplay between the size of the saccade, the manner in which the verbal command is given, and the degree of salience of the targets to the patient, among other factors, will trigger clinically significant variations in performance that the clinician needs to observe and record. The NSUCO Oculomotor Test can be used to quantify the performance of the saccades, while making observations of the patient's ability, accuracy, and associated head and body movement.

SOME SPECIAL TESTS

In some instances, it may not be possible to elicit eye movements with the above approach and it might be necessary to further investigate patients' visual abilities. The optokinetic nystagmus (OKN) and vestibular ocular reflex (VOR) tests may be helpful in these situations. The OKN uses unique aspects of the human visual system to trigger involuntary movement of the eyes. Nystagmus is an periodic movement of the eye, usually seen as a slow drift in one direction followed by a jump back in the other direction (4). When a patient with nystagmus is asked to look at a stripe pattern that is moving at a moderate speed from left to right or right to left, the eyes will follow for a while with the lines and then will jump quickly back in the opposite direction.

The OKN drum (Fig. 18-3) is held by the handle so that the stripes are vertical and then the drum is rotated slowly. If the drum is rotated too quickly, then a patient will see the whole drum as a gray blur and will not track it. It can be difficult to use the OKN drum to observe a patient's eye movements without the patient fixating on the clinician's face instead of the drum. A patient often will see the clinician's head begin to come out from behind the drum before the eye movement can be observed. It takes practice and sometimes cunning to clearly observe eye movements before the patient switches to look directly at the clinician. Once the nystagmus movements are seen, it is important to rotate the drum in the opposite direction to make sure that the observed movements are symmetric. The periodic nature of the movement will be in the opposite direction, but the movements should be similar in amount as long as the drum is turning at the same velocity.

Asymmetries between the eyes may be seen in three different ways. First, there might be asymmetry between the eyes at the same time; both eyes are expected to move exactly in a yoked manner. Second, a clinician might see asymmetry between the total movement patterns when rotating the drum one way versus the other. Here, the asymmetry might be that the eyes travel further in one direction during the following phase or that they don't follow at all unless the drum is slowed a considerable amount relative to the other direction.

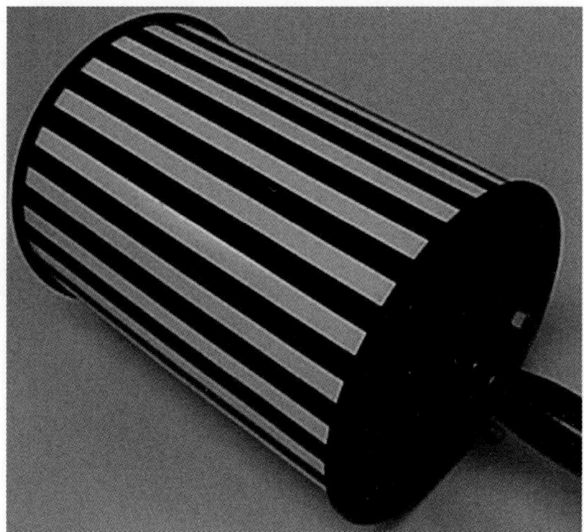

FIGURE 18-3. OKN drum used for the testing of OKN nystagmus. This is available from Bernell, item number DAL300.

Third, there might be asymmetry between the directions of movements when the patient is tested monocularly. Asymmetries, particularly in the "into-out" versus the "out-to-in" directions, are expected prior to 3 months of age but should equalize between 3 to 6 months of age. There has been some discussion that faulty development of symmetries in OKN tested monocularly during this time frame might be related to the development of strabismus (5). If any of these asymmetries are present, the clinician may consider referring the patient for a neurologic evaluation.

The VOR works in several ways to help stabilize fixation on a target when a person's head moves side to side. The eye movements that compensate for head rotations are triggered by the semicircular canals of the inner ear. There are extensive connections throughout the oculomotor control system that allow the VOR to work appropriately (4). In patients who can understand the instruction to keep their eyes on a target, it may be possible to observe the VOR directly by putting the patient in a chair that turns and quickly rotating the chair one way and then the other way, watching to what degree they can maintain fixation on the target.

The VOR is particularly useful with infants and toddlers. Neural systems, when saturated over an extended period of time, will recalibrate rather rapidly so that when the stimulation is removed, a rebound or opposite effect is viewed. The clinician hugs the child face-in and supports the head well. While seated on a stool that will twirl easily, the clinician then begins spinning rapidly anywhere from five to eight times around and then stops abruptly. The child is then tipped over out of the hugged-in position, generally into their parent's lap and the eyes are observed immediately. The eyes should move into a nystagmus pattern, similar to that described in the OKN section above. However, the eye movements will decay over a short period of time as the system recalibrates to the nonspinning condition. Once the child has recovered fully, the procedure should be repeated with the spinning in the opposite direction. Any asymmetries noted should be recorded. Any significant asymmetry noted may be referred for further evaluation if no explanation is known.

TESTING

Table 18.2 provides a partial list of oculomotor tests used, but is by no means exhaustive. Because of the nature of working with patients with special needs, many patients may not be able to complete the formal tests in the following list and the clinician will have to rely exclusively on that which has already been presented. Table 18.2 also provides some the pros and cons of each test. Many of these tests are discussed in detail in Chapter 16, Comprehensive Examination Procedures.

TREATMENT

The treatment of oculomotor dysfunction follows long-established principles of optometric vision therapy. The acquisition of oculomotor skills follows the principles of general development and learning. Several cognitive theories, including an almost purely Piagetian perspective and modern learning theory, influence the tactics used in therapeutic intervention. In general, the basis for the therapeutic approach does not affect the procedures or activities performed; the differences are at the meta- or explanatory levels.

Effective therapy relies on a clinician's knowledge of developmental sequences. In treatment, a child must solve a series of problems that move along the developmental continua. A clinician must present a task that is at just the right level for the child to benefit from the activity. Vygotsky (6) coined the phrase "zone of proximal development (ZPD)," which essentially is the junction between the skills a child can achieve alone, unaided and automatically, from the skills a child has yet to acquire. The challenge for a clinician is to continually match the demands of tasks presented to a child with a level that is just inside that child's ZPD.

The optometric profession has a universal set of 400+ activities. At the surface, many of the activities look substantially different from one to the other, and individual optometrists use different subsets of activities as core treatment procedures. Because of the variability in optometrists' use of treatment methods, an outsider looking in might conclude that the discipline of optometric vision therapy is fractured and that no consistent theory exists. This could not be further from the truth. At a meta level, it becomes clear that optometrists applying principles of vision therapy address a limited number of visual abilities, oculomotor skills being a major one, similarly but with different targets and at different levels of development. Thus, the similarities among the disparate methodologies appear as a coherent field. The challenge for newcomers to the field is to recognize the need to shift to the meta levels of analysis and thinking.

SIGNAL-TO-NOISE RATIOS—THE KEY

Essentially, a clinician may only manipulate two aspects of an activity: the relative amounts of signal and noise. The signal is what the child must attend, and the noise is everything else. If a child is not capable of looking at a target and is not achieving a particular task, then the task is likely outside the child's ZPD. To shift the task's demand downward along the developmental axis, the signal may be increased or the noise decreased. If the child is already capable of easily performing the task, then the signal may be decreased and the noise increased. These principles will be illustrated using an optometric vision therapy procedure known as "Eye Control," but the concepts are applicable to all optometric vision therapy activities.

Eye Control The procedure known as "Eye Control" emerged from several legacy approaches to working with oculomotor dysfunctions but was codified by the late Robert A. Kraskin, OD (7). In the optometric vision therapy protocols that are part of the Optometric Extension Program—Clinical Curriculum, eye control is in the treatment protocol for all diagnoses. The stated purpose of the activity is

> *To provide the patient with the opportunity to have the necessary meaningful experience to learn to use the eyes free of the rest of the body (no movement in the rest of the body), through the full range of possible movements.*

In the basic eye control procedure, a Wolff wand (a small steel ball on a metal rod that is used as a fixation target) is held very close to the face in four different positions in front of each eye. The patient looks directly at the wand and sees his or her reflection. The patient must feel his or her eyes in these extreme positions of gaze and must follow the positions with only eye movement (Fig. 18-4).

TABLE 18.2 Benefits and Limitations for Tests Used to Assess Oculomotor Skills

Performance Test	Visual Abilities Assessed	When Done: Triggering Observations	Benefits/Pros	Limitations/Cons
King-Devick Saccadic Test	Eye movements for reading, left–right top–down sequencing, rapid automated naming	Age 5.5 and up with some type of complaint related to school or reading performance	Very fast Easy to grade Norms from age 6 to 14 Easy to relate to public Can give in a tiered fashion (can stop as soon as difficulties have been identified)	Must know number names Must be verbal
Classic Version Groffman Visual Tracing Test NOTE: There is a new version of this test but the original is strongly recommended	Sustained visual attention Visual concentration Figure-ground Visual tracking Eye movements for handwriting	Age 5.5 and up with some type of complaint related to school or reading performance Handwriting problems Visual attention problems Attention Deficit Disorder (ADD)/attention deficit hyperactivity disorder (ADHD) in history	Easy to administer, grade, and relate to the public Two forms are available allowing testing with and without lenses with the ability to compare scores directly	Child can go into overload on this test. This is diagnostic but must be ready to stop if they move into "flight." Less useful for patients who score below age 7 or above age 12
Wold Sentence Copy Test	Copying skills Pencil grip/writing posture observation Use of space and spatial organization Fine visual–motor development	Age 6.5 and up with some type of complaint related to school or reading performance Whenever copying from the blackboard is mentioned in the history	Can be stopped at any time Allows for the observation of many aspects of visual development and posture.	Can go on for a long time if some children are made to finish the entire sentence
Developmental Eye Movements	Eye movements for reading, left–right top–down sequencing Rapid automated naming	Recommended later in a VT program in cases where most things seem to be improving but the times on the NYSOA KD test remain slow and there appears to be some difficulty in oral reading or rapid automated naming	Yields information similar to the KD. May give additional insights into rapid automated naming and a possible language and/or visual–language integration role in causing the learning problems.	Takes longer to do than the NYSOA KD test. Requires some calculations to be done to derive scores. Entire test must be completed to yield scores, therefore is time consuming
NSUCO Oculomotor Test	Pursuit and saccadic eye movements	This can be done as a frontline standard test for all patients to look at eye movements to a target in space.	Is a standardized test that is easy to teach and easy to do clinically and should facilitate intra- and interprofessional communication	Requires the clinician to scale all parts to derive a score. Therefore, this may not be suitable for children with very poor oculomotor skills.
Developmental Test of Visual Perception II Eye–Hand Coordination Subtest	Eye–hand coordination Sustained visual attention Vigilance	Whenever handwriting or copying from the blackboard is mentioned in the history as a problem	Easy to administer Easy to relate to public Can document difficulty with a score rather than a judgment of their penmanship Fine grading scale allows for good pre- and postmeasurement documentation	Takes long to grade the test

(*Continued*)

TABLE 18.2 Benefits and Limitations for Tests Used to Assess Oculomotor Skills *(Continued)*

Performance Test	Visual Abilities Assessed	When Done: Triggering Observations	Benefits/Pros	Limitations/Cons
Beery Developmental Test of Visual–Motor Integration	Visual perception Spatial organization Eye–hand coordination	Used if Wold is not used and good for lower-level performers on paper-and-pencil tasks	Tightly standardized data and useful to communicate with educators or other care providers	Difficult to communicate to the public interpretation of results. Takes a long time to do. Difficult to factor out the degree to which a problem with manipulating a writing implement might be causing the difficulty.
ReadAlyzer—Visagraph Infrared Eye Movement Recording	Visual mechanics for reading; fixations, regressions, average duration of fixation, reading speed	Used when there are any complaints about reading and the patient reads at least at a third-grade level or higher Used with many head injured patients as well	Powerful demonstration tool Gives finely graded performance statistics from which goals for treatment can be set Good for before and after measures Device is self-calibrating and does the analysis itself. Report graphs are easy to understand	Must be done correctly. Some aspects of the test have been built up to be more than the device is actually capable of measuring. Be careful to not get drawn into these overly high levels of complication.
3, 6, and 12 piece form puzzles	Visual perception Visual problem solving Eye–hand coordination Degree of visually guided behavior	Useful for a younger population (late 2 to age 5)	To observe eye–hand coordination and visual memory, laterality and directionality, form perception and lead-support use of hands Good communication tool	Poorly standardized Too highly dependent on observation skills of the tester

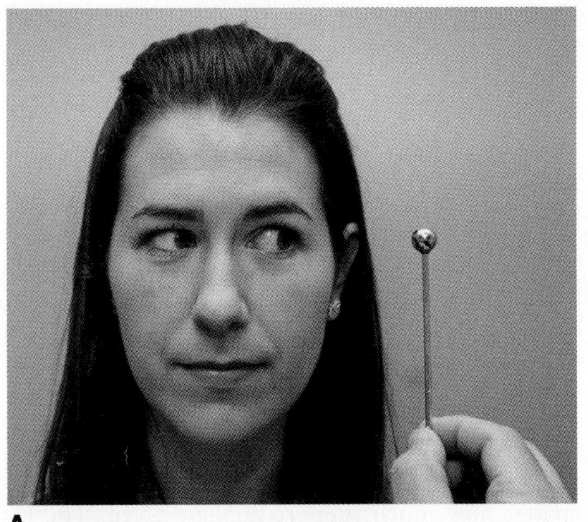

A

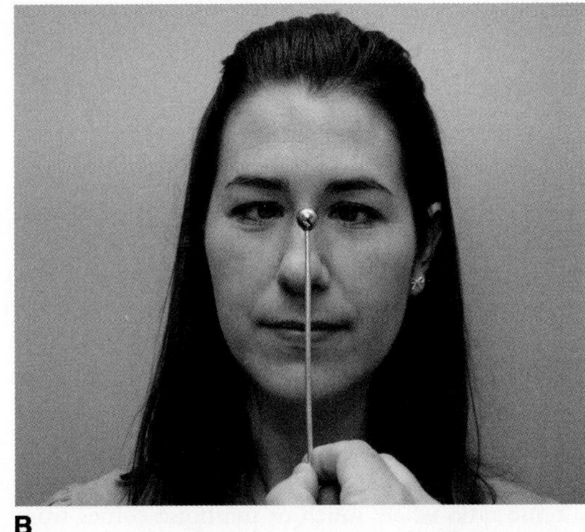

B

FIGURE 18-4. **A:** In the picture on the left, the Wolff wand is to the patient's extreme left and both eyes are stretched far to her left and locked on the target. **B:** The picture at the right shows the Wolff wand now directly in the center with extreme convergence being demonstrated. Note that the patient has maintained nearly perfectly a steady head position.

With most patients who require optometric vision therapy, treatment can begin at this demand level. However, with most special needs patients, this would be far too difficult a task, because they might not be able to lock onto the Wolff wand or to prevent head movement as the wand is moved. The next section provides guidance on how to modify the eye control procedure up and down the developmental demand axis by altering the signal-to-noise ratio.

INCREASING SIGNAL

The Wolff wand is a highly reflective ball bearing on the end of a metal rod. Despite its conspicuousness, a patient requires a good bit of visual attention to fixate on it. The following is a list of attributes that can be modified to increase the signal:

- Make the object bigger
- Make the object brighter: shine lights onto it or replace it with a light itself (Kraskin (7))
- Make the object intermittent: blink or tremor
- Move the object
- Make the object emit noise

Additional examples of signal variations, going from bigger to lesser signal strength would be blinking bright light → blinking light → direct view light → indirect view light → highly reflective target with bright illumination → less reflective target with less illumination.

DECREASING NOISE

Many times, the optometrist or vision therapist becomes an integral part of the visual background for the patient during the activity. By moving into position to see a patient's eyes, a clinician becomes part of the visual background. Even the clothing a clinician wears becomes part of the noise that a patient must sift through to find and fixate on the target. For this reason, clinicians should carefully consider wardrobe selections and avoid visually noisy clothing and jewelry. For example, a striped shirt or blouse has a high chance of becoming the target rather than the Wolff wand or the light. A silver Wolff wand on the backdrop of a gray shirt would be harder to pick up than on either a solid black or white shirt.

THE BODY AS NOISE

One big source of noise in learning new motor activities is a patient's body. Many special needs patients have tremendous difficulty with body stabilization and do so with much more dynamic tension (simultaneous contraction in both the agonist and antagonist pairs). Dynamic tension and other body control problems can create a great deal of background noise against which it becomes difficult to feel eye movements. One way to help a child with excess body tension become more aware of how eye movements feel is to have the child lie down on the floor. Because the child does not have to support the body in this position, dynamic tension throughout the body reduces.

The following are intermediate steps between the extremes of lying down on the floor and standing unsupported: sitting on a chair with a supportive back, sitting on a stool with no back, sitting on a "T" seat (like a milking stool), standing with back to a wall, standing while touching a stable object, and standing unsupported in an open space. These are all methods for decreasing noise to improve the signal-to-noise ratio where much of the noise comes from tension in the patient's body.

MORPHING THE ACTIVITY

To achieve the proper signal-to-noise ratio that will make a procedure productive, the needed modifications may seem so extreme that the procedure no longer resembles the starting activity. Such a result is called morphing the activity. For example, many special needs patients will not be able to handle the demands of the eye control activity even while on their backs in a dimly lit room with a bright light as the target. To tap into a patient at this level of need, it might make sense to use the patient's hand or finger as the target. To use a patient's hand as the target, join hands with the patient, like playing "thumb war." In some instances, a penlight can be used to "light up" a patient's finger, like the scene in the movie *E.T.* By using a part of the patient's body as the target, the patient gets the additional kinesthetic feedback about where to look. Practically, using the patient's hand as a target works well when the clinician's right hand holds the patient's right hand while the clinician uses the left hand to stabilize the patient's head, even if the patient is lying on the floor. Over time, as the support from the hand on the head or the use of the light is withdrawn, the patient will acquire the ability to fixate and stay locked on the target. Once a patient's level is identified, the patient can often move to greater a development demand rather rapidly. The challenge is to continually move up and down the developmental demands ladder to find the ZPD.

GRADIENTS

One final challenge to mention is that of gradients. Often, when an optometrist or therapist is initially learning an activity, they identify several discrete steps or stages for performing the activity. Later, when the activity is used with a special needs patient, the novice therapist might get stuck in the following trap: the patient can perform well at a given level of demand, but the next level of demand is simply too hard, no matter how much support they are given. The key challenge for the therapist is to discover how to break the one large step down into several smaller steps that can be managed. To do so requires manipulation of the signal-to-noise ratios at a finer and finer degree of granularity and then moving up and down the finer gradients with patients. Table 18.3 indicates the gradients used in the therapy room in regard to treating oculomotor dysfunction.

CONCLUSION

At first, a clinician might fear that the needs of these patients might be too complex or might require a higher level of skill and ability. In reality, the demands of patients with special needs are at more fundamental levels of visual ability. As a clinician learns to manipulate the demand levels of the activities closer to fundamental levels of visual skill, their skill as a vision therapist will grow. In addition, these patients are often appreciative of even small gains, because seemingly small gains can cause huge changes in the quality of life for the patient and the patient's family. The quality-of-life improvement makes working with patients with special needs extremely rewarding. As oculomotor skills and abilities improve, other aspects of a patient's visual skills and abilities improve. As the primary purpose of the visual process is the direction of movement, with improved oculomotor skill comes more efficient and more accurate direction of movements with commensurate improvements in quality of life.

TABLE 18.3 Oculomotor Skills: Definitions and Associated Signs and Symptoms

Oculomotor Skills Category	Subskills	Definition	Signs and Symptoms
Fixation	• Locate	The ability to find an object	Difficulty where the visual process is primary and they would have to get information critical to learning or moving from the visual process
	• Grasp	The ability to redirect the eye to the object so that the light rays from the object fall on the fovea/macula	
	• Maintain hold	The ability to keep this alignment for longer and longer periods of time.	This would affect high spatial frequency types of information more profoundly.
Pursuits	• Simple movements to and from primary gaze in the horopter	Pursuits are to move the eyes in such a way so that the light from a moving object is kept on the fovea or macula area continuously.	Difficulty gaining knowledge from and interacting with moving objects.
	• Movements out of the horopter		This can lead to a lack of general coordination and clumsiness as well as avoidance of those activities where such interactions would normally occur.
	• Movements of different speeds		
	• Movements that stop and start		
Saccades	• Disengage	The eyes move very fast from one object in space to another or where the pursuit movement alone is not fast enough to keep up with object of regard.	Trouble shifting from one area of space to another
	• Move		
	• Engage	The saccade has discrete steps including (1) Disengage—visual attention is pulled away from the currently fixated object (2) Move—the actual shift in fixation occurs to the new object (3) Engage—visual attention is now locked onto the new target	Difficulty with sequencing activities They may perseverate on things rather than explore their visual environment as they should. In children on the autism spectrum, this could be one aspect of those that seem to get entranced in visual stimulation that is repetitive.

REFERENCES

1. Gesell A. Vision—its development in infant and child. Santa Ana: OEPF; 1998.
2. Maples WC, Ficklin T. Comparison of eye movement skills between above average and below average readers. J Behav Optom. 1990;1:87–91.
3. Maples WC, Atchley J, FicklinT. Northeastern state university college of optometry's oculomotor norms. J Behav Optom. 1992;3:143–50.
4. Ciuffreda K, Tannen B. Eye movement basics for the clinician. St. Louis: Mosby-Year Book Inc.; 1995.
5. Tychsen L. Early visual development. Normal and abnormal. London: Oxford University Press; 1993.
6. Vygotsky L. Mind in society. The development of higher psychological processes. Cambridge: Harvard University Press; 1978.
7. Kraskin RA. Vision training in action. Santa Ana: Optometric Extension Program Foundation; 1965–1968.

CHAPTER 19

Erin Jenewein, OD, MS, FAAO
Kelly Meehan, OD, FAAO

Diagnosis and Treatment of Binocular Vision and Accommodative Disorders

Whether a child or an adult, the visual system is used throughout the day to view targets at different distances and shift gaze between far and near. Demand depends upon lifestyle; due to an increase in the amount of near work and computer use, demand is greater than any time in the history of modern civilization. The clinical evaluation of the entire visual system, including both the accommodative and vergence systems, is an essential part of diagnosing visual dysfunction (1).

During an eye examination, the measurement of accommodative ability is important particularly for those with developmental disabilities, as reduced accommodation is a frequent occurrence within this population (2). Studies have shown that accommodative dysfunction has been reported in 60% to 80% of patients with binocular vision problems (3). Up to 80% of patients with Down syndrome and 53% of patients with cerebral palsy have accommodative deficits (2,4). Decreased visual acuity, high refractive error, strabismus, and nystagmus are often seen in patients with developmental disabilities. These conditions contribute to impaired visual development and may also occur concurrently with accommodative problems (4).

A proper analysis of the vergence system in all patients is also important. Vergence anomalies often manifest in patients with symptoms of asthenopia, fatigue, eyestrain, headache, diplopia, sleepiness, or difficulty concentrating (5). A study of university students showed that the most common symptoms associated with binocular vision disorders were eyestrain, asthenopia, or headache (6). In this study, 32.3% of the students studied presented with an accommodative or nonstrabismic binocular vision disorder, with approximately 15% of patients suffering from a vergence anomaly (6). Another study by Lara et al. found an incidence of 22.3%, with 14.3% of patients suffering from a binocular disorder (7). Even though there have been few papers citing the incidence of nonstrabismic vergence anomalies in patients with special needs, with such a high incidence in the general population, it is important to test for these anomalies in all patients.

Accommodation and vergence are synergistic. Testing the binocular visual system involves creating stress on the visual system during the examination to help evaluate the relationship between accommodation and vergence. These measurements may fluctuate at the end of the day due to fatigue, and are influenced by the size of the target, the patient's effort, and the speed of measurement (8). Often, anomalies of vergence and accommodation present together. It is not uncommon to see a vergence anomaly secondary to an accommodative problem, or vice versa.

The significant prevalence of binocular vision disorders combined with the impact on learning and development make the proper diagnosis of these disorders a concern for all optometrists (9). The vergence and accommodative systems are linked and are dependent on one another for proper function (10). Ocular discomfort, fatigue, and eyestrain are common symptoms among today's population. These symptoms may develop due to the visual system being unable to perform the appropriate vergence and accommodative response for a specific task (9). In young patients and patients with special needs that may not complain of asthenopia, the avoidance of near tasks is a common symptom that can be associated with accommodative and vergence disorders. A proper case history, including patient complaints and symptoms, is the first important step to the proper diagnosis of a binocular vision disorder (9). Treatment of these disorders can range from the use of lenses to optometric vision therapy (OVT). The basis of treatment is generally linked to the severity of patient symptoms. With proper diagnosis and treatment, patients with binocular vision problems can show improvements of both visual comfort and performance.

DIAGNOSIS

The Accommodative System In the visual system, accomodation is a "complex response to a combination of visual, mechanical, and psychological stimuli" (4). An accurate accommodative response is necessary to shift focus from distance to near. Accommodation is achieved by contraction of the ciliary muscle (11), which relaxes tension on the zonular fibers (12). This relaxation causes an increase in the power of the lens (11) and continues until the near image is clear (13). The first classifications of the accommodative anomalies were by Duane in 1915 (14). Accommodative dysfunction is commonly classified into four categories:

1. Accommodative insufficiency (AI)
2. Accommodative excess (AE)
3. Accommodative infacility
4. Ill-sustained accommodation

Diagnosis of Accommodative Dysfunction Testing procedures for accommodative dysfunction include measurement of accommodative amplitude, monocular and binocular facility testing using flippers, monocular estimation method (MEM), fused crossed cylinder (FCC)/binocular crossed cylinder, and negative relative accommodation (NRA)/positive relative accommodation (PRA). The most widely used measurement of accommodative amplitude is the subjective push-up method. This procedure requires a patient to report when a near target becomes blurred (2). Wick and Hall (15) studied the relationships between the three areas of accommodation, amplitude, facility, and lag. They found that it is impossible to predict the results of one test based on the results of another. When accommodative dysfunction is suspected, a complete assessment of all three areas is necessary (15).

When testing patients with intellectual disabilities, Nott dynamic retinoscopy or the MEM may be the preferred methods for evaluating accommodative posture. Nott retinoscopy is an objective technique shown to provide valid and repeatable measures in both typically developed children and those with disabilities (16). A study by Goss et al. (17) suggested that although Nott and MEM retinoscopy techniques yield similar values in most individuals, in patients with a high lag of accommodation, the Nott method had a lower measurement than MEM. This should be considered when using these methods to determine add power.

Anomalies of the Accommodative System

Accommodative Insufficiency Accommodative insufficiency is defined as "a condition in which the patient has difficulty stimulating accommodation" (5). This diagnosis is given when a patient exhibits an accommodative amplitude lower than expected for the patient's age (5). Hofstetter's formula can be used to determine this normative age value. This formula states that the lower limit is equal to 15 – (0.25 × age of patient) (18). An abnormal accommodative amplitude measurement is any value 2D or more below the lower age limit (5).

Symptoms of AI are variable. Some of the more common complaints include blur, asthenopia, headaches, eyestrain, double vision, reading problems, fatigue, difficulty changing focus from one distance to another, and sensitivity to light (19) (Table 19.1). Additionally, patients with AI may also complain of blur with prolonged near work, a result of fatigue of the fast accommodative mechanism (9).

The classic clinical sign of AI is a reduced accommodative amplitude. Additionally, any test that involves stimulating accommodation or a minus lens, such as PRA testing and monocular and binocular accommodative facility testing, may be reduced in a patient with AI (5). Patients with AI may also exhibit a lag (or a higher plus value) with MEM retinoscopy and the FCC test (5).

Accommodative Excess (Spasm) Patients with AE have trouble relaxing their accommodation, and therefore have more difficulty with plus lenses. Common complaints include asthenopia and headaches while performing near tasks and blurred vision (5) (Table 19.2). Common signs of AE are

TABLE 19.1 Signs and Symptoms of Accommodative Insufficiency

Symptoms

These symptoms are generally related to the use of the eyes for reading or other near tasks:

Long-standing
Blurred vision
Headaches
Eyestrain
Reading problems
Fatigue and sleepiness
Loss of comprehension over tine
A pulling sensation around the eyes
Movement of the print
Avoidance of reading and other close work

Signs

Direct measures of accommodative stimulation

Reduced amplitude of accommodation
Difficulty clearing −2.00 with monocular accommodative facility
High MEM retinoscopy finding
High fused cross-cylinder finding

Indirect measures of accommodative stimulation

Reduced positive relative accommodation
Difficulty clearing −2.00 with binocular accommodative facility
Low base-out to blur finding at near

Scheiman M, Wick B. *Clinical management of binocular vision.* Philadelphia: Lippincott Williams & Wilkins; 2002, with permission.

fluctuating visual acuities and low acceptance of plus lenses resulting in a relative lead for MEM findings (more minus power) and a low NRA value. Patients with AE may have difficulty with plus lenses during monocular and binocular accommodative facility testing.

Accommodative Infacility Patients with accommodative infacility have difficulty changing accommodative posture from near to distance quickly (5). Symptoms generally include blur when changing focus from near to distance, blurry vision, and eye strain (5) (Table 19.3). Patients with accommodative infacility will typically have difficulty with both plus and minus lenses during accommodative testing, resulting in reduced NRA and PRA findings. The most common tests for diagnosing this condition are monocular and binocular accommodative facility. In patients with accommodative infacility, both tests are usually reduced.

Ill-sustained Accommodation Patients with ill-sustained accommodation will commonly have no complaints early in the day but will manifest

TABLE 19.2 Signs and Symptoms of Accommodative Excess

Symptoms

These symptoms are generally related to the use of the eyes for reading or other near tasks:

Long-standing
Blurred vision worse after reading or other close work
Headaches
Eyestrain
Difficulty focusing from far to near
Sensitivity to light

Signs

Direct measures of accommodative relaxation

Difficulty clearing +2.00 with monocular accommodative facility
Low MEM retinoscopy finding

Indirect measures of accommodative relaxation

Reduced NRA
Difficulty clearing +2.00 with binocular accommodative facility
Low fused cross-cylinder finding
Low base-in to blur finding at near

Scheiman M, Wick B. *Clinical management of binocular vision.* Philadelphia: Lippincott Williams & Wilkins; 2002, with permission.

TABLE 19.3 Symptoms and Signs of Accommodative Infacility

Symptoms

These symptoms are generally related to the use of the eyes for reading or other near tasks:

Long-standing
Blurred vision, particularly when looking from near to far or far to near
Headaches
Eyestrain
Reading problems
Fatigue and sleepiness
Loss of comprehension over time
A pulling sensation around the eyes
Movement of the print
Avoidance of reading and other close work

Signs

Direct measures of accommodative facility

Difficulty clearing −2.00 and +2.00 with monocular accommodative facility

Indirect measures of accommodative facility

Reduced positive relative accommodation and NRA
Difficulty clearing −2.00 and +2.00 with binocular accommodative facility
Low base-out and base-in to blur finding at near

Scheiman M, Wick B. *Clinical management of binocular vision.* Philadelphia: Lippincott Williams & Wilkins; 2002, with permission.

TABLE 19.4 Signs and Symptoms of Accommodation Ill-Sustained

Symptoms
Blurred near vision
Discomfort and strain associated with near tasks
Fatigue associated with near-point tasks
Difficulty with attention and concentration when reading
Signs
Normal accommodative amplitude if administered just one; the amplitude decreases if repeated five to ten times
Low positive relative accommodation
Fails monocular and binocular accommodative facility with minus lenses; the performance will decrease over time
Esophoria at near
High MEM and fused cross-cylinder

[a]Taken (Scheiman M, Wick B. *Clinical management of binocular vision.* Philadelphia: Lippincott Williams & Wilkins; 2002, with permission.)

symptoms after prolonged near work. In patients with ill-sustained accommodation, amplitude values will appear normal if administered once, but may decline with repeated testing. Signs of ill-sustained accommodation are similar to those seen in AI (Table 19.4).

The Vergence System A response by the vergence system consists of input from four different types of vergence: tonic vergence, disparity vergence, accommodative vergence, and proximal vergence. Tonic vergence is created by baseline neural input from the midbrain (21), and it creates the patient's ocular alignment at distance. Tonic vergence makes the ocular position relatively more "eso" in posture than the physiologic resting position (22). Disparity or fusional vergence is driven by retinal disparity between two eyes (21). The goal of the fusional vergence system is to maintain a single image on the retina. Within the fusional vergence system, there is fast fusional vergence, which is responsible for quick movements to regain binocularity, and slow fusional vergence, which is responsible for maintaining a vergence posture over time (21). The slow fusional vergence system is responsible for maintaining binocularity during sustained near work. Any abnormality in the function of this system can lead to near-point symptoms (23). Accommodative vergence is a vergence movement that is stimulated by the accommodative system (22). When accommodation is stimulated, this type of vergence moves the eyes together to converge. Proximal vergence occurs because an object is in close proximity to the patient (21,22). This type of vergence can cause an increase in eso posture when a phoria measurement is taken using the phoropter.

Diagnosis of Vergence Dysfunction The first step in evaluating the vergence system is determining the phoria measurement. The phoria can be determined through both objective and subjective methods. Patients with special needs, or younger patients, may have difficulty responding to subjective testing; objective testing may be more appropriate. Alternating cover test is an objective method used to determine the phoria, while von Graefe phorias, modified Thorington technique/Howell card, and Maddox rod are examples of subjective methods. When determining a subjective phoria measurement, the modified Thorington technique and the Maddox rod may be more appropriate when examining a patient with special needs, as both tests are done out of the phoropter. A study by Lyon et al. (24) found that using the modified Thorington technique to assess the phoria was successful in 96% to 98% of first- and fourth-grade students.

Testing fusional vergence amplitude is important in diagnosing a deficiency in the vergence system. Fusional vergence amplitudes allow us to calculate how much vergence reserve the patient has to compensate for the phoria. The most common method for measuring fusional vergence ranges is using Risley prisms in the phoropter, although the step vergence method may be more appropriate for testing patients with special needs. This method is performed in free space, giving the patient peripheral cues during testing (24,25). The other advantage to this method is that it is an objective test, and thus can be performed on patients that may have difficulty verbalizing what they are seeing (25). Step vergence measurements are different than smooth vergence measurements, and practitioners should not compare the test results (26). The method of vergence testing, therefore, should remain consistent from examination to examination.

The near point of convergence (NPC) can be easily measured either subjectively or objectively and is a simple and quick test to perform. For patients with special needs, an objective measurement of the NPC may be more appropriate. The NPC can be measured using either an accommodative target, such as a fixation stick with a letter, or a nonaccommodative target, such as a penlight. In prepresbyopic patients, the accommodative system has an influence on the NPC, so it should be noted that using an accommodative target will yield a closer NPC (27,28). It has been suggested that in symptomatic patients that have an NPC within normal ranges, repeating the NPC with a nonaccommodative target may yield a more receded NPC (28).

Vergence facility will often elicit a binocular problem in patients that have otherwise normal values on binocular vision testing. Although this test is useful in determining binocular dysfunction in symptomatic patients with normal fusional vergence range values (29), it may be difficult to perform on patients with special needs. In order to obtain results in patients with poor comprehension of the task or poor verbal skills, it may be necessary to objectively monitor the patient's qualitative responses rather than relying on numeric values.

Normally, the patient's binocular system converges at near and diverges at distance to maintain a single, fused image. Anomalies of the vergence system can include difficulty with converging at near or diverging at distance or an excess of convergence at near or divergence at distance. Often, the anomalies of the vergence system are organized by their accommodative convergence to accommodation ratio (AC/A ratio), which measures the link between the accommodative and vergence systems (5). A high AC/A ratio is reflective of a strong link between accommodation and vergence, while a low AC/A ratio shows a relatively lower influence of accommodation on the vergence system. The different anomalies of the vergence system can thus be categorized into high AC/A conditions, low AC/A conditions, and normal AC/A conditions.

High AC/A Conditions Convergence excess is a condition in which the distance deviation is generally small or orthophoric with a large near esophoric or esotropic deviation. The near angle of deviation should exceed the distance angle of deviation by approximately 10 prism diopters (30). Patients may also exhibit poor negative fusional vergence ranges at near and a high AC/A ratio (5). A study of college students found the incidence of convergence excess to be 1.5% (6), while another study by Lara et al. (7) found the incidence to be 4.5% in a clinic population.

Divergence excess (DE) can be caused either by a true excess in the divergence system at distance or by an excess of accommodative vergence at near (31). An excess of accommodative vergence at near causes a condition called simulated divergence excess, which is actually basic exophoria (or tropia) with an excess of convergence at near. These two types of exophoria can be differentiated by monocularly occluding the patient for 1 hour followed by measuring the deviation at near (32). The deviation can also be measured while the patient views through +3.00 lenses at near; if the patient's near deviation increases (to within 10 diopters of the near deviation), a simulated divergence excess is diagnosed (33).

Low AC/A Conditions Convergence insufficiency (CI) is a decrease in convergence, or positive relative vergence, resulting in a decrease in normal binocularity at near (34,35). Patients with this condition are often symptomatic, complaining of headache, diplopia at near, and asthenopia when reading (35). Convergence insufficiency is the most common vergence disorder. Reported incidence ranges from <1% to >50% of patients, depending on the criteria used and the population studied (6,7,36–38). Generally, the incidence of CI has been reported to be around 4% to 6% of the population (36–38). Convergence insufficiency has been shown to have a higher prevalence in patients with attention deficit hyperactivity disorder (ADHD) (39) since these patients scored higher on the convergence insufficiency symptom survey (CISS) (40). Children with CI were found to have a higher number of behaviors found in patients with ADHD as compared to children without CI (39). A study of patients on the autism spectrum (41) showed a reduced NPC in 33% of patients with lower functioning autism; however, further studies are needed to determine the incidence of CI in this population.

When diagnosing CI, it is important to test the accommodative system as well. Patients with poor accommodative ability, or AI, may also exhibit poor convergence and exophoria at near. The constant drive of the vergence system on the accommodative system creates fatigue, resulting in an exophoric posture at near and reduced NPC (42). This condition is known as pseudo-CI. It can be clinically distinguished from true CI by the presence of a weak accommodative system and improvement of convergence with low-powered plus lenses at near (5).

Diagnosing CI begins with testing the NPC, which is reduced in patients with this condition.

The NPC break value used to accurately diagnose CI has been shown to be anywhere from 5 to >10 cm (37,43–45). A study on treatment of CI by the Convergence Insufficiency Treatment Trial (CITT) study group used a break of ≥6 cm as one of the diagnostic criteria (43). Other diagnostic criteria used by the CITT study group included an exodeviation that was 4 prism diopters greater at near than distance, and an insufficient positive fusional vergence system (43). Along with clinical signs, patient symptoms are also important in this diagnosis. The CITT study group developed the CISS to identify patients that have CI (vs. normal binocular vision) based on the patient's and parent's responses to different questions (32). Both adults and children with CI scored significantly higher, and thus were significantly more symptomatic than patients with normal binocular vision (46–49). This survey was also found to be an accurate indicator of CI independent of examiner bias, meaning that it can be used in a clinical setting to accurately predict patients with CI versus those with normal binocular vision (47). Although young children or patients with special needs may not be able to complain of symptoms related to CI, it is important to note whether or not the patient has a history of avoiding near activities (34).

Divergence insufficiency (DI) is a condition in which patients have a larger esophoria or esotropia at distance than at near and a low negative fusional vergence ranges at distance (5,50). Often, patients are orthophoric at near, with an esodeviation at distance. Generally, DI is more common in elderly patients and can progress slowly as the patients age (51). In a study of patients with DI by Jacobson, 95% of the patients studied were over 50 years of age (50). When evaluating patients with DI, it is important to rule out any underlying neurologic cause of this condition. Divergence insufficiency can be caused by conditions such as Graves disease, pseudotumor cerebri, hydrocephalus, brainstem stroke, meningitis, brain tumors, temporal arteritis, progressive supranuclear palsy, and Chiari 1 malformation (50–52). Jacobson found that primary DI was mostly seen in elderly patients that had a viral prodrome or minor head injury, and 40% of the patients had a resolution of their diplopia after 5 months (50). Although a concomitant deviation is generally found in primary DI, mild forms of Graves disease have been shown to cause concomitant DI (51).

Normal AC/A Conditions Basic exophoria is a condition in which the distance and near phoria are equal, and the patient has poor positive fusional vergence ability at both distance and near (5). A study by Porcar et al. (6) found the incidence of basic exophoria to be 3.1% in a population of college students. In patients with basic esophoria, the near and distance phoria measurements are approximately equal, and the patient will also exhibit poor negative fusional vergence abilities (5). Porcar et al. (6) found the incidence of basic esophoria to be 1.5%, less common than basic exophoria.

With fusional vergence dysfunction (FVD), accommodative and phoria testing is normal, but the patient has reduced positive and negative fusional vergence ranges (5). Patients presenting with this condition can easily go undiagnosed (5,53), and thus it is important to include vergence facility testing for all symptomatic patients that have normal phorias and accommodative systems. A study by McDaniel et al. (54) showed that vergence ranges and vergence facility measurements do not always correlate, and thus it is important to perform vergence facility in patients that have symptoms when all other binocular testing appears normal (39). Fusional vergence dysfunction has been found to have an incidence of 1.5% and is less common than other vergence disorders (6).

TREATMENT

Lens Therapy The treatment of both accommodative and vergence disorders involves the sequential management of correction of ametropia, added lenses and OVT. Uncorrected refractive error, particularly hyperopia, astigmatism, and low degrees of anisometropia, can result in accommodative fatigue and other symptoms that are associated with a binocular vision disorder (5). Prescribing the appropriate distance optical correction is therefore the first line of treatment for all patients. The optimal refractive end point is reached when a patient has a prescription with the least minus or plus power that achieves the best corrected visual acuity. It is important to remember that this correction may have an effect on the accommodative and vergence systems, and correction alone may eliminate symptoms.

After the distance vision is properly corrected, additional plus lenses for near should be the next consideration. After analyzing the near-point data, a potential add may be needed to decrease symptoms and the demand on the binocular system. The amount of plus needed can be determined by following the formula ([NRA + PRA]/2). Monocular estimation method can be used to refine this result, paying special attention to whether a lag or lead is present. If a lead is present then the near addition lens power should be reduced, and conversely, a lag would indicate that near plus should be increased.

Near lenses will be most useful for patients that have trouble stimulating accommodation and are the first line of treatment in AI, ill-sustained accommodation, and pseudo-CI. Convergence excess can also be successfully treated with near addition lenses, particularly in patients with this condition that have a high AC/A ratio (30). Using the AC/A ratio may be helpful in selecting the correct near addition lens in patients with CE to reduce the patient's esophoria at near.

It has been shown that underaccommodation is common among patients with disabilities, particularly Down syndrome (55). Although the etiology of this decrease in accommodation is unknown, bifocal spectacles have been shown to induce accurate accommodation, improving near focusing in school-aged children with Down syndrome (20). Patients with special needs can benefit from a bifocal prescription if additional plus at near is indicated. It has been shown that children with Down syndrome are more likely to use the near portion of the bifocal when the bifocal segment is placed at the mid-pupil (20).

Although plus lenses are more commonly used in lens therapy for binocular vision disorders, minus lenses may also be used to treat specific conditions. Patients with true DE can be treated with minus lenses. Overminusing a patient with DE (by way of the CA/C ratio) can be used to increase accommodation and thus increase fusional convergence (5,33). This treatment is generally used in patients that are too young (5) or unable to participate in active OVT.

Prism Therapy Prism correction may be successful in patients that have anomalies of the vergence system. Two methods that are commonly used to calculate the amount of prism needed are Sheard's and Percival's criterion. For Sheard's criterion, the calculated prism correction needed can be expressed by the formula correcting prism needed = 2/3 phoria − 1/3 compensating fusional vergence blur finding. The formula used to calculate prism needed based on Percival's criterion is P = 1/3 (greater blur value, either base-in or base-out) − 2/3 (lesser blur value, either base-in or base-out) (5).

Base-out prism can be used to successfully treat patients with basic esophoria. Base-out prism at near can be used in patients with CE that cannot be fully corrected with near addition lenses and OVT. In patients with DI, the use of base-out prism is the initial treatment (5).

Base-in prism is used to treat patient with basic exophoria, CI and DE. Although relieving prism is not the first-line treatment for CI (45), one study found that base-in relieving prism significantly reduced the asthenopia associated with CI in presbyopic patients wearing progressive addition lenses (56). A study by Scheiman et al., however, found that base-in prism did not alleviate symptoms in children with CI (57).

Optometric Vision Therapy After appropriate optical correction and additional plus lenses have been prescribed if needed, an OVT program may help improve vergence and accommodative skills and reduce asthenopia associated with these visual disorders. The appropriate program must be tailored to each individual patient, with consideration for their symptoms, needs, and goals.

While therapy is the first line of treatment for AE and accommodative infacility, it can also have a positive effect on patients with AI and ill-sustained accommodation. Optometric vision therapy for AI should concentrate on increasing accommodative amplitude and facility, and is often used in conjunction with plus lenses at near. For patients with AE, plus lenses are not appropriate, and OVT is the only modality that will help the patient learn to relax his or her accommodation. In patients with accommodative infacility, OVT improves the speed and flexibility of their accommodative system.

Office-based vision therapy was shown to be the most effective treatment for CI in children (43,58). Although pencil push-ups have long been one of the most popular techniques given to patients with CI (59), a study by Scheiman et al. showed that pencil push-ups do not produce significant improvements in clinical signs or symptoms of CI (60). It is important to note that while patients were undergoing office-based vision therapy for CI, clinical signs improved before patients noted a decrease in symptoms of CI. This study also recommended at least 12 weeks of therapy for optimal results from vision therapy for this condition (61). Patients that were successful after 12 weeks of office-based vision therapy were shown to remain symptom free for 1 year after treatment (62).

Surgery Individuals with special needs are often not ideal candidates for surgical intervention. Many have cardiac, respiratory, or other neurologic or systemic conditions that would make surgery more of a risk. For this reason, many ophthalmic surgeons may shy away from offering this form of intervention and treatment. For patients with vergence disorders that cannot be treated with lenses, OVT, or prism correction, surgery may be indicated. For patients with DE, if the angle of deviation is large and/or the patient has not had success with other treatment modalities, then a surgical consult is indicated (5,33). For patients with DI, a bilateral medial rectus recession has been shown to be a successful treatment in elderly patients with a slowly progressive condition (51). Up to one-third of the individuals who have strabismus surgery will require a second surgery, and of those, up to an additional one-third may need a third surgery.

Treatment of all binocular vision disorders, including lenses, prisms, and OVT, is not age restrictive. Optometric vision therapy can be successful at any age, with the proper patient motivation and dedication. In some cases, the best treatment includes a combination of lenses, prisms, and/or OVT. Review Chapter 25, Optometric Management of Functional Vision Disorders for a more detailed review of the treatment for the conditions discussed above. When choosing a treatment modality, it is important to keep the patient's needs, goals, and abilities in mind.

REFERENCES

1. Garcia A, Cacho P, Lara F. Evaluating relative accommodations in general binocular dysfunctions. Optom Vis Sci. 2002; 79:779–87.
2. Woodhouse J, Meades J, Leat S, et al. Reduced accommodation in children with Down syndrome. Invest Ophthalmol Vis Sci. 1993;34:2382–7.
3. Hodoka S. General binocular dysfunction in an urban optometry clinic. J Am Optom Assoc. 1985;56:560–2.
4. McClelland J, Parks J, Jackson A, Saunders K. Accommodative dysfunction in children with cerebral palsy: A population-based study. Invest Ophthalmol Vis Sci. 2006;47: 1824–9.
5. Scheiman M, Wick B. Clinical management of binocular vision. Philadelphia: Lippincott Williams & Wilkins; 2002.
6. Porcar E, Martinez-Palomera A. Prevalence of general binocular dysfunctions in a population of university students. Optom Vis Sci. 1997;74:111–3.
7. Lara F, Cacho P, Garcia A, et al. General binocular disorders: prevalence in a clinic population. Ophthalmic Physiol Opt. 2001;21:70–4.
8. Feldman J, Cooper J, Eichler R. The effect of stimulus parameters (size, complexity, depth, and line thickness) on horizontal fusion amplitudes in normal humans. Binoc Vis Eye Muscle Surg Q. 1998:23–30.
9. Cooper J, Burns C, Cotter S, et al. Optometric clinical practice guideline care of the patient with accommodative and vergence dysfunction. St. Louis: American Optometric Association; 2006.
10. Schor C, Ciuffreda K. Vergence eye movements: basic and clinical aspects. Boston: Butterworth-Heinemann Publishing; 1983.
11. Kaufman P, Alm A. Adler's Physiology of the Eye. St. Louis: Mosby; 2003.
12. Schwartz S. Visual Perception a clinical orientation. New York: McGraw-Hill; 2004.
13. Benjamin W. Borish's Clinical Refraction. Philadelphia: W.B. Saunders Company; 1998.
14. Duane A. Anomalies of accommodation clinically considered. Trans Am Opthalmol Soc. 1915;1:386–400.
15. Wick B, Hall P. Relation among accommodative facility, lag, and amplitude in elementary school children. Am J Optom Physiol Opt. 1987;64:593–8.
16. Leat S, Gargon J. Accommodative response in children and young adults using dynamic retinoscopy. Optahlmic Physiol Opt. 1996;16:375–84.
17. Goss D, Groppel P, Dominguez L. Comparison of MEM retinoscopy and Nott retinoscopy and their interexaminer repeatabilities. J Behav Optom. 2005;6:149–55.
18. Carlson NB, Kurtz D, Heath DA. Clinical procedures for ocular examination. Stanford: Appleton and Lang; 1996.
19. Daum KM. Accommodative dysfunction. Doc Ophthalmol. 1983;55:177–98.
20. Stewart RE, Woodhouse M, Trojanowska LD. In focus: The use of bifocal spectacles with children with Down's Syndrome. Ophthalmic Physiol Opt. 2004;25:514–22.
21. Ciuffreda K, Barry T. Eye movement basics for the clinician. St. Louis: Mosby; 1995.
22. Grosvenor T. Primary care optometry. 4th ed. Woburn: Butterworth-Heinemann; 2002.
23. Rosenfield M. Tonic vergence and vergence adaptation. Optom Vis Sci. 1997;74:303–28.
24. Lyon D, Goss D, Horner D, et al. Normative data for modified Thorington phorias and prism bar vergences from the Benton-IU study. Optometry. 2005;76:593–9.
25. Wesson M. Normalization of prism bar vergences. Am J Optom Physiol Opt. 1982;59:628–34.

26. Antona B, Barrio A, Gonzalez E, Sanchez I. Repeatability and agreement in the measurement of horizontal fusional vergences. Ophthalmic Physiol Opt. 2008;28:475–91.
27. Rosenfield M, Ciuffreda K, Ong E. Vergence adaptation and the order of clinical vergence range testing. Optom Vis Sci. 1995;72:219–23.
28. Scheiman M, Gallaway M, Frantz K, et al. Nearpoint of convergence: test procedure, target selection, and normative data. Optom Vis Sci. 2003;80:214–25.
29. Gall R, Wick B, Bedell H. Vergence facility: establishing clinical utility. Optom Vis Sci. 1998;75:731–42.
30. Arnoldi K. Convergence excess: characteristics and treatment. Am Orthopt J. 1999;49:37–47.
31. Kushner B, Morton G. Distance/near difference in intermittent exotropia. Arch Ophthalmol. 1998;116:478–86.
32. Kushner B. Diagnosis and treatment of exotropia with a high accommodation convergence – accommodation ratio. Arch Ophthalmol. 1999;117:221–4.
33. Burian H. Exodeviations: their classification, diagnosis and treatment. Am J Ophthalmol. 1966;62:1161–6.
34. Cooper J, Duckman R. Convergence insufficiency: incidence, diagnosis, and treatment. J Am Optom Assoc. 1978;49:673–80.
35. Lavrich J. Convergence insufficiency and its current treatment. Curr Opin Ophthalmol. 2010;21:356–60.
36. Rouse M, Hyman L, Hussein M. Frequency of convergence insufficiency among fifth and sixth graders: The Convergence Insufficiency and Reading Study (CIRS) group. Optom Vis Sci. 1998;75:643–9.
37. Rouse M, Hyman L, Hussein M, Solan H. Frequency of convergence insufficiency in optometry clinic settings: The Convergence Insufficiency and Reading Study (CIRS) group. Optom Vis Sci. 1998;75:88–96.
38. Borsting E, Rouse M, DeLand P, et al. Association of symptoms and convergence and accommodative insufficiency in school-age children. Optometry. 2003;74:23–34.
39. Borsting E, Rouse M, Chu R. Measuring ADHD behaviors in children with symptomatic accommodative dysfunction or convergence insufficiency: a preliminary study. 2005;76:599–2.
40. Rouse M, Borsting E, Mitchell G, et al. Academic behaviors in children with convergence insufficiency with and without parent-reported ADHD. Optom Vis Sci. 2009;86:1169–77.
41. Milne E, Griffiths H, Buckely D, et al. Vision in children and adolescents with autistic spectrum disorder: evidence for reduced convergence. J Autism Dev Disord. 2009;39:965–75.
42. Rutstien R, Duam K. Exotropia associated with defective accommodation. J Am Optom Assoc. 1987;58:548–54.
43. CITT Study Group. Randomized clinical trial of treatments for symptomatic convergence insufficiency in children. Arch Ophthalmol. 2008;126:1336–49.
44. Hayes G, Cohen B, Rouse M, et al. Normative values for the nearpoint of convergence of elementary schoolchildren. Optom Vis Sci. 1998;75:506–12.
45. Maples W, Henes R. Near point of convergence norms measured in elementary school children. Optom Vis Sci. 2007;84:224–8.
46. Borsting E, Rouse M, DeLand P. Prospective comparison of convergence insufficiency and normal binocular children on CIRS symptoms surveys. Optom Vis Sci. 1999;76:221–8.
47. Borsting E, Mitchell G, Cotter S, et al. Validity of the convergence insufficiency symptom survey: a confirmatory study. Optom Vis Sci. 2009;86:357–63.
48. Rouse M, Borsting E, Mitchell G., et al. Validity and reliability of the revised convergence insufficiency symptoms survey in adults. Ophthalmic Physiol Opt. 2004;24:384–90.
49. Borsting E, Rouse M, Mithcell G, et al. Validity and reliability of the revised convergence insufficiency symptom survey in children aged 9 to 18 years. Optom Vis Sci. 2003;80: 832–8.
50. Jacobson D. Divergence insufficiency revisited: natural history of idiopathic cases and neurologic associations. Arch Ophthalmol. 2000;118:1237–41.
51. Bothun E, Archer S. Bilateral medial rectus muscle recession for divergence insufficiency pattern esotropia. J AAPOS. 2005;9:3–6.
52. Pokharel D, Siatkowski R. Progressive cerebellar tonsillar herniation with recurrent divergence insufficiency esotropia. J AAPOS. 2004;8:286–7.
53. Amster D. Fusional vergence dysfunction: a case report. J Behav Optom. 2008;19:59–62.
54. McDaniel C, Fogt N. Vergence adaptation in clinical vergence testing. Optometry. 2010;81:469–475.
55. Haugen O, Hovding G, Lundstrom I. Refractive development in children with Down's Syndrome; a population based, longitudinal study. Br J Ophthalmol. 2001;85:714–9.
56. Teitelbaum B, Pang Y, Krall J. Effectiveness of base in prism for presbyopes with convergence insufficiency. Optom Vis Sci. 2009;86:153–6.
57. Scheiman M, Cotter S, Mitchell L, et al. Randomised clinical trial of the effectiveness of base-in prism reading glasses versus placebo reading glasses for symptomatic convergence insufficiency in children. Br J Ophthalmol. 2005;89: 1318–23.
58. Scheiman M, Rouse M, Kulp M, et al. Treatment of convergence insufficiency in childhood: a current perspective. Optom Vis Sci. 2009;86:420–8.
59. Scheiman M, Cooper J, Mitchell G, et al. A Survey of treatment modalities for convergence insufficiency. Optom Vis Sci. 2002;79:151–7.
60. Scheiman M, Mitchell G, Cotter S, et al. A randomized clinical trial of vision therapy /orthoptics versus pencil pushups for the treatment of convergence insufficiency in young adults. Optom Vis Sci. 2005;82:583–95.
61. Scheiman M, Kulp M, Cotter S, et al. Vision therapy/orthoptics for symptomatic convergence insufficiency in children: treatment kinetics. Optom Vis Sci. 2010;87:593–603.
62. CITT Study Group. Long-term effectiveness of treatments for symptomatic convergence insufficiency in children. Optom Vis Sci. 2009;86:1096–103.

CHAPTER 20

Yin C. Tea, OD, FAAO
Jacqueline Rodena, OD

Diagnosis and Treatment of Strabismus and Amblyopia

Patients with special needs are at greater risk for ocular and vision problems including strabismus and amblyopia than the rest of the population. Yet, research and surveys have shown that their eye care needs are often not met (1). This need not be the case. Eye care providers are well versed in the diagnosis, treatment, and management of binocular vision disorders. However, determining the diagnosis and providing the most appropriate treatment plan can be complicated by physical or cognitive restrictions. A few modifications to the traditional examination, including test environment, sequence, and the techniques themselves, combined with a close evaluation of what makes a particular patient unique, will allow the practitioner to accurately and successfully evaluate even the most challenging cases. (See Chapter 16, Comprehensive Examination Procedures, for more information regarding examination techniques.)

Objective testing methods become invaluable when examining patients with special needs. Treatment goals should take into consideration the day-to-day needs and physical or mental abilities of each unique patient. Tailoring treatments and recommendations so they are specific to each patient will greatly impact and improve their individual quality of life.

EPIDEMIOLOGY OF STRABISMUS AND AMBLYOPIA IN SPECIFIC POPULATIONS

Down Syndrome Strabismus appears in approximately half the Down syndrome (DS) population. Stephen et al. (2) reported that 47% of strabismus in patients with DS was found in patients younger than 5 years old. Haugen and Hø′vding (3) reported a 42% incidence of strabismus in a population-based, longitudinal study. Out of the 25 patients who manifested strabismus, 21 patients had esotropia, whereas only 2 had exotropia and only 2 had vertical strabismus (3). The mean age of onset was approximately 4 years (54 ± 35 months) (3). Although the prevalence of strabismus is much higher in patients with DS, the incidence of infantile esotropia in both populations is similar (1%–2%) (3). Normally, infantile onset is the more common presentation of esotropia; however, in the DS population, acquired esotropia is more common (3). This finding has been used to support the hypothesis that there might be a faulty emmetropization process in children with DS (4). Since it is more common for children with DS to have acquired strabismus rather than infantile strabismus, they should have a history of positive alignment with normal binocular stimulation during early visual development, allowing for the potential of restoring normal functional binocularity with treatment.

The challenge of obtaining clinical data in some patients with special needs makes it difficult for researchers to determine the frequency or presence of amblyopia when these numbers can be dependent upon accurate visual acuity measures. Therefore, reports of amblyopia in children with DS are limited. Haugen and Hø′vding reported that they were only able to test visual acuity in 15 out of 25 patients (3) with strabismus. They reported that five to six patients were suspected of having amblyopia. A recent study reported the presence of amblyopia in DS patients to be as high as 22% due to strabismus, high bilateral refractive errors, or anisometropia (5).

The presence of strabismus may have a negative impact on learning. Merrick and Koslowe (6) reported a significant portion of patients with DS and strabismus were found to have moderate to severe learning disabilities. The children with mild learning difficulties did not manifest strabismus. Although strabismus is likely only one of many contributing factors complicating the visual world of these patients, this difference in the performance of patients with strabismus in comparison to those without highlights the importance of binocularity. (See Chapter 4, Down Syndrome, for further details concerning DS.)

Cerebral Palsy Cerebral palsy (CP) is classified using the Gross Motor Function Classification System (GMFCS), which has five levels (7). The GMFCS rates the motor function of patients with CP independent of the type of CP. Ghasia et al. (8) studied children with various severities of CP, diagnosed using the GMFCS definition, and evaluated whether the different categories had any differences in visual dysfunction. The prevalence of horizontal strabismus was significant for all the GMFCS levels. Primary esotropia was the most common type of strabismus with a 2.2:1 ratio when compared to primary exotropia. The percentage of primary esotropia was 60% to 70% in levels 1 and 2 but dropped to 40% in levels 4 and 5. Thirty-two percent of the esotropia observed in levels 1 and 2 was purely refractive in etiology. These deviations were correctable with spectacle treatment and intermittent in frequency. The other 68% were diagnosed with infantile esotropia. Constant esotropia was seen in 90% of children in levels 3 to 5. Vertical deviations were prevalent in 50% of the children throughout levels 1 to 4.

Dyskinetic strabismus is a unique finding associated with patients who have CP. Fluctuation between esotropia and exotropia under similar accommodative conditions along with a slow tonic deviation comparable to a vergence movement is the hallmark sign of a dyskinetic strabismus (9). As the patient ages, exotropia becomes more common. There appears to be a correlation between dyskinetic strabismus and the athetoid category of CP (9). Dyskinetic strabismus was seen in only the most severe type of CP (8).

The reported prevalence of strabismus in patients with CP ranges from 15% to 69% (10–14, 17). Esotropia was the more common type of strabismus with a reported prevalence between 30% and 70% (8, 10–12, 14–17) as opposed to only 8% to 37% for exotropia (8, 10, 12, 14–17). The prevalence of vertical deviations is between 3% and 52% (14–16). The average age of onset was approximately 1.36 years (14). A high percentage of strabismus in patients with CP was paralytic in nature (17%) (16).

In summary, the prevalence of strabismus in children with milder forms of CP is similar to that found in neurologically normal children within the general population, 1% to 4% (14–16). In contrast, children with severe forms of CP have a higher prevalence of strabismus with associated features neurologically normal children generally do not present with, such as high myopia and dyskinetic strabismus (8).

Visual acuity testing can be limited by impairments in the physical ability to point or match targets, speech disability, restricted gaze, and trunk and/or head control limitation. When quantitative visual acuity data is difficult to confirm or cannot be obtained, a child may be incorrectly labeled as visually blind. Ghasia et al. studied the ability to obtain visual acuity measures using optotype testing in patients with CP. They found that 94% of patients who were diplegic, 75% of patients who were hemiplegic, and 48% of patients who were quadriplegic were able to perform this type of testing (21).

Amblyopia has been found in 6% to 71% of patients with CP (10, 12, 15–17). This definition includes organic as well as functional amblyopia caused by anisometropia or strabismus. Scheiman looked at optometric findings in patients with CP and found unilateral amblyopia in 20% and bilateral amblyopia in 11% (17). Patients regarded as level 1 on the GMFSC have the highest motor function, while level 5 is the most limited. Strabismic amblyopia was found in 70% of children in levels 1 and 2 (8). Contrary to what might be expected, the authors reported a lower prevalence of amblyopia in the more severely affected children in levels 3 to 5. They speculated that this could be due to the difficulty in obtaining visual acuity and a higher frequency of dyskinetic strabismus found at the higher levels. The fluctuation in the magnitude and frequency of the deviation with dyskinetic strabismus explains how this type of strabismus is less of an amblyogenic factor than a constant unilateral strabismus (9). Strabismic amblyopia was found more commonly in children diagnosed with the physiologic subtype spastic CP (8). Amblyopia secondary to anisometropia was found more often in children classified into the mixed category (dyskinetic, athetoid, hypotonic, and ataxic CP) (8). Ghasia et al. generalized that children with diplegic and spastic-type CP tended to be hyperopic and esotropic in addition to having the highest prevalence of stereopsis and fusion (8). Additionally, children with quadriplegic and mixed-type CP often presented with high myopia, cerebral visual impairment, dyskinetic strabismus, and severe gaze dysfunction (8). (See Chapter 3, Cerebral Palsy, for further details concerning CP.)

Fragile X Syndrome The reported prevalence of strabismus associated with Fragile X syndrome (FXS) was 30% to 40% (22, 23). A study by Hatton et al. (24) looking at the ocular status of males with FXS found a much lower prevalence of 8%. Esotropia was found to be the most common condition (50%–70%) (22, 23). One published case report described a female with FXS who had refractive anisometropic amblyopia (25). Maino et al. (26) reviewed the eye examination findings in one family where all three children were diagnosed with FXS. Although neither parent had strabismus, all three children presented with esotropia. (See Chapter 5, Fragile X Syndrome, for further details concerning FXS.)

Prader-Willi Syndrome Strabismus is the most common ocular finding associated with patients who have Prader-Willi syndrome (PWS). Hered et al. (27) found strabismus present in 54% of patients diagnosed with PWS. In the patients with strabismus, 48% presented with esotropia. Amblyopia was found in 24% of the patients (27).

Spina Bifida (Meningomyelocele) with and without Hydrocephalus Vision problems associated with meningomyelocele, or spina bifida, were not documented in the literature before the 1960s. One explanation is that the improvement in modern medicine has enabled children with these diagnoses to survive long enough to manifest ocular or visual problems. Strabismus is the most common condition found in this population. The prevalence of strabismus in children with meningomyelocele ranged from 30% to 61% (28–36). These studies revealed a high correlation of strabismus in children who were diagnosed with meningomyelocele and hydrocephalus. Rothstein et al. found strabismus in 23 out of the 52 (34%) (28) cases that had meningomyelocele and hydrocephalus. Although most studies reported similar findings, Clements and Kaushal (37) found a high prevalence of strabismus (50%) even in children who had meningomyelocele without hydrocephalus. Biglan reported that the predominant type of strabismus was esotropia: 114 out of 183 patients (63%) presented with the deviation (29). Similar percentages were found by Paysse et al. with 28 out of 43 children (65%) having esotropia (32). A-pattern deviations were mostly found in children with exotropia (39%). Biglan (35) suggested that this finding was acquired in association with hydrocephalus. Another finding caused by increased intracranial pressure secondary to shunt malfunction was bilateral sixth cranial nerve (CN) palsy. In a longitudinal study, Biglan found 22 patients (29) presenting with this condition. He explained that as intracranial pressure increased, there was higher probability that the sixth CN would be affected (29).

The prevalence of amblyopia in patients with meningomyelocele was reported to be 16% (51 out of 298) (29) although the different types of amblyopia were not separated. These children were successfully treated with amblyopia therapy even when mild forms of optic atrophy were diagnosed (29). Cortical blindness, or decreased vision secondary to infarction of the visual cortex, was only documented in 2 out of 298 cases (29).

Autism Limited literature is available discussing ocular alignment in patients with autism. Scharre and Creedon looked at several visual aspects in children with autism. They found 21% and 18% of the 34 children having an eye turn in the distance and near, respectively. All cases were intermittent and a greater frequency of exotropia than esotropia was documented (38). A study by Miller et al. (39) looking at thalidomide-affected patients found autism in four out of the five patients who were severely intellectually disabled. They reported that three out of four of these patients also had a horizontal noncomitant deviation (39). For more information on autism, see Chapter 8, Autism.

ETIOLOGY OF STRABISMUS AND AMBLYOPIA IN SPECIAL NEEDS POPULATION

A comprehensive understanding of the etiology of all types of strabismus has yet to be discovered. Several risk factors have been identified: maternal smoking (40,41) and perinatal risk factors such as the presence of congenital abnormalities, low birth weight (41, 42), prematurity, and large head circumference (43). The presence of strabismus sometimes indicates the presence of other abnormalities. Any infant with the rare finding of a large constant exotropia should be carefully evaluated for other congenital abnormalities (42).

Genetics has been identified as one etiology in the development of strabismus. Twin studies provide strong support for the role of genetic inheritance. The prevalence of strabismus in monozygotic twins is significantly greater than they are for dizygotic twins (44). Podgor et al. (45) found a strong familial aggregation among siblings who had esotropia. The probability that asibling manifested esotropia was more than doubled if the other sibling also had esotropia (45). Exotropia, on the other hand, showed familial aggregation in multiple births. The chance of a sibling having exotropia increased by a factor of 17 if any of the other siblings had exotropia (45).

A review article by Schiavi (46) suggested that one contributing cause for the concomitant strabismus found in many patients with DS could be brain damage. The basis for this conclusion is that exodeviations are often found in association with abnormal neurologic findings. Erkkilä et al. found that more than half of the CP children studied had a congenital exodeviation (16). However, despite the high prevalence of exotropia in children with DS when compared to the general population, esotropia is still found more often than exotropia. Haugen and Høvding (3) even argued that since their study showed that exodeviation was rare in patients with DS, brain damage should not be considered one of the major etiologic factors. They proposed instead that the frequent finding of accommodative weakness, frequently found in children with DS, was a more likely cause. The suggested mechanism was that a manifest esotropia was due to excess accommodative effort expended in compensation for an underlying accommodative weakness. However, since accommodative weakness is also found in children with DS who did not have strabismus, there might be other contributing factors. Enzyme-reduced activity of choline acetyltransferase and acetylcholinesterase was found by Yates et al. (47) in the brains of three patients with DS. The parasympathetic system using these enzymes is crucial to its function, and thus Haugen and Høvding (3) suggested that weak accommodation may be an element in the general malfunction of the system. Some other suggestions for the etiology of strabismus were weak fusional capacity (48), hypotonia (49), and accommodation–convergence dysfunction (50).

Pigassou-Albouy and Fleming (51) proposed that the development of strabismus in patients with CP was due to lesions in the mesencephalic oculomotor center. They explained that this subcortical mechanism helps cortical reflexes like binocular motor coordination and binocular vision develop so that damage to this area might lead to strabismus (51). Amblyopia in children with CP is considered to be partly functional but also caused by neurologic lesions to the subcortical motor centers (51).

Creel et al. (52) used visual evoked potentials to show that patients with PWS, hypopigmentation, and strabismus had a misrouting of ganglion fibers at the optic chiasm. Hered et al. (27) speculated that patients with PWS have narrow bifrontal diameters and small pupillary distances which might have a role in their development of strabismus. However, radiologic studies of the orbit were not available to confirm this. They also suggested that strabismus could be related to the infantile hypotonia and refractive error.

DIAGNOSIS OF STRABISMUS

Ocular alignment can be measured using several methods. The cover test has long been held as the gold standard for evaluating the presence and magnitude of a strabismus or phoria. If a reliable cover test is still not feasible, useful information can be garnered through the Hirschberg, Brückner, and Krimsky tests. These procedures are covered in depth in Chapter 16, Comprehensive Examination Procedures.

Esotropia Esotropia is a manifest inward deviation of one or both eyes. It is often divided into two general categories based on time of onset. It is classified as either early onset, infantile esotropia (before 1 year), or acquired esotropia (after 1 year). Infantile esotropia is a broad term used to describe a heterogeneous group of esotropes that onset within the first year of life (53). Infantile esotropia includes congenital esotropia, nonaccommodative infantile esotropia, accommodative infantile esotropia, paralytic esotropia, and esotropia associated with central nervous system abnormalities.

The reported prevalence of childhood esotropia ranges between 1% and 6% (54–61). Mohney (62) conducted a prospective observational case series of 221 children and found the most common etiology was accommodative. Either pure or partial accommodative esotropia was documented in 117 of 221 children (52.9%). Central nervous system defects were associated with 38 of 221 subjects (17.2%). Of these 38 children, 32 presented with congenital primary central nervous system disorders including CP (n = 10), nonspecific developmental delay (n = 7), and autism (n = 3). Spasmus nutans, DS, and Arnold-Chiari malformation were associated with only two cases each.

In a retrospective study, Greenberg et al. (63) reported findings similar to those reported by Mohney for the most common etiologies. The highest incidence of esotropia in the cohort was also accommodative esotropia, found in 179 out of 385 cases (46.5%). Documented central nervous system impairment was identified in 44 (11.4%) children (CP, n = 9; nonspecific developmental delay, n = 8; and DS, n = 8).

The most current research does not support the widespread belief that congenital esotropia is the most common form of childhood esotropia (62,63). Mohney suggested that the complexity of treating infantile esotropia might exaggerate the apparent incidence of the condition since only 12 (5.4%) children in his study had infantile esotropia. Esotropia associated with central nervous system defect was more common (17.2%), while the incidence of accommodative esotropia was over 10 times greater (52.9%) (62). Greenberg et al. found the incidence of congenital esotropia to be only 8.1%, while the incidence of accommodative esotropia was 46.5%. The incidence of esotropia associated with central nervous system disorder was 11.4% (63).

Congenital (Infantile) Esotropia Traditionally, infantile esotropia was described as having a large, constant deviation that rarely resolved on its own (64). Recent observational studies have found that some cases of infantile esotropia did spontaneously resolve and that the presentation of infantile esotropia is more varied in size and character than previously thought (65). Spontaneous resolution generally occurred in patients with smaller magnitude deviations and an intermittent or variable frequency of strabismus. Patients with stable esotropia >40 prism diopters had a very low likelihood of spontaneous resolution. In some populations, such as patients with DS, the prevalence of infantile versus acquired esotropia differs from what is found in the standard population. In general, infantile esotropia is more common than acquired esotropia. The reverse is true in the DS population. An equal prevalence and higher frequency of infantile esotropia is found associated with DS in comparison to the general population, but there is a higher frequency of acquired esotropia associated with DS (8). Cerebral palsy (8) and meningomyelocele (28, 29) were also associated with infantile esotropia.

Accommodative Esotropia Accommodative esotropia is used to describe overconvergence produced by accommodative effort, whether due to uncorrected hypermetropia or a high accommodative convergence–to-accommodation (AC/A) ratio (66). Accommodative esotropia typically onsets between 2 and 3 years of age, although it has a reported onset as early as 4 months of age and as late as 7 years of age (53, 67, 68). The onset is usually gradual with intermittent frequency. If left untreated even for a relatively short period of time, the deviation can become constant and amblyopia can result. Donahue (69) reported that this could occur within just a few weeks after the initial onset of an intermittent strabismus. Visual acuity is generally good with the potential for normal correspondence when treated since normal binocular vision is usually present prior to the onset of strabismus.

Patients with pure refractive accommodative esotropia will manifest moderate hyperopic refractive errors. A patient with a high AC/A ratio might present with esotropia despite a very low refractive error and vice versa for those with a low AC/A ratio. The deviation associated with accommodative esotropia is usually intermittent and moderate in size with a tendency to be equal at distance and near. In comparison, esotropia caused by a nonrefractive accommodative etiology will manifest a greater deviation at near than far. The deviation is usually moderate in size and intermittent but can be constant at near. Amblyopia is uncommon.

Some of the special needs populations that have been documented to have accommodative esotropia are patients with DS (70–72), meningomyelocele (29), and PWS (27). The terms "hypoaccommodation" and "accommodative weakness" are also used to describe a defective accommodative process that occurs in patients with DS (3). This is the main reason why a bifocal spectacle correction is highly recommended for this population.

Classification of Esotropia Duane's classification system (73) provides a simple method of identifying deviations by comparing the distance and near magnitudes. Convergence excess esotropia describes a strabismus where the near esodeviation is greater than the distance deviation. These patients manifest a high AC/A ratio. Basic esotropia occurs when the esodeviation is roughly the same at all distances. These patients generally have normal AC/A ratios. Divergence insufficiency presents when an esodeviation is greater at distance than it is at near. These patients will have a low AC/A ratio. Basic esotropia was found to be the most predominant type of strabismus in Asian patients with DS (80).

Exotropia A manifest outward deviation of the eyes is defined as exotropia. The general pediatric population has a 1% to 2% prevalence of exotropia (42). Although most of the special populations have a trend in esotropia, as mentioned earlier, exotropia usually manifests intermittently in most of these groups. Phillips et al. (74) concluded that intermittent exotropia that increases during near fixation is linked with neurologic conditions in children.

Congenital (Infantile) Exotropia Congenital or infantile exotropia is defined with the following characteristics: idiopathic, large angle, and constant frequency observed within the first 6 to 12 months of their life (75). In the general pediatric population, it is rarely seen, as the prevalence is 0.1% (76). Hunter et al. (75) observed infants that initially presented with intermittent exotropia but a few months later would change to a large and constant exotropia. They suggested that intermittent and constant exotropia observed in the same infant are "variable expressions of the same disease." In CP patients, more than half of the children with exotropia were considered congenital in nature in one study (16).

Classification of Exotropia Duane (73) also categorized exotropia with the following terms defined. Convergence insufficiency exotropia is defined as having the near exodeviation greater than distance with a low AC/A ratio. Basic exotropia is where the exodeviation is roughly the same at all distances along with a normal AC/A ratio. Divergence excess presents with an exodeviation greater at distance versus near with a high AC/A ratio.

In order to provide the best treatment options for the patient, true divergence excess and simulated or pseudo divergence excess (77) must be differentiated. Burian and Spivey (78) used the Duane's classification and modified it to what has become the current standard. A simulated divergence excess has not been completely dissociated and therefore presents as a smaller deviation at near than the true exodeviation angle. Burian (79) differentiated pseudo divergence excess by the deviation at near increasing after prolonged monocular occlusion. These patients with pseudo divergence excess were diagnosed by Brown using another method that involved seeing an increased near exotropia while wearing +3.00 lenses.

Haugen and Høvding (3) found 2 of 25 strabismic patients with DS to have intermittent exotropia. Kim and Hwang (80) found that in Asian patients with DS, 75% of them had the basic type of exotropia. In a longitudinal study by Biglan, children with meningomyelocele showed a slightly higher prevalence of constant exotropia in comparison to intermittent exotropia. Most of the patients with exotropia in this study were considered to have a basic exotropia. One patient had a true divergence exotropia that remained after prolonged occlusion and use of +3.00 lenses. In the study completed on autism by Scharre and Creedon (38), all six patients with exotropia demonstrated intermittent frequency. Hatton et al. (24) diagnosed one case of intermittent exotropia in a male with FXS.

Microtropia or Monofixation Syndrome Patients with microtropia generally present with good cosmetic alignment despite reduced visual acuity and limited sensory function. Clinical findings include many, if not all, of the following: constant, small angle esodeviation of 10 or less prism diopters, anomalous correspondence, eccentric fixation, reduced acuity, and gross stereopsis without appreciation of global stereopsis although peripheral fusion is present (81–85). Microtropia can also result secondary to postsurgical infantile esotropia (86) or develop in patients with accommodative esotropia over several years. Esotropia is associated with several special needs populations, so the presence of microtropia in these patients may be secondary to elective strabismus surgery for a larger initial deviation.

Vertical Deviations A hypertropia or hypotropia is usually associated with a concurrent horizontal deviation. A study by White and Brown (87) discovered that 37% of patients with a horizontal strabismus had a related vertical deviation. It is rare that an isolated vertical deviation of same magnitude occurs in all gazes. Caputo et al. (88) found that 6 of the 107 patients with DS and strabismus had a hypertropia. In children with CP, it was noted that 52% had a vertical deviation (16). This included children who had an inferior oblique overaction or superior oblique overaction.

Bielschowsky (89) classified vertical deviation into five groups: (a) concomitant verticals, (b) paretic verticals, (c) dissociated vertical deviations (DVDs), (d) overacting inferior oblique, and (e) combined verticals. Caloroso and Rouse (90) further classified vertical deviation into four categories: (a) primary vertical: vertical deviation that the direction and magnitude are still present whether the eyes are strabismic or nonstrabismic alignment; (b) secondary vertical: vertical deviation that is only present when eyes are strabismic and nonexistent in nonstrabismic alignment; (c) variable vertical: a significant fluctuation in magnitude of a vertical deviation despite the direction remaining the same; and (d) DVD: a hyper deviation that manifests in each eye under dissociated conditions.

Dissociated Vertical Deviation A DVD is a spontaneous deviation upward that presents when a patient is fatigued or under dissociated conditions, such as when one eye is occluded during a cover test or when the light reaching one eye is minimized with a red lens or translucent occluder. With a DVD, each eye elevates under occlusion as the other eye fixates. In contrast, in a left hypertropia, the right eye fixates while the left eye elevates. Then when the left eye fixates, the right eye depresses. A DVD can be present with a normal binocular system but is mostly associated with infantile esotropia (91). Commonly, it is diagnosed bilaterally with asymmetrical deviation (92). The magnitude of the nonfixating eye is commonly bigger and can increase with prolonged occlusion. When a DVD is seen monocularly, it is usually seen in conjunction with deep amblyopia and sensory heterotropia. DVDs are commonly found in patients with CP (8) and PWS (27).

A and V Patterns A- and V-pattern deviations are terms used to describe vertically noncomitant deviations that match the corresponding alphabetical letter. In an A-pattern deviation, the eyes are relatively converged in upgaze and diverged in downgaze. An A-pattern esotropia will manifest a larger-sized esodeviation in superior gaze than in inferior gaze, whereas an A-pattern exotropia will present with a larger exodeviation in inferior gaze than in superior gaze. A V-pattern esotropia will present with a larger deviation in inferior gaze versus superior gaze, while a V-pattern exotropia will show larger deviation in superior gaze than inferior gaze (Fig. 20-1). Patients may present with abnormal head posture to compensate for the noncomitant deviation. Patients with an A-pattern esotropia or a V-pattern exotropia may tip their heads back in order to maintain their eyes in relative downgaze where the magnitude of their deviation is minimized. Conversely, patients with an A-pattern exotropia or a V-pattern esotropia will prefer to depress their heads downward in order to keep their eyes in relative upgaze.

A significant portion of children with special needs that present with A-pattern exodeviations have meningomyelocele (39%) (29). There is strong association between A-pattern strabismus and patients that have a superior oblique muscle overaction (93). Biglan (29) noted that the etiology of A-pattern deviations might be due to the presence of hydrocephalus instead of spina bifida. The study reviewed CT scans of the orbit and midbrain and found the structures of the orbit to be similar to normal patients. They also found that patients with hydrocephalus and A-pattern deviation had orbits similar to hydrocephalus patients without A-pattern deviation. The scans also revealed a vertical distortion or "beak" deformity of the rostral portion of the midbrain. This midbrain location controls vertical gaze. The term "sunsetting sign" refers to the absence of upward gaze. Biglan suggested that in "sunsetting," it is the most severe presentation while milder vertical gaze difficulties may present as an A-pattern deviation. In a study by Hiles et al. (70), A- and V-pattern deviations were commonly found in patients with DS. The patterned deviation seen most in this population is A-pattern esotropia.

Paralytic Strabismus Books and literature interchangeably use the terms *paresis* and *paralysis*. However, paresis is defined as a partial motor paralysis. Patients who develop paralytic strabismus will typically present with complaints of recent onset diplopia. This is true in patients with special needs even though communication of the visual distortions they are experiencing might be difficult for some of these patients. Objective tests like the Parks 3 step can isolate and identify the problematic extraocular muscle.

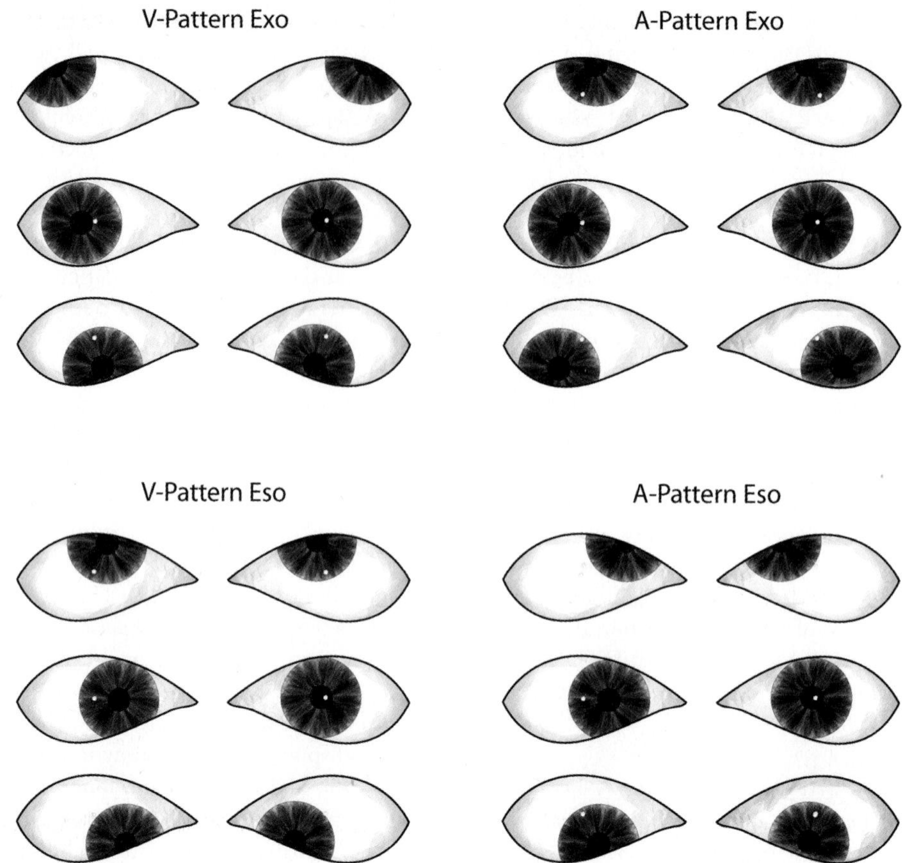

FIGURE 20-1. Representation of the eyes in A- or V-pattern esotropia or exotropia. Illustration courtesy of Gregory M. Fecho, OD.

A simple method to test the function of the extraocular muscles in patients with special needs is to see if the oculocephalic reflex or doll's head phenomenon occurs during the doll's head test. As the head is moved side to side or vertically, the eyes should move in the opposite direction of the rapid head turn and return to midline. Other than the few special needs conditions like DS where the diagnosis may be evident after birth, most of the other conditions referenced above may not be diagnosed until the child reaches toddler age. Therefore as an infant, the doll's head test can assess the integrity of the vestibulo-ocular response system. If it is noticed that this eye phenomenon does not occur, a brainstem defect may be indicated.

Cranial Nerve VI Palsy Patients with CN VI palsy will present with a face turn toward the affected side, esotropia in primary gaze, and limited abduction of the affected eye. Rush and Young (94) found CN VI palsies to be the most common (42%) of all CN palsies found in adults. They also stated that the etiologies of acquired CN VI palsy in adults of the general population included: undetermined (30%), vascular (18%), trauma (17%), neoplasm (15%), or aneurysm (4%). To the contrary, Robertson et al. (95) found the etiologies of acquired CN VI palsy in children in the general population were neoplasm (40%), trauma (20%), and inflammation (17%).

Cranial nerve VI palsy has been reported in patients with CP (16) and meningomyelocele (29). All of the patients with meningomyelocele had an acquired CN VI palsy secondary to increased intracranial pressure due to a shunt malfunction. It is critical to detect the signs of CN VI palsy in these patients as it may be an indication of shunt issues and necessitate a referral back to the neurologist.

Cranial Nerve III Palsy Patients with a complete CN III palsy present with exotropia and hypotropia (eye is down and out), ptosis, and a pupil that is fixed and dilated. Most cases of complete CN III palsy are of vascular origin and require emergency treatment. A CN III palsy that may be due to a deficiency of specific isolated muscle is usually rare and of congenital origin. Hiles et al. (70) reported several cases seen in patients with DS but did not describe the involved muscles or if a congenital or an acquired form. Cranial nerve III palsies will have variable presentations depending upon the specific muscles involved.

Cranial Nerve IV Palsy Patients with a CN IV palsy will present with a hypertropia of the involved eye, absent depression in adduction, chin depression, and a head tilt away from the involved side. In adults (when acquired), the most common etiology is "unknown" but 32% is secondary to trauma. In children, a CN IV palsy are typically congenital in nature (60%). Cranial nerve IV palsy has been reported in patients with DS (3) and CP (16).

TREATMENT OF STRABISMUS

Treatment options for strabismus in the special needs population are much like they are for the general population with modifications made to address special attentional, physical, or cognitive limitations. Treatment options consist of refractive error correction, prism, patching, optometric vision therapy, and surgery. Strabismic amblyopia can be more difficult to treat than refractive amblyopia without strabismus due to the abnormal conditions that often develop in association with an eye turn, such as suppression, eccentric fixation, and anomalous correspondence.

Treatment for Infantile Esotropia If the strabismus develops early during infancy, the patient will most likely lack the ability for normal sensory motor fusion. Nevertheless, refractive correction should be prescribed when an accommodative component to the esotropia is present, if acuity is improved in a significant manner, or when refractive error is outside of the expected range for the patient's age. The prism is often ineffective with infantile esotropia when sensory motor fusion is not possible. The prognosis of optometric vision therapy will vary depending on the ability of the patient to actively participate and engage in the therapy procedures prescribed. Patching therapy may not be feasible in patients with tactile sensitivities. Surgery might provide a reasonable cosmetic cure with limited or no improvements in binocular function.

Treatment for Accommodative Esotropia

If an accommodative strabismus is refractive in nature, correction of the refractive error is the treatment of choice. If there is a nonrefractive accommodative component to the strabismus, the patient will manifest a greater magnitude of esotropia at near than at distance due to a high AC/A ratio. These patients require a near prescription in addition to any distance correction needed. Patients with accommodative esotropia generally have normal sensory motor fusion potential and good alignment with spectacle correction alone. Mohney et al. (96) found with long-term follow-up that the majority of children with accommodative esotropia who are treated with spectacles continue to require optical correction into their second decade of life. When prescribing bifocals for children, the bifocal segment (seg) height should be placed significantly higher than that typically used for an adult. For instance, if a child is of preschool age or younger, consider bisecting the pupil. If the patient is in the earlier grades, placing the seg at the edge or middle of the iris is desirable. For older children, a seg height should be placed no lower than the bottom of the iris. When placing the bifocal in such a manner, this ensures that the patient will actually use, and therefore benefit from, the added plus power.

Treatment for Exotropia Treatment for exotropia is often sought for cosmetic alignment since most cases of exotropia present intermittently so that sensory fusion is present when aligned without amblyopia. Treatment consists of surgery, overcorrecting minus lenses, relieving prism, part-time occlusion, and optometric vision therapy. There is currently no clear consensus as to which treatment works most effectively and when a particular treatment should be prescribed (97).

Strabismus Surgery Strabismus surgery is often necessary when a constant deviation is too large for a patient to overcome using fusional vergence or when an intermittent deviation is too frequent or large for the patient to be able to maintain fusion with reasonable comfort. Strabismus surgery is often sought as a cosmetic cure since it does not necessarily result in functional improvement or binocularity. Patients that cannot be managed successfully with optical treatment or optometric vision therapy may also require surgery. Studies have shown that patients with early surgery for infantile strabismus have better potential for demonstrating some level of binocularity (98). It is not unusual for multiple ocular surgeries to be necessary to align the eyes.

Outcomes for Treatment of Strabismus in the Special Needs Population Little is written on the success of strabismus treatments for patients with special needs. Standard accommodative esotropia treatment with hyperopic correction and bifocals had successful results in patients with DS (47). Strabismus surgery followed with standard surgical tables were found to have good postoperative alignment during the following 6 months in children with DS (85.7%) (71). Patients with CP who were recommended surgery reflected a conservative approach due to older ages undergoing surgical management but had satisfactory alignment results (15). In this same study, Hiles et al. looked at several treatments for accommodative esotropia (using lenses, miotics, and surgery). Thirty-three of the forty-six patients were prescribed lenses, and ten of these patients were given bifocals. Miotics were given to 18 patients as primary treatment or together with their spectacles. Lastly, two of these patients had surgery. In 80% of patients with CP, orthophoria within 10 prism diopters was demonstrated. Those with exotropia and treated with surgery were within 10 diopters of orthophoria in 86% of the patients.

A study conducted by Lo Cascio (99) looked at optometric vision therapy on patients with CP. He selected the patients based on motivation of the patient and parents, whether a patient had a minimal specified-level verbal communication, adequate attention span, and ability to perform preliminary manual and eye–hand coordination activities. Although five of the nine patients demonstrated no improvement in the magnitude of the strabismus, one patient significantly improved in esotropic magnitude, two patients had short-term improvement, and one patient manifested a phoria at the end of treatment. In comparison, a retrospective study on patients with CP who underwent surgical correction found that over time, the tropia increased in magnitude.

DIAGNOSIS OF AMBLYOPIA

Amblyopia is a binocular vision disorder that results in a unilateral or bilateral best-corrected acuity worse than 20/20 in the absence of a pathologic etiology (100). Additionally, one or more of the following amblyogenic factors must be present prior to age 6 or 8 years in order for amblyopia to develop: anisometropia, bilateral isometropia, astigmatism of significant amounts, a history of image deprivation, or a constant unilateral strabismus (100). Amblyopia is the most common cause of unilateral vision loss in patients 20 to 70+ years of age (101). In patients under the age of 20, amblyopia is responsible for more vision impairment than trauma and all other ocular disease (102, 103). The assessment of visual acuity in patients with special needs is discussed in detail in Chapter 16, Comprehensive Examination Procedures.

Refractive Amblyopia Refractive amblyopia is caused by an amblyogenic amount of uncorrected refractive error present during early childhood years. The most common cause is uncorrected unequal refractive error between the two eyes known as anisometropia. Although uncorrected high bilateral refractive error can also cause amblyopia, the amount of ametropia necessary to cause amblyopia differs depending on the type of refractive error and whether the error is found unilaterally or bilaterally. The American Optometric Association provides guidelines for the amounts of uncorrected refractive error that would be amblyogenic if left uncorrected before age 6 or 8 years (102) (Table 20.1).

Strabismic Amblyopia Strabismic amblyopia is a decrease in vision due to a constant, unilateral strabismus that onsets during the early childhood years. If the strabismus is intermittent or alternating, the

TABLE 20.1 American Optometric Association Guidelines Related to the Level of Refractive Error as an Amblyogenic Factor

Isometropic Amblyopia	Potential Amblyogenic Refractive Error (Diopters)
Astigmatism	>2.50 D
Hyperopia	>5.00 D
Myopia	>8.00 D
Anisometropic Amblyopia	**Potential Amblyogenic Refractive Error (Diopters)**
Astigmatism	>1.50 D
Hyperopia	>1.00 D
Myopia	>3.00 D

child will rarely be amblyopic since each eye is able to receive visual stimulation at one time or another. The most common cause for strabismic amblyopia is infantile esotropia. These patients often have constant strabismus and poor prognosis for normal sensory motor fusion. Exotropia in patients tends to be intermittent, so amblyopia is less likely.

Deprivation Amblyopia Deprivation amblyopia occurs when there is a history of image degradation during the critical years of vision development. Congenital cataracts are a common cause of this type of amblyopia. Vision loss associated with deprivation amblyopia tends to be more severe with a poorer prognosis than in refractive or strabismic amblyopia.

TREATMENT OF AMBLYOPIA

A common misconception is that amblyopia treatment is not effective after 7 or 8 years of age. The time frame prior to this age was known as the critical period. This particular myth has resulted in countless patients going without treatment for a condition that might have otherwise been corrected. For decades, the literature has reported case series and clinical studies documenting vision improvement with treatment in older children and even adults with amblyopia. In a large sample, multicentered randomized clinical trials, the Pediatric Eye Disease Investigator Group showed that acuity improvement occurred in 25% of patients age 7 to 12 years and 23% of patients age 13 to 17 years (104). Additionally, acuity improvements were seen in 53% of patients when treated with 2 to 6 hours of occlusion, even when amblyopia had previously been treated. In the older age group, 13 to 17 years old, 47% of the patients showed improvement with occlusion if they had not been treated before. However, in patients with a history of past amblyopia treatment, further occlusion appears to be of little or limited additional benefit beyond spectacle correction alone (105). Nevertheless, vision loss from amblyopia does not have a set age for which treatment is no longer effective. Every patient deserves the option of treatment no matter what age they are.

Refractive Correction Refractive correction is a critical first step in the treatment of amblyopia, especially when the etiology is refractive in nature. In patients with anisometropic amblyopia, it is best to correct for the difference between the two eyes so that under- or overcorrection is equal in each eye. Correcting for the anisometropia ensures that the two eyes receive equal accommodative stimulus and the clearest retinal image possible.

In a study evaluating the effectiveness of refractive correction alone for the treatment of previously untreated anisometropic amblyopia in children age 3 to <7 years, 77% of patients showed improvement by greater than two lines (106). Amblyopia was resolved in 27% of the patients. The cases that resolved with spectacles alone tended to be those with moderate amblyopia.

Refractive correction alone is the primary treatment for bilateral refractive amblyopia, whether the cause is bilateral hyperopia, myopia, or astigmatism. Treatment of bilateral refractive amblyopia with spectacle correction improved binocular acuity to 20/25 or better within 1 year in most patients <10 years old (107). The probability of binocular visual acuity of 20/25 or better was 21% at 5 weeks, 46% at 13 weeks, and 74% at 52 weeks.

Occlusion Treatment with Patching Patching treatment has been the mainstay of amblyopia treatment for centuries. Patching of the better-seeing eye allows the amblyopic eye a chance to receive visual stimulation without competition or inhibition from the dominant eye. Failure of vision to improve is often due to lack of compliance. Atropine penalization is an excellent treatment option for these patients who are unable or unwilling to be patched. Atropine treatment works by preventing accommodation in the better-seeing eye so that the amblyopic eye is able to take over. Randomized clinical trials have demonstrated that both patching or atropine produced similar improvements in acuity when used for treating moderate amblyopia (20/40–20/80) in children <12 years of age (108, 109).

In patients with moderate amblyopia, 2 hours of daily patching produced improvement in acuity similar to 6 hours of daily patching for moderate amblyopia in children <7 years of age (110). Two hours of daily patching produced only modest improvements in patients with moderate to severe amblyopia (111). In children age 3 to 7 years with severe amblyopia (worse than 20/80), 6 hours of patching produced similar acuity improvement to full-time patching (112). Although occlusion produced faster initial results when patching was used versus atropine, this effect difference did not persist. By about 6 months, the amount of vision improvement was equal for the two treatment groups (112). Atropine treatment works best in patients with moderate to high hyperopia and moderate amblyopia.

Patients with CP who were diagnosed with amblyopia and were treated with occlusion therapy had a 52% success rate in reaching acuities within two lines of each eye and had central steady fixation with each eye (15). A slightly higher percentage of success (60%) was seen in patients with meningomyelocele who attained visual acuities within a difference of one line of acuity between the eyes (29).

Occlusion Treatment with Atropine The recommended treatment dose when prescribing atropine penalization is one drop of 1% atropine sulfate ophthalmic solution in the better-seeing eye once a day, two times a week. Studies show that atropine instilled over the weekend produced improvement in vision similar to daily atropine in patients with moderate amblyopia (113). An important consideration when prescribing atropine is that the constant blur of the nonamblyopic eye at near can be detrimental to a child's academic performance. This is of less concern in a nonreading patient or in a younger age group, but the blur at near should be addressed if the patient is regularly reading or writing. Near readers or bifocals may be prescribed for the child to use for classroom and homework.

Erkkilä et al. used a short-term cycloplegic, like cyclopentolate hydrochloride, as occlusion treatment in patients with CP (16). Almost half of these patients alternated fixation independently or achieved symmetric acuities. This treatment was preferred over the intensive all day patching because it was less obstructive to their daily lives.

Stability of Treatment Effect Regression after successful treatment for amblyopia occurred in about 25% of young children (<7 years old) within the first year following cessation of treatment (114). In older children (7–12 years old), vision improvement was sustained for at least one year following cessation of occlusion treatment (105). Reinstating occlusion treatment in all patients who demonstrate regression is recommended.

Discontinuing patching after successful acuity improvement has been done either gradually or all at once by different clinicians. Studies show that the manner in which treatment is discontinued has an effect on the risk of regression. In patients with severe amblyopia who were initially treated with more than 6 hours of daily patching, regression occurred in 42% of patients when patching time was not reduced prior to cessation (114). Regression occurred in only 14% of patients when treatment was reduced to 2 hours prior to cessation. It is therefore recommended that clinicians gradually reduce the amount patching time in patients receiving >6 hours of daily patching once the desired acuity level is reached.

Optometric Vision Therapy Active optometric vision therapy can be used to enhance passive treatment options such as spectacle correction or occlusion. The goal of optometric vision therapy is to normalize sensory motor function and eliminate competitive inhibition of the dominant eye toward the amblyopic eye. Optometric vision therapy is most effective when the patient can be actively engaged, maintain some level of cognitive and visual attention, and have the ability to follow verbal instructions or copy demonstrated behavior. This may not be possible in some patients with special needs. Further discussion of optometric vision therapy for patients with special needs is presented in Chapter 25, Optometric Management of Functional Vision Disorders.

CONCLUSION

In summary, strabismus and amblyopia are quite significant issues in patients with special needs. Potentially, with early intervention, these patients are capable of achieving or maintaining binocularity. Standard treatments for amblyopia and strabismus should be recommended in spite of cognitive or physical disability. Although careful attention should be paid to those patients who have tactile sensitivities or have limited mobility, this should not deter the eye care provider from treating these patients. The key to success of these treatments is for the patients, parents, caregivers, therapists, and optometrists to begin with a positive approach, follow through with determination, be creative when obstacles like a child not wanting to patch occurs, and continuously educate that although these patients have a disability they can still have success with these treatments.

REFERENCES

1. Woodhouse JM, Adler P, Duignan A. Vision in Athletes with intellectual disabilities: the need for improved eyecare. J Intellect Disabil Res. 2004;48:736–45.

2. Stephen E, Dickson J, Kindley AD, Scott CC, Charleton PM. Surveillance of vision and ocular disorders in children with Down syndrome. Dev Med Child Neurol. 2007;49:513–5.
3. Haugen OH, Høvding G. Strabismus and binocular function in children with Down syndrome. A population-based, longitudinal study. Acta Ophthalmol Scand. 2001;79:133–9.
4. Cregg M, Woodhouse JM, Stewart RE, et al. Development of refractive error and strabismus in children with Down syndrome. Invest Ophthalmol Vis Sci. 2003;44:1023–30.
5. Tsiaras WG, Pueschel S, Keller C, Curran R, Giesswein S. Amblyopia and visual acuity in children with Down's syndrome Br J Ophthalmol. 1999;83:1112–4.
6. Merrick J, Koslowe K. Refractive errors and visual anomalies in Down syndrome. Downs Syndr Res Pract. 2001;6(3):131–3.
7. Gross Motor Function Classification System. Available from: www.motorgrowth.canchild.ca/en/GMFCS/resources/GMFCS-ER.pdf. Last accessed April 25, 2011.
8. Ghasia F, Brunstrom J, Gordon M, Tychsen L. Frequency and severity of visual sensory and motor deficits in children with cerebral palsy: gross motor function classification scale. Invest Ophthalmol Vis Sci. 2008;49:572–80.
9. Buckley E, Seaber, JH. Dyskinetic strabismus as a sign of cerebral palsy. Am J Ophthalmol. 1981;91:652–7.
10. Guibor GP. Some eye defects seen in cerebral palsy with some statistics. Am J Phys Med. 1953;32:342–7.
11. Breakey AS. Ocular findings in cerebral palsy. Arch Ophthalmol. 1955;53:852–6.
12. Altman HE, Hiatt RL, Deweese MW. Ocular findings in cerebral palsy. South Med J. 1966;59:1015–8.
13. Schrire L. An ophthalmological survey of a series of cerebral palsy cases. S Afr Med J. 1956;30:405–7.
14. Levy NS, Cassin B, Newman M. Strabismus in children with cerebral palsy. J Pediatr Ophthalmol. 1976;13:72–4.
15. Hiles DA. Results of strabismus therapy in cerebral palsied children. Am Orthop J. 1975;25:46–55.
16. Erkkilä H, Lindberg L, Kallio AK. Strabismus in children with cerebral palsy. Acta Ophthalmol Scand. 1996;74:636–8.
17. Scheiman M. Optometric findings in children with cerebral palsy. Am J Optom Physiol Opt. 1984;61:321–3.
18. Stidwell D. Epidemiology of strabismus. Ophthalmic Physiol Opt. 1997;17:536–9.
19. Friedman DS, Repka MX, Katz J, et al. Prevalence of amblyopia and strabismus in White and African-American children aged 6 through 71 months: the Baltimore Pediatric Eye Disease Study. Ophthalmology. 2009;116(11):2128–34.
20. Aring E, Grönlund MA, Andersson S, et al. Strabismus and binocular functions in a sample of Swedish children aged 4–15 years. Strabismus. 2005;13:55–61.
21. Ghasia F, Brunstom J, Tychsen L. Visual acuity and visually evoked responses in children with cerebral palsy: Gross Motor Function Classification Scale. Br J Ophthalmol. 2009;93:1068–72.
22. Maino DM, Wesson M, Schlange D, et al. Optometric findings in the Fragile X syndrome. Optom Vis Sci. 1991;68(8):634–40.
23. Storm RL, PeBenito R, Ferretti C. Ophthalmologic findings in the Fragile X syndrome. Arch Ophthalmol. 1987;105:1099–102.
24. Hatton DD, Buckley E, Lachiewicz A, et al. Ocular status of boys with Fragile X syndrome: a prospective study. J AAPOS. 1998;2:298–302.
25. Amin VR, Maino DM. The Fragile X female: a case report of the visual, visual perceptual, and ocular health findings. J Am Optom Assoc. 1995;66:290–5.
26. Maino DM, Schlange D, Maino JH, et al. Ocular anomalies in fragile X syndrome. J Am Optom Assoc. 1990;61:316–23.
27. Hered RW, Rogers S, Zang YF, et al. Ophthalmologic features of Prader-Willi syndrome. J Pediatr Ophthalmol Strabismus. 1988;25:145–50.
28. Rothstein TB, Romano PE, Shoch D. Meningomyelocele-associated ocular abnormalities. Trans Am Ophthalmol Soc. 1973;71:287–95.
29. Biglan AW. Ophthalmologic complications of meningomyelocele: a longitudinal study. Trans Am Ophthalmol Soc. 1990;88:389–462.
30. Gaston H. Does the spina bifida clinic need an ophthalmologist? Z Kinderchir. 1995;40:46–50.
31. Gaston H. Ophthalmic complications of spina bifida and hydrocephalus. Eye. 1991;5:279–90.
32. Paysse EA, Khokhar A, Brady McCreery KM, et al. Upslanting palpebral fissures and oblique astigmatism associated with a-pattern strabismus and overdepression in adduction in spina bifida. J AAPOS. 2002;6:354–9.
33. Rothstein TB, Romano PE, Shoch D. Meningomyelocele. Am J Ophthalmol. 1974;77:690–3.
34. Caines E, Dahl M, Holmström G. Longterm oculomotor and visual function in spina bifida cystic: a population-based study. Acta Ophthalmol Scand. 2007;85:662–6.
35. Biglan AW. Strabismus associated with meningomyelocele. J Pediatr Ophthalmol Strabismus. 1995;32:309–14.
36. Harcourt RB. Ophthalmic complications of meningomyelocele and hydrocephalus in children. Br J Ophthalmol. 1968;52:670–6.
37. Clements DB, Kaushal K. A study of the ocular complications of hydrocephalus and meningomyelocele. Trans Ophthalmol Soc UK. 1970;60:383–90.
38. Scharre JE, Creedon MP. Assessment of visual function in autistic children. Optom Vis Sci 1992;69:433–9.
39. Miller MT, Strömland K, Gillberg C, et al. The puzzle of autism: an ophthalmologic contribution. Trans Am Opthalmol Soc. 1998;96:369–85.
40. Torp-Pederson T, Boyd HA, Poulsen G, et al. In-utero exposure to smoking, alcohol, coffee, and tea and risk of strabismus. Am J Epidemiol. 2010;171:868–75.
41. Chew E, Remaley NA, Tamboli A. Risk factors for esotropia and exotropia. Arch Ophthalmol. 1994;112:1349–55.
42. O'Connor AR, Stephenson TJ, Johnson A, et al. Strabismus in children of birth weight less than 1701 g. Arch Ophthalmol. 2002;120:767–73.
43. Torp-Pederson T, Boyd HA, Poulsen G, et al. Perinatal risk factors for strabismus. Int J Epidemiol. 2010;39;1229–39.
44. Paul TO, Hardage LK. The heritability of strabismus. Ophthalmic Genet. 1994;15:1–18.
45. Podgor MJ, Remaley NA, Chew E. Associations between siblings for esotropia and exotropia. Arch Ophthalmol. 1996;114:739–44.
46. Schiavi C. Comitant strabismus. Curr Opin Ophthalmol. 1997;8:17–21.
47. Yates CM, Simpson J, Maloney AF, Gordon A, et al. Alzheimer-like cholinergic deficiency in Down syndrome. Lancet. 1980;2:979.

48. Jaeger EA. Ocular findings in Down's syndrome. Trans Am Ophthalmol Soc. 1980;78:808–45.
49. Eissler R, Longenecker LP. The common eye findings in mongolism. Am J Ophthalmol. 1962;54:398–406.
50. Fanning GS. Vision in children with Down's syndrome. Aust J Optom. 1971;54:74–82.
51. Pigassou-Albouy R, Fleming A. Amblyopia and strabismus in patients with cerebral palsy. Ann Ophthalmol. 1975;7:382–7.
52. Creel DJ, Bendel CM, Wiesner GL, et al. Abnormalities of the central visual pathways in Prader-Willi syndrome associated with hypopigmentation. New Engl J Med. 1986;314:1606–9.
53. Coats DK, Avilla CW, Paysse EA. Early-onset refractive accommodative esotropia. J AAPOS. 1998;2:275–8.
54. Jakobsson P, Kvarnstrom G, Abrahamsson M, et al. The frequency of amblyopia among visually impaired persons. Acta Ophthalmol Scand. 2002;80:44–6.
55. Graham PA. Epidemiology of strabismus. Br J Ophthalmol. 1974;58:224–31.
56. Friedmann L, Biedner B, David R, et al. Screening for refractive errors, strabismus and other ocular anomalies from ages 6 months to 3 years. J Pediatr Ophthalmol Strabismus. 1980;17:315–7.
57. Thompson JR, Woodruff G, Hiscox FA, et al. The incidence and prevalence of amblyopia detected in childhood. Public Health. 1991;105:455–62.
58. Holmes JM, Beck RW, Repka MX, et al.; Pediatric Eye Disease Investigator Group. The Amblyopia Treatment Study visual acuity testing protocol. Arch Ophthalmol. 2001;119:1345–53.
59. Kornder LD, Nursey JN, Pratt-Johnson JA, et al. Detection of manifest strabismus in young children. 1. A prospective study. Am J Ophthalmol. 1974;77:207–10.
60. Friedman Z, Neumann E, Hyams SW, et al. Ophthalmic screening of 38,000 children, age 1 to 2 1/2 years, in child welfare clinics. J Pediatr Ophthalmol Strabismus. 1980;17:261–7.
61. Stayte M, Johnson A, Wortham C. Ocular and visual defects in a geographically defined population. Br J Ophthalmol. 1990;74:465–8.
62. Mohney BG. Common forms of childhood esotropia. Ophthalmology. 2001;108:805–9.
63. Greenberg AE, Mohney BG, Diehl NN, et al. Incidence and type of childhood esotropia: a population based study. Ophthalmology. 2007;114:170–4.
64. Costenbader FD. Symposium: infantile esotropia. Clinical characteristics and diagnosis. Am Orthopt J. 1968;18:5–10.
65. Pediatric Eye Disease Investigator Group. Spontaneous resolution of early-onset esotropia: experience of the congenital esotropia observational study. Am J Ophthalmol. 2002;133:109–18.
66. Baker JD, Parks MM. Early-onset accommodative esotropia. Am J Opthalmol. 1980;90:611–8.
67. Parks MM. Abnormal accommodative convergence in squint. Arch Opthalmol. 1958;59:364–80.
68. von Noorden GK. Binocular vision and ocular motility: theory and management of strabismus. 5th ed. St Louis: Mosby; 1996.
69. Donahue SP. Clinical practice. Pediatric strabismus. N Engl J Med. 2007;356(10):1040–7.
70. Hiles DA, Hoyme SH, McFarlane F. Down's syndrome and strabismus. Am Orthop J. 1974;24:63–8.
71. Yahalom C, Mechoulam H, Cohen E, et al. Strabismus surgery outcome among children and young adults with Down syndrome. J AAPOS. 2010;14:117–9.
72. Akinci A, Oner O, Bozkurt OH, et al. Refractive errors and strabismus in children with down syndrome: a controlled study. J Ped Ophthalmol Strabismus. 2009;46:83–6.
73. Duane A. A new classification of the motor anomalies of the eye based upon physiological principles, together with their symptoms, diagnosis, and treatment. Ann Ophthalmol Otolaryngol. 1896;5:969–1008.
74. Phillips PH, Fray KJ, Brodsky MC. Intermittent exotropia increasing with near fixation: a "soft" sign of neurological disease Br J Ophthalmol. 2005;89:1120–2.
75. Hunter DG, Kelly JB, Buffenn AN, Ellis FJ. Long-term outcome of uncomplicated infantile exotropia. J AAPOS. 2001;5:352–6.
76. Biglan AW, Davis JS, Cheng KP, et al. Infantile exotropia. J Pediatr Ophthalmol Strabismus. 1996;33:79–84.
77. Von Noorden GK. Divergence excess and simulated divergence excess: diagnosis and surgical management. Doc Ophthalmol. 1969;26:719–28.
78. Burian HM, Spivey BE. The surgical management of exodeviations. Trans Am Ophthalmol Soc. 1964;62:276–305.
79. Burian HM. Selected problems in the diagnosis and treatment of the neuromuscular anomalies of the eyes. In: Curso Internacional de Oftalmologia. Vol 2. Barcelona, Spain: Publicaciones del Instituto Barraquer; 1958:456–67.
80. Kim U, Hwang J-M. Refractive errors and strabismus in Asian patients with Down syndrome. Eye. 2009;23:1560–4.
81. Helveston EM, von Noorden GK. Microtropia: a newly defined entity. Arch Ophthalmol. 1967;78:272–81.
82. Lang J. Microtropia. Arch Ophthalmol. 1969;81:758–62.
83. Parks MM. The monofixation syndrome. Trans Am Ophthalmol Soc. 1969;67:609–57.
84. Lang J. Management of microtropia. Br J Ophthalmol. 1974;58:281–92.
85. Setayesh AR, Khodadoust AA, Daryani SM. Microtropia. Arch Ophthalmol. 1978;96:1842–7.
86. von Noorden GK. A reassessment of infantile esotropia: XLIV Edward Jackson Memorial Lecture. Am J Ophthalmol. 1988;105:1–10.
87. White JW, Brown HW. Occurrence of vertical anomalies associated with convergent and divergent anomalies. Arch Ophthalmol. 1939;21:999–1009.
88. Caputo AR, Wagner RS, Reynolds DR. Down syndrome: clinical review of ocular features. Clin Pediatr. 1989;28:355–8.
89. Bielschowsky A. Disturbances of the vertical motor muscles of the eyes. Arch Ophthalmol. 1938;20:175–200.
90. Calorosos EE, Rouse MW. Clinical management of strabismus. Boston: Butterworth-Heinemann; 1993;279–90.
91. Kutluk S, Avilla CW, von Noorden GK. The prevalence of dissociated vertical deviation in patients with sensory heterotropia. Am J Ophthalmol. 1995;119:744–7.
92. von Noorden GK. Current concepts of infantile esotropia (Bowman lecture). Eye. 1998;2:343–57.
93. Rabinowicz IM. Visual function in children with hydrocephalus. Trans Ophthalmol Soc UK. 1974;94:353–65.
94. Rush JA, Younge BR. Paralysis of cranial nerves III, IV, and VI. Arch Ophthalmol. 1981;99:76–9.

95. Robertson DM, Hines J, Rucker CW. Acquired sixth-nerve paresis in children. Arch Ophthalmol. 1970;83:574–9.
96. Mohney BG, Lilley CC, Green-Simms AE, et al. The long-term follow-up of accommodative esotropia in a population-based cohort of children. Ophthalmology. 2010;118: 581–5.
97. Hatt S, Gnanaraj L. Interventions for intermittent exotropia. Cochrane Database Syst Rev. 2006;3:CD003737.
98. Birch EE, Stager DR. Long-term motor and sensory outcomes after early surgery for infantile esotropia. J AAPOS. 2006;10:409–13.
99. Lo Cascio GP. Treatment for strabismus in cerebral palsy. Am J Optom Physiol Opt. 1987;64(11):861–5.
100. Ciuffreda KJ, Levi DM, Selenow A. Amblyopia. Boston: Butterworth-Heinemann; 1991:1–64.
101. National Eye Institute. Visual acuity impairment survey pilot study. Bethesda: NEI; 1984.
102. AOA. Optometric clinical practice guideline: care of the patient with amblyopia. St. Louis: American Optometric Association; 1994.
103. Evens L, Kuypers C. The incidence of functional amblyopia in Belgium. Bull Soc Belge Ophtalmol. 1967;147:445–9.
104. Pediatric Eye Disease Investigator Group. ATS3—randomized trial of treatment of amblyopia in children aged 7–17. Arch Ophthalmol. 2005;123:437–47.
105. Pediatric Eye Disease Investigator Group. ATS3 follow-up—stability of visual acuity improvement following discontinuation of amblyopia treatment in children aged 7 to 12 years. Arch Ophthalmol. 2007;125:655–9.
106. Pediatric Eye Disease Investigator Group. ATS5 secondary—treatment of anisometropic amblyopia in children with refractive correction. Ophthalmology. 2006;113:895–903.
107. Pediatric Eye Disease Investigator Group. ATS7—treatment of bilateral refractive amblyopia in children 3 to <10. Am J Ophthalmol. 2007;144:487–96.
108. Pediatric Eye Disease Investigatory Group. ATS1—a randomized trial of atropine vs patching for treatment of moderate amblyopia in children. Arch Ophthalmol. 2002;120:268–78.
109. Pediatric Eye Disease Investigatory Group. ATS9—Patching vs atropine to treat amblyopia in children age 7–12 years. Arch Ophthalmol. 2008;126(12):1634–42.
110. Pediatric Eye Disease Investigatory Group. ATS2B—a randomized trial of patching regimens for treatment of moderate amblyopia in children. Arch Ophthalmol. 2003;121:603–11.
111. Pediatric Eye Disease Investigatory Group. ATS5 primary—a randomized trial to evaluate 2 hours of daily patching for strabismic and anisometropic amblyopia in children. Ophthalmology. 2006;113:904–12.
112. Pediatric Eye Disease Investigatory Group. ATS2A—a randomized trial of prescribed patching regimens for treatment of severe amblyopia in children. Ophthalmology. 2003;110:2075–87.
113. Pediatric Eye Disease Investigatory Group. ATS4—a randomized trial of atropine regimens for treatment of moderate amblyopia in children. Ophthalmology. 2004;111:2076–85.
114. Pediatric Eye Disease Investigatory Group. ATS2C—risk of amblyopia recurrence after cessation of treatment. J AAPOS. 2004;8:420–8.

CHAPTER 21

Deborah M. Amster, OD, FAAO, FCOVD

Diagnosis and Treatment of Vision Information Processing Disorders

INTRODUCTION

Learning-related vision problems encompass deficits in two broad visual system components: visual efficiency and visual information processing (1). Visual efficiency includes the essential visual neurophysiologic process of visual acuity (and refractive error), accommodation, vergence (fusion), and ocular motility/tracking. These topics are discussed in Chapter 17, Diagnosis and Treatment of Refractive Error; Chapter 18, Diagnosis and Treatment of Oculomotor Dysfunction; Chapter 19, Diagnosis and Treatment of Binocular Vision and Accommodative Disorders. Visual information processing involves higher-level brain functions, including the non-motor aspects of visual perception and cognition, and their integration with the motor, auditory, language, and attention systems (1). This is the focus of this chapter. Visual information processing skills, also referred to as visual-perceptual skills, need to be considered when working with the patient with special needs. It has been clearly demonstrated that these skills are related to learning readiness and academic achievement in children (1–7).

Perception refers to the active process of locating and extracting information from the environment, as well as interpreting it to direct meaningful action. It is a core process in cognition and the acquisition of knowledge (2). In contrast to perception, learning is the process of acquiring information through experience and storing information. Learning facilitates the perceptual process since the acquired and stored information is used as a model against which the environmental information is measured (2). Thinking, or the manipulation of information to solve problems, is facilitated by the ability to perceive (extract) information easily (2). According to Johnson and Mykleburst (3), "visual perception may be viewed as a bi-directional bridge between functional vision and cognition." They proposed that learning occurs at a number of levels and proceeds from sensation to perception, imagery, language, symbolization, and finally conceptualization (3). Interruption of this hierarchy at any level jeopardizes functioning at more advanced cognitive levels. It is perception that is basic to learning and thinking (2).

According to Gibson (4), the perceptual systems, or modalities used for the perceptual process, include the basic orientating, haptic (proprioception and touch), taste-smell, auditory, and visual systems. Gesell and Birch believe that even though there is partial overlap and interaction of the various systems, in order to function at maximum capacity and efficiency, it is necessary for an individual to become visually dominant.

ASSOCIATION BETWEEN VISION INFORMATION PROCESSING AND LEARNING

Vision information processing anomalies and learning disabilities have been linked to each other for decades. It has been proposed that adequate conceptual development is dependent on adequate perception (2). Kephart, in particular, felt that perceptual and motor development form the basis for behavior, language, and conceptual learning. Along with Piaget, they felt that motor development preceded perceptual development (2). The earliest demonstrations of intelligent behavior are motor in nature and are present before language. It is necessary for a sound motor foundation to exist for cognitive development to take place. Kephart conceptualized seven developmental stages that a normal child progresses through as the child develops increasingly effective and efficient strategies for information processing (2). The initial stage is at the level of proprioceptive or internal bodily awareness and the final stage is thinking ability, which transcends motor and perceptual cues. His seven developmental stages include the motor stage, motor perceptual stage, perceptual motor stage, perceptual stage, perceptual conceptual stage, conceptual stage, and conceptual perceptual stage (2). Based on these theories, it makes sense that individuals with conditions such as cerebral palsy (CP) would be at significant risk for developing visual-perceptual motor difficulties as their motor development is compromised.

Several researchers have related visual perception to learning disabilities through the use of experimental studies. For instance, through a meta-analysis of 161 studies, Kavale (5) found that visual-perceptual skills are important correlates of reading achievement and they should be considered among the complex of factors related to the prediction of reading ability. A variety of visual-perceptual skills were investigated and included visual discrimination, visual form constancy, visual figure ground, visual closure, visual memory, visual spatial relationships, visual–motor integration, and visual–auditory integration (Table 21.1). Although each skill was significantly associated with reading achievement, visual memory and visual discrimination showed a stronger relationship with reading ability than the other perceptual skills (5).

Robertson and Zaborske-Roy (6) have postulated that since 80% of what is learned is typically received through the visual sensory channel, it seems logical to reason that the ability to perceive and remember what was seen is a skill directly related to learning. A strong correlation between visual memory and reading and visual memory and spelling was found, even for those children functioning at a higher level than expected for their age. They believe that "it seems logical that if a child is to progress from early phonetic stages of sounding out each word as he reads, to a more advanced level of reading fluently words grouped in sentences/paragraphs, visual memory would be a contributing factor. However, it should be emphasized that visual memory is only one skill that is part of the reading process."

Brooks and Clair (7) found in a group of educable mentally handicapped children that visual figure-ground perception is related to reading at the readiness and first reader level, indicating a need for research on the use of visual figure-ground training procedures for children who cannot read. They also found a relationship between IQ and visual figure-ground perception.

While the ability to integrate information from one modality, or intramodally, is usually deficient in the leaning disabled individual, it is the individual's deficient ability to integrate information from different sensory modalities, or intermodally, that may be more significant. In particular, visual–motor and auditory integration have been most important (2). For instance, Kulp (8) showed the presence of a significant relationship between visual analysis/visual fine motor/visual–motor integration skills and reading, writing, math, and spelling performance in children of average school-related cognitive ability. Performance on the Beery Visual Motor Integration (Beery VMI) Test was significantly correlated with reading achievement teacher ratings in 7- and 8-year-olds, with math and writing achievement in 7-, 8- and 9-year–olds, and with spelling achievement in 8- and 9-year-olds. In addition, Mattison et al. (9) analyzed visual–motor problems in children with learning disabilities and found subjects had significantly more trouble than normal children with design copy tasks with simultaneous visuomotor components.

Williams (10) found that improved performance on visual–verbal tasks, which involve the rapid retrieval of verbal labels for visually presented stimuli (and are dependent on rapid visual processing), "reduces frustration, has a salutary effect on a child's reading fluency, and increases their interest in reading." They reported that naming speed (the ability to name an array of numbers, letters, objects, or colors presented in sequence while timed) was a necessary skill and had a high correlation with reading performance.

Solan (11) demonstrated among a group of normally achieving fourth and fifth graders that in the performance of written arithmetic, visual–spatial skills (see Table 21.1) had a significantly greater impact than those that were verbal in nature. In the performance of mental arithmetic, verbal skills appeared to have a greater influence than spatial skills. He stressed that visual–spatial and perceptual skills and verbal skills are essential for both written and mental arithmetic. He emphasized the importance of visualization,

TABLE 21.1 Visual-perceptual Skills

Visual-perceptual Skill Category	Visual-perceptual Subskill	Definition	Signs and Symptoms of Specific Deficiencies
Visual Spatial Skills	Bilateral Integration	The ability to be aware of and use both sides of the body separately and simultaneously	Delayed development of gross motor skills, decreased coordination, balance, and ball-playing skills, confusion of right and left, letter reversal errors of writing and reading, inconsistent directional attack when reading, inconsistent dominant handedness, and difficulty in tasks requiring crossing of the midline (1)
	Laterality	The ability to be internally aware of and identify right and left on oneself	
	Directionality	The ability to interpret right and left directions in external visual space, including orientational specificity of written language symbols	
Visual Analysis Skills	Visual Discrimination	The ability to perceive dominant features in different stimuli	Delayed learning of the alphabet (letter identification), poor automatic recognition of words (sight word vocabulary), difficulty performing basic mathematics operations, confusion between similar looking words (apparent letter transpositions), difficulty spelling nonregular words, difficulty with classification of objects on the basis of their visual attributes (e.g., shape, size), and decreased automatic recognition of likenesses and differences of visual stimuli (1)
	Visual Spatial Relations	The ability to perceive the position of objects in space	
	Visual Figure Ground	The ability to distinguish an object from irrelevant background stimuli	
	Visual Memory	Either the ability to recall a dominant feature of a stimulus or the ability to recall the sequence of visually presented stimuli	
	Visual Form Constancy	The ability to recognize an object regardless of orientation and location	
	Visual Closure	The ability to recognize a complete feature from fragmented stimuli	
Visual Integration Skills	Visual–Motor Integration	The ability to integrate vision with body movements	Difficulty copying from the chalkboard, writing delays, mistakes, and confusions, letter reversals and transpositions when writing, poor spacing and organization of written work, misalignment of numbers in columns when doing math problems, poorer written spelling than oral spelling, poor posture when writing, exaggerated paper rotations when writing, and awkward pencil grip (1)
	Visual–Auditory Integration	The ability to match serially presented visual stimuli with auditory counterparts	Difficulty with sound symbol associations, difficulty with spelling, and slow reading (1).
	Visual–Verbal Integration	The rapid retrieval of verbal labels for visually presented stimuli	Difficulty learning the alphabet (letter identification), difficulty with spelling, faulty sight word vocabulary (word recognition), and slow reading (1)

directionality, receptive and expressive language skills, and auditory and visual sequential memory on mental arithmetic. When performing written arithmetic, visual discrimination and form constancy are important. Some factors that are relevant to both are auditory–visual integration and auditory and visual memory.

While the incidence and prevalence of these disorders has not been specifically reported in the special needs population, several studies have indicated their presence. For instance, visual-perceptual problems are common in children with CP and can affect children's reading ability and learning (see Chapter 3, Cerebral Palsy) (12). Due to the fact that many patients with CP, which primarily involves the motor system, are born prematurely, any task that engages motor input and/or output will be affected (2). Adequate motor abilities are essential for us to explore our world and interact with our environment so we may learn, grow, and develop. Children with CP have many learning-related visual processing deficiencies in the areas of bilateral integration, laterality/directionality, and visual–motor/fine motor skills (2). Although visual-perceptual deficiencies in diplegic children born preterm may be partially attributed to sensory vision loss and fine manipulation difficulties, they may also be related to difficulties with eye movements and in using anticipatory control to process information (13). Dysfunction in visual analysis skills, specifically in discrimination, closure, form constancy, figure ground, spatial relationships, and memory, is also seen (14). Interestingly, when assessing mental imagery abilities in adolescents with spastic diplegic CP, it was suggested that CP was not systemically associated with visual imagery deficits, but that the presence or absence of these deficits depended on the existence of associated perceptual deficits (15). In addition, although a significant improvement in visuomotor skills was not observed, there was a significant improvement in visuoperceptual skills seen in individuals with CP when given a task that was presented with reversed color figure ground (16). Auditory–visual processing anomalies may be present in those with CP (2).

Children with Down syndrome also demonstrate visual, auditory, and motor perceptual abnormalities (see Chapter 4, Down Syndrome) (2). It has been shown that while spatial short-term memory capacity is similar to age matched normal children, as memory load increases or when visual and spatial demands are combined, performance is impaired (17).

Females with Fragile X syndrome have been shown to experience visual information processing problems that include difficulties in visuoconstruction of spatial designs, visual–motor planning, and integration (2,18). In addition, female carriers of the Fragile X full mutation have been shown to be at risk for difficulties in the areas of visual discrimination, visual memory, visual form constancy, visual figure ground, and visual closure (Chapter 5, Fragile X Syndrome) (19).

Individuals with autism spectrum disorder (ASD) experience difficulty in developing adequate visual–spatial skills such as body awareness, body location in space, relating objects to self and others, and visual logical reasoning. They often compensate by relying on tactile or kinesthetic feedback (20). Visual completion or visual closure has been found to be reduced in children with pervasive developmental delay. The ability to visually complete partly occluded shapes and use contextual influences has been demonstrated to be weaker, particularly as shapes become more complex (21). Interestingly, enhanced discrimination, detection, and memory for visually simple patterns in ASD may account for superior performance in individuals that are high functioning on tasks involving pattern recognition as it relates to maps, either in recognizing or memorizing landmarks or in detecting the similarity between map and landscape features (22). Those with ASD, attention deficit disorders, and Fragile X syndrome have also been reported to have difficulty integrating visual information with information from other senses (23).

In addition, individuals with ASD seem to uniquely demonstrate altered processing of faces and emotional expression, as evidenced by behavioral and neuroimaging studies (24). As face processing is an emergent and developmental skill that relies on early exposure to faces, it may be that central nervous system abnormalities in individuals with ASD hinder their ability to attribute social meaning to faces, thereby limiting subsequent opportunity to develop normal face processing abilities (24). Studies also indicate that face processing differences in individuals with ASD may be due to brain-based visual-perceptual impairment as opposed to social deficiency (25). Review of visual scan paths of adults with ASD demonstrated that they tend to view the core areas of the face displaying emotional expression (eyes, nose, and mouth) less often than they do other areas of the face. They also demonstrated deficient emotion recognition, especially fear (26). In addition, when assessing facial emotion, autistic individuals were less likely to use information from the eye region and more likely to use information from the mouth region (see Chapter 8, Autism) (27).

DIAGNOSIS OF VISUAL INFORMATION PROCESSING DYSFUNCTION

Visual processing problems include delays or deficits in visual–spatial orientation, visual analysis (which encompasses motor–visual perception), and visual integration skills (auditory–visual, visual–motor, and visual–verbal). Clinically, norm-referenced tests are used to assess these abilities. Qualitatively, behavioral observations, such as attention to task, ability to understand instruction sets, cognitive style, problem-solving ability, frustration tolerance, and excessive motor ability, may provide supplemental information that is important for diagnosis and treatment (1).

The diagnosis of visual information processing disorders begins when the patient presents for the initial evaluation. It is essential that prior to specific visual-perceptual testing, a comprehensive eye and vision examination be performed to rule out any disorders of visual efficiency, uncorrected refractive conditions, and eye health that may be contributory. Information concerning the patient's day-to-day function and visual needs may be gathered through case history and direct observation. As children with special needs are evaluated by several professionals, each with his or her own area of expertise, information regarding any previous assessments or therapy will be necessary to have the best understanding of your patient's abilities (2). The types of evaluations often performed include medical, neurologic, audiologic, occupational therapy, physical therapy, psychoeducational, speech and language, and visual (2). In addition, to specifically determine if visual information processing testing is warranted, it may be helpful for patients and/or their caregivers to fill out an intake symptom checklist, such as the College of Optometrists in Vision Development Quality-of-Life Survey and the Convergence Insufficiency Symptom Survey, that includes possible signs and symptoms of such deficits. Refer to Table 21.1 for signs and symptoms of specific visual processing deficiencies.

When evaluating the visual information processing skills of individuals with special needs, it is important to realize that although they may have limitations specific to their condition, many are able to perform the tests typically used to assess the average school-aged child. Table 21.2 describes one such sample battery that may be used.

TABLE 21.2 Visual Information Processing Tests

Visual Processing Skill	Visual Processing Subskill	Test
Visual–Spatial Skills	Gross Motor/Bilateral Integration Laterality Directionality	Standing Angels Chalkboard Circles Piaget L/R Awareness Test Gardner: Matching Gardner: Execution Gardner: Recognition Jordan Left–Right Reversals
Visual Analysis Skills	Visual Discrimination	TVPS: Visual discrimination or MVPT: Visual discrimination
	Visual–Spatial Relations	TVPS: Visual–spatial relations or MVPT: Spatial relations
	Visual Figure Ground	TVPS Visual figure ground or MVPT: Figure ground
	Visual–Spatial Memory	TVPS: Visual memory or MVPT: Visual memory
	Visual Form Constancy	TVPS: Visual form constancy
	Visual Sequential Memory	TVPS: Visual sequential memory
	Visual Closure	TVPS: Visual closure or MVPT: Visual closure
Visual Integration Skills	Visual–Motor Integration	Developmental Test of Visual–Motor Integration (Beery VMI) Wold Sentence Copy
	Auditory–Visual Integration	Birch Belmont Auditory Visual Integration Test TAPS: Digits forward
	Visual–Verbal Integration/Perceptual Speed/Automaticity	Developmental Eye Movement Test (DEM): Vertical subtest
	Visualization	TAPS: Digits backward

There are several advantages to using the Test of Visual-Perceptual Skills (TVPS) on those individuals with special needs. The TVPS evaluates seven aspects of visual processing including visual memory and visual figure ground in a multiple-choice format. A primary advantage is that more than one response mode may be used, as the child may identify his or her answer choice by pointing or indicating the number of his or her choice verbally or by any other means that is understood by the examiner (28). This test has been shown to be useful and reliable in evaluating the perceptual skills of children specifically with CP (12,14), as it eliminates the need for a motor response that is often impaired in these individuals.

The Developmental Test of Visual-Motor Integration (Beery VMI) is useful in evaluating visual–motor integration skills in special populations in that it is age normed for children as young as one year old and assesses abilities from marking and scribbling to imitating and/or copying more complex designs. It also contains supplemental tests that enable assessment of visual-perceptual and motor components separately (29).

Another test inventory that some have found useful in evaluating individuals of with special needs is the Wachs Analysis of Cognitive Structures (WACS). It is used to determine a child's cognitive development in terms of body and sense thinking, as described by Piaget and further elaborated on by Furth and Wachs (30). Although designed to evaluate children from 3 to 6 years of age, if used in a patient who is developmentally delayed, it can provide information concerning your patient's developmental age. The WACS is composed of 15 tests, divided into four subtests. The test is used to show the existence and quality of (a) cognitive schemes for discrimination of same/not same qualities from visual and hand information seeking; (b) schemes for appropriate hand manipulation of objects or construction of design from actual models; (c) schemes for the manipulation of graphic imagery, where the model is a sign for the object, not the object itself; and (d) schemes for action through body movement and imitation. Taken all together, these schemes define body and sense thinking as measured by the child's ability to perform various nonverbal activities. The purpose of the WACS is toward determination of structures of intelligence within the child rather than just a quantitative measure of the external manifestations of isolated actions (31).

TREATMENT OF VISION INFORMATION PROCESSING DISORDERS

Studies that have focused on the treatment of specific visual-perceptual skills in the areas of visual–spatial, visual analysis, and visual–motor integration in underachieving children have demonstrated improvement not only in these skill areas but also in academic performance (2). Prior to initiating any therapy regimen, however, many factors specific to the individual such as feasibility and motivation need to be taken into account. Realistic goals and expectations need to be determined. For instance, if determined by Intelligence Quotient (IQ) testing that an individual has below average potential, a processing skill may improve from very weak to a higher level of very weak or to weak and may never reach average levels after therapy. It is important to emphasize the desire for progress, not perfection.

Table 21.3 highlights the goals and various optometric vision therapy techniques specific to each of the visual processing disorders. In addition, specific therapy programs, such as the program detailed in Wachs and Furth's *Thinking Goes to School*, have been used to address deficits in visuospatial and visuomotor processing skills in some patients (20,30).

The use of lenses and prisms to improve visual processing and integration skills is used in conjunction with active optometric vision therapy, or as a substitute when participation is not possible due to a multitude of reasons. For instance, yoked prisms have been used with patients with ASD to cause a shift in sensory and motor organization in the cortex (32) and have been shown to improve orientation, posture, and visual–motor skills, particularly in ball-catching skills (33–35). The use of low plus lenses with a small amount of vertical yoked prism has been shown to improve spatial awareness, orientation, and body posture (36,37). It has been postulated that this creates the need to reorganize visual function, affecting visual–motor and visual sensory processes (38). The use of red/green glasses with white targets has been well received in patients with ASD exhibiting sensory problems (33). In addition, colored overlays have been demonstrated to increase reading speed in ASD individuals and may provide a useful support during reading for these children (39).

TABLE 21.3 Goals and Activities for Developing Visual-perceptual Skills

Visual–spatial Skills

Bilateral Integration

Goal: Develop the patient's motor planning ability by performing isolated, simultaneous, and sequential movements of the two sides of the body (2).

Activities:

Angels in the snow, chalkboard circles/squares, paper crunches, ball bounce, alternate hop, jumping jacks, balance activities, Randolph shuffle, slap tap

Laterality

Goal: Develop the patient's internal awareness of how the right side is different from the left side into concepts the patient can express orally (2)

Activities:

Simon says, ball bouncing, angels in the snow, Randolph shuffle, slap tap, circle square, SUNY hands/hands and feet, floor map

Directionality

Goal: Develop the ability to use directional concepts to make right and left judgments of objects and spatial orientation of linguistic symbols in external space (2)

Activities:

Simon says, floor map, Kirshner arrows, directional triangles, stickman, computer directionality, b, d, p, q sheets, recognition of reversal worksheets

Visual Analysis Skills

Visual Discrimination

Goal: Develop the ability to be aware of the distinctive features of forms, including size, shape, color, and orientation (2)

Activities:

Parquetry blocks/tangrams, geoboard, perceptives cards, same/different worksheets

Visual Figure Ground

Goal: Develop the ability to attend to a specific feature or form while maintaining an awareness of the relationship of this form to the background information (2)

Activities:

Visual tracing, parquetry blocks, geoboard, where's Waldo, hidden pictures, Michigan tracking, word searches

Visual Memory

Goal: Develop the patient's short-term memory abilities (2)

Activities:

Parquetry blocks with memory, geoboard with memory, tachistoscope, flash cards, visual memory game, visual memory workbooks, visual sequential beading patterns

Visual Closure

Goal: Develop the patient's ability to be aware of clues in the visual array that allow him or her to determine the final precept without the necessity of all of the details being present (2)

Activities:

Parquetry blocks, perceptives cards, dot to dots, computer visual closure, computer visual thinking, visual closure worksheet

Visualization

Goal: Develop the patient's ability to recall visually presented material and manipulate these images mentally (2)

Activities:

Parquetry blocks/parquetry blocks with rotation, geoboard, tachistoscope, floor map, golf game visualization, space/size matching, computer visual thinking, spelling word visualization, visualization directionality workbook, drawing pictures with eye closed, feely bag/tactilo

Visual–Motor Integration Skills

Goal: Develop patient's ability to integrate visual information processing skills with the fine motor system in order to reproduce complex visual patterns (2). This includes the following: (a) general eye–hand coordination, (b) efficient visual–motor ergonomics, (c) accurate and rapid visually guided fine motor control, and (d) ability to plan visually guided motor actions in order to reproduce complex spatial patterns (2).

Activities:

Bean bag toss, Marsden ball bunting, bead stringing, lite brite, pegboard, stick in straw, dive bombing, X and O tracing, haptic writing, mazes, dot to dots, talking pen, computer visual–motor integration, Rosner dots, geoboard, parquetry blocks, puzzles

CONCLUSION

The failure to diagnose visual information processing disorders can negatively affect an individual's quality of life, academic achievement, employment, and learning opportunities. Self-esteem and peer relationships will be hindered as well. Ultimately, society must face the challenge of providing financial and service resources. Optometrists, as members of the multidisciplinary team, must diagnose and assist in treating learning-related vision problems whether with optometric vision therapy, performance lenses and prisms, or by referring our special needs patients for evaluation and comanagement by other specialists.

REFERENCES

1. Optometric clinical practice guideline: care of the patient with learning related vision problems. St. Louis: American Optometric Association; 2000. Available from: http://www.aoa.org/documents/CPG-20.pdf. Accessed February 1st 2011.
2. Scheiman MM, Rouse MW, editors. Optometric management of learning related vision problems. St. Louis: Mosby Elsevier; 2006.
3. Johnson DJ, Mykleburst HR. Learning disabilities: educational principles and practices. New York: Grune & Stratton, 1983.
4. Gibson JJ. The senses considered as perceptual systems. Boston: Houghton Mifflin, 1966.
5. Kavale K. Meta-analysis of the relationship between visual perceptual skills and reading achievement. J Learn Disabil. 1982;15(1):42–51.
6. Robertson KL, Zaborske-Roy L. The relationship of academic achievement to visual memory. J Optom Vis Dev. 1988;49:12–5.
7. Brooks CR, Clair TN. Relationships among visual figure ground perception, word recognition, IQ, and chronological age. Percept Mot Skills. 1971;33:59–62.
8. Kulp MT. Relationship between visual motor integration skill and academic performance in kindergarten through third grade. Optom Vis Sci. 1999;76(3):159–63.
9. Mattison RE, McIntyre CW, Brown AS, Murray ME. An analysis of visuo-motor problems in learning disabled children. Bulletin of the Psychonomic Society. 1986;24:51–54.
10. Williams GJ. The clinical significance of visual-verbal processing in evaluating children with potential learning related visual problems. J Optom Vis Dev. 2001;32:107–10.
11. Solan HA. The effect of visual spatial and verbal skills on written and mental arithmetic. J Am Optom Assoc. 1987; 58(2):88–94.
12. Tsai L-T, Lin K-C, Liao H-F, et al. Reliability of two visual perceptual tests for children with cerebral palsy. Am J Occup Ther. 2009;63:473–80.
13. Fedrizzi E, Anderloni A, Bono R, et al. Eye movement disorders and visual perceptual impairment in diplegic children born preterm: a clinical evaluation. Dev Med Child Neurol. 1998;40:682–8.
14. Menken C, Cermak SA, Fisher A. Evaluating the visual perceptual skills of children with cerebral palsy. Am J Occup Ther. 1987;41(10):646–51.
15. Courbois Y, Coello Y, Bouchart I. Mental imagery abilities in adolescents with spastic diplegic cerebral palsy. J Intellect Dev Disabil. 2004;29(3):226–38.
16. Marozas DS, May DC. Effects of figure-ground reversal on the visual-perceptual and visuo-motor performances of cerebral palsied and normal children. Percept Mot Skills. 1985;60:591–8.
17. Visu-Petra L, Benga O, Tincas I, et al. Visual-spatial processing in children and adolescents with Down's syndrome: a computerized assessment of memory skills. J Intellect Disabil Res. 2007;51(12):942–52.
18. Cornish KM, Munir F, Cross, G. The nature of the spatial deficit in young females with Fragile-X syndrome: a neuropsychological and molecular perspective. Neuropsychologia. 1998;36(11):1239–46.
19. Block SS, Brusca-Vega R, Pizzi WJ, et al. Cognitive and visual processing skills and their relationship to mutation size in full and permutation female Fragile X carriers. Optom Vis Sci. 2000;77(11):592–9.
20. Coulter RA. Understanding the visual symptoms of individuals with autism spectrum disorder (ASD). Optom Vis Dev. 2009;40(3):164–75.
21. de Wit T, Schlooz W, Hulstijn W, et al. Visual completion and complexity of visual shape in children with pervasive developmental disorder. Eur Child Adolesc Psychiatry. 2007;16(3):168–77.
22. Caron MJ, Mottron L, Rainville C, et al. Do high functioning persons with autism present superior spatial abilities? Neuropsychologia. 2004;42:467–81.
23. Allison CL, Gabriel H, Schlange D, et al. An optometric approach to patients with sensory integration dysfunction. Optometry. 2007;78:644–51.
24. Sasson NJ. The development of face processing in autism. J Autism Dev Disord. 2006;36(3):381–94.
25. Behrmann M, Thomas C, Humphreys K. Seeing it differently: visual processing in autism. Trends Cogn Sci. 2006;10(6):258–64.
26. Pelphrey KA, Sasson NJ, Reznick JS, et al. Visual scanning of faces in autism. J Autism Dev Disord. 2002;32(4):249–61.
27. Spezio ML, Adolphs R, Hurley R, et al. Abnormal use of facial information in high-functioning autism. J Autism Dev Disord. 2007;37:929–39.
28. Martin NA. Test of Visual perceptual skills. 3rd ed. Novato: Academic Therapy Publications; 2006.
29. Beery KE, Beery NA. The Beery Buktenika Developmental Test of Visual Motor Integration (Beery VMI): manual. 5th ed. NCS Pearson, Inc. Minneapolis, MN; 2004.
30. Furth H, Wachs H. Thinking goes to school. New York: Oxford University Press; 1975.
31. Wachs H, Vaughan LJ. Wachs analysis of cognitive structures manual. Huntingtown: Western Psychological Services; 1977.
32. Kaplan M, Edelson SM, Selp JL. Behavioral changes in autistic individuals as a result of wearing ambient transitional prism lenses. Child Psychiatry Hum Dev. 1998;29(1):65–76.
33. Rose N, Torgerson NG. A behavioral approach to vision and autism. Optom Vis Dev. 1994;25:269–75.
34. Streff J. Optometric care for a child manifesting qualities of autism. J Am Optom Assoc. 1975;46(6):592–7.

35. Carmody DP, Kaplan M, Gaydos AM. Spatial orientation adjustments in children with autism in Hong Kong. Child Psychiatry Hum Dev. 2001;31(3):233–47.
36. Press LJ. Physiological effects of plus lens application. Am J Optom Physiol Opt. 1985; 62(6):392–7.
37. Eubank TF, Ooi TL. Improving visually guided action and perception through the use of prisms. Optometry. 2001;72:217–27.
38. Kraskin RA. Lens power in action. Santa Ana: Optometric Extension Program, Inc.; 2003.
39. Ludlow AK, Wilkins AJ, Heaton P. The effect of coloured overlays in reading ability in children with autism. J Autism Dev Disord. 2006;36(4):507–16.

CHAPTER 22

William Kress, OD
Andrew Rixon, OD, FAAO
John Neal, OD

Diagnosis and Treatment of Commonly Diagnosed Ocular Health Anomalies

The diagnosis and management of congenital and acquired ocular conditions are discussed in this chapter. The topic itself is broad and beyond the scope of this chapter alone. As such, some of the more common congenital malformations and acquired disease processes found in patients with special needs are listed. The following compilation focuses on the identification of the disease process or congenital malformation, the expected associated ocular and systemic findings, and the management options from both an acute and chronic care standpoint.

HERPES VIRUS

Herpes zoster is a viral disease that affects both children and adults. Once a patient is infected with the varicella zoster virus, which is responsible for "chicken pox," the virus is carried in a latent form, which can then reactivate later in life to cause herpes zoster. The clinical signs and symptoms of the two infections are very different from one another despite having the same agent at the root of the infection.

The varicella zoster virus is related to the herpes simplex group of viruses. It is spread through direct contact with the affected areas of skin as well as through the respiratory system. Once inside the host, the virus is dealt with by the body's immune system. However, a latent form of the virus remains dormant in the dorsal root ganglion of the host (1). The reactivation of this latent virus is responsible for the presentation of herpes zoster later in life. Initially, the virus infects the host cells in a child. In an immune-competent child, this most commonly produces a mild skin reaction with associated itching. However, in an immune-compromised child, the virus can be lethal with its initial presentation (2).

Due to its multiple routes of transmission, the varicella zoster virus has a high level of infectivity. The virus is found worldwide and is prevalent from one generation to the next. No seasonal incidence has been noted nor does infection occur in epidemics. Incidence of the disease is highest among those individuals over the age of 55 (3). However, the disease can occur in immune-compromised patients regardless of age. This puts the special needs population at increased risk due to the fact that this patient base may have other health concerns that strain the body's immune system.

Herpes zoster can present in a number of different ways and in varying magnitude. Skin vesicles begin to appear after the initial reactivation of the virus. The time that passes between reactivation and the appearance of skin lesions is variable from patient to patient. Upon reactivation, the dormant viral particles begin to replicate in the cell bodies of the spinal root ganglion and subsequently travel down the axons to affect the skin within the distribution of that specific ganglion (4). This area is known as a dermatome. Only one dermatome at a time is affected without lesions crossing the midline. The affected dermatome will develop numerous blister-like vesicles filled with a serous fluid material. Over time, these vesicles will harden and scab over. This process usually occurs over the course of 7 to 10 days and most commonly results in scarring and discoloration of the skin in the affected area. The presence of these vesicles in a banded pattern makes the diagnosis of herpes zoster simple. Before these vesicles appear, the diagnosis is more difficult to make. The symptoms are commonly general and nonspecific in nature. They include fever, general malaise, and sometimes a tingling or throbbing sensation in the area that later becomes affected by the skin vesicles (5). It should be noted that herpes zoster infections in children are commonly painless (6). However, if the infection appears on the head, there is concern that the eye can become involved. Vesicles appearing on the nose are referred to as "Hutchinson's sign" and indicate that ocular involvement is much more likely (Fig. 22-1). Once the eye is involved in the infection, it is referred to as herpes zoster ophthalmicus (HZO) (7).

The predominant symptom of a herpes zoster infection is pain. Pain is commonly present from the beginning of the infection and only subsides after the infection is cleared. In some individuals, the pain persists even after the infection has subsided. This phenomenon is referred to as postherpetic neuralgia. Pain is usually managed by the patient's primary care physician and can include many different medications including opioids (8).

Management of the disease is comprised of antiviral therapy and sometimes steroid treatment. Antibiotic ointment may also be used to prevent a secondary skin infection in the affected area. The most commonly used antiviral medications include Acyclovir, Valacyclovir and Famciclovir. Acyclovir is dosed at 800 mg five times a day for 7 to 10 days. Steroid treatment, if administered, is aimed at reducing the inflammation caused by the virus, thus reducing pain (8).

Patients presenting with HZO are at risk for serious ocular sequelae. While the skin lesions appear to be identical to those that appear on the trunk, a new set of issues arise once the ocular structures are involved. Treatment of the ocular tissue is mainly aimed at controlling the inflammation and the subsequent damage it causes. Patients with HZO are at risk for trabeculitis, pesudodendrites, and neurotrophic keratitis.

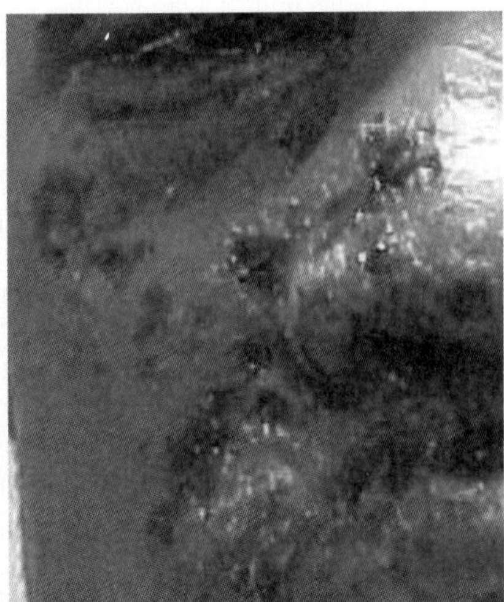

FIGURE 22-1. Herpes zoster (Hutchinson's sign). Photo courtesy of Andrew Gurwood, O.D., F.A.A.O. (See also Color Section.)

Trabeculitis is an inflammation of the tissues that comprise the trabecular meshwork. If the inflammation is severe enough, the intraocular pressure (IOP) can spike and place the patient at risk for secondary glaucoma. The treatment for trabeculitis secondary to HZO is aggressive topical steroid therapy (qid-q2h) and a topical IOP-lowering medication such as a beta-blocker, alpha agonist, or carbonic anhydrase inhibitor. The patient should be monitored in-office until the IOP is at an acceptable level. Follow-up period varies, and the severity of the initial IOP spike should be taken into account (9).

Pseudodendrites appear as elevated patches of epithelium that stain with rose bengal. These lesions usually appear during the acute event, but may surface weeks later. Either spontaneous resolution or progression is possible. If progression occurs, the anterior stroma may become involved and the practitioner may detect infiltrates. These findings usually resolve spontaneously within a few weeks (9).

Neurotrophic keratitis is the result of decreased corneal sensitivity secondary to corneal nerve damage. The resultant hypothesia can lead to epithelial erosion with subsequent ulceration and potentially perforation. Treatment options available to the practitioner include a bandage contact lens and potentially a complete or lateral tarsorrhaphy (9).

DIABETES MELLITUS

Diabetes mellitus (DM) is a chronic, systemic disease that affects the vascular system. The disease process arises when the pancreas cannot produce enough insulin, or when the body cannot effectively use the insulin it produces to take up glucose from the bloodstream into the surrounding tissue. A combination of these two etiologies may also exist at various levels. Nonetheless, the poor regulation of and chronic elevated levels of glucose in the bloodstream may eventually lead to vascular compromise, surrounding tissue malnutrition, and eventual death of that tissue.

The current estimated number of individuals worldwide with DM is approximately 220 million (10). Approximately 2 million American adolescents, or 1 out of every 6 children, aged 12 to 19 are overweight and have pre-DM. Type 1 and type 2 DM accounts for approximately 8% to 10% and 90% cases, respectively. Type 1 is characterized by little to no production of endogenous insulin by the β-cells of the pancreas. Proposed etiologies include viral prodrome, idiopathic nature, and an autoimmune response. Type 2 is characterized by a decrease in peripheral insulin receptor sensitivity and/or concomitant insulin secretion deficiency. Obesity is a major risk factor in the development of type 2 DM. Adolescent conditions such as autism, Down syndrome, and other intellectual/developmental disabilities have been found to have an increased incidence of obesity and therefore an associated increased risk for the development of DM (11–13).

To eye care professionals, diabetic retinopathy is a concerning ocular condition associated with DM (14). Retinopathy presents with varying degrees of clinical findings and may or may not affect the measured visual acuity of the patient (Fig. 22-2). Retinopathy is caused by vascular breakdown and the subsequent compromise to tissue perfusion/nutrition. Long-term effects can be subtle, but compromise to the retinal tissue is cumulative. The severity of the ocular findings dictates the appropriate follow-up time frame and/or treatment intervention. Treatment in most cases is a dilated fundus exam looking for the progression of retinopathy culminating in neovascularization and/or the presence of macular edema that would affect visual acuity. In each case, the treatment option is to decrease retinal hypoxia and vascular permeability. Specific laser procedures used to decrease retinal hypoxia aid in the resolution of both neovascularization and retinal edema. Pan-retinal photocoagulation (PRP) is a procedure in which patches of peripheral retina are ablated in hope of decreasing retinal oxygen demand, which can cease the progression of retinal neovascularization (Fig. 22-3). Focal laser procedures in the macula can decrease retinal edema caused by vascular hyperpermeability. Some retinal specialists are using intraocular injections of either a steroid suspension, such as Triamcinolone, or an anti-vascular endothelial growth factor medication, such as Ranibizumab or Bevacizumab, in the treatment of diabetic macular edema. Preservation of central and peripheral vision is the primary goal of all eye care professionals, with maintenance of ocular health paramount.

A common part of the aging process, cataract formation, is accelerated in individuals with DM. Duration of DM and higher levels of HbA_{1c} are major modifiable risk factors for the incidence of cataract formation and progression. Diabetes mellitus can also play a role in extraocular muscle palsies. Typically, these individuals have other underlying comorbidities for vasculopathy such as hypertension, atherosclerosis, and high cholesterol. Complications involving the extraocular muscles (EOM) may involve either the third, fourth, or sixth cranial nerves. Rarely will simultaneous EOM palsies or pupillary involvement exist. Such presentation should warrant consideration for imaging and cautious follow-up testing. Resolution of EOM palsies secondary to DM

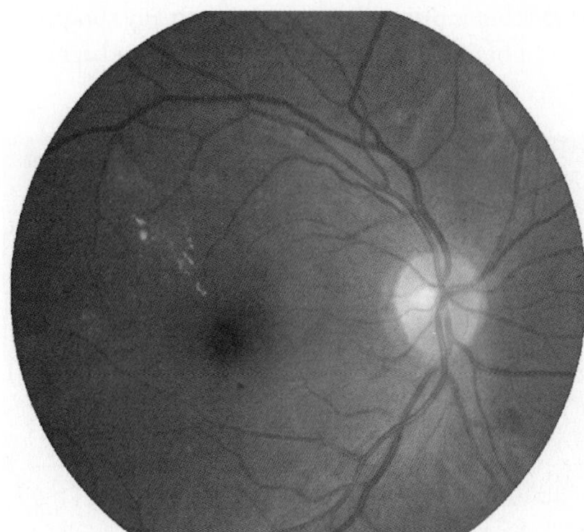

FIGURE 22-2. Diabetic retinopathy. Note the dot hemorrhages and exudates surrounding the macula. (See also Color Section.)

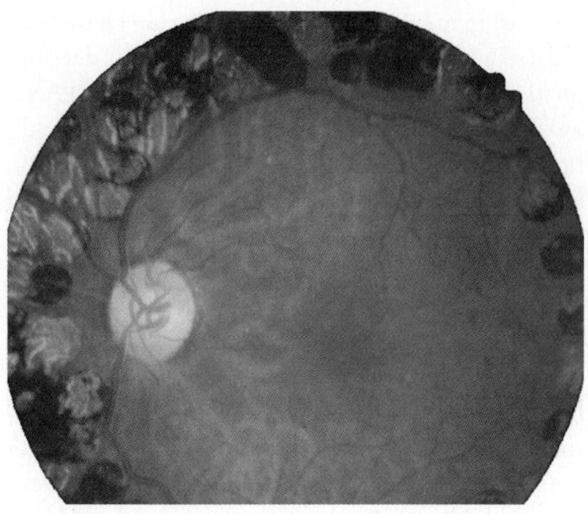

FIGURE 22-3. Pan-retinal photocoagulation for diabetic retinopathy. (See also Color Section.)

typically occurs within 3 to 6 months of onset and may be either complete or incomplete.

Dry eye syndrome (DES) is a relatively common diagnosis for both diabetic and nondiabetic patients. Studies show at least 50% of DM patients have either symptomatic or asymptomatic DES. Both lacrimal gland integrity and corneal sensitivity are shown to be affected by diabetic neuropathy. Treatment options for DES will vary depending upon the severity of presentation and patient symptoms. Artificial tear drops are a good start for those patients with a mild presentation or mild symptoms. A thorough evaluation of the underlying ocular cause will ultimately lead to a correct diagnosis and management plan, as DES may be a result of a host of other ocular and systemic conditions.

Diabetes mellitus can be a threatening systemic condition, including a significant threat to vision. Yearly ocular examinations are recommended for all diabetic patients and should include a comprehensive evaluation of the retina. Retinal vascular evaluation plays a crucial role in the management of patients with diabetes and can give practitioners a view of the vascular health in vivo.

MICROPHTHALMIA/ANOPHTHALMIA

Anophthalmia and microphthalmia are rare congenital defects of the globe that stem from disruptions in embryonic development, primarily development of the optic vesicles (15). Etiologies are multifactorial with prenatal environmental issues, genetic and unknown causes all implicated (16). Several genes involved in microphthalmia/anophthalmia have been isolated and are principally related to ocular development and brain development. They include PAX6, SOX2, PAX2 and SHH, and CHX10. The conditions can be unilateral or bilateral and may occur in isolation or as part of a syndrome (17). The combined birth prevalence of these conditions is as great as 30 per 100,000 population, with microphthalmia reported in up to 11% of blind children (18). Anophthalmia refers to the complete absence of the globe in the presence of an intact ocular adnexa (eyelids, conjunctiva, and lacrimal apparatus). Microphthalmia is defined as a globe with a total axial length that is at least two standard deviations below the mean for the child's age. Accordingly, axial length <21 mm in an adult eye or 19 mm in a 1-year-old substantiates a diagnosis of microphthalmos (19).

Classification of microphthalmia depends on the anatomical appearance and extent of axial length reduction. It may be broken down into simple, complex, and severe forms (17). Simple microphthalmia refers to an eye with reduced axial length that is nonetheless anatomically intact (Fig. 22-4). The reduced axial length is typically mild and may exist in patients with high hyperopia or microcornea. A subset of patients with posterior microphthalmos, a form of simple microphthalmia, can have significant vision loss due to posterior segment abnormalities (20). Nanophthalmos is a subtype of microphthalmos involving microcornea, axial length <18 mm, and high hyperopia. Angle closure glaucoma is not uncommon. Complex microphthalmos refers to an eye with anterior and/or posterior segment dysgenesis in the context of mild, moderate, or severe reduction in axial length. Severe microphthalmia refers to a globe where the corneal diameter is <4 mm and the axial length is <10 mm at birth or <12 mm after age 1. The globe is often not easily discerned on examination and is often confirmed to exist through imaging studies, which reveal the presence of ocular tissue remnants (17).

The diagnosis of anophthalmia/microphthalmia is made by clinical observation, diagnostic imaging, and if necessary electrodiagnostic testing. A-scan is used to measure total axial length. B-scan evaluates the internal structures of the globe and is useful in ruling out posterior segment dysgenesis (17). Neuroimaging, preferably MRI with its higher resolution and lack of radiation, is useful for more in-depth analysis of the orbital contents, optic nerve, and EOMs but is primarily used to rule out any abnormalities in brain development (16,17). Electrodiagnostic

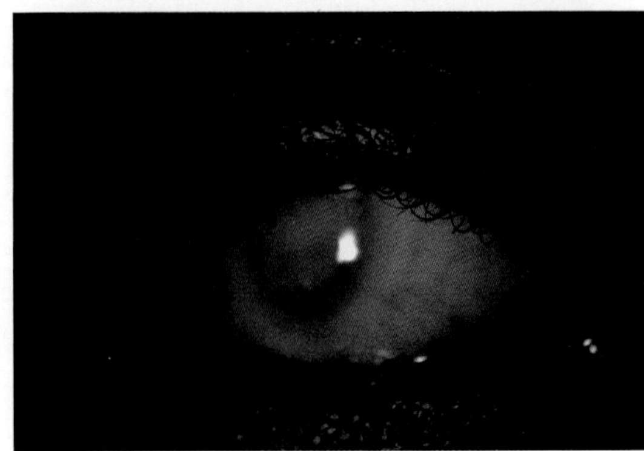

FIGURE 22-4. Simple microphthalmia with corneal opacification. (See also Color Section.)

testing, specifically flash and pattern Visual Evoked Potential, can be used to determine the presence of vision, establish a level of acuity, and determine the extent of optic nerve dysfunction (16).

There is a spectrum of disease that exists between these two conditions with over 50% of these cases having associated systemic abnormalities (16). There are many syndromes involving both ocular and systemic manifestations with a wide range of severities present (17). Many of these syndromes with their associated ocular and systemic abnormalities are described in Table 22.1.

A team approach to diagnosis and management is recommended, especially given the wide range of systemic anomalies that can be associated. The initial assessment is likely to be carried out in the immediate neonatal period by the pediatrician. Depending on the initial presentation, coordination of care with an optometrist or pediatric ophthalmologist for further testing is recommended. That provider should perform the necessary confirmatory testing, establish and maximize the visual potential, and prescribe protective eyewear as indicated (16). Additionally, early socket expansion by an ocular prosthetic specialist should be considered in cases of anophthalmia or severe microphthalmia (16). Subsequently, triage as necessary to other health care professionals including nephrology, audiology, genetic counseling, ocularist, occupational therapy, physical therapy, speech pathology, and child psychiatry/psychology should occur. The previous list is not exhaustive, and the necessity of referral beyond pediatrics, optometry, and ophthalmology is entirely dependent on the extent of diseases associated with the condition present.

BLEPHARITIS

Blepharitis is an inflammation of the eyelids and one of the most common external disease conditions found in both normal and special populations (Fig. 22-5). The prevalence of blepharitis has been reported to be as great as 50% in patients with Down syndrome (21). The disease can be acute and unilateral, but is generally chronic, intermittent, and bilateral. Blepharitis has been historically classified according to the region of the eyelid margin involved and is divided into anterior and posterior forms (22). Anterior blepharitis is the inflammation of the eyelashes and follicles, while posterior blepharitis involves the meibomian glands. There is often some overlap between the regions (23). There are multiple etiologies responsible for this condition, which can be narrowed to infectious or noninfectious. Infectious etiologies commonly result in bacterial colonization, mainly by *Staphylococcus*. Noninfectious etiologies can be related to seborrheic dermatitis, rosacea, and allergy to medication (24). The diagnosis of blepharitis begins with a thorough history addressing possible patient symptoms of itching, burning, tearing, and crusting. The patient is to be assessed grossly ruling out any obvious dermatologic issues. They are then examined under the slit-lamp biomicroscope, specifically observing the eyelashes, lid margin thickness, and vascularization. Expression of the meibomian

TABLE 22.1 Ocular and Systemic Abnormalities Associated with Microphthalmia and Anophthalmia

Syndrome	Ocular (Micro/Anophthalmia)	Systemic Manifestations
SOX2 anophthalmia syndrome	Anophthalmia, Microphthalmia	Hypothalamic–pituitary abnormalities, growth failure, developmental delay, seizures, esophageal atresia
Renal-coloboma syndrome	Microphthalmia	Renal hypoplasia
CHARGE syndrome	Microphthalmia	Heart defects, choanal atresia, retarded growth and development, ear anomalies, deafness
Gorlin syndrome	Microphthalmia	Medulloblastoma, basal cell carcinoma
Fanconi anemia	Microphthalmia	Bone marrow failure, breast cancer, growth retardation, café au lait spots, hearing loss, thumb and kidney abnormalities
Holoprosencephaly 2	Microphthalmia	Hypotelorism, microcephaly, craniofacial abnormalities
Walker-Warburg syndrome	Microphthalmia	Developmental delay, muscular dystrophy, hydrocephalus, agyria, epilepsy
Oculofacialcardiodental syndrome	Microphthalmia	Mental retardation, heart defects, dental and facial abnormalities
Fraser syndrome	Microphthalmia	Genital and kidney abnormalities, finger webbing

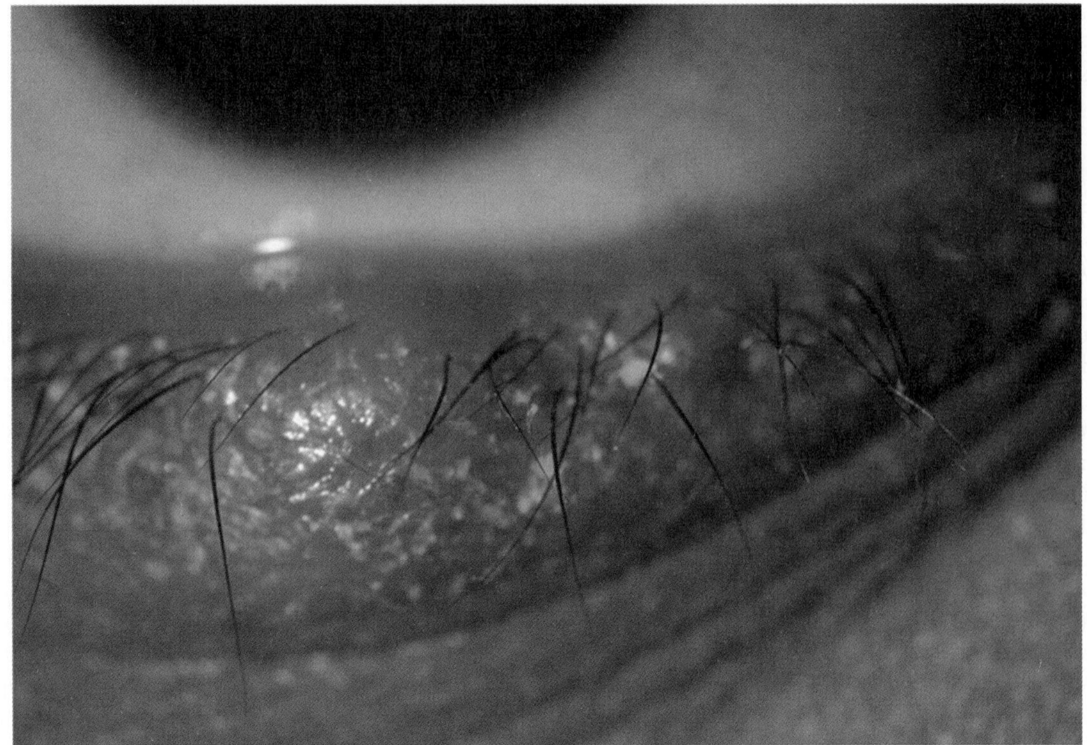

FIGURE 22-5. Anterior blepharitis and small chalazion. (See also Color Section)

glands and evaluation of the secretion should occur. Treatment will depend on the diagnosis and may involve topical and systemic antibiotics, topical corticosteroids and immunomodulators, lid scrubs, warm compresses, and in-office therapeutic expression of the meibomian glands (22). Direct management should be by an optometrist or ophthalmologist and may involve dermatology if the blepharitis is suspected to be associated with a skin condition.

OCULAR SURFACE ISSUES

There are multiple congenital and acquired lid and facial abnormalities that are associated with conditions often present when dealing with special needs patients (Table 22.2). It is imperative that these abnormalities not only be diagnosed correctly but that appropriate treatment and management be taken. In many of these cases, the anatomical features lead to ocular surface abnormalities. These ocular surface issues may include exposure keratopathy, superficial punctate keratitis, epiphora, corneal desiccation, and corneal ulceration. Ultimately, diagnosis is made by gross observation ruling out such issues as lid colobomas, ectropion, entropion, ablepharon, blepharophimosis, epiblepharon, and incomplete closure (19). Symptoms associated with these abnormalities may be elicited from verbal patients and may include itching, burning, tearing, and foreign body sensation. Although cosmetic issues are a significant concern, it is important that the primary focus be preservation or enhancement of the functional aspects of the eyelids and subsequently protection of the underlying ocular surface. These considerations will provide direction as to whether conservative or aggressive management is necessary.

The mainstay of conservative treatment in ocular surface disorders is lubrication. The amount of surface exposure will dictate whether a mild, moderate, or highly viscous lubricant is used. Artificial tears such as Systane, Optive, or Genteal Mild can be prescribed at a minimum of four times a day, more often as needed. Recommendations of Refresh Celluvisc or Genteal Gel for nighttime use may be appropriate, as these

TABLE 22.2 Congenital and Acquired Lid and Facial Abnormalities that Are Associated with Ocular Surface Disease

Condition	Lid Condition	Treatment
Treacher-Collins	Lid coloboma	Lubrication, occlusion, eyelid reconstruction
Down syndrome	Ectropion	Lubrication, taping, lid surgery
CN VII palsy	Entropion	Lubrication, taping, lid surgery
	Blepharophimosis	Lid surgery (if visual axis obstructed)
	Lid retraction	Observation, lubrication, lid surgery
	Incomplete closure, ectropion	Lubricants, taping at night, occlusion, tarsorrhaphy, surgery
	Epiblepharon	Lubrication, surgery (rare)
	Ablepharon	Surgical lid reconstruction

highly viscous materials will provide longer-lasting coverage. Conservative treatment may also involve taping of the eyelid to reduce surface exposure.

If conservative management is not an option, the patient should be referred to a pediatric ophthalmologist to evaluate the value of surgical repair or reconstruction. It is often preferable to delay surgical intervention until early childhood when the tissues are larger and the repair simpler (19). Extreme surface disease can lead to the loss of corneal integrity resulting in scar formation and ultimately, decreased vision. The long-term functional prognosis depends on early diagnosis and intervention. If no intervention occurs, the long-term psychosocial and societal loss of productivity can be substantial.

CONJUNCTIVITIS

Conjunctivitis, which can occur at any age, is an inflammation or infection of the thin, clear tissue layer covering the sclera and the inside of the eyelids. There are multiple causes including allergy, viral, bacterial, fungal, and mechanical irritation. The patient typically presents with one or a combination of the following symptoms: itching, burning, photophobia, excessive tearing, mucus discharge, decreased visual acuity, pain/discomfort, and red eye. The patient may have associated rhinitis, history of a recent upper respiratory infection (URI) or cold/flu, and skin lesions. To correctly diagnose and properly manage these patients, the true etiology must be determined. This section focuses primarily on common pediatric causes of conjunctivitis, the signs and symptoms, and the appropriate treatment plans based upon the diagnosis.

Viral Conjunctivitis Viral conjunctivitis can affect individuals of any age, and the specific etiology may vary across age groups. Included in the etiologic subgrouping of viral conjunctivitis are adenovirus, herpes simplex virus, varicella zoster virus, human immunodeficiency virus, and rubella virus.

From a pediatric standpoint, adenovirus is a common cause of conjunctivitis. The ocular subtypes of adenoviral conjunctivitis include epidemic keratoconjunctivitis ("pink eye") and pharyngoconjunctival fever, which is determined by the serotype of the infecting virus and associated findings. Patients with adenoviral conjunctivitis may present with morning crusting of the eyelids, hyperemia, itching, chemosis, and tearing that initially occur unilaterally, but may be bilateral by the time of the visit. The individual may report a recent history of a cold, URI, fever, headache, sore throat, or being exposed to someone else with these symptoms. They will likely have some form of lymphadenopathy, so the clinician should check the preauricular or submandibular nodes for swelling/tenderness to help confirm the diagnosis. Careful examination of the inferior and superior palpebral conjunctiva may show a follicular reaction. The course of the conjunctivitis will vary. Typically the symptoms are worse 3 to 5 days after the initial infection and will dissipate in 7 to 14 days. More complicated cases may take up to 2 to 3 weeks for complete resolution.

Management consists of thorough patient education on appropriate hygiene, especially during the first 7 to 10 days when the viral shedding makes the condition highly contagious. Patients should avoid rubbing their eyes or around their eyes. Thorough hand washing with antibacterial soap is encouraged. The patient should avoid sharing washcloths, towels, and other materials that they may come in contact with. Over-the-counter artificial tear drops and cool compresses can provide some relief in mild cases. The eyelids should be kept clear of mucus or other debris with a soapy washcloth. More complex forms of adenoviral conjunctivitis may spread to the cornea (keratoconjunctivitis) causing ocular pain and/or photophobia. Based on slit-lamp exam findings, there may be corneal epithelial compromise, in which case the patient should be placed on a regimen of preservative-free artificial tears and an ocular antibiotic drop, such as Polytrim or Tobramycin four times a day, as prophylactic coverage until the epithelial disruption subsides.

More complex cases may present with corneal subepithelial infiltrates areas of inflammatory cellular migration in response to the virus. Subepithelial infiltrates typically occur within 7 to 10 days of the initial infection and may cause moderate to severe pain, tearing, and photophobia. The pain may be severe enough that the patient has a protective ptosis, causing them to keep their eyes closed. Management of these cases will include a topical steroid drop (Pred Forte or Lotemax) four times a day or steroid/antibiotic combination drop (Tobradex or Zylet) taken anywhere from four times a day, up to every 2 hours while awake based on severity of signs and symptoms. In addition, artificial tears and cool compresses are used.

Although the majority of adenoviral conjunctivitis cases are relatively self-limiting, the health care professional should be aware of all potential treatment options. These options will frequently consist of some form of palliative care for much of the pediatric "pink eye" cases. Patient education is necessary, and emphasis on the contagious nature of the condition is of utmost importance.

Allergic Conjunctivitis Allergic conjunctivitis is the one of the most common forms of conjunctivitis. It can occur in isolation or with concurrent systemic allergies. Over the past decade, the estimated prevalence of allergic rhinitis, a common presenting diagnosis to most primary health care professionals, has continued to increase from 10% of the population in 1970 to 30% of adults and 40% of children in 2000. The severity ranges from mild to debilitating (25). Allergic rhinitis and conjunctivitis typically go hand in hand; allergic conjunctivitis may appear in 80% to 90% of cases of allergic rhinitis (26).

Allergic conjunctivitis can be broken down into the following subtypes: seasonal allergic conjunctivitis (SAC), perennial allergic conjunctivitis, giant papillary conjunctivitis, vernal keratoconjunctivitis, and atopic keratoconjunctivitis. Approximately 50% of allergic conjunctivitis cases are considered SAC. This form is associated with the changing of seasons and the associated allergens. Perennial allergic conjunctivitis is commonly caused by irritating household and food products such as feathers, dust mites, dander, and peanuts. Giant papillary conjunctivitis is associated with persistent mechanical trauma to the conjunctiva and is commonly associated with contact lens wear. Vernal keratoconjunctivitis predominantly affects teenage boys in warmer, dry climates and is a chronic condition with relatively severe symptoms. Atopic keratoconjunctivitis is associated with atopic dermatitis and commonly appears in patients with a family history of allergies.

Patient symptoms range from asymptomatic with mild to moderate anterior ocular presentations to symptomatic without ocular presentations to severe ocular presentations and symptoms. Itching is the hallmark symptom of allergic conjunctivitis and is likely the chief complaint. Many patients present with similar symptoms and findings as viral conjunctivitis, including morning crusting of the eyelids, erythematous papillae on the inferior and superior palpebral conjunctiva, hyperemia, puffiness (chemosis), tearing, and ropy mucus discharge. Pain and photophobia may be present, especially in those with associated corneal compromise. Assessing the onset of the condition can be helpful, as well as determining the potential for recurrence or causative factors. Of course the patient should be questioned about associated rhinitis, sinusitis, and respiratory issues.

Management will depend on the severity of the presentation. Milder presentations can be managed with the daily use of artificial tears to wash away allergens in the tear film, as well as cool compresses to alleviate chemosis and hyperemia and improve comfort. Prescription medications such as steroids (Pred Forte, Lotemax), antihistamines (Elestat, Alaway), mast cell stabilizers (Alamast, Alocril, Crolom), and antihistamine/mast cell stabilizer combination drops (Patanol, Bepreve, Zaditor) work well on acutely symptomatic or chronic ocular allergies. Systemic anti-inflammatory, steroid, or antihistamine medication can be used concurrently with topical treatment, or as stand-alone therapy in those with recurrent and significant ocular and systemic allergy symptoms. Oral antihistamine treatment can be considered by both eye care professionals and general physicians as a first-line-therapy for some forms of allergic conjunctivitis as prophylaxis, including those with milder presentations of SAC.

It is important to note that oral antihistamines can exacerbate dry eye symptoms.

Allergic conjunctivitis is potentiated by a host of causative factors. The chronic nature of allergic conjunctivitis can be bothersome to some patients, and preventative management plays an important role in patient care. Ultimately, the goal is to eliminate and/or decrease exposure to these factors and maintain a level of comfort for the patient that is acceptable.

Bacterial Conjunctivitis Bacterial conjunctivitis is a broad-based subject. This section focuses primarily on those bacterial infections common to newborns and infants. Bacterial conjunctivitis is initiated by an infectious component and often also involves the corneal surface. Bacterial conjunctivitis has more sight-threatening potential than viral or allergic conjunctivitis, especially if treatment is delayed or does not control the infecting agent.

When bacterial conjunctivitis inflicts newborns, the physician must be first concerned with those conditions associated with sexually transmitted diseases, such as chlamydia and gonorrhea. *Chlamydia trachomatis* and *Neisseria gonorrhoeae* are transmitted from mother to newborn during vaginal childbirth. It is possible that the mother is completely asymptomatic at the time. Due to the overlap in ophthalmic signs, chlamydial and gonococcal conjunctivitis can be hard to differentiate. It is important to recognize that the incubation period for chlamydia is typically longer than gonorrhea, therefore gonorrhea may present at 3 to 5 days following birth and chlamydia will appear 5 to 12 days following birth. If unsure, cultures should be ordered to ensure appropriate treatment. Both forms may present with associated systemic conditions, including pneumonia, ear infections, and digestive tract colonization.

Chlamydia has been reported as the most common infectious agents in the United States with an estimated incidence of 6.2 per 1,000 live births (27). Infections involving chlamydia (inclusion conjunctivitis) may present with mild ocular hyperemia, significant ocular and lid hyperemia, chemotic eyelids, and the presence of a purulent ocular discharge. It is possible to find pseudomembrane formation of the palpebral conjunctiva. Sight-threatening ocular complications arise when eyelid scarring and corneal involvement in the form of pannus occurs (trachoma). Treatment options for newborns and infants primarily include oral and topical Erythromycin. Topical treatment alone is inadequate in the treatment of this infection. Oral Doxycycline is another preferred option for the treatment of chlamydial conjunctivitis for adults or children >8 years of age.

Gonococcal ophthalmia neonatorum has an estimated incidence of 3 per 1,000 live births in the United States (27). Infections involving gonorrhea typically present more severely than those caused by chlamydia. Moderate to severe hyperemia, chemosis, and significant purulent discharge are common signs. Similar to chlamydial conjunctivitis, pseudomembranes may also form. If left untreated or not treated aggressively, ocular manifestations such as diffuse corneal epithelial edema or corneal ulceration may progress to perforation and endophthalmitis leading to blindness or loss of the eye. The corneal anatomy lends it to be an effective barrier to most infectious agents; however, *Neisseria gonorrhoeae* has the ability to quickly penetrate all layers of this barrier and enter the eye. Therefore, treatment should be initiated quickly in light of diagnostic signs, cultures, or even as prophylaxis if the diagnosis is delayed. Options may include intravenous Penicillin G, or for Penicillin-resistant strains the treatment of choice is a combination of topical Erythromycin and an intramuscular or intravenous dose of a third-generation Cephalosporin. During active purulent ocular discharge, the eyes should be flushed with saline solution until the discharge completely resolves.

Current medical practice in the United States involves the prophylactic treatment of newborns with antibiotic eye drops. The class of medication used will vary based on physician preference, but may include aminoglycosides, fluoroquinolones, povidone–iodine, or combination therapies. This discussion on causes of ophthalmia neonatorum is limited and focused on specific bacterial causative agents. Potential etiologies not discussed include the following differential diagnoses: herpes simplex, congential nasolacrimal duct obstruction, chemical agents, orbital or preseptal cellulitis, dacryocystitis, and other bacterial etiologies, such as *Pseudomonas* and *Staphylococcus*.

SUBCONJUNCTIVAL HEMORRHAGE

Subconjunctival hemorrhage is a relatively benign, self-limiting condition in which there is a compromise to the integrity of the vascular structure located in the potential space between the conjunctiva and sclera (Fig. 22-6). The etiology in most cases is an increase in arterial perfusion pressure secondary to straining or overexertion (i.e., Valsalva). This is typically found in association with systemic hypertension and/or atherosclerosis. Similar to integumentary ecchymosis, subconjunctival hemorrhage may also be associated with trauma of the surrounding tissue. Other causes include clotting disorders, anemia, orbital or conjunctival neoplasms, and ocular surgical procedures. Subconjunctival hemorrhage may also be caused by and/or exacerbated by systemic medications such as Warfarin, acetylsalicylic acid (aspirin), and vitamins A and D. If the cause is not able to be determined, it is referred to as idiopathic.

Pertinent questioning for a presenting subconjunctival hemorrhage includes duration, recurrence, potential for systemic diagnoses, and any history of trauma or straining. Patients may be completely asymptomatic and be aware of the hemorrhage based solely on appearance or have a mild ocular irritation. Diagnosis is made on gross observation or slit-lamp evaluation of the anterior segment. The sclera will have a focal or diffuse area of bleeding overlying its surface. The hemorrhage is isolated to the subconjunctival space, and even a small amount of blood may be alarming to the patient. If trauma is the suspected etiology, a dilated fundus exam should be performed to rule out posterior segment involvement. Treatment is palliative, and the patient should be reassured that the hemorrhage will resolve over a period of 1 to 2 weeks; longer if they are taking Warfarin or aspirin. If ocular irritation is present, the patient should be asked to use artificial tears to lubricate the ocular surface and provide comfort. Cool compresses are used initially to facilitate vasoconstriction and prevent further leakage. One to two days following the hemorrhage, the patient should begin to use warm compresses to facilitate vasodilation and reabsorption.

Recurrent subconjunctival hemorrhages may warrant a closer evaluation and systemic workup focusing on potential hematologic etiologies. Conditions that may present as recurrent subconjunctival hemorrhage include conjunctival neoplasms, bleeding disorders, and leukemia. If the patient presents with concurrent eye movement restriction, proptosis, or eye pain, imaging of the orbit and cavernous sinus should be performed to rule out space-occupying lesions.

KERATOCONUS

Keratoconus is an ocular condition characterized by progressive, asymmetric, and bilateral thinning of the inferior and inferior–central cornea (Figs. 22.7 and 22.8). Progressive corneal thinning causes visual acuity reduction secondary to high myopia, irregular astigmatism, corneal steepening, and aberrations and can lead to corneal stromal scarring. The onset of keratoconus may begin as early as adolescence and can continue into middle-age adulthood. There appears to be a strong predilection for the development of keratoconus in individuals with Down syndrome. A reported incidence between 5.5% and 15% in Down syndrome patients is considerably higher than the incidence of approximately 5 per 10,000 (0.05%) in the general population (28). The exact etiology of keratoconus remains unknown. Proposed mechanisms include genetics, inherent biochemical processes, biomechanical factors (i.e., eye rubbing), and related syndromes and diseases (Down syndrome, connective tissue disorders, atopy, and mitral valve prolapse).

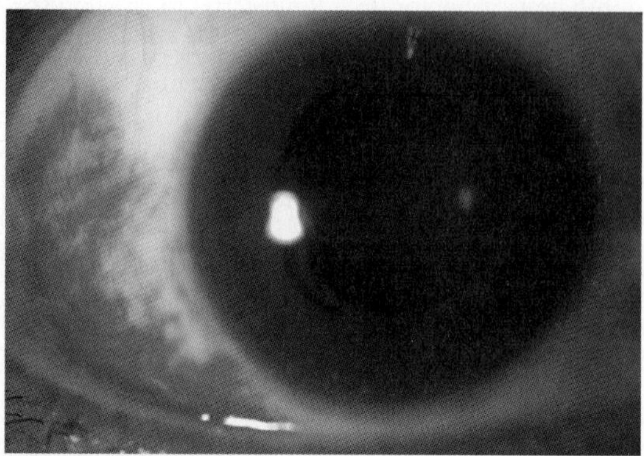

FIGURE 22-6. Subconjunctival hemorrhage. (See also Color Section.)

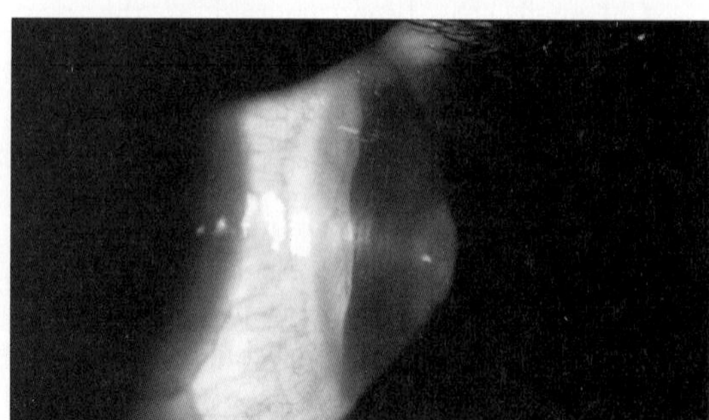

FIGURE 22-7. Advanced keratoconus with central corneal steepening. Photo courtesy of Stephen Byrnes, O.D. (See also Color Section.)

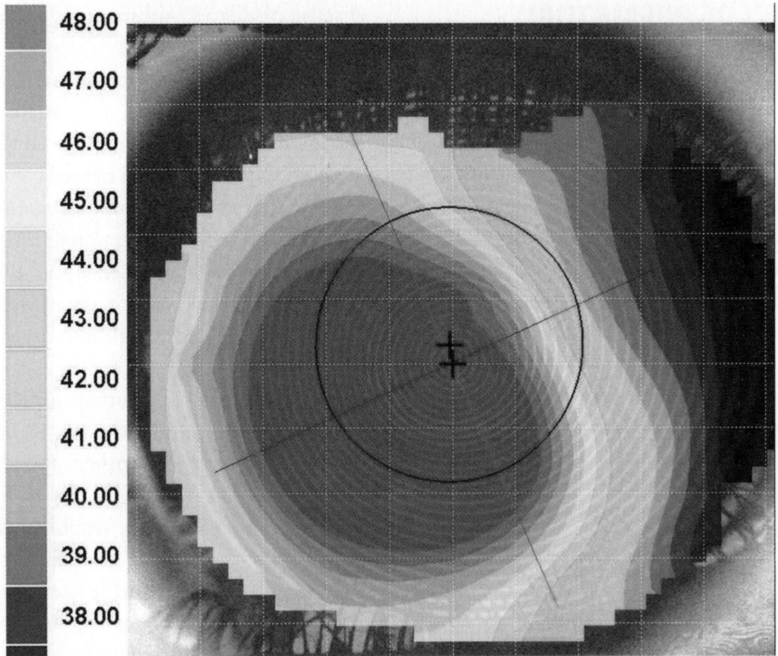

FIGURE 22-8. Keratoconus as viewed on a corneal topography map. Photo courtesy of Daniel Fuller, O.D. (See also Color Section.)

As keratoconus may be a slowly progressive disease process, the diagnosis may go undetected for decades. In milder cases, the individual may be completely asymptomatic and forego regular ocular exams. A typical first-time presentation to the eye care provider in which the patient is symptomatic will yield a complaint of progressive worsening of distance vision. In more advanced cases, the patient may complain of glare, photophobia, monocular diplopia, and even ocular pain.

For the eye care professional, determination of the refractive error and examination of anterior segment are crucial in making a diagnosis of keratoconus. A thorough refractive exam will reveal irregular astigmatism on keratometry and refraction as well an abnormal "scissoring reflex" on retinoscopy. Slit-lamp examination of the anterior segment may yield the following: noticeable thinning in the central and inferior mid-peripheral aspect of the cornea, a Fleischer ring (iron deposits in a ring pattern in the corneal basal epithelium), Vogt's striae (vertical linear "stress line" signs found on the corneal stroma), Munson's sign (outward bulging of the lower lid during patient down gaze), and in severe cases, painful corneal hydrops (breaks in Descemet's membrane allowing fluid into the corneal stroma).

The treatment options for keratoconus are dictated by the severity of refractive and corneal findings and the overall affect on vision and ocular comfort. Treatment options include spectacle or contact lens correction in the majority of cases. If the corneal astigmatism becomes significant and vision cannot be corrected to a satisfactory point for the patient with spectacles or soft contact lenses, then the eye care professional may need to fit a rigid, gas-permeable contact lens. Other treatment options include corneal collagen cross-linking (a procedure exposing the cornea to riboflavin and ultraviolet A in hopes to stabilize the progressive thinning of the stroma), INTACS (a plastic polymer inserted into the corneal stroma that decreases surface steepness and changes refractive error, including astigmatism), and a host of corneal transplant procedures, each identified by the depth and types of corneal tissue transplanted.

Keratoconus can be a debilitating condition from both a visual and ocular health standpoint. However, the vast majority of cases can simply be managed with spectacle or contact lens correction, improving the overall quality of life for the patient. Individuals at risk should have an eye examination once a year to assess the potential for keratoconus and subsequent progression.

RETINOPATHY OF PREMATURITY

Retinopathy of prematurity (ROP) is a vasoproliferative disease process affecting preterm and low-birth-weight infants (Fig. 22-9). The retinal vasculature develops at various stages throughout gestation, and prematurity places the infant at risk for incomplete retinal vascularization. The visual outcome of ROP patients may range from no affect at all to total blindness. The location, severity, extent of the retinal disease, and degree of prematurity all place the infant at risk for visual morbidity.

Infants at greatest risk and those who should be carefully screened for ROP (29):

- Birth weight <1,500 g (3.3 lbs)
- Gestational age of 32 weeks or less (as defined by the neonatologist)
- Selected infants with a birth weight between 1,500 and 2,000 g
- Gestational age of more than 32 weeks with an unstable clinical course (required cardiorespiratory support, prolonged exposure to supplemental oxygen)

The International Classification of ROP is used to document retinal findings and includes (30) (a) the location of retinal involvement by zone, (b) the extent of retinal involvement by clock hour, (c) the stage or severity of retinopathy at the junction of the vascularized and avascular retina, and (d) the presence or absence of dilated and tortuous posterior pole vessels (plus disease).

Ablative therapies of retinal tissue using either indirect laser photocoagulation or cryotherapy are treatment options commonly used. These techniques are used to reduce retinal hypoxia and the stimulation for vascular proliferation, associated retinal fibrosis, and subsequent tractional retinal detachment. Treatment, which is based upon ROP classification and the potential risk for the aforementioned complications, is typically initiated within 72 hours of diagnosis.

Pediatricians and other health care practitioners that care for infants with ROP must be aware of the potential for other visual complications. Nearsightedness (myopia), visual field loss, retinal detachments, glaucoma, strabismus, and cataracts may be associated with this disorder and the invasive treatments used to preserve ocular integrity. Amblyopia may develop secondary to either a significant intereye difference in refractive error and/or strabismus. In advanced cases where vision loss may be due to severe ROP or secondary to the treatment of the retinal findings, an individual may need more than spectacle correction to meet visual demands. For instance, a child that is having difficulty at school and/or is considered legally blind may benefit from a low-vision consult. In this setting, the task-specific needs of the patient can be addressed, including tinted glasses to reduce glare/photophobia, reading

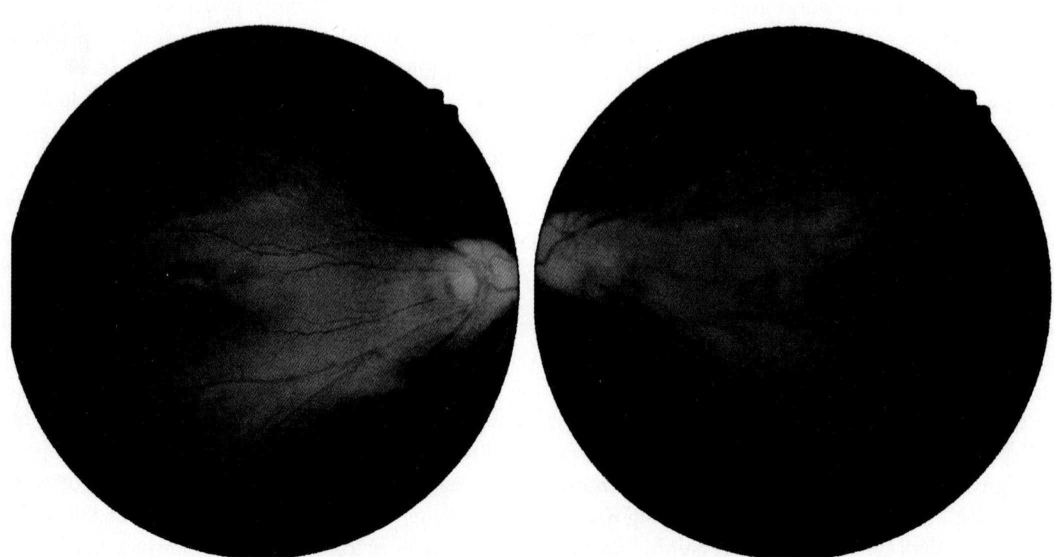

FIGURE 22-9. Retinopathy of prematurity. (See also Color Section.)

aids, and portable electronic devices to help the student see the blackboard or computer.

OPTIC NERVE HYPOPLASIA

Optic nerve hypoplasia (ONH) is the most common congenital optic disc anomaly encountered in pediatric ophthalmic practice. A nonprogressive condition of variable presentation, it is a major cause of visual impairment and blindness in children (31). Visual acuities can range from normal to profound vision loss, involvement can be unilateral or bilateral, and it may or may not be associated with neurologic, developmental, behavioral, or endocrine issues (32). This condition is histologically characterized by a subnormal amount of retinal ganglion cells and axons in the retinal nerve fiber layer and optic nerve (33). Although there are multiple proposed etiologies for ONH, all are proposed to alter normal embryonic development (34). Clinically, the optic nerve appearance can range from total aplasia to having only subtle abnormalities. The nerves can be as small as one-third to one-half their normal size or could be unchanged. Smaller nerves are often circumscribed by a yellowish halo and dark ring of pigment. This is known as the "double-ring sign" (35). The outer retina, retinal pigment epithelium, and choroid are usually normal. There is no gender, racial, or socioeconomic predilection (36).

There are many conditions associated with congenital ONH (Table 22.3). Children with ONH are frequently first-born infants of young mothers, with up to 51% of cases involving mothers in the 10-to-19-year age group (37). Diabetic mothers, alcohol, tobacco, and drug use during pregnancy, as well as pre- and perineonatal complications are all associated (38). Patients may have a wide range of developmental and behavioral issues including autism, attention deficit-hyperactivity disorder, and severe intellectual disability. Central nervous system issues such as cephalic disorders, periventricular leukomalacia, cerebral atrophy, absence of the septum pellucidum, and agenesis of the corpus callosum can all be associated. Neurologic issues such as cerebral palsy, intellectual disability, fetal alcohol syndrome, and epilepsy may be present. Although very rare, there have been reported cases of craniopharyngioma and optic glioma associated. Endocrine issues such as hypopituitarism resulting in hypothyroid, growth hormone deficiency, and diabetes insipidus may be present (32). Other ocular associations include albinism, aniridia, optic disc and chorioretinal colobomas, high myopia, Duane retraction syndrome, retinal vascular tortuosity, and nystagmus (33).

The ocular diagnosis of congenital ONH is not in principal, complicated. The diagnosis may be difficult when the optic disc is only slightly reduced in size or when central visual acuity is normal or only minimally decreased (38). Posterior pole photographs should be taken for documentation purposes and to measure the disc–macula distance to disc diameter ratio (DM:DD) (Fig. 22-10). This ratio can be estimated using the formula: DM/DD = (half the

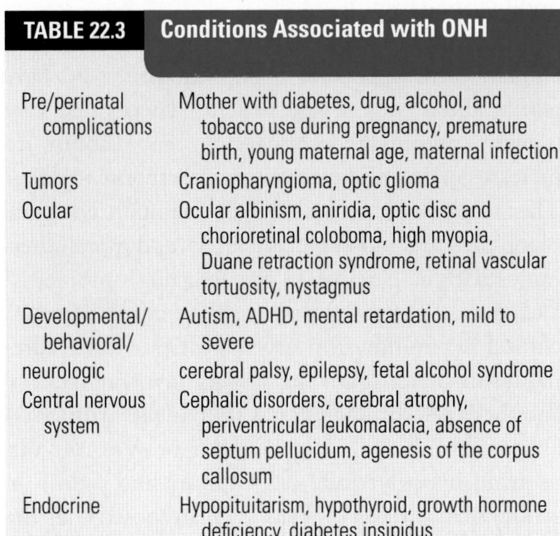

TABLE 22.3 Conditions Associated with ONH

Pre/perinatal complications	Mother with diabetes, drug, alcohol, and tobacco use during pregnancy, premature birth, young maternal age, maternal infection
Tumors	Craniopharyngioma, optic glioma
Ocular	Ocular albinism, aniridia, optic disc and chorioretinal coloboma, high myopia, Duane retraction syndrome, retinal vascular tortuosity, nystagmus
Developmental/ behavioral/ neurologic	Autism, ADHD, mental retardation, mild to severe cerebral palsy, epilepsy, fetal alcohol syndrome
Central nervous system	Cephalic disorders, cerebral atrophy, periventricular leukomalacia, absence of septum pellucidum, agenesis of the corpus callosum
Endocrine	Hypopituitarism, hypothyroid, growth hormone deficiency, diabetes insipidus

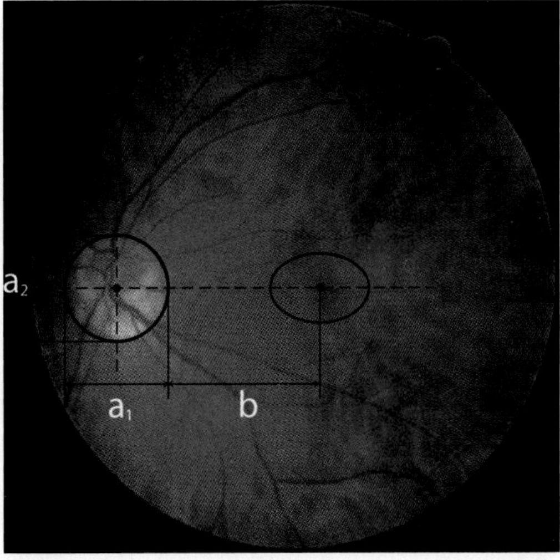

FIGURE 22-10. Optic nerve hypoplasia classification. Photo courtesy of Andrew Gurwood OD, FAAO Artwork courtesy of Susan Doyle. (See also Color Section.)

horizontal disc diameter (a1) + the distance between the fovea and the temporal disc margin (b))/the mean disc diameter. The mean normal ratio is 2.64. Studies have shown a ratio of >3.00 to be highly suggestive of ONH (39). Utilization of this formula is easier when the case is unilateral as a specific normal ratio can be established from the other eye for comparison.

In children presenting for the first time to the optometrist's office, it is imperative to make an accurate diagnosis of ONH. If in-office diagnosis is difficult for the optometrist due to the patient's age or level of cooperation, a referral to pediatric ophthalmology for an examination under sedation or under anesthesia is warranted. Once the diagnosis is confirmed, referral to pediatric neurology for evaluation and radiologic studies would be mandated, given the potential for neurologic issues. The results of neuroimaging would then dictate whether consultation with pediatric endocrinology is necessary. Optometric management will depend on the presentation and may involve a range of therapies including occlusion therapy in a unilateral case with amblyopia to the use of low-vision devices in a moderate to severe bilateral presentation. Given the possible neuropsychiatric and behavioral issues associated with ONH, childhood psychiatry/psychology may need to be involved. Additionally, specialists in the areas of orientation and mobility, occupational therapy and speech pathology may need to be involved depending on the severity of the overall presentation. Given the wide array of ocular and systemic associations a patient with ONH may manifest, these patients may be managed by anywhere from a small team of doctors to a large group of specialists. Appropriate referral and good communication among all team members is required to best attend to the possibly complex needs of the patient.

SEPTOOPTIC DYSPLASIA/ DEMORSIER SYNDROME

Septooptic dysplasia (SOD) is characterized by ONH and a combination of absent septum pellucidum, thinning or agenesis of the corpus callosum, and/or dysfunction of the hypothalamic–pituitary axis (40,41). Up to 30% of patients display all three manifestations (42). Optic nerve hypoplasia is the most prevalent finding, followed by pituitary hypofunction (41). Although most cases are sporadic, mutations within the HESX1 gene, essential for the formation of the pituitary and development of the forebrain, have been implicated (42–44). Visual acuity and laterality will depend on the extensiveness of the ONH and may range from normal to no light perception and may be unilateral or bilateral. Signs related to decreased visual acuity may include absent fixation, searching nystagmus, visual inattentiveness, or strabismus (45).

The etiology and pathogenesis of SOD is multifactorial, as it is associated with a number of environmental factors and a broad spectrum of neurologic defects (35). Associated central nervous system malformations may include schizencephaly, cortical heterotropia, and encephalomalacia. Most cases are sporadic, but familial cases associated with autosomal-recessive inheritance have been described (35). Absence of the septum pellucidum, which separates the two lateral ventricles and provides adhesion of the corpus callosum to the fornix, would suggest the possibility of neurologic impairment, learning disability, and intellectual disability (35). However, research indicates that lack of a septum pellucidum does not predispose a patient with SOD to any of the above (46). Given that up to 62% of SOD patients manifest dysfunction of the hypothalamic–pituitary axis, many of these patients may have endocrine disorders (45). Specific dysfunctions include cortisol insufficiency, growth hormone insufficiency, thyroid-stimulating hormone, and adrenocorticotropic hormone deficiencies. Accordingly, patients with SOD in many cases need a full endocrinology workup because of the hormone deficiencies that may occur. The diagnosis of SOD requires an MRI specifically looking at the visual pathway, the hypothalamus–pituitary region, the septum pellucidum, and corpus callosum, as well as ruling out the presence of other midline abnormalities (47).

There have been reports of sudden death in children with SOD and hypopituitarism who have febrile illness (48). These patients deteriorated very quickly, presumed secondary to an inability to increase corticotrophin secretion in response to stress. This resulted in an inability to maintain adequate blood pressure, blood glucose levels, and overall thermoregulation. Notable to the referring optometrist and surgical ophthalmologist is the finding that subclinical hypopituitarism can manifest as acute adrenal insufficiency following surgery involving general anesthesia. Accordingly, in SOD patients with operable strabismus, the surgeon must be very cautious to avoid hypoglycemia, dehydration, and a drop in serum cortisol levels. It has been proposed that the surgeon should consider perioperative corticosteroids to avoid the highly rare but aforementioned adrenal insufficiency that resulted in these deaths (48). Management of SOD is similar to that of ONH and depends on the expression of the condition. The specialties that may be involved are pediatrics, optometry, ophthalmology, endocrinology, neurology, radiology, childhood psychiatry/psychology, speech pathology, orientation and mobility, and occupational therapy. This team is by no means exclusive, and additional members should be included by the primary provider according to the needs of the individual patient.

CONCLUSION

The management of pediatric special population ocular health covers a broad range of congenital and acquired conditions. Although these are only a few of the ocular conditions a health care provider may encounter, it is likely that they will see one or more of during the care of their special needs patients. Identification is not only vital for the preservation of vision and overall ocular health but can also be important in uncovering previously unknown associated systemic conditions. Caring for a patient with special needs becomes more than just a single provider's role; multidisciplinary care is not only suggested but is required.

REFERENCES

1. Johnson RW, Dworkin, RH. Treatment of herpes zoster and post-herpetic neuralgia. Br Med J. 2003;326:748–50.
2. Abendroth A, Arvin AM. Immune evasion as a pathogenic mechanism of varicella zoster virus. Semin Immunol. 2001;13:27–39.
3. Apisarnthanarak A, Kitphati R, Tawatsupha P, et al. Outbreak of varicella-zoster virus infection among Thai healthcare workers. Infect Control Hosp Epidemiol. 2007;28:430–4.
4. Kennedy PG. Varicella-zoster virus latency in human ganglia. Rev Med Virol. 2002;12:327–34.
5. Peterslund NA. Herpes virus infection: an overview of the clinical manifestations. Scand J Infect Dis. 1991;80:15–20.
6. Dworkin RH, Johnson RW, Breuer J, et al. Recommendations for the management of herpes zoster. Clin Infect Dis. 2007; 44(Suppl 1):S1–26.
7. Shaikh S, Ta CN. Evaluation and management of herpes zoster ophthalmicus. Am Fam Physician. 2002;66:1723–30.
8. Baron R. Post-herpetic neuralgia case study: optimizing pain control. European. J Neurol 2004;11(Suppl 1):3–11.
9. Yanoff M, Duker J. Ophthalmology. St. Louis: Mosby; 2004.
10. World Health Organization. Available from: http://www.who.int/mediacentre/factsheets/fs312/en/index.html. Last accessed February 2011.
11. Emerson E. Overweight and obesity in 3- and 5-year old children with and without developmental delay. Public Health. 2009;123:130–3.
12. Rimmer JH, Yamaki B, Lowry BM, et al. Obesity and obesity-related secondary conditions in adolescents with intellectual/developmental disabilities. J Intellect Disabil Res 2010; 54:787–94.
13. Bergholdt R, Eising S, Nerup J, et al. Increased prevalence of Down's Syndrome in individuals with Type I diabetes in Denmark: a nationwide population-based study. Diabetologia. 2006;49:1179–82.
14. PubMed Health. Diabetic Retinopathy. Available from: http://www.ncbi.nlm.nih.gov/pubmedhealth/PMH0002192 Last Accessed February, 2011.
15. Fuhrmann, S. Eye Morphogenesis and Patterning of the Optic Vesicle. Curr Top Dev Biol. 2010;93:61–84.
16. Ragge NK, Subak-Sharpe ID, Colin JRO. A practical guide to the management of anophthalmia and microphthalmia. Eye. 2007;21:1290–300.
17. Bardakjian T, Weiss A, Schneider A. Anophthalmia/Microphthalmia Overview. GeneReviews-NCBI Bookshelf. NIH. Available from: http://www.ncbi.nlm.nih.gov/books/NBK1378/ Last accessed December 13, 2010.
18. Verma, A, Fitzpatrick D. Anophthalmia and microphthalmia. Orphanet J Rare Dis. 2007;2: Available from: http://www.ojrd.com/content/2/1/47 Last accessed December 13, 2010
19. Taylor D, Hoyt C. Pediatric Ophthalmology and Strabismus. 3rd ed. Philadelphia: Elsevier Saunders; 2005. p. 193.
20. Khairallah M. Posterior segment changes associated with posterior microphthalmos. Ophthalmology. 2002;109:569–74.
21. Creavin A, Brown R. Ophthalmic Abnormalities in Children with Down Syndrome. J Pediatr Ophthalmol Strabismus. 2009;46:76–82.
22. Jackson, Bruce. Blepharitis: current strategies for diagnosis and management. Can J Ophthalmol. 2008;43:170–9.
23. Bernardes TF, Bonfioli AA. Blepharitis. Semin Ophthalmol. 2010;25:79–83.
24. Rapuano C, Luchs J, Kim T. Anterior Segment. The Requisites in Ophthalmology. St.Louis: Mosby; 2000. p. 41–43.
25. Dykewicz MS, Fineman S, Skoner DP, et al. Diagnosis and management of rhinitis: complete guidelines of the joint task force on practice parameters in Allergy, Asthma, and Immunology. American Academy of Allergy, Asthma, and Immunology. Ann Allergy Asthma Immunol. 1998;81:478–518.
26. Singh K, Axelrod S, Bielroy LJ. The epidemiology of ocular and nasal allergy in the United States, 1988–1994. J Allergy Clin Immunol. 2010;126:778–783.e6.
27. Jatla KK, Enzenauer RW, Zhao F. Conjunctivitis, neonatal. Available from: http://emedicine.medscape.com/article/1192190-overview. Last accessed December, 2010.
28. Global Keratoconus Foundation. Available from: http://kcglobal.org/content/view/14/26/. Last accessed November, 2010.
29. American Academy of Pediatrics. Policy statement: screening examination of premature infants for retinopathy of prematurity. Pediatrics. 2006;117:572–6.
30. An international committee for the classification of retinopathy of prematurity. The international classification of retinopathy of prematurity revisited. Arch Ophthalmol. 2005;123:991–9.

31. Brodsky M. Septo-optic dysplasia: a reappraisal. Semin Ophthalmol. 1991;6:227–32.
32. Marsh-Tootle W, Alexander L. Congenital optic nerve hypoplasia. Optom Vis Sci. 1994;71:174–81.
33. Lambert S, Hoyt C, Narahara M. Optic nerve hypoplasia. Surv Ophthalmol. 1987;32:1–9.
34. Hellstrom A. Optic nerve morphology may reveal adverse events during prenatal and perinatal life-digital image analysis. Surv Ophthalmol. 1999;44:S63–S73.
35. Campbell CL. Septo-optic dysplasia: a literature review. Optometry 2003;74:417–26.
36. Tornqvist K, Ericsson A, Kallen B. Optic Nerve hypoplasia: risk factors and epidemiology. Acta Ophthalmol Scand. 2002;80:300–4.
37. Tait PE. Optic nerve hypoplasia: a review of the literature. J Vis Impairm Blind. 1989;207–11.
38. Wakakura M, Alvarez E. A simple clinical method of assessing patients with optic nerve hypoplasia. The disc-macula distance to disc diameter ration (DM/DD). Acta Ophthalmol. 1987;65:612–7.
39. Alvarez E, Wakakura M, Khan Z, et al. The disc-macula distance to disc diameter ratio: a new test for confirming optic nerve hypoplasia in young children. J Pediatr Ophthalmol Strabismus. 1988;25:151–4.
40. Egan R, Kerrison J. Survey of genetic neuro-ophthalmic disorders. Ophthalmol Clin North Am. 2003;16:595–605.
41. Birkebaek, NH, Patel L, Wright NB, et al. Endocrine status in patients with optic nerve hypoplasia: relationship to midline central nervous system abnormalities and appearance of the hypothalamic–pituitary axis on magnetic resonance imagine. J Clin Endocrinol Metab. 2003;88:5281–6.
42. Thomas P, Dattani MT, Brickman JM, et al. Heterozygous HESX1 mutations associated with isolated congenital pituitary hypoplasia and septo-optic dysplasia. Hum Mol Genet. 2001;10:39–45.
43. Dattani, MT, Martinez-Barbera JP Thomas PQ, et al. Mutations in the homeobox gene HESX1/Hesx1 associated with septo-optic dysplasia in human and mouse. Nat Genet. 1998;19:125–33.
44. McNay DEG, Turton JP, Kelberman D, et al. HESX1 mutations are an uncommon cause of septooptic dysplasia and hypopituitarism. J Clin Endocrinol Metab. 2007;92: 691–7.
45. Anderson M. Monocular nystagmus with sectoral optic nerve hypoplasia in a patient with septo-optic dysplasia. Clin Exp Optom. 2009;92:38–41.
46. Brodsky W, Brodsky MC, Griebel M, et al. Septo-optic dysplasia: the clinical insignificance of an absent septum pellucidum. Dev Med Child Neurol. 1993;35:490–501.
47. Brodsky MC, Glasier CM. Optic nerve hypoplasia: clinical significance of associated central nervous system abnormalities on magnetic resonance imaging. Arch Ophthalmol. 1993;111:66–74.
48. Brodsky MC, Conte F, Taylor D, et al. Sudden death in septo-optic dysplasia. Arch Ophthalmol. 1997;115:66–70.

CHAPTER 23

Scott B. Steinman, OD, PhD, FAAO, FCOVD-A
Maryke Nijhuis Neiberg, OD, FAAO

Special Assessment Procedures

Patients with special needs often require alternative examination techniques as they may not be verbal or understand clinical psychophysical tests. When psychophysical and eye movement testing is possible, the Test of Variables of Attention (TOVA) and the Visagraph/ReadAlyzer eye movement recorders may supplement standard clinical testing. For those patients for whom psychophysical testing is not possible, electrodiagnostic procedures alone will yield meaningful clinical data that will allow for proper treatment to be provided. Electrodiagnostic testing may also avoid the "sensory overload" of a standard optometric examination.

VISAGRAPH/READALYZER

Patient with special needs are often at risk for learning problems (1). Visual-perceptual tests may show areas of visual perception deficit that can contribute to learning problems, while oculomotor-related learning problems can be revealed by directly measuring reading eye movements. The Visagraph (Taylor and Associates) was one of the first commercially available reading eye movement measurement devices but had an imprecise infrared recording system that simply displayed the reading eye movements without analyzing them. The newer Visagraph III uses a more sensitive infrared recording device that records horizontal eye movements as the patient reads paragraph-sized reading passages. Like its predecessor, the Visagraph III analyzes fixation and saccade parameters (2). The ReadAlyzer (Compevo AB) utilizes the same hardware and software, as Compevo also developed the Visagraph III system used by Taylor and Associates.

The ReadAlyzer/Visagraph analysis includes measures such as the number of fixations in a standardized reading passage, the average fixation duration in milliseconds, the number of regressions (backward saccades), span of recognition (number of letters processed during each fixation, but it does not take into account the overlapping letters processed by successive fixations), and the reading speed in words per minute.

Special needs and other reading-disabled patients, when compared to normal children of the same age, exhibit an increased number of regressions, inaccurate return sweeps, and diminished reading speed (3). In language-auditory reading disability, the reading performance improves as the grade level of the reading material is reduced, while in visuospatial reading disability the reading performance stays the same no matter what the grade level of the reading material. It's important to note that the underlying mechanisms of reading disabilities may be multifactorial, including phonologic deficits, attention deficits, and abnormal fixation eye movement signals.

TEST OF VARIABLES OF ATTENTION

The TOVA (the TOVA Company) is a computer-based assessment of attention usually used to diagnose attention deficit disorder rather than specific visual attention disorders. For example, visual attention is reduced in strength as well as the extent of the visual field over which it has an excitatory effect in reading-disabled subjects (4). In addition, sustained visual attention is inhibited, reducing the ability to analyze text and reducing the time available to the individual to process information (4).

The TOVA is designed to appear to be a simple computer game to the patient and has been used for even very young children (age 4) (5). It is therefore suitable for use in special populations. The program measures responses to either visual shapes or auditory tones, and the results are compared to age-matched normal subjects' responses.

The visual component of the TOVA uses both a target to be attended (a large light gray square containing a smaller black square at its top) and a nontarget (a large square containing a smaller square at its bottom) to be ignored. The task is to press a handheld button as quickly as possible only when the target appears, but not when the nontarget is presented. This is similar to the target versus nontarget conditions used in visual search research (6). In the first part of the test, the target appears infrequently (22% of the presentations), while in the second part, the target appears frequently (78%). The entire test takes 23 minutes with equally split halves. The manipulation of the frequency of target appearance would be expected to change the patient's willingness to say "yes, the target is present" (7). The auditory portion of the test is performed the same way but with the target being a high-pitched tone and the nontarget being a low-pitched tone.

The output of these tests are response time (the reaction time in msec), "d" (the signal detection measure of visibility), commission errors (false alarms for the nontarget), omission errors (incorrect rejections of the target), post-commission response times (how much a previous error changes the reaction time), anticipatory responses (when the patient guesses rather than waiting to make a cognitive decision), and, of course, the attention deficit hyperactivity disorder (ADHD) score that compares performance relative to age-matched normals.

The TOVA concentrates on the ability to engage attention and to make a cognitive decision of whether a target or nontarget was presented. While these are important for the diagnosis of ADHD, the TOVA does not measure all aspects of attention, omitting many that would be very important in patients with special needs. For example, the ability to engage, lock, disengage, and move attention is especially important for the initiation of saccadic eye movements. In fact, a saccadic eye movement cannot be made at all without attention being shifted first (4). The ability to divide attention, allocate attention to a specific part of the visual field, and to ignore multiple distracters is important for learning environments.

OPHTHALMIC ULTRASOUND

Ultrasonography can reveal congenital anatomical abnormalities in the structure of the eye and orbit, as well as anatomical changes secondary to disease or injury. It is a noninvasive test requiring little cooperation that can be easily administered to special populations.

A-scan ultrasound directs ultrasound pulses from its probe in a single direction and measures the time needed for a reflection of that pulse to be received by a transducer in the probe. This time is converted to a distance from the probe at which the reflection occurs at the interface between various ocular structures. The plot presented to the clinician shows the location of the reflective surfaces (in depth) and the degree of sound reflection at each surface. (Fig. 23-1) A-scan ultrasonography is therefore a powerful tool for determining position and thickness of the crystalline lens and the axial length of the eye (8). It can be used both to determine the strength of the intraocular lens implant needed after cataract extraction and to confirm the degree of posterior staphyloma progression in axial myopia.

B-scan ultrasonography is the technique known more widely by clinicians. The B-scan probe contains a pulser that is swept in an arc across the width of the probe. The net result is a two-dimensional plot of sound reflection amplitude (as brightness of the plot) as a function of the two-dimensional position of the reflecting surface. The plot therefore takes a cross section of the globe, looking more like an anatomical drawing of an eye than does an A-scan. Depending on the probe ultrasound frequency, the eye or the orbit can be selectively visualized. While the corneal structure cannot be seen in a common B-scan, the posterior lens surface, retinal surface, and contour of the optic nerve can be seen. Figure 23-2 shows a posterior staphyloma as visualized by a B-scan ultrasound. More advanced ultrasound units can show a three-dimensional reconstruction of the eye.

B-scan ultrasonography can reveal the presence of vitreous bleeding, membranes or traction, or retinal detachment behind a dense cataract (Fig. 23-3). More importantly, it can help the clinician to differentiate between retinal masses that look similar (malignant melanoma, metastatic carcinoma, hemangioma, and subretinal hemorrhage). By reducing the gain of the transducer, one can detect the highly sound-reflective calcium infiltrates of optic nerve head drusen. Following trauma, an intraocular foreign body, subluxated crystalline lens, vitreous hemorrhage, or retinal detachment, can be detected using a B-scan.

OCULAR IMAGING

Any additional information that can be objectively obtained from those with special needs during the

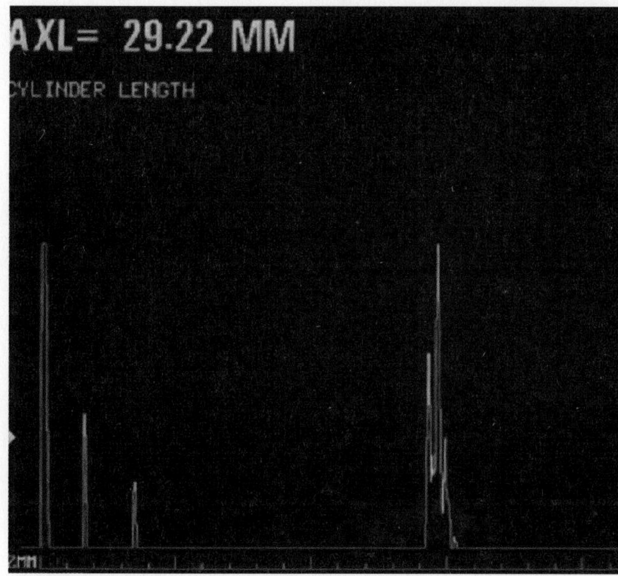

FIGURE 23-1. A-scan ultrasound in axial myopia. The normal axial length of the human eye is approximately 25 mm. In this myopic eye, the axial length is 29.22 mm.

optometric routine adds enormous diagnostic value. Issues like compliance and safety are always paramount but even more so in this population. Young children and our patients with special needs are not always very compliant when asked to stay still for a short while and may move around too much to obtain good ocular images. In some cases, unexpected movement could be dangerous to the child. In most cases, the natural squirming is just frustrating in our quest to collect usable images. Sedation may be considered when essential measurements and imaging may be required. Magnetic resonance imaging (MRI), computed tomography (CT), and radiographs may be required to image the orbit and orbital contents.

The procedures selected should preferably be simple, easily administered, produce very little discomfort, and should not intimidate the child or patient. Testing in free space, without cumbersome equipment, is usually the most productive method.

BRÜCKNER IMAGING

The most simplistic and least invasive of the ocular imaging techniques is the Brückner Test. The test is used to screen for strabismus, anisometropia, media opacities, and posterior pole abnormalities in infants, young preverbal children, and special populations.

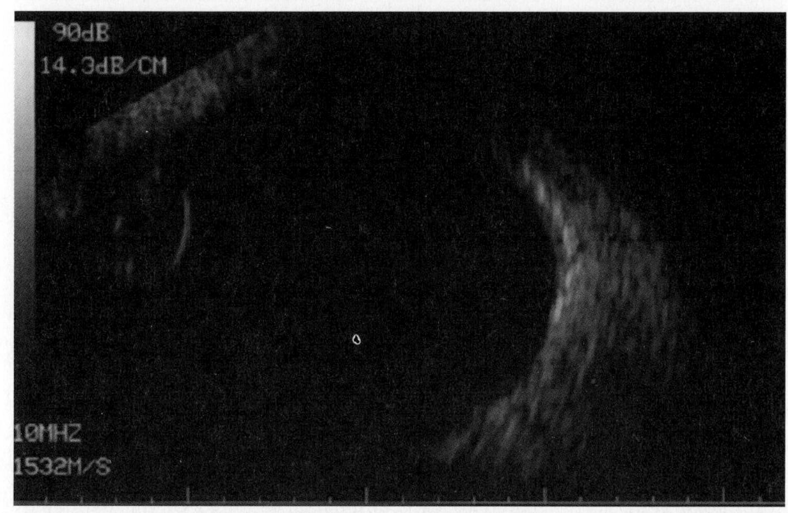

FIGURE 23-2. B-scan ultrasound of a patient with posterior staphyloma. Note the outward bulging of the retina and sclera.

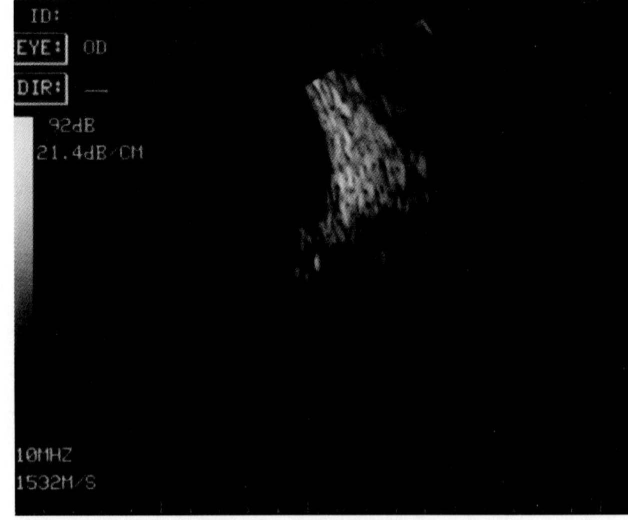

FIGURE 23-3. B-scan ultrasound of a retinal detachment. The free-floating retina can be seen in front of the round choroid and scleral surfaces

Using a direct ophthalmoscope to illuminate the eyes from a distance of approximately 1 m, the coaxial fundus reflex can be examined, preferably with nondilated pupils (9,10). A +1.00 diopter lens can be dialed into the ophthalmoscope to give a clear view of the patient's pupils at this distance. When both eyes are fixating, the reflexes should be equally bright. The darker red reflex indicates the fixating eye, and the whiter, lighter, or brighter reflex indicates the nonfixating eye. This procedure is covered in more detail elsewhere in this chapter as well as in Chapter 16, Comprehensive Examination Procedures.

This setup can be modified by introducing a camera to allow quantifiable imaging of the subject's pupils. In an experiment by Miller et al. (10), the minimum brightness that could be observed and quantified was within 0.5 degrees of central fixation, while the maximum brightness appeared at 5 degrees of eccentricity. The images can be stored and compared to monitor changes while active treatment is occurring.

PHOTOSCREENERS

Photoscreeners objectively screen for amblyogenic risk factors in children (11). The newer generation of photoscreeners use digital image technology instead of photographic film as the recording media. They are an effective and portable tool used to screen for amblyopia and small angle strabismus at vision screenings. Video photorefractors are also available, such as the Fortune Optical VRB-100 (Fortune Optical, Padova, Italy) video photorefractor (12).

SLIT LAMP BIOMICROSCOPY

Conventional imaging with a slit lamp may be useful if clear images can be obtained. The images can be evaluated at the examiner's leisure without the patient having to sit still for an extended period of time. Image capture–assisted software attached to the slit lamp has made the process significantly easier as images or video can be captured in real time while the patient is being examined and easily replayed for further evaluation.

ULTRAWIDE FIELD IMAGING SYSTEMS

The ultrawide field imaging system by Optos (Optos plc, Scotland SC139953) produces full color, high-resolution images that encompass a large area of the fundus measuring approximately 200 internal degrees (Figs. 23-4 and 23-5). The Optos, two low-powered lasers that the retina simultaneously and allows views of the retinal layers. The lasers are a green laser of 532 nm and a red laser of 633 nm. Once the image is captured, the software allows analysis by magnification and adjustment of brightness and contrast for enhancement. Measurements and annotations on the images themselves are also possible. The screening plane is an ellipsoidal mirror that places the image at the plane of the patient's iris (13). The Optomap image is taken with an undilated eye, increasing compliance in children and patients with special needs. The fixation target is large and easy to explain to the patient. The capture procedure is rapid, and compared to the compliance required of the patient by

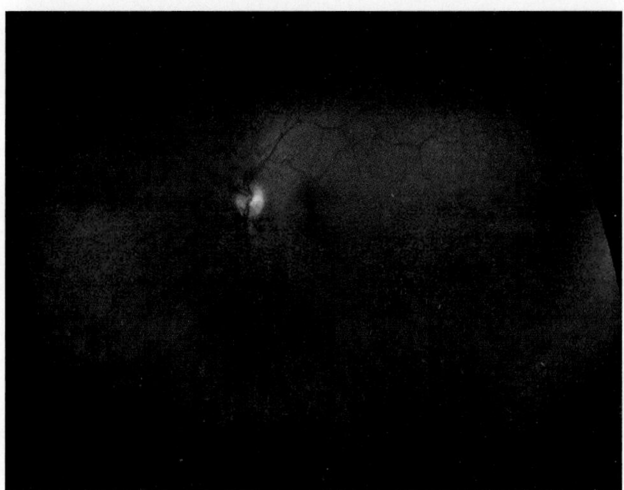

FIGURE 23-4. This picture represents a normal fundus as seen with the Optos "Optomap." (See also Color Section.)

traditional ophthalmoscopy, it is an excellent screening tool that can be used to speedily asses the patient's retinal health. The captured image can be stored and maintained as a baseline (14). The eyepiece must remain free of all dust to avoid artifact and this can sometimes be problematic. On occasion, the patient's lashes may interfere, causing an otherwise good image to not be useful. In these cases, the lids can be retracted using a cotton-tipped applicator, improving the area of retina visualized (15).

The Optomap by Optos is highly specific and moderately sensitive to lesions posterior to the equator but has low sensitivity for lesions anterior to the equator (14). According to a 2009 study, the Optomap is successful at detecting detachments but does not accurately detect retinal holes and tears (16). Optomap interpreters may on occasion miss findings such as white without pressure, lattice degeneration, paramacular drusen, and pigmentary changes at the fundus (17). In consideration of our special populations, lack of pigment may be an important clinical diagnostic tool in patients with Sjögren-Larsson syndrome, an autosomal recessive hereditary disorder with congenital ichthyosis, spastic diplegia or tetraplegia, and mental retardation. These patients have a characteristic macular dystrophy, reduced acuity, and photophobia and should be evaluated with care using the most appropriate procedures (18).

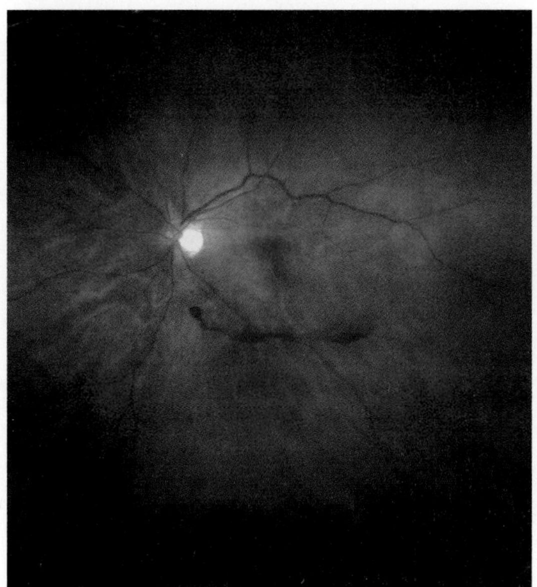

FIGURE 23-5. An Optos image showing a large floater following a complete posterior vitreous detachment. (See also Color Section.)

One of the yet untapped areas of potential use of the Optos is the application in telemedicine or remote medicine. The procedure can be performed by a trained layperson and interpreted off-site. The images from the Optos Panoramic 200, which are nonmydriatic images, can be used effectively in at-risk populations to assess diabetic retinopathy and clinically significant macular edema and therefore may be used in telescreening programs in such cases (16,19).

OPTICAL COHERENCE TOMOGRAPHY

Optical coherence tomography (OCT) was introduced to clinical practice in 1997 and has evolved to include tomography of the anterior chamber and Fourier-domain OCT (20). Traditional time-domain technology was originally capable of capturing 100 axial scans per second with 10 μm resolution. New Fourier-domain technology is capable of capturing 26,000 axial scans per second with a 5 μm resolution (21).

The principle of OCT is based on measuring the time delays of light returning from various depths in the tissues of the eye. A coupler splits the light from the light source to the reference mirror and the eye. The light source consists of a wide band of wavelengths that allows short coherence length and high depth resolution. The reflections are then combined and the delay between the reference mirror and the eye measured by interferometry. Each cycle produces an axial or a scan. In time-domain OCT, the reference mirror moves with each cycle or scan, while Fourier-domain OCT allows the reference mirror to remain stationary (21). This improvement allows faster scan acquisition and improved resolution, reducing artifacts induced by the patient's eye movements (21). The purpose of the OCT is to detect abnormalities in the retina in three broad categories: thickness, morphology, and reflectivity characteristics of the tissue.

The optic nerve head scan pattern was the earliest application of the OCT used for the diagnosis of glaucoma (21) (Fig. 23-6). The application of this technology is widely used to follow specific conditions such as diabetic retinopathy, age-related macular degeneration, and glaucoma (Fig. 23-7). Abnormal

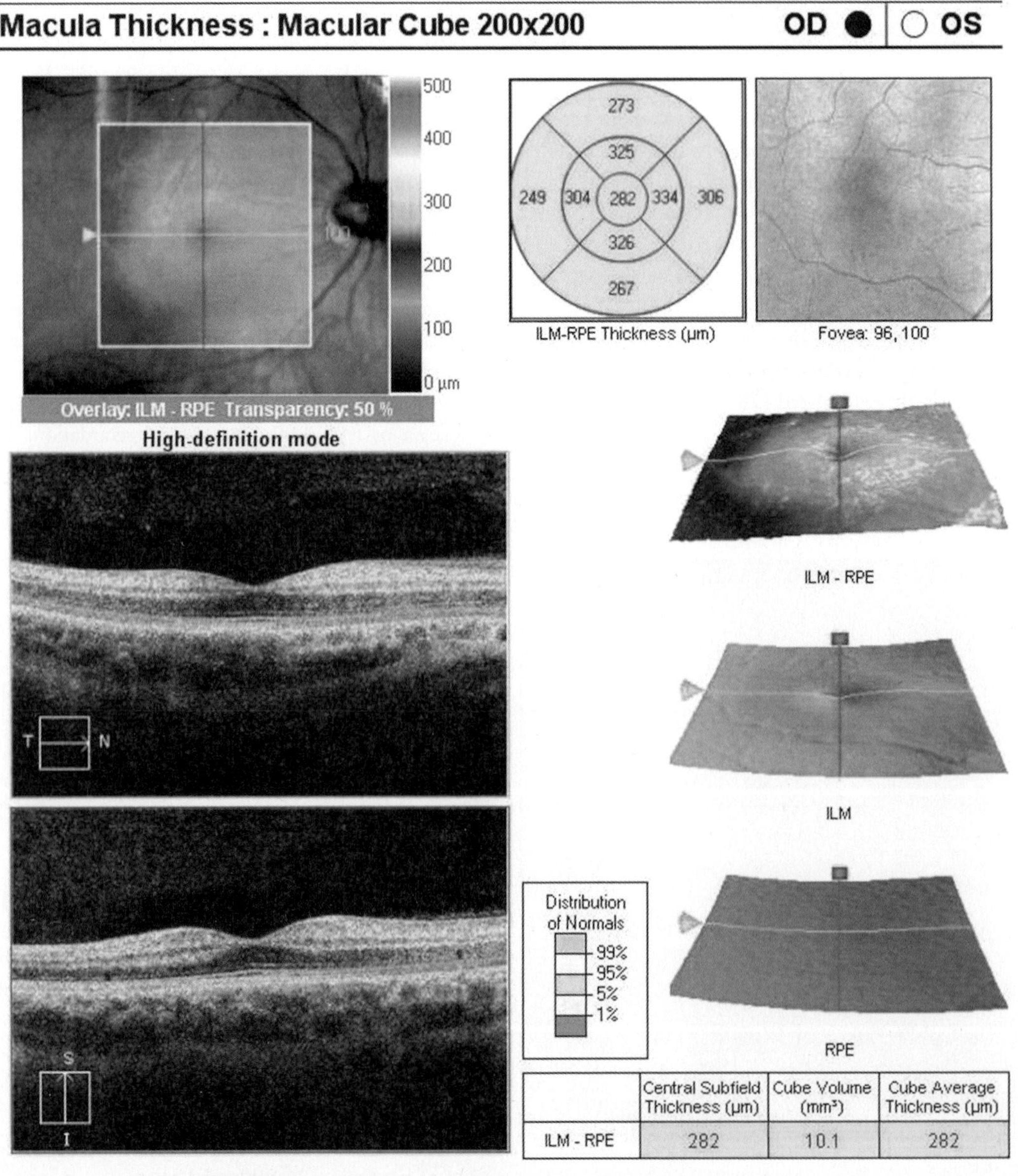

	Central Subfield Thickness (µm)	Cube Volume (mm³)	Cube Average Thickness (µm)
ILM - RPE	282	10.1	282

FIGURE 23-6. A normal OCT of the macular region. (See also Color Section.)

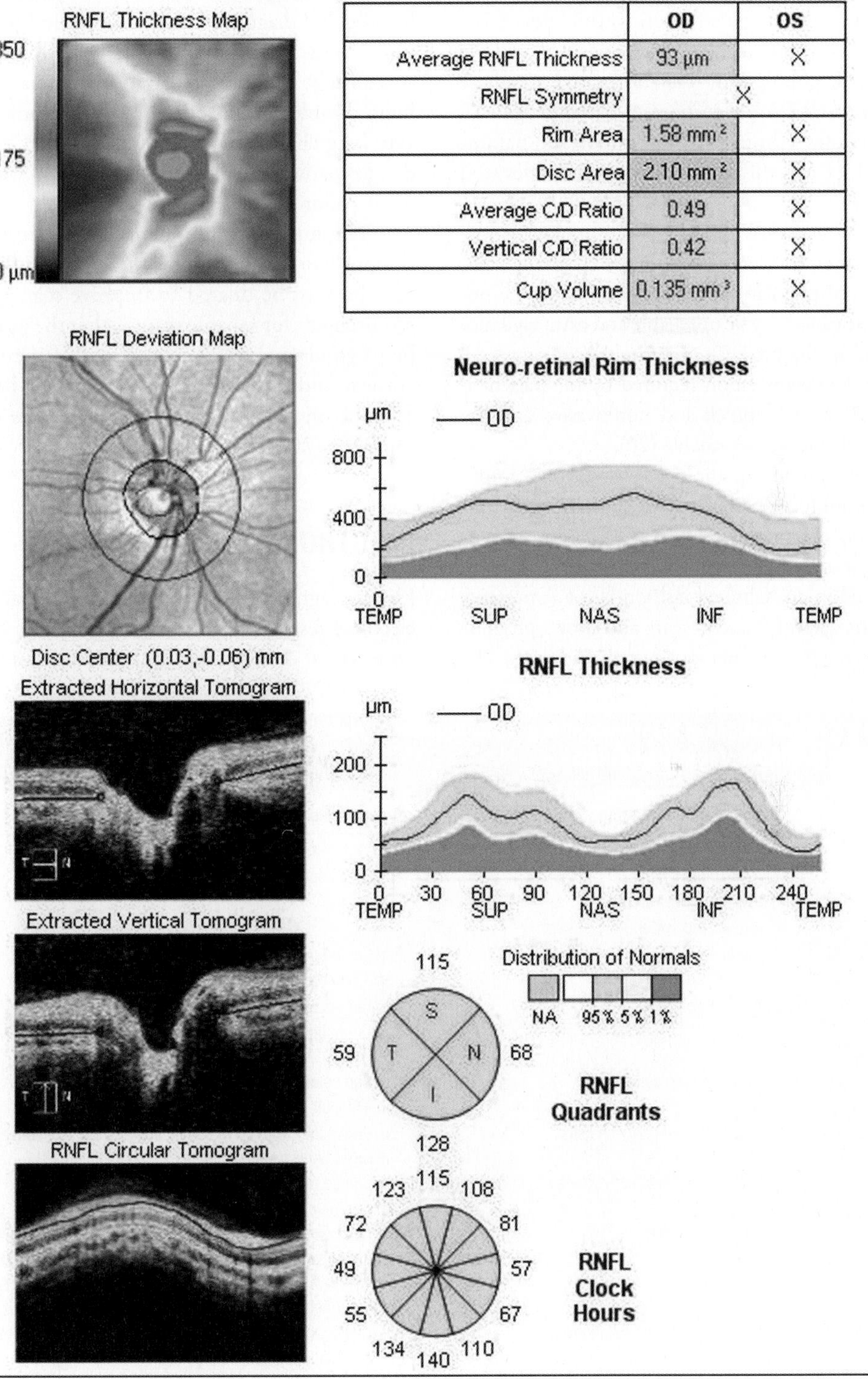

	OD	OS
Average RNFL Thickness	93 µm	X
RNFL Symmetry	X	
Rim Area	1.58 mm²	X
Disc Area	2.10 mm²	X
Average C/D Ratio	0.49	X
Vertical C/D Ratio	0.42	X
Cup Volume	0.135 mm³	X

FIGURE 23-7. A normal OCT of the optic nerve head. (See also Color Section.)

scans are best interpreted in conjunction with dilated fundus exam and fluorescein or indocyanine green angiography (20).

A normative database for retinal thickness exists for comparison, but regrettably it does not include the pediatric population. The normative database specific to the RTVue incorporates patients aged 18 to 82, includes ethnicity as an important parameter but does not differentiate between males and females (21).

Optical coherence tomography technology is ideally not used as a screening tool but is especially valuable in special populations where visual fields are not always obtainable, may be unreliable and extra vigilance is indicated in the presence of pathology or suspected pathology. The cooperation required by the patient is minimal. The test is quick and noninvasive and the results are reliable and repeatable (20).

Certain unique pathologic conditions found more commonly in patients with special needs may be effectively diagnosed using the OCT. Hunter syndrome or mucoploysaccharidoses type II, A and B, are inherited in an X-linked fashion. Type A presents between the ages of 2 and 4 years and shows progressive involvement of the nervous system and body. The OCT shows loss of photoreceptors outside the fovea and cystoid spaces within the inner nuclear ganglion cell and outer nuclear layers of the retina and could be used as a diagnostic tool in subclinical forms (22). Optic nerve atrophy in adrenoleukodystrophy was successfully demonstrated by OCT. This is a metabolic disorder characterized by the accumulation of very long chain fatty acids in all tissues. Optic nerve demyelination can be seen with MRI, while optic nerve pallor can be seen clinically (23).

The minimum pupil size for obtaining a scan is approximately 3 mm; therefore, small pupils may have to be dilated to improve scan quality. A requirement for reliable scans is that the optic media be of good quality. The condition of the tear film, cornea, and lens can affect the images negatively. Silicone oil in the vitreal chamber makes the scans unusable (20).

ELECTRORETINOGRAM

Electrodiagnostic tests are procedures that measure electrical responses from visual neurons in the retina up to visual cortex. Table 23.1 summarizes the stages

TABLE 23.1 Applications of Electrodiagnostic Tests Relative to Neurons Stimulated and Advantages/Disadvantages

Test	Stage of Visual System	Advantages/Disadvantages
Flash ERG	A wave: photoreceptors B wave: bipolar cells (Photopic: cone system) (Scotopic: rod system)	Pro: Very clean and repeatable Con: Does not reflect ganglion cell disorders or local lesions
Bright Flash ERG	Same as Flash ERG	Pro: Can be used in the presence of ocular media opacities Con: Can overestimate retinal function
Focal ERG	Same as Flash ERG	Pro: Can record from local retinal areas Con: Stimulator is monocular indirect ophthalmoscope, which is no longer manufactured
Pattern ERG	Retinal ganglion cells	Pro: Can be used to test glaucoma Con: Difficult to record
Multifocal ERG	Bipolar cells and ganglion cells	Pro: Can record from up to 256 focal areas and from several retinal neuron types
Flash VEP	Striate cortex, optic nerve transmission to cortex	Pro: Can be recorded in infants Con: Striate cortex responds better to patterns than flashes of light
Pattern VEP	Same as Flash VEP	Pro: Can test acuity, refraction, color vision, abnormal routing of optic nerve fibers, and response to contrast in unresponsive patients Con: Requires fixation and active attention
Binocular Beat VEP	Binocular striate cortical neurons	Pro: Can quantify degree of binocular summation, even in infants Cons: Difficult to find vendors
Sweep VEP	Same as Pattern VEP	Pro: Can be recorded quickly even on infants, can predict posttherapy acuity Cons: Requires fixation and attention

of the visual system targeted by these different tests and the pros and cons of using electrodiagnostic tests.

The electroretinogram (ERG) measures the functional integrity of the retina. It is therefore most useful as an adjunct test for the differential diagnosis of retinal disorders including hereditary chorioretinal dystrophies such as retinitis pigmentosa (RP). It can also detect other night-blinding disorders, cone dystrophies, the toxic effects of medications such as chloroquine on the retina, or the deleterious effects of intraocular foreign bodies.

The full-field ERG (standard or flash ERG) is the summated or pooled activity of the entire retinal area stimulated by a flash of light (24). The light flashes are diffused with a matte white Ganzfeld bowl to ensure even illumination spread out across the entire retina (25). A contact lens electrode is used in the form of either a scleral contact lens with a wire embedded within it or the standard Burian-Allen electrode with a wire surrounding a smaller contact lens with an attached lid speculum. The lid speculum serves not only to keep the patient's eyelids from blinking as a stimulus light flash is triggered but is also a reference electrode against which the corneal electrode's signal is compared. The Burian-Allen electrode is favored in children due to both the increased accuracy of the ERGs and the presence of the lid speculum. However, smaller electrode sizes are needed in pediatric patients.

The flash ERG is composed of several different components called "waves," but only two of these waves are clinically significant. The first is the a-wave, a negative voltage change that originates from the photoreceptors. It is followed by the positive b-wave, the largest component of the ERG. The b-wave originates from both bipolar cell activation and ionic exchange between the bipolar and Müller cells (26). Flash ERG recordings, showing the a-wave and b-wave, can be seen in Figures 23-8A and 23-8B.

There are two types of photoreceptors in the retina that convert light energy into electrical activity, cones and rods. Cones are specialized for collecting the high levels of light present in daylight, while rods are activated during low light situations such as nighttime. The photoreceptors are followed by bipolar cells, which transmit the photoreceptor signal to retinal ganglion cells. It is the axons of the retinal ganglion cells that exit the eye via the optic nerve. Their signal travels to the visual cortex.

The standard flash ERG may be recorded in two basic ways: photopic (light adapted), which preferentially activates cone photoreceptors and their associated bipolar cells (Fig. 23-8A), and scotopic (dark

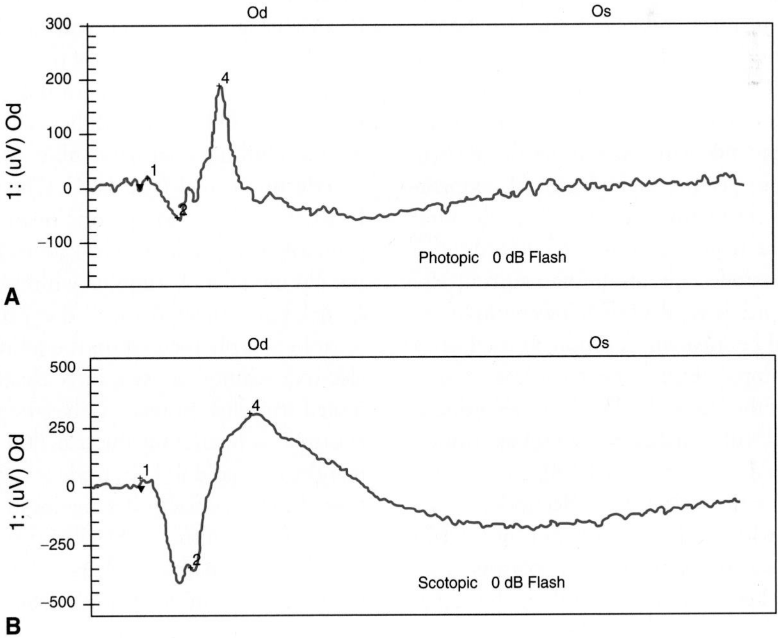

FIGURE 23-8. The normal electroretinogram as recorded by the LKC Technologies electrodiagnosis system. **A:** The photopic (light-adapted) ERG, with its negative a-wave and positive b-wave. **B:** The scotopic (dark-adapted) ERG. The scotopic ERG is larger in amplitude and longer in implicit time than the photopic ERG.

adapted), which stimulates rod photoreceptors and rod bipolar cells (27) (Fig. 23-8B). Classically, these were recorded in different manners. The photopic ERG was recorded with a bright background light to bleach out the rods and therefore inactivate them and a bright red stimulus light since cones are more responsive to red than are rods. For a scotopic ERG, the recording is performed in complete darkness after 30 to 40 minutes of dark adaptation, rendering the rods their most sensitive and inactivating cones. A dim blue flash is used, to which rods are more sensitive (28). More recently, the International Society for Clinical Electrophysiology of Vision standard for recording ERGs (29) suggests using only white stimulus flashes, recording photopic ERGS with a bright white flash in the presence of a background light (see Fig. 23-8A) and scotopic ERGs with dim white flashes following dark adaptation (see Fig. 23-8B).

The scotopic ERG is larger in amplitude and slower (i.e., has a longer implicit time) than the photopic ERG because the human eye contains more rods than cones, but rods respond more slowly (30). By recording photopic and scotopic ERGs, we can diagnose diseases that selectively attack the cone and rod systems, respectively. The full-field ERG is therefore especially useful in the diagnosis of outer retinal diseases such as rod-cone degenerations. The prototypical rod-cone degeneration is RP. Retinitis pigmentosa can be distinguished from other rod disorders by the fact that not only are both photopic and scotopic ERGs abnormal, although rod ERGS are more so, but the ERGs also show a delayed implicit time (31).

In many patients with special needs, it may not be possible to get the high degree of cooperation needed to record with an ocular electrode. Oral sedation might be required, as in ERG recording in infants. Skin electrodes are an alternative if all else fails, but they typically yield a much lower amplitude ERG and should be used with caution. If used, they should be monitored during the recording session for movement of the electrode. The ERG recordings, whether recorded with contact lens or skin electrodes, must be compared to age-matched ERGs from normal children using the same type of electrode.

In patients with reduced penetration of light to the retina, such as in dense cataracts, corneal scarring, or vitreous hemorrhages, not only is the retina less visible upon ophthalmoscopy but the standard ERG flash stimulus may not yield a significant retinal response. Here, we use what is called the bright flash ERG, which is a highly intense light flash that can penetrate media opacities. While it is possible to get false positives on this test, the bright flash ERG can be valuable in determining whether or not cataract or vitreoretinal surgery is warranted.

One disadvantage of the standard full-field ERG is that it is a measure of the summated activity across the entire retina and therefore is not affected significantly by damage to a local retinal region. For example, a full-field ERG can be within normal limits with substantial damage to the macula (24). A specialized type of flash ERG, the focal ERG, uses a localized light stimulus embedded within a monocular indirect ophthalmoscope so that it may be directed at a local lesion (32). Only this small stimulated retinal area contributes to the focal ERG, and therefore the focal ERG can localize retinal lesions, ranging in size from a few degrees to about 15 degrees in such disorders as sector RP (32). Because the American Optical (AO) monocular indirect ophthalmoscope is no longer manufactured, fewer and fewer clinics offer this service. The recent VERIS multifocal ERG, invented by Erich Sutter (Electro-Diagnosis Inc.), overcomes the global nature of the flash ERG. It records individual local ERGs from up to 256 retinal locations simultaneously, yielding a visual field–like plot of ERGs (33). While originally a research tool, it is gaining clinical acceptance in adult populations. Unfortunately, it requires too much cooperation and steady fixation to be a viable test for patients with special needs.

A second disadvantage of the standard flash ERG is that it reflects the activity of the outer retina, photoreceptors, and bipolar/Müller cells. A blind patient with a nonfunctional nerve fiber layer can still yield a perfectly normal flash ERG. The pattern ERG or PERG (34), however, has origins in the inner retina, primarily the ganglion cells. Pattern ERGs use a temporally modulated stimulus with a constant average spatial luminance. Because the patterned stimulus must be sharply focused on the retina, a contact lens electrode cannot be used; these electrodes blur a patterned stimulus. Instead, a silver-impregnated thread electrode is floated on the tear film at the lower lid margin, or a gold foil electrode is tucked beneath the lower lid. These electrodes are not in the optical path.

The stimulus, a black-and-white grating or checkerboard pattern, changes stimulus contrast, reversing back and forth while the average brightness does not change. Ganglion cells are especially sensitive to temporal changes in contrast so the pattern ERG can be used in the diagnosis of inner retinal diseases. In addition, the use of a patterned stimulus biases the PERG to responses from the central visual field. However, while the PERG requires active fixation and accommodation as in the visual evoked potential (VEP) (see below), to keep the pattern stimulus clear in the central visual field, an electrode on the surface of the eye is still required. In many patients with special needs, it is not possible to get the high degree of cooperation needed to record while awake with an ocular electrode, necessitating the use of sedation. Skin electrodes cannot be used for the PERG because the signal is small even with ocular electrodes. Therefore, while a valuable test, PERGs cannot be used practically on patients with special needs.

VISUAL EVOKED POTENTIAL

The VEP provides a measure of the integrity of the macula, optic nerve, and visual cortex, although it is used clinically primarily as a test of optic nerve function (35). Visual evoked potentials are cortical potentials elicited by visual stimulation that are very small, in the range of a few microvolts in amplitude. They must be detected within a background of strong cortical activity from the rest of the brain, the electroencephalogram, which, for the purposes of our clinical testing, is considered unwanted "noise" that must be removed by special techniques such as signal averaging and filtering. The active electrode for VEP recording is positioned on the scalp over the posterior pole of the occipital lobe, where the striate cortex (also called area V1), the first visual cortical area, lies (Fig. 23-9). There are a greater number of visual cortical neurons in V1 dedicated to the macular (or central) region of the visual field, and this foveal representation is situated at posterior pole of the striate cortex. Therefore, the standard VEP is almost entirely a response to macular stimulation and can be affected by both macular and optic nerve disorders.

Visual evoked potential recordings require patient cooperation, attention, and fixation on the stimulus computer monitor. Decreased attention will reduce the VEP amplitude or yield an unrecordable response. Likewise, poor fixation or inaccurate accommodation can impair the response (36). Therefore, the child must be actively engaged by directing his or her attention to the monitor screen. When recording from children or special needs patients, an assistant should constantly observe the patient's fixation while the doctor is observing the VEP trace. The most important tests for the population in question and the disorders one needs to rule out should be performed first before the child's attention can no longer be maintained. The VEP recordings should be compared to the norms for the age range of that patient.

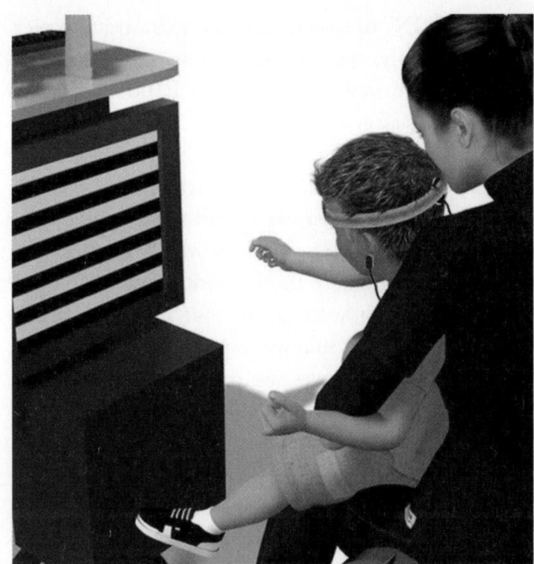

FIGURE 23-9. Recording the VEP in a toddler with the Diopsys Enfant electrodiagnostic system. The toddler sits in the parent's lap, while older children may sit in the chair by themselves. The active electrode is on the back of the head, on the midline 1 cm above the inion. This is the scalp location above the posterior pole of striate cortex (area V1). Reference electrodes are placed elsewhere on the head. Here, one ear-clip electrode serves as the reference electrode, while another serves as an electrical ground for safety. The toddler is watching a computer monitor screen with contrast-reversing bars, such as those used in the sweep VEP. (Courtesy of Barbara Steinman, OD., PhD.)

Aside from the ability to record VEPs from both flash and patterned stimuli, different types of clinical VEPs are distinguished according to the stimulation rate. Transient VEPs are produced by a stimulus that may be either patterned (e.g., reversing checks or gratings) or nonpatterned (flashes) at slow temporal frequencies of no more than four stimulus changes per second. Patterned stimuli are preferred because of the selectivity of visual cortex to patterned stimuli instead of diffuse light. If a patient has nystagmus, contrast-reversing stimuli cannot be used. A pattern appearance/disappearance stimulus must be used instead.

The slow rate of stimulation of the transient VEP allows the separation of numerous component waves that occur at different implicit times after each stimulus contrast reversal, and which arise from different regions of the brain from the lateral geniculate nucleus (LGN) to striate cortex to extrastriate cortex (37). Clinically, we are most concerned with the major positive wave, named P1 or P100, indicating that it occurs after a delay of about 100 ms following visual stimulation (Fig. 23-10). P1 has its origin from electrical generator sites in the striate cortex. With more rapid stimulation, we record what is called the steady-state VEP, a less complex waveform than the transient VEP because the individual waves "blend" together, yielding a waveform that resembles a distorted sine wave. While we lose the ability to examine the individual waves, we can perform frequency analysis (Fourier analysis).

Visual evoked potentials are typically used in conjunction with flash ERGs and PERGs to localize the disease process in the visual pathways. The combination of these tests can determine if a disorder is resulting from a pathologic process involving the retinal pigment epithelium, photoreceptors, bipolar cells, ganglion cells, optic nerve, or striate cortex. For example, optic neuritis (inflammation of the optic nerve) is characterized by a normal ERG, a normal PERG if no retrograde degeneration has occurred, and a severely abnormal VEP. Visual evoked potentials are very important in the diagnosis of multiple sclerosis (MS) in patients with optic neuritis (38). Patients with MS affecting the visual system will exhibit VEPs with increased implicit time of the P1 wave, with latencies from 120 up to even 200 ms, effectively doubling the transmission time of visual information to the striate cortex. Patients with optic atrophy exhibit reductions in the VEP amplitude, while the ERG amplitude is normal.

Visual evoked potentials can also be used to diagnose disorders due to their anatomical effects on the wiring of the optic pathways. In albinism, the proportion of optic nerve fibers crossing through the optic chiasm to the contralateral hemisphere of the brain versus those passing straight through to the ipsilateral hemisphere is altered. This is revealed in the VEP by a differential amplitude of VEPs recorded from each eye alone at electrodes on either side of the occipital lobe (39). In cortical vision impairment, the VEP can provide both diagnostic and prognostic information (40,41).

Recent research has focused on a specific pathway within the visual system called the magnocellular or M pathway that may contribute to reading disabilities. This pathway is responsible for seeing gross shape, fast motion, directing tracking eye movements, and activating rapid (transient) visual attention. There is some evidence that the VEP is affected in reading-disabled patients, although research in this area is sparse. Khaliq et al. (42) studied slow learners in comparison to normal learners and noted that the N75 component of the VEP was delayed. They attributed this delay to abnormalities in the LGN through which visual information passes on its way

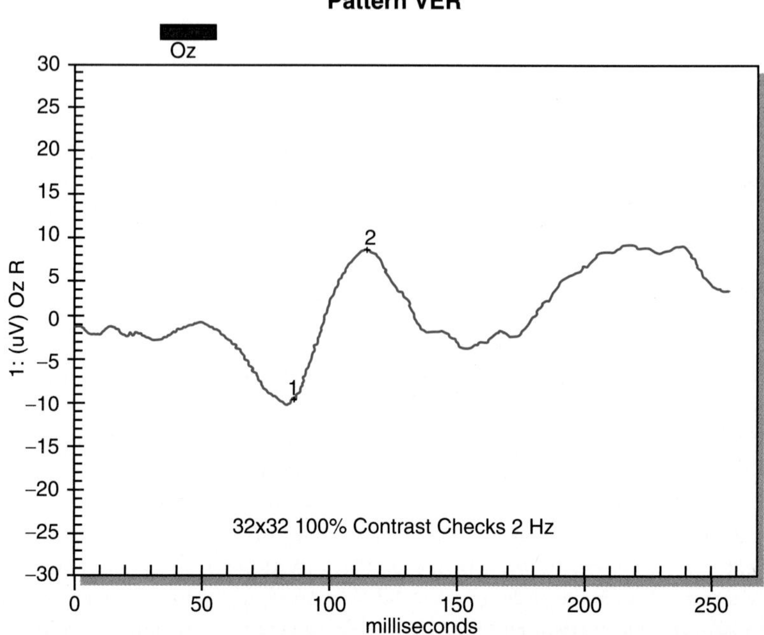

FIGURE 23-10. The normal pattern VEP. This plot depicts a VEP trace in response to a pattern-reversal checkerboard.

to the visual cortex. The authors then state that their data is consistent with an magnocellular (M) pathway deficiency at the level of the LGN or visual area V1. This study is flawed by its inclusion of low IQ subjects in the reading-disabled group while the normal group had normal IQs. In addition, their data does not lead to the conclusion that the magnocellular pathway is inhibited.

More convincing evidence for the role of the magnocellular pathway in reading disability comes from the VEP study by Lehmkuhle et al. (43). They surrounded a counterphase reversing sine-wave grating with a uniform field. Reading-disabled subjects showed a delayed VEP compared to normal subjects when the grating's frequency was low, but not when it was high, an indication that the magnocellular system is involved in reading-disabled subjects. Then, they surrounded a low spatial frequency reversing grating with a high-frequency flickering field, which preferentially inhibits the M pathway. The VEPs to this stimulus showed no further delay in reading-disabled subjects, only the amplitude was affected. The results can be interpreted as showing that the M pathway is already inhibited in reading-disabled subjects, and further inhibition of the M neurons has no additional effect. The role of the magnocellular pathway in reading disability is corroborated by research on transient visual attention (4,44).

The degree of binocular summation is reduced in infants and children with amblyopia or at risk of developing amblyopia. Special populations such as patients with cerebral palsy have an increased incidence of strabismus and amblyopia relative to normal patients (45). While clinicians typically measure binocular summation by comparing the monocular VEP amplitude to the binocular VEP amplitude, this is an incorrect and misleading technique. In normal individuals, the binocular VEP can be larger, equal to, or smaller than monocular VEPs, depending on the check size and contrast-reversal rate used (46). The same variability is seen in amblyopes (47). This makes it impossible to discern whether binocular summation is occurring or not in a given patient. Therefore, it is impossible to diagnose amblyopia with this technique. However, improvement of the binocular VEP relative to the monocular VEP can be assessed within patients. For example, the degree of improvement of the binocular VEP can be determined as a function of prism strength or lens power, allowing the clinician to confirm the optimal prism or lens to apply.

To accurately assess the degree of binocular summation, a specialized VEP called the binocular "beat" VEP must be used (48). Here, slightly different temporal frequencies of flicker are presented to the two eyes via LED goggles. The VEP recording is Fourier analyzed. In all patients, the VEP response contains the original stimulus frequencies, but in patients with binocular summation, two additional frequencies known as the "beat" frequencies appear. These are the sum and difference of the original frequencies. For example, if flicker of 20 Hz is shown to one eye and 18 Hz to the other eye simultaneously, all patients' VEP recordings will have frequency components of 20 and 18 Hz. Patients with binocular summation will also have VEP "beat" frequencies of 2 Hz and 38 Hz. The weaker the "beat" responses, the less the binocular summation. Because the flicker can penetrate the eyelids of even sleeping, noncooperative infants, it is an excellent test for binocular summation for patients with special needs. Only a few electrodiagnostic equipment manufacturers, such as Metrovision in France, offer binocular beat VEP capabilities.

Amblyopia, a cortically based disorder, is characterized by a normal flash ERG response, a normal pattern ERG, and an abnormal VEP, indicating reduced acuity in the amblyopic eye and reduced binocular summation. Amblyopia also affects the ability of the affected eye to process luminance contrast, which results in a reduction in the slope of the plot of VEP amplitude as a function of contrast relative to that of a normal eye (49).

If different sizes of stimuli are presented over time with a steady-state VEP (the "sweep" VEP), specialized tasks such as determining visual acuity in infants and children can be performed (50). Sometimes the sweep VEP is the only method that can be used to determine visual acuity in multiply handicapped children. Recently, it has been discovered that the sweep VEP can be used to determine the prognosis for the treatment of amblyopia (51) (Fig. 23-11).

CONCLUSION

Patients with special needs present with challenge to standard clinical eye examinations. However, these need not prevent the clinician from obtaining additional diagnostic data through the use of special testing. The techniques outlined in this chapter can help diagnose and quantify attention and reading deficits, as well as ocular and visual system diseases. Clinicians should consider making these tests available to their patients.

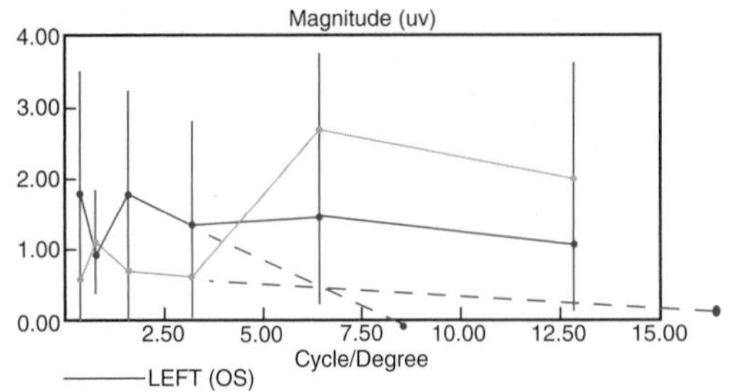

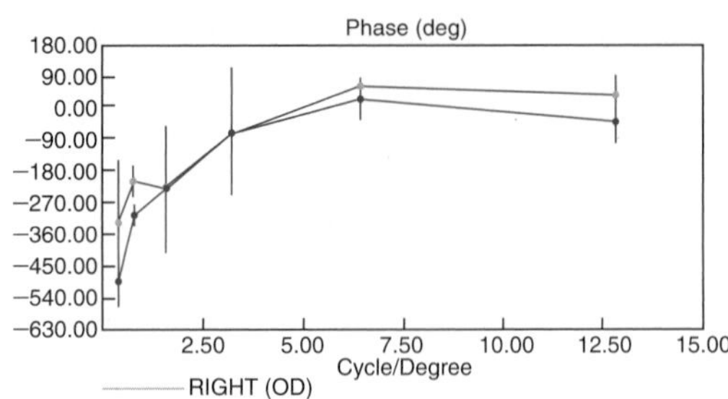

Significant differences: 0.4: 2.44 0.8: 4.67 1.6: 0.75 3.2: 0.36 6.4: 2. 12.9 1.92 Test Date: 8/19/2010 10:31:54
Print Date: 8/19/2010 10:31:58

OD 16.50 cpd = 20/36
OS 8.66 cpd = 20/69

FIGURE 23-11. Sweep VEP in an amblyopic child. The psychophysical visual acuities in this child were OD 20/25, OS 20/100. The sweep VEP-derived visual acuities indicate that the left eye's visual acuity can be improved to at least 20/69 by vision therapy.

REFERENCES

1. Han Y, Ciuffreda KJ, Kapoor N. Reading-related oculomotor testing and training protocols for acquired brain injury in humans. Brain Res Brain Res Protoc. 2004;14:1–12.
2. Tannen BM, Ciuffreda KJ. A Proposed addition to the standard protocol for the Visagraph II eye movement recording system. J Behav Optom. 2007;18:143–7.
3. Ciuffreda KJ, Tannen B. Eye movement basics for the clinician. St. Louis: Mosby; 1995.
4. Steinman SB, Steinman BA, Garzia RP. Vision and attention II: is visual attention a mechanism through which a deficient magnocellular pathway might cause reading disability? Optom Vis Sci. 1998;75:674–81.
5. Leark RA, Greenberg LM, Kindschi CL, et al. Test of variables of attention continuous performance test. The TOVA Company. 2007.
6. Duncan J, Humphreys GW. Visual search and visual similarity. Psychol Rev. 1989;96:433–58.
7. Green DM, Swets JA. Signal detection theory and psychophysics. New York: Wiley; 1966.
8. Coleman DJ, Silverman RH, Lizzi FL, et al. Ultrasonography of the eye and orbit. 2nd ed. Philadelphia: Lippincott Williams & Wilkins; 2006.
9. Carlson NB, Kurtz D. Clinical procedures for ocular examination. 3rd ed. New York: Mc Graw-Hill; 2003.
10. Miller JM, Hall HL, Greivenkamp JE, et al. Quantification of the Bruckner test for strabismus. Invest Ophthalmol Vis Sci. 1995;36:897–905.
11. Matta NS, Arnold RW, Singman EL, et al. Comparison between the PlusoptiX and MTI Photoscreeners. Arch Ophthalmol. 2009;127:1591–5.
12. Cooper CD, Gole GA, Hall JE, et al. Evaluating photoscreeners II: MTI and fortune videorefractor. Aust N Z J Ophthalmol. 1999;27:387–98.
13. Optos Available from: www.Optos.com. Last Accessed December 1st, 2010
14. Mackenzie PJ, Russell M, Isbister CM, et al. Sensitivity and specificity of the Optos Optomap for detecting peripheral retinal lesions. Retina. 2007;27:1110–24.
15. Cheng SC, Yap MK, Goldschmidt E, et al. Use of the Optomap with lid retraction and its sensitivity and specificity. Clin Exp Optom. 2008;91:373–8.
16. Khandhadia S, Madhusudhana KC, Kostakou A, et al. Use of Optomap for retinal screening within an eye casualty setting. Br J Ophthalmol. 2009;93:52–5.
17. Neubauer AS, Kernt M, Haritoglou C, et al. Nonmydriatic screening for diabetic retinopathy by ultra-widefield scanning laser ophthalmoscopy (Optomap). Graefes Arch Clin Exp Ophthalmol. 2008;246:229–35.
18. Van der Veen RL, Fuijkschot J, Willemsen MA, et al. Patients with Sjögren-Larsson syndrome lack macular pigment. Ophthalmology. 2010;117:966–71.
19. Kernt M, Pinter F, Hadi I, et al. Diabetic retinopathy: comparison of the diagnostic features of ultra-widefield scanning laser ophthalmoscopy Optomap with EDTRS 7-field fundus photography. Ophthalmologe. 2011;108:117–23.
20. Brancato R, Lumbroso B. Guide to optical coherence tomography interpretation. Italy: Innovation News Communication; 2004.
21. Weinreb RN, Varma R. RTVue Fourier-Domain Optical Coherence Tomography Primer Series Vol III Glaucoma. Available from: http://www2.opto.com.br/imgs/downloads/1281618551_glaucomaprimerreva.pdf. Last Accessed December, 2010.
22. Yoon MK, Chen RW, Hedges TR, et al. High-speed, ultrahigh resolution optical coherence tomography of the retina in Hunter's syndrome. Ophthalmic Surg Lasers Imaging. 2007;38:423–8.
23. Grainger BT, Papchenko TL, Danesh-Meyer HV. Optic nerve atrophy in adrenoleukodystrophy detectable by optic coherence tomography. J Clin Neurosci. 2010;17:122–4.
24. Armington JC. The electroretinogram. New York: Academic Press; 1974.
25. Holopigian K, Hood D. Electrophysiology. Ophthalmol Clin N Am. 2003;16:237–51.
26. Dick E, Miller RE, Bloomfield S. Extracellular K+ activity changes related to electroretinogram components: II. Rabbit (E-type) retinas. J Gen Physiol. 1985;85:991–31.
27. Sieving PA, Murayama K, Naarendorp F. Push-pull model of the primate photopic electroretinogram: a role for

hyperpolarizing neurons in shaping the b-wave. Vis Neurosci. 1994;11:519–32.
28. Granit R. Sensory mechanisms of the retina. London: Oxford University Press;1947.
29. Marmor MF, Zrenner E. Standard for clinical electroretinography. Doc Ophthalmol. 1995;89:199–210.
30. Gouras P, MacKay C. Adaptation effects on the electroretinogram. In: Heckenlively JR, Arden GB, editors. Principles and practice of clinical electrophysiology of vision. St. Louis: Mosby; 1991. p. 391–5.
31. Berson EL, Rosen JB, Simonoff EA. Electroretinographic testing as an aid in detection of carriers of X-chromosome-linked retinitis pigmentosa. Am J Ophthalmol. 1979;87:460–8.
32. Lyons JS, Sapper DJ. Evaluation of the LKC stimulator for focal ERG testing. Doc Ophthalmol. 2001;103:163–73.
33. Sutter EE, Tran D. The field topography of ERG components in man: I. the photopic luminance response. Vis Res. 1992;32:433–46.
34. Marmor MF, Holder GE, Porciatti V, et al. Guidelines for basic pattern electroretinography. Doc Ophthalmol. 1996; 91:291–8.
35. Odom JV, Bach M, Barber C, et al. Visual evoked potentials standard. Doc Ophthalmol. 2004;108:115–23.
36. Harter MR, Salmon LE. Intra-modality selective attention and evoked cortical potentials to randomly presented patterns. Electroencephalogr Clin Neurophysiol. 1972;32:605–13.
37. DiRusso F, Martinez A, Sereno MI, et al. Cortical sources of the early components of the visual evoked potential. Hum Brain Mapp. 2002;15:96–111.
38. Halliday AM, McDonald WI, Mushin J. Delayed visual evoked response in optic neuritis. Lancet. 1972;1:982–5.
39. Apkarian PA, Reits D, Spekreijse H, et al. A decisive electrophysiological test for human albinism. Electroencephalogr Clin Neurophysiol. 1983;55:513–31.
40. Grant DB, Hertle RW, Quinn GE, et al. The visual-evoked response in infants with central visual impairment. Am J Ophthalmol. 1993;116:437–43.
41. Taylor MJ, McCulloch DL. Prognostic value of VEPs in young children with acute onset of cortical blindness. Pediatr Neurol. 1991;7:111–5.
42. Khaliq F, Yumnam A, Vaney N. Visual evoked potential study in slow learners. Indian J Physiol Pharmacol. 2009;53:341–6.
43. Lehmkuhle S, Garzia RP, Turner L, et al. A defective visual pathway in children with reading disability. New Engl J Med. 1993;328:989–96.
44. Steinman BA, Steinman SB, Lehmkuhle S. Transient visual attention is dominated by the magnocellular stream. Vis Res. 1997;37:17–23.
45. Erkkilä H, Lindbrtg L, Kallio AK. Strabismus in children with cerebral palsy. Acta Ophthalmol Scand. 1996;74:636–8.
46. Apkarian PA, Nakayama K, Tyler CW. Binocularity in the human evoked potential: Facilitation, summation and suppression. Electroencephalogr Clin. Neurophysiol. 1981;51:32–48.
47. Apkarian PA, Levi D, Tyler CW. Binocular facilitation in the visual-evoked potential of strabismic amblyopes. Am J Optom Physiol Opt. 1981;58:820–30.
48. Baitch LW, Levi DM. Binocular beats: psychophysical studies of binocular interaction in normal and stereoblind humans. Vis Res. 1989;29:27–35.
49. Levi DM, Harwerth RS. Contrast evoked potentials in strabismic and anisometropic amblyopia. Invest Ophthalmol Vis Sci. 1978;17:571–5.
50. Tyler CW, Apkarian P, Levi DM, et al. Rapid assessment of visual function: an electronic sweep technique for the pattern visual evoked potential. Invest Ophthalmol Vis Sci. 1979;18:703–13.
51. Ridder WH III, Rouse M. Predicting potential acuities in amblyopes: predicting post-therapy acuity in amblyopes. Doc Ophthalmol. 2007;114:135–45.

CONFLICT OF INTEREST Dr. Steinman is a scientific consultant for Diopsys Inc., manufacturers of VEP recording systems for pediatric and special populations.

CHAPTER 24

Dominick M. Maino, OD, MEd, FAAO, FCOVD-A
Robert Donati, PhD
Yi Pang, OD, PhD
Stephen Viola, FAAO, PhD
Susan R. Barry, PhD

Neuroplasticity

A sea change, a change of such magnitude that it transforms the very nature of a subject, is now occurring in the field of neuroscience. For the past half century the adult human brain was thought to be largely hardwired and incapable of significant plasticity. Today, that mindset is being overturned. Our brains are dynamic, continually changing, and capable of reorganization, recovery, and rehabilitation throughout life.

Chakraborty et al. note that the current science of neuroplasticity shows us a "phenomenon where different stimuli leads to an increase or decrease in the number of brain cells and remodeling of synapses." Neuroplasticity research has "... established beyond doubt that instead of being a static cell mass, our brain is actually a dynamic system of neural network that has the capability of significant growth under favorable circumstances...." (1).

The brain is not just a stagnant, nonpliable, round mass, submersed in a fluid and surrounded by a durable case. It is not finished in its development once we reach adulthood. The brain changes over time, and with that change, end organs such as the eye (and its very function) can be cortically changed, show improvement after insult and injury, and be remediated and enhanced. Up until very recently, many optometrists and the majority of ophthalmologists were unwilling to accept this conceptual sea change when just about all other professionals, scientists, and lay individuals appeared to have gotten the message (2–5).

Optometrists and ophthalmologists, who have dismissed the possibility of neuroplasticity in their adult and elderly patients, often cite the work of Wiesel and Hubel (6) for justification. This justification rests on the misinterpretation of critical periods, periods of sensitivity, and mistaken concepts of neuroplasticity. They may also demonstrate a lack of knowledge of the underlying triggers and mechanisms for neuroplasticity. As a result, effective treatments for many disorders, including amblyopia, have been delayed or dismissed outright.

CRITICAL PERIODS, PERIODS OF SENSITIVITY AND NEUROPLASTICITY

The critical period has been defined by Hensch as "a strict time window during which experience provides information that is essential for normal development and permanently alters performance" (7). Sengpiel defines it as "...a time during early postnatal life when the development and maturation of functional properties of the brain, its 'plasticity,' is strongly dependent on experience or environmental influences" (8). Despite subtle differences in the various definitions, the critical period is thought to be a period, usually early in an individual's life, when neuronal circuitry is particularly sensitive to outside environmental influences.

These definitions of the critical period were born out of the early monocular deprivation studies by Hubel and Weisel (6,9,10) in which one eyelid of cats and monkeys was sutured shut at various times in the life cycle in order to observe the effects on the visual circuitry. The major finding of these studies was that monocular deprivation during very early life causes functional blindness in the deprived eye, despite the fact that the retina of this eye was fully functional after reopening the eye.

These experiments provided carefully recorded and detailed physiologic and anatomic data which had an enormous impact on how we viewed the adult brain. The data implied that the brain was responsive to environmental stimuli in early life in order to adapt to real-life conditions. After this critical period however, plasticity supposedly ended. Interpretations from these experiments were then generalized to the development of a wide variety of situations.

Little attention however was drawn to the fact that the manipulation performed in Hubel and Wiesel's monocular deprivation experiments—the removal of all form vision in one eye in early infancy—was an extreme measure. Indeed, Hubel and Wiesel designed their monocular deprivation experiments specifically to serve as a model of deprivation amblyopia, such as occurs with a congenital cataract of one eye. However, this condition is very rare. Most people develop amblyopia, not through a congenital cataract, but as a result of strabismus or anisometropia. As a result, they have not been deprived of all form vision in one eye since the beginning of life. Thus, the changes observed in the brains of cats and monkeys following monocular deprivation may not be found in the brains of people with the most common forms of amblyopia (11), and the impact of a presumed critical period on visual plasticity in human amblyopia is not known.

Moreover, the use of caged animals in laboratory experiments may have impeded recognition of the substantial plasticity present in the adult mammalian brain. Current scientific research indicates that brain plasticity is dramatically enhanced in enriched environments, increased by physical exercise, and substantially reduced by stress (12–14). Yet, most neurobiological experiments have made use of caged animals that live in deprived, sedentary, boring, unnatural, and stressful environments. Indeed, a 2007 paper indicates that the effects of early monocular deprivation on visual outcomes in rats can be reversed in adulthood by exposing these lab animals to enriched environments (15).

Furthermore, the concept of a critical period does not imply that all neuroplasticity ends after a certain age. The critical period should have a beginning of strong plasticity in response to a sensory experience, a well-defined time period when initiation of plasticity occurs readily and a time of reduced sensitivity when plasticity to the same stimulus no longer happens (at the same level). Although plasticity occurs over an individual's lifetime, different types of plasticity dominate during certain periods of one's life and are less prevalent during other periods. According to Hooks and Chen (16), the phases of plasticity that define the critical period are as follows:

1. **The precritical period**: The initial formation of neuronal circuits that is not dependent on visual experience
2. **The critical period**: A distinct onset of robust plasticity in response to the visual experience when the initially formed circuit can be modified by experience
3. **Closure of the critical period**: After the end of the critical period, the same visual experience no longer elicits the same degree of plasticity

A number of active inhibitory factors may play a role in the closure of the critical period (17). One such inhibitory system involves myelin and Nogo-A (Nogo)-66 receptor (NgR) signaling (18). Nogo is a myelin-associated protein found in oligodendrocytes, while NgR is found on the neuron. Binding of Nogo to the NgR activates a signaling cascade in the neuron that leads to growth cone collapse and inhibition of axonal sprouting, which are very important in neuroplasticity. By knocking out the NgR gene in mice, McGee et al. (18) were able to prevent the closure of the critical period for ocular dominance determination in the visual cortex by allowing plasticity to continue beyond the normal time frame. There are other factors such as tissue plasminogen activator, extracellular matrix proteins, and NMDA receptors that may play a role in the closure of the critical period, but a description of these mechanisms is beyond the scope of this discussion (8,11,12).

Hooks and Chen (16) also state that the timing of the above may be as critical as the cellular mechanisms underlying the critical period. All must be in place anatomically, developmentally, and neurologically *and* at the right time for the maximum end result to occur. They have also reviewed animal studies that show that the critical period of onset and closure are not set at various fixed ages of the animal, but can be changed and/or regulated by physiological and molecular manipulation, interference, and enhancement. While the authors write that the same degree of plasticity may not be available after the closure of the critical period, they do not say that varying degrees of neuroplasticity under the right circumstances cannot occur at some point in the individuals' life. This is an important and critical concept so that our sea change perspective on neuroplasticity can take place.

The *sensitive period* is somewhat different than the critical period in that it begins and ends gradually (not abruptly like the critical period) and provides a time line for maximum sensitivity to stimuli. Critical periods may be viewed as sensitive periods when certain experiences provide essential information for normal development and alter performance in what may be a permanent manner (19). According to Knudsen, a sensitive period cannot open until the following three conditions are met (19).

1. The information provided to the circuit must be sufficiently reliable and precise.
2. The circuit must contain adequate connectivity, including both excitatory and inhibitory connections, to process the information.
3. It must have activated mechanisms that enable plasticity, such as the capacity for altering axonal or dendritic morphologies, for making or eliminating synapses, or for changing the strengths of the synaptic connections.

Sensitive periods may affect how subcortical regions of the visual system develop. Sensitive periods in visual development may also have strong parallels to that of cortex development (7). This period of synaptic refinement spans the time of initial eye opening, but it is spontaneous retinal activity, not vision, driving the resultant changes. The concept of a sensitive period also does not imply that neuroplasticity ends after a certain age. When a sensitive period ends, plasticity may still occur, but extra energy is required for that circuit to maintain a less stable pattern of connectivity (14). There is a growing body of evidence to support the concept that neuroplasticity and growth are possible for not only the young (20) but also seniors (21).

NEUROPLASTICITY AND THE BRAIN

From a cellular point of view, the closure of the critical period may be conceived as a transition point in development when a balance between inhibition and excitation has been established in the maturing brain. From a functional point of view, the closure of the critical period may occur when the brain no longer changes in response to any strong and repetitive stimulus. As we mature, we develop habits, ways of moving and perceiving, that become entrenched. These habits will change only in response to behaviorally important stimuli (22–24) and following specific training and experience. Plasticity in the adult brain requires active learning, self-awareness, and motivation. The stroke patients who recover best are those who take control of their own rehabilitation. These are the patients who plan out how they will use the weakened limb in daily tasks, keep a diary of their actions, and solve problems as they occur (25,26). Promoting plasticity in the adult brain is not a passive process.

Some forms of adult learning may require neurogenesis or the birth of new nerve cells throughout life. Just as it was difficult for many scientists and physicians to give up the dogma of irreversible critical periods, it took more than half a century for neuroscientists to recognize neurogenesis in the mammalian and human brain. Since the neuron has a very complicated structure, it seemed unlikely that it would undergo cell division to form daughter cells. As early as 1962, however, Joseph Altman documented the birth of new neurons in the rat brain, and these new cells derived not from mature neurons, but from neuroblasts or progenitor cells (27). Altman's research as well as that of others on neurogenesis was ignored until recently.

In order for some forms of adult learning, memory and mood regulation to take place, neurogenesis may be necessary. Adult neural stem and/or progenitor cells are now known to continuously generate new neurons throughout life in various areas of the mammalian central nervous system (28,29). Neurogenesis is increased by physical exercise, learning, and enriched environments and decreased by stress (12–14). The birth of new neurons has been demonstrated not just in mice and monkeys but in humans as well (30). Newborn neurons may contribute to new circuits, synaptic plasticity, new memories, and new behaviors.

Neurogenesis however does not underlie all forms of neuronal plasticity. There is evidence, for example, of neuronal structural changes that occur in the dendritic spines of neurons found in specific regions of adult mouse visual cortex (31). In this study, Hofer et al. demonstrate that rearrangement of the intracortical connections via the dendritic spines may be a mechanism that contributes to experience-dependent plasticity that is independent of new cell growth. These spines and their specific arrangement can also embody the history of previous adaptations by these neural circuits. So it may not only be the generation of new spines but their specific arrangement that determines the efficacy of plasticity in a given cortical circuit.

While genetics certainly play a role in establishing the brain's plasticity, the environment also exerts heavy influence in maintaining it. Even in adulthood, the rat brain reacts to the stimulation of environmental enrichment with an increase in spines and a lengthening of dendrites (32). However, this is somewhat smaller than during early postnatal development and becomes smaller with advancing age (33). This is to be expected as the size of dendrites and the maturation of synapse have generally reached a stable level in adulthood. The environmental enrichment effects are detected in a number of cortical areas, but not in all. Furthermore, there appear to be differences in male rats, compared to female rats. The greatest differences are found in the hippocampal dendrites of female rats and in the occipital cortical dendrites of male rates (34).

Changes in the strength of individual synapses and in the balance of excitation and inhibition also have enormous effects on plasticity (35). These changes may be necessary for changes in cortical maps. For example, extensive use of the index finger, such as occurs when an individual learns to read Braille, will expand the territory for the index finger on sensorimotor maps in the brain (36), and these changes may be mediated by changes in synaptic weights. Changes at the molecular level can influence plasticity as well. Beck and Yaari (37) reviewed data that suggested that alterations in voltage and Ca^{++} gated ion channels change the functional properties of neurons and impart an intrinsic plasticity independent of any neurogenesis. In fact, these authors think that intrinsic plasticity may be involved in certain central nervous system disorders such as Parkinson disease, schizophrenia, and phantom limb sensation.

Additional evidence for cortical plasticity is the result of changes observed in the anatomy and structure of adult brains. One study that taught individuals how to juggle noted that the juggler group demonstrated a significant expansion of gray matter in the midtemporal area and in the left posterior intraparietal sulcus of the cortex after only a few practice sessions. The investigators found a close relationship between the changes in gray matter and improvement in juggling performance. Since nonjugglers showed no change in gray matter over the same period, these changes were specific to the training (38). In another study that looked at brain volume of experienced typists, it was noted that long-term bimanual training increases gray matter volume in adults as well (39). This means that learning not only affects function but also structure in the adult brain.

Chemical, monoaminergic, and cholinergic transmitter maturation continues into adulthood (40–45), and for the roles of dopamine, noradrenalin, and serotonin, a mature pattern can be expected to emerge in early adulthood (46,47). As a consequence, maturation of receptors for several transmitters on cortical neurons occurs throughout puberty and early adulthood (48). These observations are important because liberation of these neurotransmitters by brainstem and basal forebrain neurons onto cortical cells may facilitate and strengthen the plastic changes at cortical synapses that occur with learning and training (49).

Ge et al. (50) state that, "Adult brains exhibit significant plasticity for life-long learning." Neuroplasticity does not consist of a single type of morphologic change but rather includes several different processes that occur throughout an individual's lifetime. The phrase "life-long learning" should now take on new significance for optometrists. Adults can learn throughout their life cycle. This means that we can make a considerable difference in the lives of all our patients including adults and those with special needs.

NEUROPLASTICITY AND REHABILITATION

Neuroplasticity is critical for the damaged or disabled brain. Without neuroplasticity, lost functions could never be regained, nor could disabled processes ever hope to be improved. Plasticity allows the brain to rebuild the connections that, because of trauma, disease, or genetic misfortune, have resulted in decreased abilities. Neuroplasticity allows us to compensate for damaged or dysfunctional neural pathways.

Scientists have identified four patterns of plasticity (51). First is the situation in which healthy cells surrounding an injured area of the brain change their function, even their shape, so as to perform the tasks of the injured area. This process is called *functional map expansion*. The second mechanism involves brain cells reorganizing existing synaptic pathways. This form of plasticity is known as a *compensatory masquerade*. It allows already-constructed pathways that are near a damaged area to respond to changes in the body's demands caused by lost function in some other area.

These two mechanisms rely on synaptic changes mentioned earlier and may underlie some of the recovery of function following stroke (52). A third neuroplastic process, *homologous region adaption*, allows an entire brain area to take over functions from another distant brain area (one not immediately neighboring the compensatory area, as in function map expansion) that has been damaged. And finally, neuroplasticity can occur in the form of *cross-model reassignment*. This allows one type of sensory input to entirely replace another damaged one. Cross-model reassignment allows the brain of a blind individual, while learning to read Braille, to rewire the sense of touch so that it replaces the responsibilities of vision in the brain areas linked with reading. It is one, or a combination, of these neuroplastic responses that allow for rehabilitation.

Kleim and Jones (53) in their paper *Principles of Experience-Dependent Neural Plasticity: Implications for Rehabilitation after Brain Damage* lists 10 key principles that should be followed to take advantage of any neuroplasticity present and to improve function. These principles include the following:

1. **Use it or lose it** (if you do not drive specific brain functions, functional loss will occur)
2. **Use it and improve it** (therapy that drives cortical function enhances that function)
3. **Specificity** (the therapy you choose determines the resultant plasticity and function)
4. **Repetition matters** (plasticity that results in functional change requires repetition)
5. **Intensity matters** (induction of plasticity requires the appropriate amount of intensity)
6. **Time matters** (different forms of plasticity take place at different times during therapy)
7. **Salience matters** (it has to be important to the individual)
8. **Age matters** (plasticity is easier in the younger brain but possible in the adult)
9. **Transference** (neuroplasticity and the change in function that results from one therapy can augment the attainment of similar behaviors)
10. **Interference** (plasticity in response to one experience can interfere with the acquisition of other behaviors)

Scientific research supports these 10 principles. For example, our somatosensory and motor cortices contain several maps of our body, with the number of neurons devoted to a given body part directly related to the amount that it is used. If you were to learn to read Braille for example, the representation of your reading index finger on the body maps would increase (36). Thus, the principles of "use it or lose it" and "use it and improve it" make scientific sense. Studies in a wide variety of species from sea slugs to primates indicate that new long-term memories are dependent upon changes in synaptic weights, and these changes require, as indicated by principles 4 and 5, repetition and increases in stimulus intensity (35). In addition, tasks that introduce novelty and reward and are important to the individual stimulate the release of neuromodulators in the brain, and these compounds trigger, facilitate, and stabilize changes in brain circuitry (50).

These 10 principles can play a major role in how we treat our patients after the diagnosis has been made. Now that we know that even adults can exhibit neuroplasticity that can result not only in anatomical and physiologic changes in the cortex but also in functional changes in behavior; it is appropriate to review the current eye and vision care research that also supports the concept of neuroplasticity as it is applicable for clinical optometry.

NEUROPLASTICITY AND OPTOMETRY

Although the definition of neuroplasticity may change somewhat between professions and between disciplines, Trojan and Pokorny (54) have defined neuroplasticity and its various iterations in a manner that fits appropriately into the patient care schema of optometrists. They note that the mechanisms associated with neuroplasticity can be the result of natural or artificial stimuli that may occur within the individuals' internal/external environment. The end results of these stimuli on neuroplasticity can be positive (or negative) and can occur during development (evolutionary neuroplasticity), after short-term exposure (reactive plasticity), and after enduring and/or uninterrupted stimuli (adaptational plasticity). They also note that neuroplasticity can occur during functional and/or structural recovery from damaged neuronal circuits (reparation plasticity).

The term *evolutionary neuroplasticity* seems ideally suited for the developmental optometrist who specializes in child development and vision function as it changes over time either with or without intervention. *Reactive plasticity* can be thought of as the immediate effect that initial optometric treatment may have on a system. This might be reflected in the immediate but often transient change in the individual's accommodative system when the uncorrected myope initially puts on his new spectacles. *Adaptational plasticity*, on the other hand, could describe the long-term effects of in-office optometric vision therapy on disorders of the binocular vision system, while *reparation plasticity* might occur during the treatment options offered by the low vision specialist or optometrist working with those who have experienced traumatic brain injury (TBI).

As the American Optometric Association definition of optometry notes: *Doctors of optometry are the primary health care professionals for the eye. Optometrists examine, diagnose, treat, and manage diseases, injuries, and disorders of the visual system, the eye, and associated structures as well as identify related systemic conditions affecting the eye* (55). When it comes to neuroplasticity, the wording "treat, and manage ... disorders of the visual system" are particularly apt.

MANAGEMENT AND TREATMENT OF DISORDERS OF THE VISUAL SYSTEM AND NEUROPLASTICITY

So what disorders of the visual system that involve neuroplasticity are most appropriate for optometrists to treat and manage? It would appear that almost any anomaly associated with visual development, vision perception, and visual function would be potential candidates. These disorders incorporate but are certainly not restricted to

1. Refractive error development
2. Amblyopia
3. Strabismus
4. Nonstrabismic, nonamblyopic binocular vision disorders
5. Learning-related vision anomalies
6. Vision development/perception disorders
7. Vision dysfunction associated with developmental disability
8. Vision dysfunction association with acquired brain injury

REFRACTIVE ERROR DEVELOPMENT

During presentations made by Earl Smith III, OD, PhD, and Kenneth Ciuffreda, OD, PhD, at the 2007 College of Optometrists in Vision Development Annual meeting, it was apparent that neuroplasticity played a significant role in refractive error development in both Dr. Smith's animal studies (56–58) or Dr. Ciuffreda's human subject results (59–61). During their presentations, both of these distinguished researchers noted how external factors (i.e., different methods of inducing retinal defocus, for example) could have an effect on the development of refractive error and speculated on how various interventions influence the development of a variety of refractive errors (e.g., myopia).

Results from research into optometric intervention in the development of refractive error and in particular decreasing myopia progression have been mixed (62). Recent studies have been much more supportive, however. Several clinical trials and other studies have noted that an alteration in an individual's visual world with positive addition lenses or drugs can decrease the magnitude of myopia development. Bifocals have been shown to slow myopic progression in children with near-point esophoria, but not necessarily in children with exophoria (63–65). Leung and Brown (66) reported that progressive lenses significantly reduced the progression of myopia in Chinese children, while another clinical trial came to a similar conclusion for Japanese children (67). The results from the Correction of Myopia Evaluation Trial also showed reduced myopic progression for those who used progressive addition lenses (68). Atropine has been shown to reduce myopia progression as well (69). Considering the possible unwanted side effects of atropine, however, a newer M_1-specific muscarinic antagonist, pirenzepine, has been introduced. This drug has fewer side effects than atropine and has been confirmed in clinical trials to slow myopia progression by almost 50% (70,71).

As optometrists, we can and should alter refractive error development (especially myopia) by using those tools readily available to us. In the not too distant future, we would imagine that additional methodologies, lens applications, drugs, and clinical approaches will be developed as well.

AMBLYOPIA

The Pediatric Eye Disease Investigator Group (PEDIG) is a research network funded by the National Eye Institute that consists of 80 distinct sites, 132 pediatric ophthalmologists, 52 pediatric optometrists, and 11 colleges of optometry. This single entity has done more to dispel the myths and expand the science surrounding amblyopia and its treatment than any other single group in modern history.

Some eye care professionals believe that response to amblyopia treatment is unlikely after the age of 6 or 7 years, while others consider age 9 or 10 years as the upper age limit for successful treatment. One of PEDIG's most significant studies dispelled the myth that you cannot treat amblyopia in older children and young adults (those under 18 years) (72). PEDIG has reported that amblyopia improves with optical correction alone in about 25% of patients aged 7 to 17 years. For patients aged 7 to 12 years, patching and atropine can improve visual acuity even if the amblyopia has been previously treated. For patients aged 13 to 17 years, patching may improve visual acuity when amblyopia has not been previously treated (45). Neuroplasticity in the older child and younger adult (and by extrapolation the adult) allows the optometrist to treat amblyopia at any age. These studies also noted that prescribing spectacles is an important first step in the treatment of amblyopia with resolution of amblyopia in at least one-third of 3- to <7-year-old children with untreated anisometropic amblyopia (73). Another study concluded that the "treatment of bilateral refractive amblyopia with spectacle correction improves binocular visual acuity in children 3 to <10 years of age, with most improving to 20/25 or better within 1 year," (74) while it was also noted in yet another PEDIG-generated paper that strabismic amblyopia can improve and even resolve with spectacle correction alone (75). Once again, the importance of the refractive care provided by an optometrist takes center stage and demonstrates that by the judicious use of spectacles, we can alter vision function in a positive way for our patients.

The PEDIG studies support evidence that has been lurking in the scientific literature for more than half a century. In a 1957 paper, Carl Kupfer demonstrated dramatic improvements in adult amblyopes after a 4-week period of patching combined with vision therapy (76). Twenty years later, Martin Birnbaum and colleagues analyzed 23 published studies on amblyopia and noted that improvements in eyesight were seen for all ages (77). A 1992 study by Wick et al. (78) found that a combination of proper lenses, part-time occlusion, and vision therapy improved acuity in the amblyopic eye of anisometropic amblyopes. Finally, perceptual learning studies and binocular approaches to amblyopia treatment have demonstrated gains in both acuity and stereopsis in adult amblyopes (79–83).

Currently PEDIG is conducting a pilot study on the efficacy of vision therapy in amblyopia. (Other PEDIG studies have given us the evidence-based science supportive of the use of atropine (84) and reduced patching times (85) for the treatment of this disorder of the visual cortex.)

We can and should diagnose and treat amblyopia for all of our patients. Age may be a factor in how we choose to treat this disorder but should seldom dictate to us the range of treatment available to our patients. Neuro- and cortical plasticity that occurs in the adult brain suggests that our treatment options are open and will continue to grow.

STRABISMUS AND NONSTRABISMIC, NONAMBLYOPIC BINOCULAR VISION DISORDERS

Dr. Mitch Scheiman (as the primary investigator) and his Convergence Insufficiency Treatment Trial colleagues have done for the treatment of binocular anomalies what the PEDIG has achieved for amblyopia. The "Randomized Clinical Trial of Treatments for Symptomatic Convergence Insufficiency in Children" clinical trial has clearly demonstrated the superiority of in-office optometric vision therapy (along with home reinforcement) as opposed to only out-of-office therapy (86) for the treatment of convergence insufficiency and noted that vision therapy/orthoptics was more effective than pencil push-ups or placebo vision therapy/orthoptics in reducing symptoms and improving clinical signs of convergence insufficiency in children and young adults (87). Some of our colleagues (88) may continue to be bound by prior biases and beliefs that will not allow them to readily accept the results of these clinical trials (89), but the science is there. It is time to make that sea change in some areas where it is personally difficult to do so.

In 1961, William Ludlam published a study on the effects of optometric vision therapy on 149 patients with strabismus, none of whom had had surgery. After the 12-week treatment period, 75% of the patients demonstrated straight eyes and binocular vision with stereopsis (90,91). These results were confirmed by several other investigators (92,93), but with the growing momentum behind the idea of the critical period, these studies were largely ignored. In 2009, neuroscientist Susan Barry published *Fixing My Gaze*, a book which documents her experience of gaining stereopsis though optometric vision therapy despite a diagnosis of esotropia in early infancy (94). A 2011 paper by Ding and Levi (95) demonstrated acquisition of stereopsis in adult strabismics through perceptual learning. These reports indicate that an irreversible critical period for the development of stereopsis may not exist and that optometric vision therapy can be an effective treatment for strabismus.

Research at the level of the clinical trial is still needed for other disorders of the binocular visual system to support the optometric approach to treatment and the neuroplasticity that we now know to be present in patients of all ages. However, the current level of science needed to be fairly confident in our approach to patient care is sufficient until those clinical trials can be completed (96). Optometric vision therapy has a strong basis in science (97–101), and if we delay treatment, oftentimes the problems do not improve (102). Let us use optometric vision therapy appropriately while taking advantage of the neuroplasticity exhibited by our patients.

LEARNING-RELATED VISION PROBLEMS AND VISION DEVELOPMENT/PERCEPTION DISORDERS

Non-clinical trial research, thus far, supports the positive effects of vision therapy on learning-related vision problems and vision development/perception disorders. This research includes the role vision plays in reading (103–105), the effect of vergence and accommodative therapy on reading eye movements and reading speed (106), and the diagnosis and treatment of perceptual disorders and the effect of therapy on various learning anomalies (107–112). Researchers at the Center for Cognitive Brian Imaging at Carnegie Mellon University used functional magnetic response imaging to detect which parts of the brain become stronger as children with reading disabilities develop their ability to read. As reported in the journal Neuropsychologia, follow-up scans 1 year after the children received 100 hours of remediation from teachers showed increased brain activation, especially in the left parietal lobe (113).

Bowan (114) and later Lack (115) wrote responses in review articles in *Optometry* to address the misleading and false statements made in various position papers by the American Academy of Pediatrics, the American Academy of Ophthalmology, and the American Association of Pediatric Ophthalmology and Strabismus. They identified more than 1,400 references from Medline and other database sources and pertinent texts that supported optometry's role in diagnosing and treating learning-related vision problems. Even so, much more needs to be done in terms of research in this area. The current research strongly appears to favor a therapeutic approach that uses neuroplasticity to its best advantage.

VISION DYSFUNCTION ASSOCIATED WITH DEVELOPMENTAL DISABILITY

Sands et al. (116) documented the lack of published research and postgraduate education in optometry and ophthalmology in the areas of the special needs patient. Wesson and Maino (117) also noted that many barriers exist that constrain those with disability from full participation within the health care arena. These barriers include but are not necessarily limited to those created by the following:

Health Care System

1. Fragmentation of the health delivery care system
2. Poor planning
3. Excessive governmental regulation
4. Low financial rewards for health care provider
5. Excessive paperwork
6. Increased provider/patient contact time

Consumer (patient)

1. Poor ability to communicate symptoms (118,119)
2. Little health care history information
3. Complex medical/behavioral problems
4. Questions about informed consent

Health Care Provider

1. Negative attitudes
2. Architectural barriers
3. Poor transportation
4. Lack of availability of health care providers
5. Poor training of health care providers

Direct Care Provider

1. Poor training
2. Excessive paperwork
3. Crisis-oriented health care

The research that does exist concerning eye care practitioners and those with disability notes that many problems are present but can be overcome with further education of eye care professionals and a reduction of negative attitudes toward those who have a disability (120,121). There is, on the other hand, a great deal of research documenting the high level of vision and vision information processing dysfunction within this population (122–130), but few articles are available when it comes to treatment.

The research that is available in the area of treatment shows that the accommodative dysfunctions and esotropia often seen in those with Down syndrome can be treated with the application of multifocal lenses (131,132) and that the accommodative anomalies (133) in the individual with cerebral palsy can be modified through the use of optometric vision therapy (134,135), as well as the application of other therapies to improve the patients' functional vision abnormalities (136,137).

Neuroplasticity is present in those with developmental disability (although it may be different than that seen in the nondisabled) (138) and is usually noted in the outcomes of such early intervention programs as Head Start (139). The research into neuroplasticity and Down syndrome appear to be only at the genetic mouse model stage (140), while in cerebral palsy, the research is starting to include clinical trials that show movement (141) as an important aspect of neuroplastic based treatment. Neuroplasticity for those with developmental disability will play a larger and larger role in our treatment of individuals with these disorders, but a great deal of research is needed to determine how we will apply the science of neuroplasticity for these special needs patients.

VISION DYSFUNCTION ASSOCIATION WITH ACQUIRED BRAIN INJURY

Functional recovery through neuroplasticity should play a major role in the management of those with acquired brain injury. Traumatic brain injury, cerebral vascular accident, and other forms of cortical insult have a significant impact on the overall visual function of your patients. Padula (142) noted that patients with posttrauma vision syndrome exhibit

1. Exotropia (or high exophoria)
2. Accommodative dysfunction
3. Convergence insufficiency
4. Decreased blink rate
5. Spatial disorientation
6. Pursuit/saccade dysfunction (143)
7. Unstable ambient vision (magnocellular pathway)

Kapoor (144) supports these syndrome findings by showing that those with traumatic brain injury often demonstrate anomalies of accommodation, version dysfunction, vergence dysfunction (both strabismic and nonstrabismic), photosensitivity, visual field integrity anomalies, and significant ocular health problems.

We have already discussed the research conducted and treatment options available for various binocular vision problems (convergence insufficiency (86,87), amblyopia (72–85)). We have not discussed, however, if oculomotor dysfunctions can be improved for those with traumatic brain injury. Ciufredda et al. (145) concluded that *Nearly all patients in* [their] *clinic sample exhibited either complete or marked reduction in … oculomotor-based symptoms and improvement in related clinical signs, with maintenance of the symptom reduction and sign improvements at the 2- to 3-month follow-up.* [Their findings showed] *the efficacy of optometric vision therapy for a range of oculomotor abnormalities in the primarily adult, mild brain-injured population. Furthermore, it* [showed] *considerable residual neural plasticity* [present within each individual] *despite the presence of documented brain injury.*

So it appears that we can improve the oculomotor abilities of those with traumatic brain injury, but what about those oculomotor skills needed while reading and the act of reading itself? Once again Ciuffreda et al. (146) showed that with optometric vision therapy rehabilitation of reading-related oculomotor skills in brain-injured patients produced significant gains in both the subjective and objective measures used to assess oculomotor ability and reading. Han et al. (147) demonstrated that these skills appear to also transfer to the activities of daily living required by those with traumatic brain injury so that their quality of life can improve.

Can the perceptual anomalies caused by brain injury be diagnosed and treated? Cortical insult can cause many visual perceptual disturbances including

1. Agnosia (inability to understand or interpret what is seen)
2. Alexia (inability to recognize or comprehend written or printed words)
3. Aphasia (inability to understand, recognize, or comprehend the spoken word)
4. Color anomia (inability to name colors)
5. Color dyschromatopsia (inability to see colors)
6. Prosopagnosia (facial recognition problems)

7. Simultanagnosia (can only recognize one element at a time)
8. Optic ataxia (mislocalization when reaching for an object) (148)

The treatment of these perceptual disorders typically takes place in the psychologist's and/or the physiatrist's office or under the care of an occupational or physical therapist and not necessarily in the office of the optometrist. Neuroplasticity is often involved in the treatment of many of these disorders, however. After treatment, patients with prosopagnosia, for instance, show improvements in facial recognition, which is accompanied by changes in the brain as measured with functional magnetic resonance imaging (149). Treatment for alexia indicates that neuroplastic changes are involved as well (150).

IMPROVING BRAIN FUNCTION AND NEUROPLASTICITY

How does nutrition affect brain function and neuroplasticity? The belief that there are "brain foods" dates back millennia. Today we see an increasing abundance of research about the use of Omega-3 fish oils for a wide range of health and cognitive benefits. Current research on the health and cognitive benefits is still somewhat mixed (151–153), but the "gut" may still be involved in how and how well our brains function (154).

It has been shown that certain drugs can also enhance neuroplasticity. These drugs include fluoxetine (155) (an antidepressant) for the use of restoring plasticity in the adult visual cortex, particularly as a complementary treatment for amblyopia, and tianeptine (156) (another antidepressant), which seems to affect glutamate, a known mediator of neuroplasticity (157). Erythropoietin (a glycoprotein hormone) (158) and L-arginine, a precursor of creatine synthesis (159), have also demonstrated an ability to stimulate neuroplasticity, but there seems to be no "magic pill" that we can currently use for ourselves or our patients.

If there is a "magical fix" for increasing neuroplasticity, it is exercise, practice, and learning activities that are new and novel (160,161). Researcher John Ratey in his book *SPARK: The Revolutionary New Science of Exercise and the Brain* examines the science of the connection between exercise and the neuroplasticity of the brain (162). He reviews how exercise affects learning, attention, stress, depression, and more.

CONCLUSION

It is obvious that the current research supports the view that neuroplasticity, and therefore functional recovery, can occur at any age. If we are to help those with special needs, we should clinically apply those research-supported therapies that promote neuroplasticity. When we do this, all of our patients benefit.

ACKNOWLEDGMENT *The article, Maino D. Neuroplasticity: Teaching an Old Brain New Tricks. Rev Optom. 2009;46(1):62–64,66–70, served as the beginning of this greatly expanded and more inclusive chapter.*

REFERENCES

1. Chakraborty R, Chatterjee A, Choudhart S, et al. Neuroplasticity-a paradigm shift in neurosciences. J Indian Med Assoc. 2007;105:513–21.
2. Sacks O. A neurologists note book: stereo sue. Why two eyes are better than one. The New Yorker. 2006 June: 64–73.
3. Going Binocular: Susan's First Snowfall. Available from: http://www.npr.org/templates/story/story.php?storyId=5507789. Last Accessed March 23, 2011.
4. Press L. The story behind "Stereo Sue" and a world-famous neurologist's discovery of vision therapy. Optom Vis Dev. 2006;37:55–7.
5. Levin HS. Neuroplasticity and brain imaging research: implications for rehabilitation. Arch Phys Med Rehabil. 2006;87:S1.
6. Wiesel TN, Hubel DH. Single-cell responses in striate cortex of kittens deprived of vision in one eye. J Neurophysiol. 1963;26:1003–17.
7. Hensch TK. Critical period plasticity in local cortical circuits. Nat Rev Neurosci. 2005;6:877–88.
8. Sengpiel F. The critical period. Curr Biol. 2007;17:R742–3.
9. Wiesel TN, Hubel DH. Effects of visual deprivation on morphology and physiology of cells in the cat's lateral geniculate body. J Neurophysiol. 1963;26:978–93.
10. Hubel DH, Wiesel TN. The period of susceptibility to the physiological effects of unilateral eye closure in kittens. J Physiol. 1970;206:419–36.
11. Horton JC, Stryker MP. Amblyopia induced by anisometropia without shrinkage of ocular dominance columns in human striate cortex. Proc Natl Acad Sci U S A. 1993;90:5494–8.
12. van Praag H, Kempermann G, Gage FH. Running increases cell proliferation and neurogenesis in the adult mouse dentate gyrus. Nat Neurosci. 1999;2:266–70.
13. Gould E, Beylin A, Tanapat P, et al. Learning enhances adult neurogenesis in the hippocampal formation. Nat Neurosci. 1999;2:260–5.
14. Gould E, McEwen BS, Tanapat P, et al. Neurogenesis in the dentate gyrus of the adult tree shrew is regulated by psychosocial stress and NMDA receptor activation. J Neurosci. 1999;17:2492–8.

15. Sale A, Maya Vetencourt JF, Medini P, et al. Environmental enrichment in adulthood promotes amblyopia recovery through a reduction of intracortical inhibition. Nat Neurosci. 2007;10:679–81.
16. Hooks BM, Chen C. Critical periods in the visual system: changing views for a model of experience-dependent plasticity. Neuron. 2007;56:312–26.
17. Sengpiel F. Visual cortex: overcoming a No-Go plasticity. Curr Biol. 2005;15:R1000–2.
18. McGee AW, Yang Y, Fisher QS, et al. Experience-driven plasticity of visual cortex limited by myelin and Nogo receptor. Science. 2005;309:2222–6.
19. Knudsen EI. Sensitive periods in the development of brain and behavior. J Cogn Neurosci. 2004;16:1412–25.
20. Ramey CT, Ramey SL. Prevention of intellectual disabilities: early interventions to improve cognitive development. Prev Med. 1998;27:224–32.
21. Heuninckx S, Wenderoth N, Swinnen SP. Systems neuroplasticity in the aging brain: recruiting additional neural resources for successful motor performance in elderly persons. J Neurosci. 2008;28:91–9.
22. Bergan JF, Ro P, Ro D, Knudsen EI. Hunting increases adaptive auditory map plasticity in adult barn owls. J Neurosci. 2005;25(42):9816–20.
23. Bao S, Chang EF, Davis JD, et al. Progressive degradation and subsequent refinement of acoustic representations in the adult auditory cortex. J Neurosci. 2003;26:10765–75.
24. Keuroghlian AS, Knudsen EI. Adaptive auditory plasticity in developing and adult animals. Prog Neurobiol. 2007;82:109–21.
25. Taub E, Uswatte G, Mark VW, Morris DM. The learned nonuse phenomenon: Implications for rehabilitation. Eura Medicophys. 2006;42:241–56.
26. Morris DM, Taub E, Mark VW. Constraint-induced movement therapy: characterizing the intervention protocol. Eura Medicophys. 2006;42:257–68.
27. Altman J. Are new neurons formed in the brains of adult mammals? Science. 1962;135:1127–8.
28. Gage FH. Neurogenesis in the adult brain. J Neurosci. 2002;22:612–3.
29. Kemperman G, Wiskott L, Gage FH. Functional significance of adult neurogenesis. Curr Opin Neurobiol. 2004;14:186–91.
30. Eriksson PS, Perfilieva E, Björk-Eriksson T, et al. Neurogenesis in the adult human hippocampus. Nat Med. 1998;4:1313–7.
31. Hofer SB, Mrsic-Flogel TD, Bonhoeffer T, et al. Experience leaves a lasting structural trace in cortical circuits. Nature. 2009;457:313–7.
32. Uylings HBM, Kuypers K, Diamond MC, et al. Effects of differential environments on plasticity of dendrites of cortical pyramidal neurons in adult rats. Exp Neurol. 1978;62:658–77.
33. Greenough WT, Withers GS, Wallace CS. Morphological changes in the nervous system arising from behavioral experience: what is evidence that they are involved in learning and memory? In: Squire LR, Lindenlaub E, editors. The biology of memory. Stuttgart: Schattauer; 1990. p. 159–92.
34. Jurask JM. Sex differences in cognition regions of the rat brain. Psychoneuroendocrinology. 1991;16:105–19.
35. Kandel ER. In search of memory: the emergence of a new science of mind. New York: W W Norton and Co.; 2006.
36. Pascual-Leone A, Torres F. Plasticity of the sensorimotor cortex representation of the reading finger of braille readers. Brain. 1993:116:39–52.
37. Beck H, Yaari Y. Plasticity of intrinsic properties in CNS disorders. Nat Rev Neurosci. 2008;9:357–69.
38. Draganski B, Gaser C, Busch V, et al. Neuroplasticity: changes in grey matter induced by training. Nature. 2004;427:311–2.
39. Cannonieri GC, Bonilha L, Fernandes PT, et al. Practice and perfect: length of training and structural brain changes in experienced typists. Neuroreport. 2007;18:1063–6.
40. Herlenius E, Lagercrantz H. Development of neurotransmitter systems during critical periods. Exp Neurol. 2004;190:S8–21.
41. Lewis DA, Sesack SR. Dopamine systems in the primate brain. In: Bjorklund A, Hokfelt T, Bloom FE, editors. Handbook of clinical neuroanatomy. New York: Elsevier; 1984. p. 263–375.
42. Uylings HBN, Delalle I. Morphology of neuropeptide Y-immunoreactive neurons and fibers in human prefrontal cortex during prenatal and postnatal development. J Comp Neurol. 1997;379:541–50.
43. Delalle I, Evers P, Kostovic I, et al. Laminar distribution of neuropeptide-Y immunoreactive neuron in human prefrontal cortex during development. J Comp Neurol. 1997;379:523–40.
44. Uylings HBN, Delalle I, Petanjek A, et al. Structural and immunocytochemical differentiation of neurons in prenatal and postnatal human prefrontal cortex. Neuroembryology. 2002;1:176–86.
45. Kostovic I, Lukinovic N, Judas M, et al. Structural basis of the developmental plasticity in the human cerebral cortex: the role of the transient subplate zone. Metab Brain Dis. 1989;4:17–23.
46. Goldman-Rakic PS, Brown RM. Postnatal development of monoamine content and systhesis in the cerebral cortex of rhesus monkeys. Dev Brain Res. 1982;4:339–49.
47. Kalsbeek A, DeBruin JPC, Feenstra MGP, et al. Age-dependent effects of lesioning the mesocortical dopamine system upon prefrontal cortex morphometry and PFC-related behaviors. Pro Brain Res. 1990;85:257–83.
48. Cooper JR, Bloom FE, Roth RH. The biochemical basis of neuropharmacology. New York: Oxford University Press; 2002.
49. Gu Q. Neuromodulatory transmitter systems in the cortex and their role in cortical plasticity. Neuroscience. 2002;111:815–35.
50. Ge S, Yang CH, Hsu KS, et al. A critical period for enhanced synaptic plasticity in newly generated neurons of the adult brain. Neuron. 2007;54:559–66.
51. Huang JC. Neuroplasticity as a proposed mechanism for the efficacy of optometric vision therapy and rehabilitation. J Behav Optom. 2009;20:95–9.
52. Xerri C, Merzenich MM, Peterson BE, Jenkins W. Plasticity of primary somatosensory cortex paralleling sensorimotor skill recovery from stroke in adult monkeys. J Neurophysiol. 1998;79:2119–48.
53. Kleim JA, Jones TA. Principles of experience-dependent neural plasticity: implications for rehabilitation after brain damage. J Speech Lang Hear Res. 2008;51:S225–39.
54. Trojan S, Porkorny J. Theoretical aspects of neuroplasticity. Physiol Res. 1999;48:87–9.
55. American Optometric Association. Available from: http://www.aoa.org/. Last accessed March 24, 2011.

56. Ramamirtham R, Kee CS, Hung LF, et al. Wave aberrations in rhesus monkeys with vision-induced ametropias. Vision Res. 2007;47:2751–66.
57. Smith EL III, Ramamirtham R, Qiao-Grider Y, et al. Effects of foveal ablation on emmetropization and form-deprivation myopia. Invest Ophthalmol Vis Sci. 200;48:3914–22.
58. Smith EL III, Kee CS, Ramamirtham R, et al. Peripheral vision can influence eye growth and refractive development in infant monkeys. Invest Ophthalmol Vis Sci. 2005;46:3965–72.
59. Ciuffreda KJ, Vasudevan B. Nearwork-induced transient myopia (NITM) and permanent myopia—is there a link? Ophthalmic Physiol Opt. 2008;28:103–14.
60. Hung GK, Ciuffreda KJ. Incremental retinal-defocus theory of myopia development–schematic analysis and computer simulation. Comput Biol Med. 2007;37:930–46.
61. Hung GK, Ciuffreda KJ. A unifying theory of refractive error development. Bull Math Biol. 2000;62:1087–108.
62. Pang Y, Maino D, Zhang G, Lu F. Myopia: can its progress be controlled? Optom Vis Dev. 2006;37:75–9.
63. Fulk GW, Cyert LA, Parker DE. A randomized trial of the effect of single-vision vs. bifocal lenses on myopia progression in children with esophoria. Optom Vis Sci. 2000;77:395–401.
64. Fulk GW. Is esophoria a factor in slowing of myopia by progressive lenses? Optom Vis Sci. 2003;80:198–9.
65. Goss DA, Jyesugi EF. Effectiveness of bifocal control of childhood myopia progression as a function of near point phoria and binocular cross cylinder. J Optom Vis Dev. 1995;26:12–7.
66. Leung JT, Brown B. Progression of myopia in Hong Kong Chinese schoolchildren is slowed by wearing progressive lenses. Optom Vis Sci. 1999;76:346–54.
67. Hasebe S, Ohtsuki H, Nonaka T, et al. Effect of progressive addition lenses on myopia progression in Japanese children: a prospective, randomized, double-masked, crossover trial. Invest Ophthalmol Vis Sci. 2008;49:2781–9.
68. Gwiazda J, Hyman L, Hussein M, et al. A randomized clinical trial of progressive addition lenses versus single vision lenses on the progression of myopia in children. Invest Ophthalmol Vis Sci. 2003;44:1492–500.
69. Shih YF, Hsiao CK, Chen CJ, et al. An intervention trial on efficacy of atropine and multi-focal glasses in controlling myopic progression. Acta Ophthalmol Scand. 2001;79:233–6.
70. Siatkowski RM, Cotter SA, Crockett RS, et al. U.S. Pirenzepine Study Group. Two-year multicenter, randomized, double-masked, placebo-controlled, parallel safety and efficacy study of 2% pirenzepine ophthalmic gel in children with myopia. J AAPOS. 2008;12:332–9.
71. Tan DT, Lam DS, Chua WH, et al. One-year multicenter, double-masked, placebo-controlled, parallel safety and efficacy study of 2% pirenzepine ophthalmic gel in children with myopia. Ophthalmology. 2005;112:84–91.
72. Scheiman MM, Hertle RW, Beck RW, et al. Randomized trial of treatment of amblyopia in children aged 7 to 17 years. Arch Ophthalmol. 2005;123:437–47.
73. Cotter SA, Edwards AR, Wallace DK, et al. Treatment of anisometropic amblyopia in children with refractive correction. Ophthalmology. 2006;113:895–903.
74. Wallace DK, Chandler DL, Beck RW, et al. Treatment of bilateral refractive amblyopia in children three to less than 10 years of age. Am J Ophthalmol. 2007;144:487–96.
75. Cotter SA, Edwards AR, Arnold RW, et al. Treatment of strabismic amblyopia with refractive correction. Am J Ophthalmol. 2007;143:1060–3.
76. Kupfer C. Treatment of amblyopia ex anopsia in adults; a preliminary report of seven cases. Am J Ophthalmol. 1957;43:918–22.
77. Birnbaum MH, Koslowe K, Sanet R. Success in amblyopia therapy as a function of age: a literature survey. Am J Optom Physiol Opt. 1977;54:269–75.
78. Wick B, Wingard M, Cotter S, Scheiman M. Anisometropic amblyopia: is the patient ever too old to treat? Optom Vis Sci. 1992;69:866–78.
79. Levi DM. Perceptual learning in adults with amblyopia: a reevaluation of critical periods in human vision. Dev Psychobiol. 2005;46:222–32.
80. Polat U, Levi DM. Neural plasticity in adults with amblyopia. Proc Natl Acad Sci U S A. 1996;93:6830–4.
81. Hess RF, Mansouri B, Thompson B. A binocular approach to treating amblyopia: antisuppression therapy. Optom Vis Sci. 2010;87:697–704.
82. Xu JP, He ZJ, Ooi TL. Effectively reducing a sensory eye dominance with a push-pull perceptual learning protocol. Curr Biol. 2010;20:1864–8.
83. Astle AT, McGraw PV, Webb BS. Can amblyopia be treated in adulthood? Strabismus. 2011;19:99–109.
84. Repka MX, Wallace DK, Beck RW, et al. Two-year follow-up of a 6-month randomized trial of atropine vs. patching for treatment of moderate amblyopia in children. Arch Ophthalmol. 2005;123:149–57.
85. Wallace DK; Pediatric Eye Disease Investigator Group, Edwards AR, et al. A randomized trial to evaluate 2 hours of daily patching for strabismic and anisometropic amblyopia in children. Ophthalmology. 2006;113:904–12.
86. Scheiman M, Mitchell GL, Cotter S, Cooper J, et al. A randomized clinical trial of treatments for convergence insufficiency in children. Arch Ophthalmol. 2005;123:14–24.
87. Scheiman M, Mitchell GL, Cotter S, Kulp MT, et al. A randomized clinical trial of vision therapy/orthoptics versus pencil pushups for the treatment of convergence insufficiency in young adults. Optom Vis Sci. 2005;82:583–95.
88. Wallace D. Treatment options for symptomatic convergence insufficiency. Arch Ophthalmol. 2008;126:1455–6.
89. Maino D. An open letter to David K Wallace MD, MPH (and other disbelievers and holders of outdated and biased opinions and beliefs). Optom Vis Dev. 2008;39:169–70.
90. Ludlam WM. Orthoptic treatment of strabismus: a study of one hundred forty nine non-operated, unselected, concomitant strabismus patients completing orthoptic training at the Optometric Center of New York. Am J Optom Arch Am Acad Optom. 1961;38:369–88.
91. Ludlam WM, Kleinman BI. The long range results of orthoptic treatment of strabismus. Am J Optom Arch Am Acad Optom. 1965;42:647–84.
92. Etting GL. Strabismus therapy in private practice: cure rates after three months of therapy. J Am Optom Assoc. 1978;49:1367–73.
93. Flax N, Duckman RH. Orthoptic treatment of strabismus. Am Optom Assoc. 1978;49:1353–61.
94. Barry SR. Fixing my gaze: A scientist's journey into seeing in three dimensions. New York: Basic Books; 2009.

95. Ding J, Levi DM. Recovery of stereopsis through perceptual learning in human adults with abnormal binocualr vision. Proc Natl Acad Sci U S A. 2011;108:E733–41.
96. Hunter D. Do we need evidence for everything? Am Orthopt J. 2010;60;59–62.
97. Ciuffreda KJ. The scientific basis for and efficacy of optometric vision therapy in nonstrabismic accommodative and vergence disorders. Optometry. 2002;73:735–62.
98. Brautaset R, Wahlberg M, Abdi S, et al. Accommodation insufficiency in children: are exercises better than reading glasses? Strabismus. 2008;16:65–9.
99. Sterner B, Abrahamsson M, Sjöström A. The effects of accommodative facility training on a group of children with impaired relative accommodation—a comparison between dioptric treatment and sham treatment. Ophthalmic Physiol Opt. 2001;21:470–6.
100. SGrisham JD, Bowman MC, Owyang LA, et al. Vergence orthoptics: validity and persistence of the training effect. Optom Vis Sci. 1991;68:441–51.
101. Maples WC, Bither M. Efficacy of vision therapy as assessed by the COVD quality of life checklist. Optometry. 2002;73:492–8.
102. Tassinari JT. Untreated oculomotor dysfunction. Optom Vis Dev. 2007;38:121–4.
103. Vidyasagar TR. Neural underpinnings of dyslexia as a disorder of visuo-spatial attention. Clin Exp Optom. 2004;87:4–10.
104. Solan HA, Shelley-Tremblay J, Hansen PC, et al. M-cell deficit and reading disability: a preliminary study of the effects of temporal vision-processing therapy. Optometry. 2004;75:640–50.
105. Solan HA, Larson S, Shelley-Tremblay J, Ficarra A, et al. Role of visual attention in cognitive control of oculomotor readiness in students with reading disabilities. J Learn Disabil. 2001;34:107–18.
106. Gallaway M, Boas MB. The impact of vergence and accommodative therapy on reading eye movements and reading speed. Optom Vis Dev. 2007;38:115–20.
107. Goss DA, Downing DB, Lowther AH, et al. The effect of HTS vision therapy conducted in a school setting on reading skills in third and fourth grade students. Optom Vis Dev. 2007;38:27–32.
108. Crutch SJ, Warrington EK. Foveal crowding in posterior cortical atrophy: a specific early-visual-processing deficit affecting word reading. Cogn Neuropsychol. 2007;24:843–66.
109. Helms D, Sawtelle SM. A study of the effectiveness of cognitive therapy delivered in a video game format. Optom Vis Dev. 2007;38:19–26.
110. Lawton T. Training direction-discrimination sensitivity remediates a wide spectrum of reading skills. Optom Vis Dev. 2007:38:33–47.
111. Goldstand S, Koslowe KC, Parush S. Vision, visual-information processing, and academic performance among seventh-grade schoolchildren: a more significant relationship than we thought? Am J Occup Ther. 2005;59:377–89.
112. Fischer B, Köngeter A, Hartnegg K. Effects of daily practice on subitizing, visual counting, and basic arithmetic skills. Optom Vis Dev. 2008:39:30–4.
113. Meyler A, Keller T, Cherkassky V, et al. Modifying the brain activation of poor readers during sentence comprehensions with extended remedial instruction: a longitudinal study of neruoplasticity. Neuropsychologia. 2008;46:2580–92.
114. Bowan MD. Learning disabilities, dyslexia, and vision: a subject review—a rebuttal, literature review, and commentary. Optometry. 2002;73:553–75.
115. Lack D. Another joint statement regarding learning disabilities, dyslexia, and vision—a rebuttal. Optometry. 2010;81:533–43.
116. Sands W, Taub M, Maino D. Limited research and education on special populations in optometry and ophthalomology. Optom Vis Dev. 2008;39:60–1.
117. Wesson M, Maino D. Oculo-visual findings in Down syndrome, cerebral palsy, and mental retardation with non-specific etiology. In: Maino D, editor. Diagnosis and management of special populations. St. Louis: Mosby-Yearbook, Inc.; 1995. p. 17–54. Reprinted Optometric Education Program Foundation, Santa Anna, CA. 2001.
118. Cui Y, Stapleton F, Suttle C. Developing an instrument to assess vision-related and subjective quality of life in children with intellectual disability: data collection and preliminary analysis in a Chinese population. Ophthalmic Physiol Opt. 2008;28;238–46.
119. Donati RJ, Maino DM, Bartell H, et al. Polypharmacy and the lack of oculo-visual complaints from those with mental illness and dual diagnosis (MI/ID). Optometry. 2009;80:249–54.
120. Maino D, Steele G, Tahir S, et al. Attitudes of optometry students toward individuals with disabilities. Optom Ed. 2002;27:45–50.
121. Maino D. Special populations in the optometric curriculum. Optom Ed. 2002;27:38–9.
122. Maino D. Overview of special populations. In: Scheiman M, Rouse M, editors. Optometric management of learning related vision problems. St. Louis: Mosby Inc.; 2006. p. 85–106.
123. McCarthy P, Maino D. Alport syndrome: a review. Clin Eye Vis Care. 2001;12:139–50.
124. Block SS, Brusca-Vega R, Pizzi WJ, et al. Cognitive and visual processing skills and their relationship to mutation size in full and permutation female fragile x carriers. Optom Vis Sci. 2000;77:592–9.
125. Maino D. The young child with developmental disabilities: An introduction to mental retardation and genetic syndromes. In: Moore BD, editor. Eye care for infants and young children. Newton: Butterworth—Heinemann; 1997. p. 285–300.
126. Amin V, Maino D. The Fragile X female: visual, visual perceptual, and ocular health anomalies. J Am Optom Assoc. 1995;66:290–5.
127. Maino DM, Maino JH, Cibis GW, et al. Ocular health anomalies in patients with developmental disabilities. In: Maino D, editor. Diagnosis and management of special populations. St. Louis: Mosby-Yearbook, Inc.; 1995:189–206. Reprinted Optometric Education Program Foundation, Santa Anna, CA. 2001.
128. Maino D, Wesson M, Schlange D, et al. Optometric findings in the fragile X syndrome. Optom Vis Sci. 1991;68:634–40.
129. Scheiman MM. Optometric findings in children with cerebral palsy. Am J Optom Physiol Opt. 1984;61:321–3.
130. Maino D, Maino J, Maino S. Mental retardation syndromes with associated ocular defects. J Am Optom Assoc. 1990;61:707–16.

131. Stewart RE, Woodhouse JM, Cregg M, et al. Association between accommodative accuracy, hypermetropia, and strabismus in children with Down's syndrome. Optom Vis Sci. 2007;84:149–55.
132. Cregg M, Woodhouse JM, Pakeman VH, et al. Accommodation and refractive error in children with Down syndrome: cross-sectional and longitudinal studies. Invest Ophthalmol Vis Sci. 2001;42:55–63.
133. McClelland JF, Parkes J, Hill N, et al. Accommodative dysfunction in children with cerebral palsy: a population-based study. Invest Ophthalmol Vis Sci. 2006;47:1824–30.
134. Duckman RH. Vision therapy for the child with cerebral palsy. J Am Optom Assoc. 1987;58:28–35.
135. Duckman R. Accommodation in cerebral palsy: function and remediation. J Am Optom Assoc. 1984:55(4);281–3.
136. Scheiman M. Understanding and managing vision deficits: a guide for occupational therapists. 2nd ed. Horofare, NJ: Slack; 2002.
137. Maino D. Binasal occlusion for the child with cerebral palsy. J Ill Optom Assoc. 1986;44:12,18.
138. Battaglia F, Quartarone A, Rizzo V, et al. Early impairment of synaptic plasticity in patients with Down's syndrome. Neurobiol Aging. 2008;29:1272–5.
139. Bonnier C. Evaluation of early stimulation programs for enhancing brain development. Acta Paediatr. 2008;97: 853–8.
140. Morice E, Andreae LC, Cooke SF, et al. Preservation of long-term memory and synaptic plasticity despite short-term impairments in the Tc1 mouse model of Down syndrome. Learn Mem. 2008;15:492–500.
141. Gordon AM, Schneider JA, Chinnan A, et al. Efficacy of a hand-arm bimanual intensive therapy (HABIT) in children with hemiplegic cerebral palsy: a randomized control trial. Dev Med Child Neurol. 2007;49:830–8.
142. Padula W. Neuro-optometric rehabilitation. Santa Ana: Optometric Extension Program Foundation; 2000:179–93.
143. Ciuffreda KJ, Kapoor N, Rutner D, et al. Occurrence of oculomotor dysfunctions in acquired brain injury: a retrospective analysis. Optometry. 2007;78:155–61.
144. Kapoor N, Ciuffreda KJ. Vision disturbances following traumatic brain injury. Curr Treat Options Neurol. 2002;4:271–80.
145. Ciuffreda KJ, Rutner D, Kapoor N, et al. Vision therapy for oculomotor dysfunctions in acquired brain injury: a retrospective analysis. Optometry. 2008;79:18–22.
146. Ciuffreda KJ, Han Y, Kapoor N, Ficarra AP. Oculomotor rehabilitation for reading in acquired brain injury. NeuroRehabilitation. 2006;21(1):9–21.
147. Han Y, Ciuffreda KJ, Kapoor N. Reading-related oculomotor testing and training protocols for acquired brain injury in humans. Brain Res Brain Res Protoc. 2004;14:1–12.
148. Zost M. Diagnosis and management of visual dysfunction in cerebral injury. In Maino D, editor. Diagnosis and management of special populations. St. Louis: Mosby-Yearbook, Inc.; 1995. Reprinted Optometric Education Program Foundation, Santa Anna, CA. 2001.
149. DeGutis JM, Bentin S, Robertson LC, et al. Functional plasticity in ventral temporal cortex following cognitive rehabilitation of a congenital prosopagnosic. J Cogn Neurosci. 2007;19:1790–802.
150. Welbourne SR, Ralph MA. Exploring the impact of plasticity-related recovery after brain damage in a connectionist model of single-word reading. Cogn Affect Behav Neurosci. 2005;5:77–92.
151. Jia X, McNeill G, Avenell A. Does taking vitamin, mineral and fatty acid supplements prevent cognitive decline? A systematic review of randomized controlled trials. J Hum Nutr Diet. 2008;21:317–36.
152. Henriksen C, Haugholt K, Lindgren M, et al. Improved cognitive development among preterm infants attributable to early supplementation of human milk with docosahexaenoic acid and arachidonic acid. Pediatrics. 2008;121:1137–45.
153. Kidd PM. Omega-3 DHA and EPA for cognition, behavior, and mood: clinical findings and structural-functional synergies with cell membrane phospholipids. Altern Med Rev. 2007;12:207–27.
154. Gomez-Pinilla F. Brain foods: the effect of nutrients on brain function. Neuroscience. 2008;9:568–78.
155. Maya Vetencourt JF, Sale A, Viegi A, et al. The antidepressant fluoxetine restores plasticity in the adult visual cortex. Science. 2008;320:385–8.
156. Kasper S, McEwen BS. Neurobiological and clinical effects of the antidepressant tianeptine. CNS Drugs. 2008;22:15–26.
157. Tartar JL, King MA, Devine DP. Glutamate-mediated neuroplasticity in a limbic input to the hypothalamus. Stress. 2006;9:13–9.
158. Adamcio B, Sargin D, Stradomska A, et al. Erythropoietin enhances hippocampal long-term potentiation and memory. BMC Biol. 2008;6:37.
159. Chilosi A, Leuzzi V, Battini R, et al. Treatment with L-arginine improves neuropsychological disorders in a child with creatine transporter defect. Neurocase. 2008;14:151–61.
160. Forrester LW, Wheaton LA, Luft AR. Exercise-mediated locomotor recovery and lower-limb neuroplasticity after stroke. J Rehabil Res Dev. 2008;45:205–20.
161. Driemeyer J, Boyke J, Gaser C, Büchel C, et al. Changes in Gray Matter Induced by Learning—Revisited. PLoS ONE 3(7): e2669. doi:10.1371/ journal.pone.0002669. www.pubmedcentral.nih.gov/picrender.fcgi?artid=2447176&blobtype=pdf. Last accessed March 23, 2011.
162. Ratey JR. SPARK: the revolutionary new science of exercise and the brain. New York: Little-Brown and Company; 2008.

CHAPTER 25

Samantha Slotnick, OD, FAAO, FCOVD
Curt Baxstrom, OD, FAAO, FCOVD, FNORA
Jason Clopton, OD, FCOVD

Optometric Management of Functional Vision Disorders

INTRODUCTION

This chapter addresses the optometric management of functional vision disorders for patients with special needs. (Information concerning the diagnosis and treatment of ocular disease and pathology can be found in Chapter 22, Diagnosis and Treatment of Commonly Diagnosed Ocular Health Anomalies.) Lenses and prisms are the primary tools by which eye care providers can facilitate binocularity, promote visual comfort, and enhance visual performance. For many eye care providers and most of the general public, spectacles are prescribed for refractive compensation (to improve the quality of the image on the retina). They may also be prescribed for therapeutic use to relieve visual stress, improve binocular performance, or shift and slant images relative to the patient's field of view. Additional options for refractive intervention include the use of contact lenses and the consideration of refractive surgery.

More active management of a patient's vision and visual development is often achieved with the therapeutic use of occlusion and in-office or home-based optometric vision therapy (OVT). If OVT is unable to achieve the desired goal of binocularity, strabismus surgery can be considered when appropriate.

SPECTACLES

A simple spectacle correction can substantially improve the quality of life of any patient (1) including those with special needs. These patients are often overlooked since they are less apt to complain (2) or to advocate for themselves. They may simply lack the frame of reference to know that their vision quality can be improved from the way they see currently. A recent study indicated that in a population of 148 adults with intellectual disabilities, 41% of subjects could have benefited from a distance spectacle prescription and 56% from a near spectacle prescription (3).

Balanced Binocular Prescription There are a number of different ways in which the term "balanced" is applied to spectacle prescriptions. In patients who have significantly reduced vision in one eye, the term "balance" is used to describe the use of a lens in front of the nonseeing eye, which is matched in power to the lens in front of the favored eye. In the context of this chapter, a "balanced" prescription refers to the best binocular prescription for the patient. This may be achieved by either balancing the accommodative demand between the two eyes or by balancing the lens power (i.e., providing equal powers) to the two eyes.

The initial refractive evaluation should objectively determine the refractive state, with traditional distance retinoscopy as a starting point. Fixation might be difficult to control. Many clinicians find it helpful to use distance moving targets, such as a video on a monitor, or even a parent/guardian displaying a variety of objects of interest. If sufficient accommodative control cannot be achieved with objects and toys at distance, cycloplegic refraction, using cyclopentolate or tropicamide, serves as a useful tool (4,5). If 1% cyclopentolate is used to achieve cycloplegia, patients with light irides should be assessed within 10 minutes of instillation for maximum cycloplegia, while patients with dark irides require 30 to 40 minutes for maximum cycloplegia (6).

Generally, where significant refractive error is present, distance correction should be prescribed to provide the least amount of refractive correction that provides the best visual acuity (7). The full amount of cylinder often is not needed and may actually be problematic for adaptation. While cylinder may provide a sharp focus on the retina, it also creates some spatial distortions, particularly at oblique axes. However, when viewing binocularly, cylinder power can be reduced without sacrificing binocular visual acuity (8). It is recommended to attempt to reduce cylinder correction in each eye under binocular viewing conditions (8). Where an accurate endpoint is difficult to obtain, a spherical equivalent is a good approximate (9).

There are some variations in prescribing patterns among eye care professionals (10–12). Optometrists and German ophthalmologists show a general trend of undercorrecting hyperopia and astigmatism (13,14). These two groups tend to fully correct differences in ametropia to achieve a binocular balance in cases of anisometropia. Members of the American Association for Pediatric Ophthalmology and Strabismus tend to have a somewhat higher threshold before prescribing for astigmatism or astigmatic anisometropia (15,16). The correction of any anisometropia and isometropia is an important factor to consider for the prevention of amblyopia (17).

Practitioners use near-point retinoscopy to compare the refractive states between the two eyes while engaged at near point (18,19). Prescribing an appropriate refractive correction for near is important for children and adults of all ages with and without disability. This is particularly important for appropriate visual development in children and improved quality of life for adults and those with developmental delay. Anomalies in accommodative function can result in differences between the distance and near refractive states (20). It should not be surprising then that some individuals may benefit from unequal near adds. Please refer to Chapter 16, Comprehensive Examination Procedures, for considerations in testing and evaluating this population.

Prescribing For Near Whether accommodative skills are insufficient, or the binocular posture is stressful without accommodative support, a near-point prescription should optimize comfort at near point. Near-point spectacles should be prescribed for use for all visual demands within arms' reach. Keep in mind that younger children have smaller arm lengths, adults come in different sizes, and patients with physical handicaps often have restrictions in movement. When prescribing for near, all of the physical attributes of the patient and their near-point demands should be taken into account. A patient's accommodative response to a lens combination can be directly observed using dynamic near-point retinoscopy rather than relying on subjective response (19,21,22).

Prescriptions for near can be issued as a single vision lens or as a bifocal/multifocal. A single vision lens for near might be the optimal way to assist an emmetropic patient, but the lens will usually blur distance vision. Special considerations should be made for communication devices and computers where patients with special needs have a relatively short working distance. Younger patients and those with special needs may find it cumbersome to repeatedly take their glasses on and off for visual demands at different distances, so bifocal/multifocal lenses should be considered as an alternative treatment modality.

Multifocal Designs Multifocal lens designs should be considered when both distance and near visual needs cannot be met with a single lens, regardless of the refractive status. Lens design choice should be based on the patients' ability to function in their environment. In a classroom setting, visual requirements at both distance and near might necessitate a multifocal design. Adult patients and patients with poor accommodative systems should be presented with the option of multifocal lenses.

Myopic children using progressive addition lenses (PALs) show no ill effect on distance visual acuity (23) and a significant decrease in myopic progression relative to myopic children wearing a fully corrected single-vision distance prescription (24). Nonpresbyopic patients with asthenopic complaints might be better served with PALs than with single-vision lenses for ease of use with all near-point activities (25). In those individuals with limited head control, one should also consider the use of a wide flat top bifocal (such as FT-35) that allows the patient to have a wider view at near with minimal head movement. The benefit of a bifocal design in patients with Down syndrome has been well documented (26–28). This may be due in part to a lack of ability to control the accommodative system neurologically, as opposed to a physiological inability to accommodate (29).

Bifocals Versus Multifocals Bifocals offer the advantage of clear distance and near vision without peripheral distortion. Patients with acquired brain injury (ABI) and vestibular disorders commonly do better without the distortion of PALs. The use of bifocals enables clinicians to prescribe precisely for the patient's needs. This may be particularly important when the doctor seeks to control the prescription to the nearest 0.125 D. The variations in refractive power over the area of a PAL are beyond the control of the prescribing doctor. Flat top bifocals provide an easy discrimination between distance and near with minimal image jump.

Round segment bifocals may be used to minimize the appearance of the segment. A digitally surfaced round segment, manufactured by Three Rivers Optical, cosmetically minimizes the appearance of the segment. This lens is similar in appearance to a progressive lens but maintains two distinct optical areas, avoiding peripheral lens distortion (30). There is some subtle distortion at the segment interface, to which patients may or may not be sensitive. The "O-Seg" minimizes the transition zone to about 1 mm, whereas the "O-Blend" softens the transition and extends it to 3 mm. In our experience, the O-Seg is most comfortable for patients.

Low Add Multifocals: Antifatigue Lenses Progressive addition lenses should be considered, particularly for presbyopic patients; however, some training time and instruction is required. They are not optimal for many young special needs patients who are capable of accommodating but demonstrate poor accommodative control. In addition, PALs may induce symptoms including disturbances in distance vision, vertigo in lateral gaze, and difficulty ascending and descending stairs (22).

In patients in need of a very low add, there are several modest PALs available which are marketed as "antifatigue" lenses. These lenses have an add of about +0.60 with some designs offering a small amount of base-in prism in the reading portion (varies by lens power) (31,32).

PRISMS

Prisms shift images and redistribute light. Prisms are often used to help a patient coordinate the eyes with reduced effort (compensatory prism). Prisms may be placed in the same orientation in front of both eyes (yoked prism). Yoked prism shifts images (left, right, up or down) to facilitate patient comfort and efficiency when performing various tasks. Prisms are also frequently used for their ability to alter the appearance of images (spatial effects of prism). For example, a small amount of base-in prism ($\frac{1}{2}^{\Delta}$ to $1\frac{1}{2}^{\Delta}$) will subtly expand the image in the horizontal plane.

Horizontal Compensatory Prism Prisms are often used to reduce the fusional demand or asthenopia experienced by patients with intermittent strabismus or a heterophoria of high magnitude. The use of horizontal prism should be considered when its use facilitates binocular alignment. This is particularly true for patients with intermittent exotropia. Historically, Sheard's* and Percival's† criteria have been used as guidelines for prescribing prism. However, their clinical validities have not been proven (33).

It is important to confirm that the patient is capable of single binocular vision before prescribing any prism for strabismus. When prism for patients with a constant esotropia or exotropia is used, it is often done in conjunction with an active OVT program.

When prescribing compensatory prism, be sensitive to the potential for differences between visual demands at distance and near. If a significant different amount of prism is needed for distance and near, either separate spectacles should be considered or a Fresnel prism may be applied to a segment of the lens, either in the bifocal portion of the spectacle lens(es) or in the distance portion.

Vertical Prism Vertical prism compensation, whether complete or partial, may enable an enhanced range of binocular function (34). If the patient has a significant vertical phoria and has not previously worn a vertical prism correction, the clinician should trial frame the prescription and reassess the near point of convergence, stereoacuity, and

*Sheard's criterion states that the fusional reserve (i.e., compensating range) should be at least twice the fusional demand (i.e., phoria).

†Percival's criterion recommends supplementing with prism in order to place a patient in the center third of the zone of clear and single binocular vision, accounting for the overall fusional range, Base-in through Base-out.

fusional vergence ranges in free space. An improvement in performance or reduction in symptoms indicates a potential benefit. The least amount of prism that gives the patient the greatest benefit should be used. An appropriate amount of prism to use as a starting point is often the recovery value obtained during infra- or supraduction of the compensating vertical range. The practitioner can also use tests of fixation disparity to determine appropriate prismatic power (35,36).

Spatial Effects Of Prism In addition to image displacement, prism also has subtle spatial effects. These spatial effects include image expansion or compression in the vertical or horizontal plane. Figure 25-1 traces parallel rays of light (from infinity) through a prism. They emerge in parallel, but both displaced (toward the base) and deflected (toward the base). This illustrates how light rays emerge from a prism with expanded space between them when viewed in the frontal plane.

Pure prisms do not change the vergence of the light. Because of the differences in path length when light travels through different parts of a prism, the image is not only displaced but slightly rotated. Figure 25-2 illustrates how a square object may be expanded and rotated when viewed through a prism.

Spatial Effects Of Vertical Prism When prescribing compensatory vertical prism, it is worth considering the spatial effects of the prism. Rather than simply splitting the prism between the lenses, consider applying the prism asymmetrically or even unilaterally, with consideration for the prismatic effects outlined in Table 25.1.

Compensatory vertical prism can be applied with consideration for its spatial effects, supporting case management. Consider the following case: A patient presents with a 4^{Δ} right hyperphoria and a strong eso tendency. With 2^{Δ} of vertical compensation, the patient experiences increased horizontal fusion ranges. Rather than split the prism to 1^{Δ}

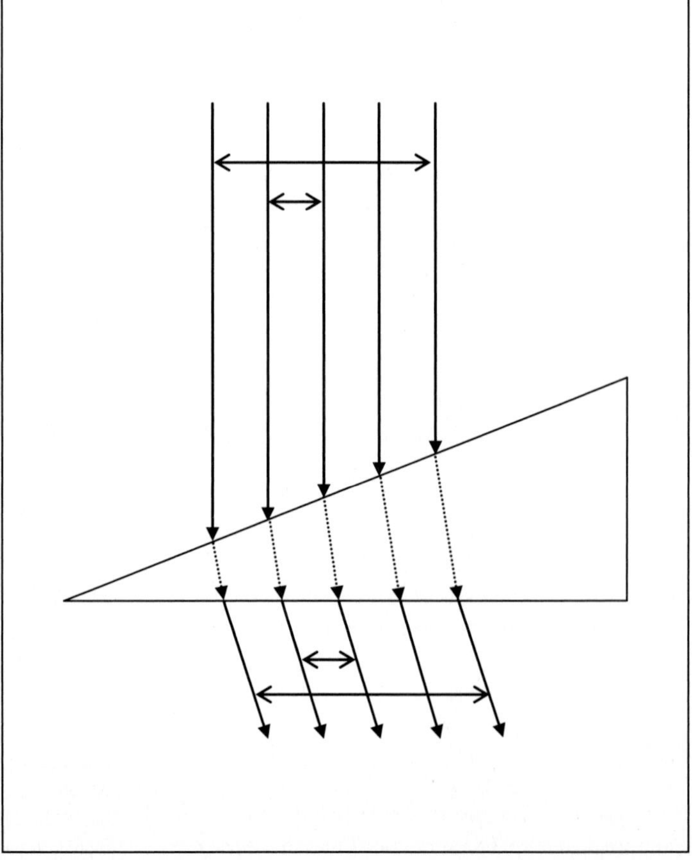

FIGURE 25-1. Prisms displace light in the direction of the base. Prisms also redistribute light, spreading the light rays farther apart: As light travels through thicker portions of prism, it moves progressively farther away from its starting point. The light rays on the left side (near the apex) are only slightly displaced. The light rays on the right side (near the base) are substantially displaced.

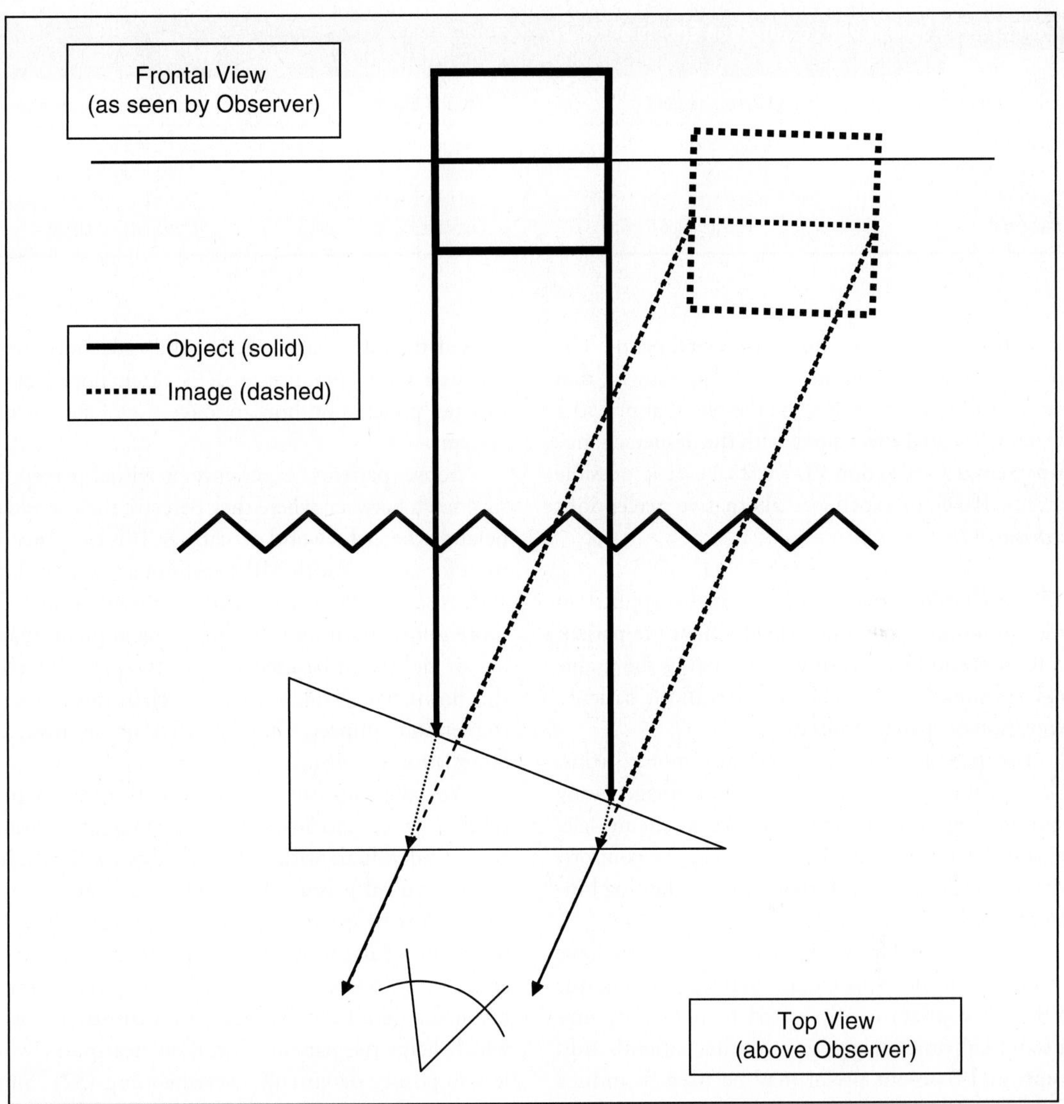

FIGURE 25-2. Prisms do not alter the vergence of light emanating from an object. Therefore, in addition to displacing the light, there is a perceived rotational effect which results from the difference in path length between the apical and basal aspects of the prism. Image is expanded horizontally; image is also rotated away from the observer at left side/ towards observer on right side.

base-down OD and 1^{Δ} base-up OS, one may take advantage of the spatial effects of base-down prism for esophoric patients. In this case, the patient may show increased comfort and performance with 2^{Δ} base-down OD (or 1.5^{Δ} base-down OD with 0.5^{Δ} base-up OS), rather than an equally split prism. When providing vertical compensation, apply the prism combination that provides a more desirable spatial effect.

Similarly, vertical prism should be applied with sensitivity to the presence of an A or V pattern strabismus. If a patient has better binocular performance in downgaze, for example, it may be best to provide vertical correction with all of the prism given monocularly as base-up, or to simply provide more base-up prism in one eye and less base-down prism in the other eye.

Spatial Effects Of Horizontal Prism Like vertical prism, prism-prescribed horizontally also has spatial effects. Some patients may be more responsive to the spatial effects of vertically oriented prism, while

TABLE 25.1 Spatial and Localization Effects of Prism

Prism Orientation	Image Displacement	Spatial Effect	Perceived Localization
Base-up	Shifts image down	Compresses visual space	Shifts images closer
Base-down	Shifts image up	Expands visual space	Shifts images further away
Base-in	Shifts image away from midline	Expands visual space	Shifts images further away
Base-out	Shifts image towards midline	Compresses visual space	Shifts images closer

others may benefit more from horizontal prism. The prism orientation (base-in, -out, -up, -down) that works best for a patient may be the one that provides the desired spatial effect along with the desired change in perceived localization (Table 25.1). It is possible for individuals to experience alternative perceptions to prism.

Yoked Prism Yoked prism may be applied in order to move images into a field which the patient finds more comfortable, or which expands the usable field of vision. It can also be used to shift the patient's perception of spatial localization (37).

For patients with noncomitant motor fields, yoked prism can be used to shift the images away from the diagnostic action field of the paretic muscle. By shifting images into a field of greater comfort, prisms can alleviate visual stress while facilitating binocularity (38).

Adults with Down syndrome appear to have a tendency to develop latent/ manifest nystagmus (39). Yoked prism is often used to reduce nystagmus by shifting images toward the patient's null point, and base-out prism may be used to induce convergence, which also can dampen the nystagmus (40–42).

Some patients may exhibit a partial visual field loss. This will often interfere with navigation, ambulation and safety. In addition, loss of a substantial portion of the visual field may cause an oculomotor dysfunction to manifest as patients avoid making saccades into their blind field. Yoked Fresnel prisms can be used over a segment of the lens (placed superiorly or laterally in the blind field) to allow access to the unseen visual field with a seeing portion of the retina. This provides an early warning system that notifies the patient that something is entering the field of view. (If the right visual field is missing, base-right prism will bring portions of the right visual field closer to view.) (43,44) With substantial amounts of visual field loss, horizontal yoked prism is used to shift images so that they are more easily accessed with lateral gaze. It is often necessary to instruct patients on how to make use of such prism systems.

Some patients experience a visual-perceptual mismatch between where they perceive their world to be and where the world actually is. It is not uncommon for patients with ABI to exhibit a visual midline shift. (See Chapter 10, Acquired Brain Injury, for more information on this topic.) Yoked prism (base-left or right) can be used to help the patient rectify this mismatch. A subtle change such as this can have tremendous impact, either positive or negative, on ambulation (45,46).

Yoked prism can also be used to create a postural shift in patients with neuromuscular limitations (individuals with cerebral palsy, for example). Vertical yoked prism when applied at near creates a subtle shift in space. In patients who have difficulty maintaining attention, base-up prism can help bring attention into down-gaze, away from visual distracters in the periphery. Base-up prism constricts space, which helps the patients find their near-point work less imposing or visually overwhelming (37). Since convergence is facilitated in down-gaze, this assists patients with convergence insufficiency as well. Yoked base-up prism has been shown to alleviate near-point asthenopia in combination with low plus lenses, greater than either prism or low-plus alone (47). Similar benefits have also been found with base-in prism, both alone and in combination with low-plus (47). Many practitioners also use yoked base-down prism to alleviate near-point asthenopia (see discussion below) (48,49). In addition, vertical prism provides spatial structure and helps a patient in organizing his or her space world. It will also reduce a tendency to tilt the head. In all cases, it is recommended that the practitioner trial frame the prism and evaluate patient response before prescribing. A stereo vision test may quickly demonstrate the value of a selected prescription (49).

Base-down prism generally provides a feeling of open space and image magnification (37). In some patients with a tendency toward accommodative or convergence excess, base-down prism alleviates visual stress (48,49). In patients who do not show sufficient plus acceptance to wear a plus add (whether children or adults), base-down prism can be used to reduce the visual demand at near by magnifying the image while shifting the image away from the patient (48,49). When the image appears larger but farther, one can sustain fixation on the image with reduced visual stress. Furthermore, patients may experience an overall body relaxation and slackening of tension when they feel they no longer have to strain to see the near-point material. This physical relaxation experienced by the patient often makes the task of sustaining near-point work more manageable (49).

With regards to patients with special needs, yoked prism is used to help optimally position themselves. Whether prisms are used to shift a patient with nystagmus toward a null point, or to facilitate upright head posture in a patient with hypotonicity, yoked prisms are valuable tools that can alleviate the amount of effort a patient must apply when performing near-point tasks. In theory, this leaves more energy available for cognitive processing.

SPECTACLE HARDWARE

Frame Design Consideration should be given to spectacle hardware (frame design and frame and lens materials) in addition to the "software" (the power of the lenses and prisms) being prescribed. Creating a pair of spectacles that can improve function and at the same time be worn comfortably is as important as prescribing the appropriate power (50). The frame should be fitted so that it locks in behind the ears, does not slide down the nose, and is not so small that the patient looks over the top of the frame rather than through the lenses (51). Frames with adjustable nose pads offer more opportunities for obtaining a comfortable fit. Frame size should also be a concern for those patients who have a head-mounted switch. Those using a head-mounted switch often need the smallest appropriate frame available so the patient does not hit the frame while moving the head and using the switch.

Eye care providers should be aware of the potential weight of the lenses, which is dependent upon the power of the lenses, the material selected, and the eye size dimensions of the frame. The weight of the finished pair of spectacles should be comfortably supported on the bridge of the nose. Larger nose pads allow for a greater contact area and greater weight distribution resulting in increased comfort (52). These concerns must be counterweighted against the particular facial contours of the patient. Small children and patients with Down syndrome often have underdeveloped nose bridges, which will influence frame selection. Special considerations for ear, nose, and facial deformities or abnormalities should be taken into account. Adaptations such as a headband or nose-pad pedestal offer the patient comfort and the use of the full visual area of the lens) (53) (Fig. 25-3).

The thickness and color of the frame should also a consideration. The frame can be used to define the visual field as noted below (54,55).

- A small frame (small eye size) is often confining for some patients, whereas others find that it alleviates the demand of taking in a larger area of information.
- A thick frame creates a greater separation between the world outside and the world inside the frame.
- A frame with a dark back-laminate can be confining. However, a dark frame with a light colored back-laminate can give the patient the freedom of choice in frame color without imposing on the visual field.
- A thin or a semi-rimless frame provides the visual correction necessary without cutting off a sense of having a large visual field that expands beyond the space of the lenses.
- Rimless frames create the most open visual field, but tend to require delicate handling to keep them in adjustment.

Special Considerations While the availability of frames that have been designed for those with special needs is somewhat limited, a line of frames has been specifically made for the different facial proportions observed in these populations in patients with poorly formed or absent nose bridges (56). These frames are reproportioned so that the temples and nose pads attach below the midline of the frame, elevating the eyewire portion of the frame (Fig. 25-4) (56).

Some children do very well with a frame that is designed to be strapped around the head rather than

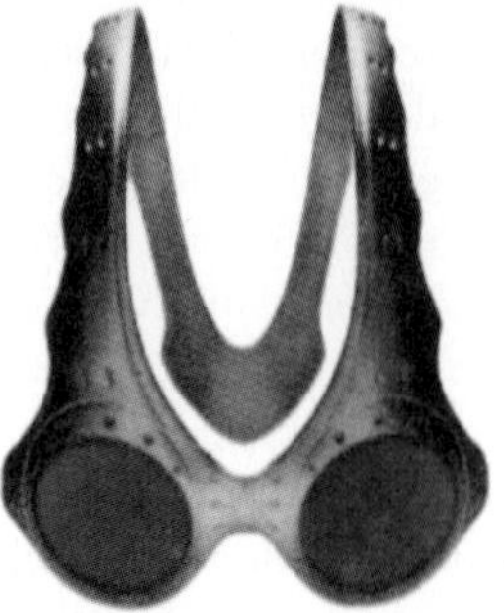

Pressure alleviation area: Ear
Options with similar concepts: Designer frames–Over The Top (www.oakley.com) RC 17S Theo GB 10 (www.theo.be)
Example: Over The Top - Courtesy of Oakley

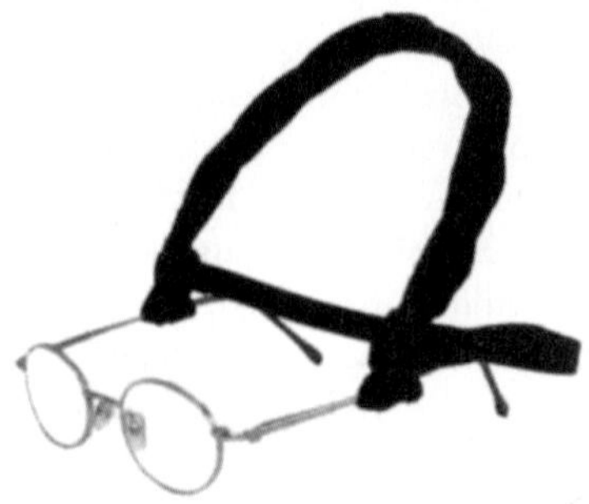

Pressure alleviation area: Ear
Options with similar concepts: Spectacle head-band (can be made with materials from a local craft store)
Example: PolyU spectacle designed headband

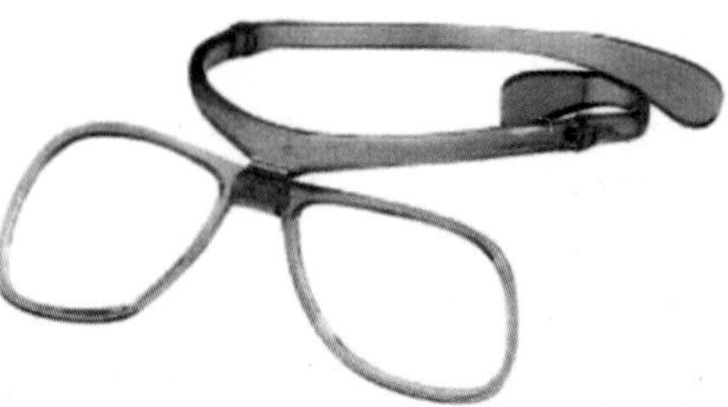

Pressure alleviation area: Ear and nose
Options with similar concepts: Temple rest frames, Weightless, Bridgeless, Multiframe, Astro II
Example: Weightless (www.franeloptical.com)

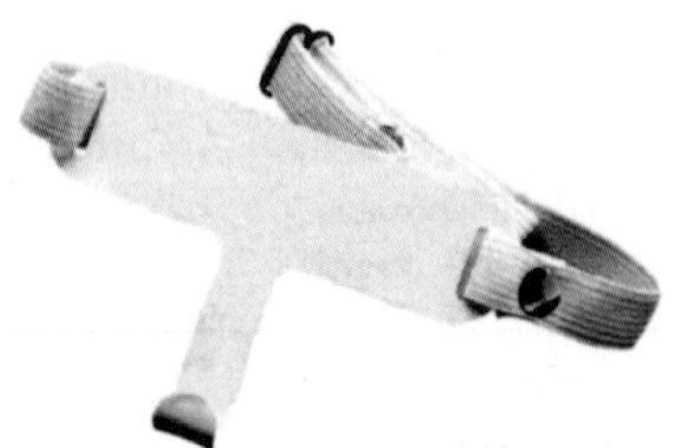

Pressure alleviation area: Nose
Options with similar concepts: Headband eyeglass suspenders–Noseguard or adhesive tape such as Micropore, Dermiclear, Blenderm
Example: Noseguard (www.franeloptical.com)

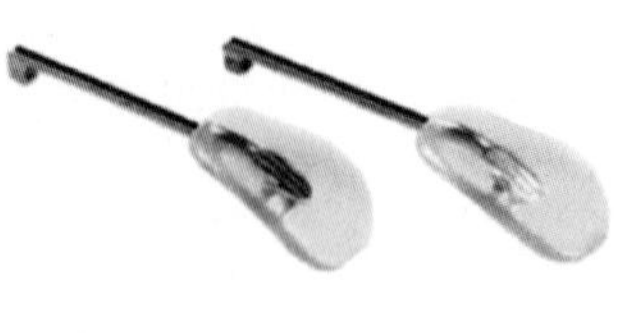

Pressure alleviation area: Nose
Options with similar concepts: Cheeklifts, Clip-on pedestals–Frame-ups (www.cosmeticpioneer.com/frameups.htm)
Example: Cheeklists

FIGURE 25-3. Options for alleviating pressure from the ears and nose for spectacle wear. Eng H, Chiu RS. Spectacle fitting with ear, nose, and face deformities or abnormalities. Used with permission from: Clin Exp Optom. 2002;85(6):389–91.

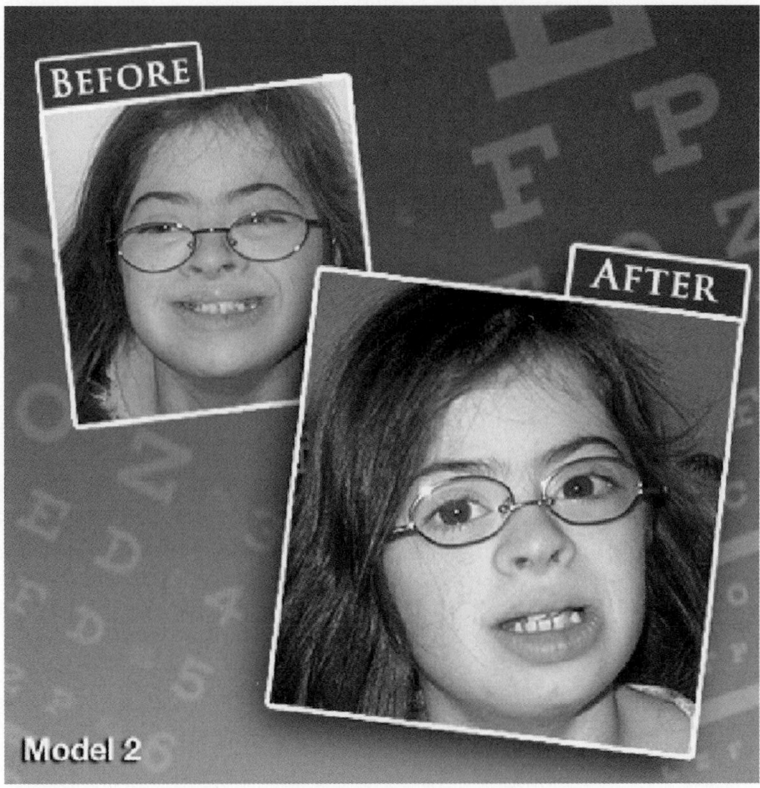

FIGURE 25-4. From Specs4Us.com, Superior Precision Eyewear for Children who are Special. (Available from: www.specs4us.com. Last Accessed October 14, 2010, used with permission.)

rest on the nose. Miraflex has expanded their line of frames to treat patients from infancy through adulthood. See http://miraflex.info for frame selection (57). These frames are made of a durable, flexible plastic with a head wrap to secure the frames in place (see Fig. 25-5). Alternatively, frames can be outfitted with Croakies to secure the frame behind the head (see Fig. 25-6).

Lens Materials For safety considerations, the lens materials of choice for children are polycarbonate and Trivex, due to their impact resistance (50,58,59). However, in patients who are particularly sensitive, polycarbonate may create some distortion and color fringe separation, which are not acceptable. Trivex offers higher optical quality (high Abbe value: lower color distortion) (60).

Plastic lenses (CR-39) may be considered in adults, particularly for glasses worn only for near-point work. However, for patient safety as well as legal considerations, it is recommended that all children's lenses be made in an approved impact-resistant material (59). See Table 25.2 below for a comparison of ophthalmic materials (61).

NONSPECTACLE REFRACTIVE AND BINOCULAR CORRECTION

For management of vision beyond spectacles, patients with special needs may benefit from the prescription of contact lenses or referral for refractive or strabismus surgery.

Contact Lenses Contact lenses remain an important management option for infants with extreme refractive errors (e.g., after removal of a congenital cataract). The primary consideration in the application of contact lenses is whether they can be safely inserted and removed with appropriate consideration of contact lens hygiene. Parents can be trained to assist with contact lenses. Specialty contact lenses are available for children with aphakia and are considered safe to use and easy to handle (62). Companies

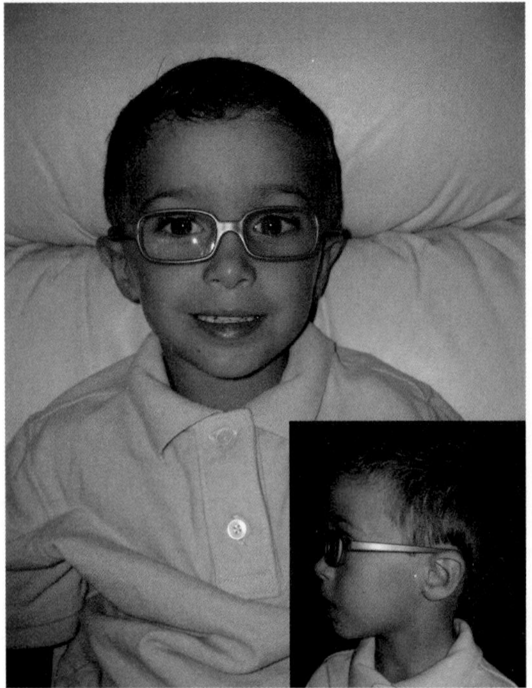

FIGURE 25-5. Miraflex frames are flexible and malleable, with an integrated strap, securing frame behind the head, rather than on the bridge of the nose.

offering such lenses include Bausch & Lomb (SilSoft), Flexlens, Alden, Continental, Kontur, and Optech (63).

Individuals with special needs can successfully wear contact lenses as long as they or their caregivers demonstrate competence inserting and removing the lenses as well as the ability to maintain their cleanliness. To reduce concerns about proper contact lens hygiene, daily disposable lenses may be preferred. However, in this population, eye care providers may not wish to offer contact lenses as an option until the request comes from the patient or their caregivers.

Refractive Surgery Refractive surgery may be an effective management option for high refractive errors in patients with motor disabilities. For example, some patients with severe cerebral palsy have great difficulty keeping their heads upright. While glasses may effectively compensate for high refractive error, the patient may not be able to control head posture well enough to view through the glasses. In such cases where glasses are not effective and contact lenses are an unsafe option, refractive surgery is a viable alternative (64).

Strabismus Surgery Treatment of strabismus (an eye turn) generally falls into two categories: cosmetic and functional. Since there are social consequences of having an obvious eye turn, patients (or parents) frequently seek treatment for cosmetic reasons (65,66). Psychosocial issues develop as patients with strabismus become sensitive to their own poor eye contact, particularly in women (67,68). Patients with strabismus are also known to struggle with job opportunities and other social situations (69,70).

When patients with strabismus are treated functionally, they learn to use information from both eyes simultaneously. This assists in the development of stereopsis (i.e., depth perception derived from a two-eye image), and also has less obvious positive impacts such as the development of spatial organization skills. This helps patients have a better sense of the world around them. In the case of patients who use wheelchairs, a better sense of spatial organization can result in greater ability to navigate space or even to communicate using directional language (e.g., "Would you please pass me the book behind and to the left of the vase?").

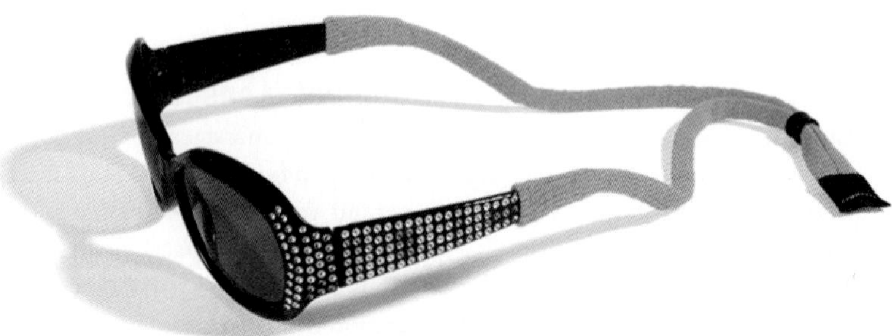

FIGURE 25-6. Croakies adjustable straps can help secure a frame onto a patient. Croakies Available from: http://croakies.com/kidsmicrosuiter.aspx. Last Accessed June 15, 2011.

TABLE 25.2 With Permission from Optometry Today

Physical Data for Typical Lens Materials

Medium	n_d	n_e	CVF	Density	UV cut-off	Abbe Number	ρ(%)
Glasses							
White crown	1.523	1.525	1.00	2.5	320	59	4.3
Light flint	1.600	1.604	0.87	2.6	334	42	5.3
1.7 glasses	1.700	1.705	0.75	3.2	340	35	6.7
	1.701	1.706	0.75	3.2	320	42	6.7
1.8 glasses	1.802	1.807	0.65	3.7	332	35	8.2
	1.830	1.838	0.63	3.6	340	32	8.6
1.9 glasses	1.885	1.893	0.59	4.0	340	31	9.4
Plastics							
CR39	1.498	1.500	1.00	1.3	355	58	4.0
INDO Superfin	1.523	1.525	0.95	1.3	350	48	4.3
Trivex	1.532	1.535	0.94	1.1	380	46	4.4
Sola Spectralite	1.537	1.540	0.93	1.2	385	47	4.5
Corning SunSensors	1.555	1.558	0.90	1.2	380	38	4.7
PPG HIP	1.560	1.563	0.89	1.2	370	38	4.8
AO Alphalite 16XT	1.582	1.585	0.86	1.3	380	34	5.1
Polycarbonate	1.586	1.589	0.85	1.2	385	30	5.2
Hoya Eyas 1.6	1.600	1.603	0.83	1.3	380	42	5.3
Polyurethanes	1.600	1.603	0.83	1.3	380	36	5.3
	1.609	1.612	0.82	1.4	380	32	5.4
	1.660	1.664	0.75	1.4	375	32	6.2
	1.670	1.674	0.74	1.4	395	32	6.3
Hoya Eyry 1.7	1.695	1.710	0.72	1.4	380	36	6.7
High index 1.71	1.710	1.715	0.70	1.4	380	36	6.9
Very high index	1.740	1.746	0.67	1.5	400	33	7.3

Jalie M, Materials for spectacle lenses. Optometry Today. 2005;(1):26–32. Used with permission.

Special considerations for the treatment of patients with special needs who also have strabismus are discussed elsewhere in this chapter. If a program of OVT does not result in the patient maintaining adequate functional control, strabismus surgery can be considered *in conjunction with a continuing vision therapy program*. Unwanted side effects of a purely surgical approach do occur with potentially detrimental results (71). Patients with neurologic disorders often require at least two surgeries to achieve alignment (72). It has also been noted that the evidence-based research that supports the use of strabismus surgery and strabismus surgery outcomes is variable (73). Patients undergoing an OVT program, on the other hand, are trained to combine information from the two eyes in an integrated way. As a result, patients who have successfully completed an OVT program for strabismus rarely require additional surgical intervention, as the impetus to reestablish an eye turn is removed.

OCCLUSION

Occlusion is the act of obscuring or blocking visual input. Occlusion methods include the use of solid, graded (as with Bangerter foils), or colored filters. Occlusion is often a beneficial tool in the treatment of many visual conditions in patients with special needs. In cases where active OVT is not possible, occlusion often provides a passive therapeutic approach (74).

This section addresses occlusion beyond the common monocular occlusion used for the treatment of amblyopia. Occlusion can be used to treat visual conditions from a variety of different causes and etiologies including eccentric fixation, strabismus, post-trauma vision syndrome (PTVS), unilateral spatial inattention, and balance problems associated with vision. These conditions affect how the individual sees and localizes space, and influences his or her posture, mobility, and various aspects of visual information processing. Occlusion is frequently used in isolation or in combination with specific lenses, prisms, and OVT. There are two main categories of occlusion: compensatory and therapeutic.

Compensatory Occlusion A compensatory approach is used to eliminate a concern that is affecting the patient's performance. An example would be the elimination of diplopia secondary to strabismus or metamorphopsia secondary to retinal disease.

Therapeutic Occlusion Therapeutic occlusion may be developmental or rehabilitative in nature. Occlusion for developmental purposes is used to enhance binocular vision outcomes. Examples include adduction deficits in bilateral exotropia or abduction deficits in infantile esotropia. Diplopia can be reduced or eliminated with this approach. Occlusion for rehabilitation is designed to help a patient recover function. Examples include patients with PTVS or those with a deficiency in visual processing (75).

There are many variables in the therapeutic use of occlusion. They include

- Mode
  - Spectacle
  - Contact lens
  - Pharmaceutical
- Form
  - Complete occlusion
  - Sectoral occlusion (e.g., nasal, binasal, slit, window) (76–78).
  - Pinhole occlusion (79)
  - Spot occlusion
- Location
  - Nasal, binasal, temporal, superior, and/or inferior
- Density
  - Opaque
  - Translucent (Bangerter foil) (80)
  - Colored (with filters)
- Size
- Duration
  - Intermittent (see Case 3, below)
  - Short-term (see Case 5, below)
  - Long-term

In many cases, the therapeutic effect may be immediate, whereas in other cases, benefits may be appreciated over time (see Case 1, below). Appropriate frame selection is critical in therapeutic occlusion. Make sure that children do not "peek" around the frame (over, under, or even through the middle by the nosepiece, which some metal frames may allow.)

Monocular Application The most common goal of monocular occlusion is the recovery of visual acuity for those with amblyopia and decreasing or eliminating strabismus. Monocular occlusion can actually be used for a variety of purposes including occlusion of the non-dominant eye (indirect occlusion), which can be beneficial in decreasing or eliminating unwanted cortical maladaptations such as anomalous correspondence (74).

Binocular Application Selective occlusion can be used in varying ways binocularly. In patients with symptoms of PTVS, binasal occlusion has been shown to decrease confusion and improve cortical processing (81). Yoked occlusion (same field of view from each eye) can also be helpful in the recovery of unilateral spatial inattention (82,83).

Occlusion may be applied binocularly to encourage a change in visual processing. Most commonly, this is accomplished when binasal occlusion is used. This occlusive technique reduces the amount of information entering an eye from the contralateral field (Fig. 25-7). This does not reduce the size of the visual field, as the temporal field from the contralateral eye still receives visual input over the same area of space. Thus, binasal occlusion *reduces the amount of binocular visual processing centrally, without reducing the size of the full visual field.*

When there is difficulty coordinating information received from the two eyes, binasal occlusion alleviates visual processing demands. It may also reduce the need to actively suppress information from one eye in the attempt to avoid visual confusion (as is often the case in strabismus). Binasal occlusion can even be applied in exotropes/high exophores and hypertropes, as it may reduce the need for suppression. Visual closure between the right eye and left eye images can support better motor coordination between the eyes, reducing an eye turn. This is illustrated in Figure 25-8.

Rethy and Rethy-Gal (84) demonstrated effective results with binasal occlusion in the treatment of

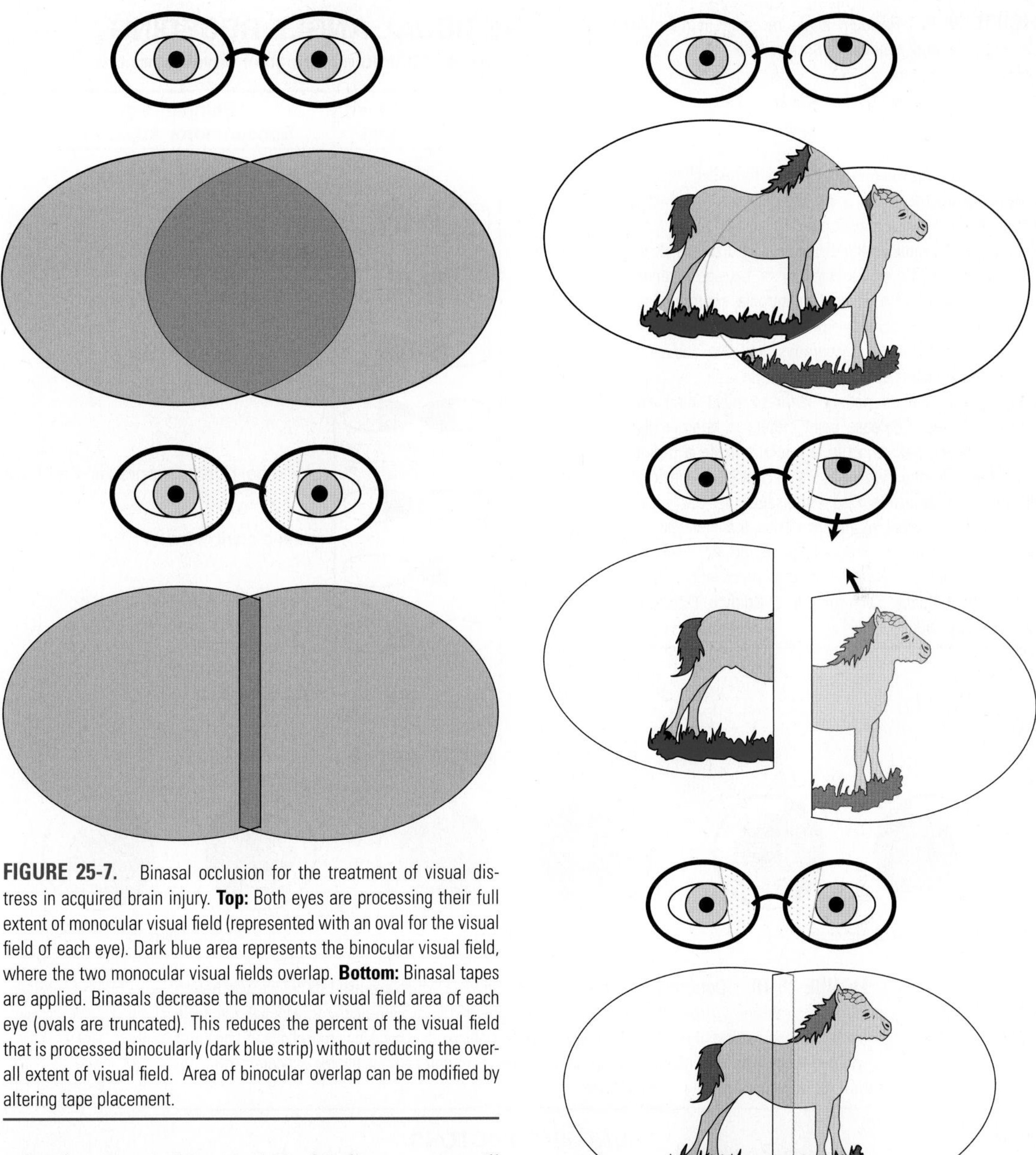

FIGURE 25-7. Binasal occlusion for the treatment of visual distress in acquired brain injury. **Top:** Both eyes are processing their full extent of monocular visual field (represented with an oval for the visual field of each eye). Dark blue area represents the binocular visual field, where the two monocular visual fields overlap. **Bottom:** Binasal tapes are applied. Binasals decrease the monocular visual field area of each eye (ovals are truncated). This reduces the percent of the visual field that is processed binocularly (dark blue strip) without reducing the overall extent of visual field. Area of binocular overlap can be modified by altering tape placement.

FIGURE 25-8. Binasal occlusion for the treatment of vertical deviations. **Top**: Left hyperexotropia. The dominant eye gets much stronger image; the image from the nondominant eye is ignored, and strabismus remains. **Middle:** Binasal occlusion is applied; the brain no longer has to choose between processing spatial information from one of two competing images. **Bottom:** Brain favors *visual closure* and enables the eyes to work collaboratively to make one composite image, removing hyper and significant exo component. Patient functions with simultaneous perception (first-degree fusion). Facilitates obtaining second- and third-degree fusion (flat fusion and stereopsis, respectively).

infantile esotropia (Fig. 25-9). In this diagram, you will see that the occlusion application was systematically modified between the right and left sectors in attempting to decrease the angle over time. This suggests that binasal occlusion should not be considered a static procedure, but rather a *dynamic* procedure with attempts to decrease the angle over time. In the case shown, the patient began with 50 prism diopters of right esotropia. By modifying the binasal occlusion, Rethy gradually helped the patient reduce the esotropia at distance to 0 by 30 weeks of treatment, leaving the patient with an esotropia manifesting only at near-point (20 prism

FIGURE 25-9. Residual angle receding in infantile esotropia. Artwork courtesy of Susan Doyle
pdpt = prism diopters
r + 50 = 50^ right unilateral esotropia
l + 20 = 20^ left unilateral esotropia
dist = distance
Table indicates application of binasal or nasal occlusion as a dynamic process which trains the patient into reducing the angle or presence of esotropia.
First 30 weeks reduced the strabismus at distance. Note the variable width and asymmetry of occlusion tapes. E.g., (weeks 1-4) with 50^ right esotropia, narrow nasal occlusion of the right side and broad nasal occlusion of the left side simultaneously encourages right eye abduction and discourages left eye cross-fixation.
Weeks 31-40 helped patient learn to build binocular function at near. "Release point" refers to nearest distance at which patient could binocularly fixate a target.
From Rethy S and Rethy-Gal S. Decreasing behavioral flexibility (of adjustment to strabismus) as the cause of resistance against treatment during the first year of life. In: Strabismus II: Proceedings of the 4th Meeting of the International Strabismological Association, 1982 Oct 25–29; Asilomar, California (Pt. 2) Orlando, FL: Grune and Stratton; 1984.

RESIDUAL ANGLE RECEDING

Phases of unfolding binocular development

Weeks of Treatment	Angle of Squint Right	Left	Remnants of Sensorimotor Adjustment
1 - 4		pdpt r + 50	Pseudoparesis of abduction
			with
5 - 8		l + 20	nystagmus
9 - 10		r + 10	
11 - 30		l + 6	microstrabismus
		dist 0	
31 -		near + 20	(blockage) due to suppression for near
34 -			release point 0.5m
36 -			" " 0.3m
38 -			" " 0.1m
40 -		near 0	no suppression

DETECTING SECTORS

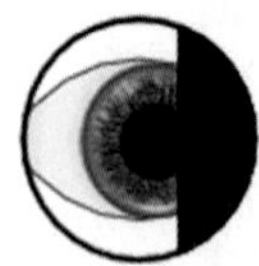
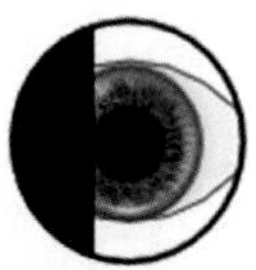

R.E. Strabismus

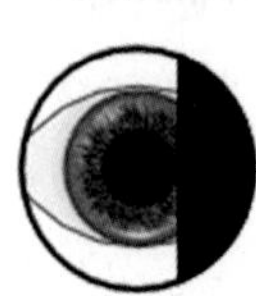
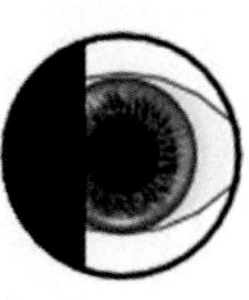

Orthophoria

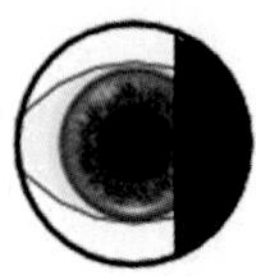
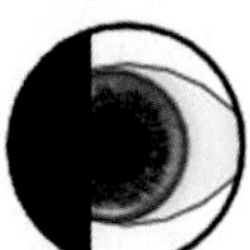

L.E. Strabismus

FIGURE 25-10. Detecting sectors are binasal occluders which are used to detect whether an infant is strabismic. Broad binasal occluders are pre-affixed symmetrically to a small spectacle frame. By comparing the infant's visible iris area behind the occlusion, the clinician can infer whether there is a monocular or alternating deviation. Symmetrically visible iris indicates orthophoria. (78) Artwork courtesy of Susan Doyle

TREATMENT SECTORS

Inferior Slit

Slits

Windows

Horizontal "V"Exercising Abduction R.E.Fixing Eye

Horizontal "V"Exercising Abduction Alternate Crossing Eye

Pupillary Screen

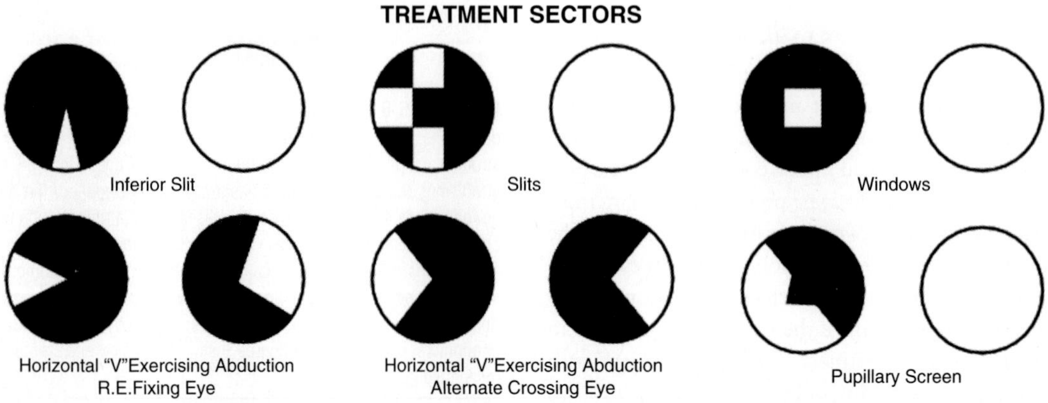

FIGURE 25-11. Treatment sectors of varying types can be used to help develop visual skills and for rehabilitation. Artwork courtesy of Susan Doyle

diopters'). He next used a single nasal sector, alternating the occlusion between the right and left eyes and eliminating the near esotropia.

Sarniguet-Badoche (78) has also found binasal occlusion to be useful in evaluating strabismic conditions (Fig. 25-10). She used variations of occlusion for many different visual conditions including cranial nerve paresis (Fig. 25-11).

OCCLUSION: CASE EXAMPLES

The following cases illustrate how occlusion can be therapeutically instituted for patients with special needs. Keep in mind that occlusion may be used alone or with other therapeutic procedures. A combination approach generally provides the best opportunity for recovery.

CASE 1: BINASAL OCCLUSION FOR INFANTILE ESOTROPIA

Infantile esotropia is a condition in which infants develop a cross fixation pattern likely secondary to an abduction deficit. This abduction deficit generally disappears by age one, but the resulting esotropia tends to persist with a cross fixation pattern. Binasal occlusion provides an opportunity for the infant to begin to break down this cross fixation pattern. The breaking down of this fixation pattern promotes alternating fixation with an improvement in the abduction deficit. This simple occlusion technique provides the infant with an opportunity to visually develop in an appropriate fashion with the right eye leading in right gaze and the left eye leading in left gaze (Fig. 25-12) (85,86).

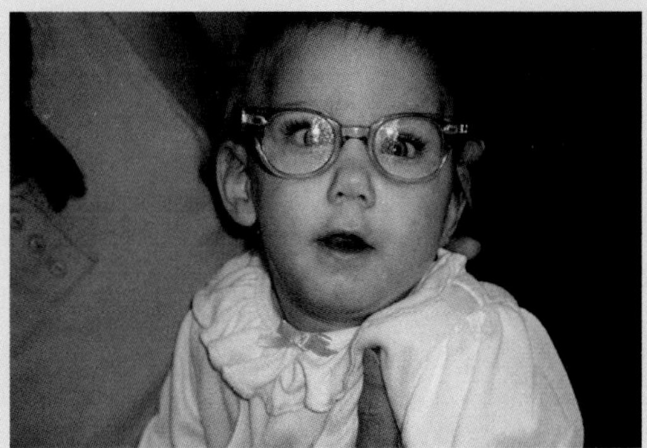

FIGURE 25-12. Binasal occlusion for infantile esotropia, encourages abduction, discourages cross-fixation.

CASE 2: BINASAL OCCLUSION FOR SPASM OF CONVERGENCE

Bilateral esotropia may result from a spasm of convergence, as opposed to an abduction deficit. In these cases, the binasal occlusion encourages abduction, decreasing any contracture of the ipsilateral medial rectus muscle. It also allows the patient to pay more attention to peripheral visual input. With frequent alternating fixation, the patient learns to lead binocular vision with the abducting eye (Fig. 25-13).

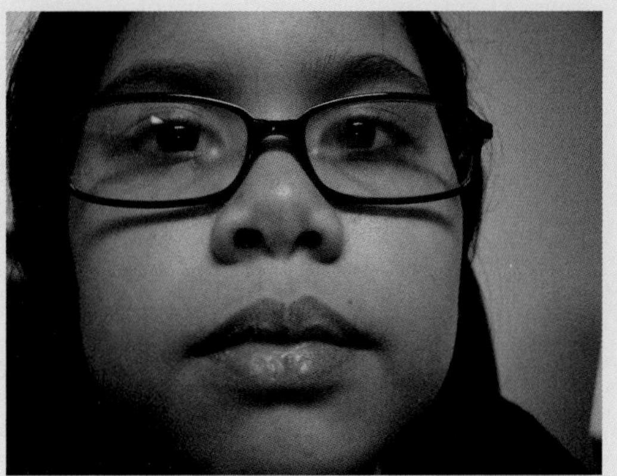

FIGURE 25-13. Binasal occlusion for spasm of convergence; guides the patient to frequently alternate fixation to break bilateral esotropia and the cross fixation pattern, while increasing peripheral awareness.

CASE 3: BITEMPORAL OCCLUSION FOR EXOTROPIA WITH ADDUCTION DEFICIT

Children with developmental delay often present with a bilateral or alternating exotropia and poor ability to adduct. The child typically uses head movement to localize objects in space. One treatment option is to develop alternating fixation with alternating occlusion. Another is to provide glasses with bitemporal occlusion, which are used for short periods of time throughout the day. This results in the patient alternately adducting an eye to localize across the midline, without needing to monocularly patch (Fig. 25-14).

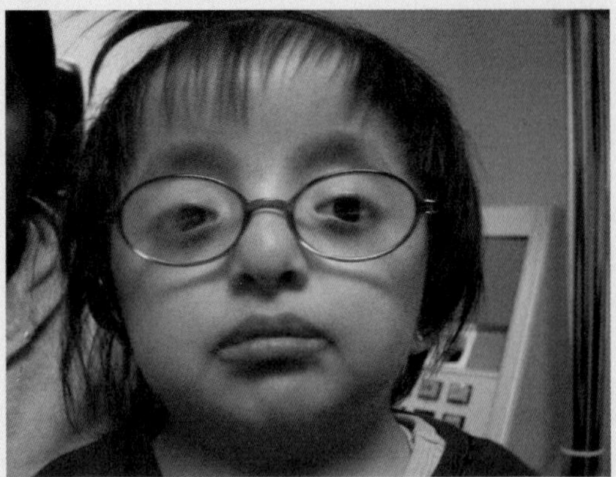

FIGURE 25-14. Bitemporal occlusion can be used to train adduction. Here, the patient adducts the right eye to primary position in order to look within unoccluded area.

CASE 4: SPOT OCCLUSION FOR SENSORY FUSION DISRUPTION SYNDROME FOLLOWING TBI

Following traumatic brain injury, some patients experience sensory fusion disruption syndrome (87,88). This is the inability to maintain fusion despite having optically aligned images. While complete occlusion is a simple option, it results in decreased peripheral input. Decreased peripheral input can negatively affect the ability to move and orient in space, and it can disrupt balance as well. By modifying the full occlusion to a spot occlusion, the patient can maintain single vision in primary gaze and off-axis viewing near that position (although they may experience diplopia in a rare extreme gaze) (Fig. 25-15). This occlusion methodology is also often beneficial for patients who participate in shooting sports when the patient has difficulty in maintaining fixation using the sighting eye.

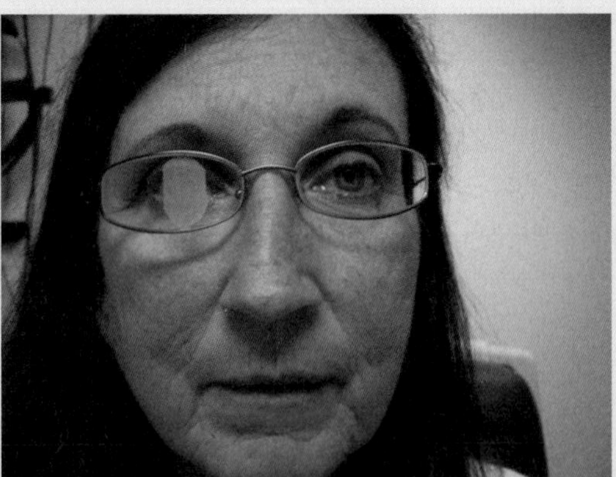

FIGURE 25-15. Spot occlusion (with Bangerter foil) removes visual confusion centrally while enabling peripheral processing.

CASE 5: PINHOLE GLASSES FOR MOTION SENSITIVITY DYSFUNCTION FOLLOWING UNILATERAL LABYRINTHECTOMY

In patients with vestibular dysfunction, motion sensitivity can be debilitating. Figure 25-16 shows a patient who had a unilateral labyrinthectomy procedure that resulted in severe motion sensitivity. With pinhole glasses, she was able to sit in a room comfortably without feeling overwhelmed by her sensitivity to motion. Once her symptoms decreased, therapy was instituted using a variety of vestibular rehabilitation techniques.

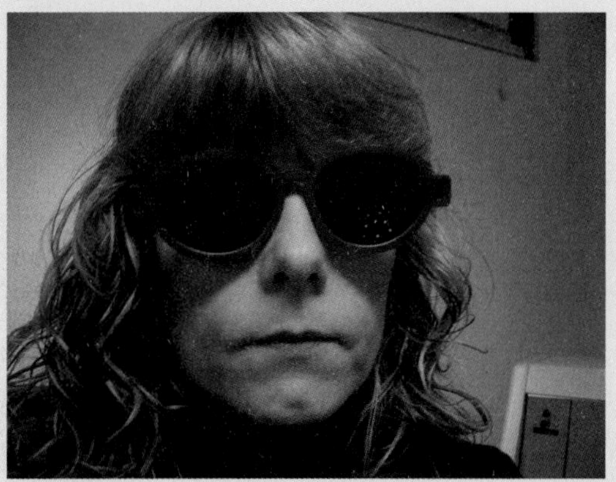

FIGURE 25-16. Pinhole occlusion reduces motion sensitivity in the patient following unilateral labyrinthectomy.

Occlusion is a useful tool for a wide variety of visual conditions. Treatment can be applied as a compensatory strategy or as a therapeutic tool. The use of monocular occlusion for amblyopia and strabismus only begins to demonstrate the potential usefulness of occlusion in helping patients with special needs. The advantage of the therapeutic application of occlusion is that it can often be used passively with patients who are not able to respond to more complicated therapeutic procedures. In addition, it is a useful way to stabilize patients without requiring them to make counterproductive visual adaptations (such as suppression or anomalous correspondence). In this way, they will be better prepared to make changes in an active OVT program at a later time.

OPTOMETRIC VISION THERAPY

This section provides an introduction to OVT along with adaptive techniques for patients with special needs. It presents a practical, developmental approach with a firm basis in neurology. Treatment interventions are provided for deficits of visual input, visual information processing, and the complex visual–motor conditions (strabismus, amblyopia) and ABI. The chapter concludes with a case study that illustrates the comprehensive application of *all* treatment modalities reviewed in this chapter.

What Is Optometric Vision Therapy?

Optometric vision therapy is a sequential program of neurosensory and neuromuscular activities individually prescribed and monitored by the optometrist to develop, rehabilitate, and enhance visual skills and visual information processing. The OVT program is based on the results of a comprehensive vision examination or consultation and takes into consideration the needs of the patient, the patient's signs and symptoms, standardized vision testing, and behavioral observations of the patient (89,90). The use of lenses, prisms, filters, occluders, activities and procedures, specialized instruments, and computer programs are all an integral part of a comprehensive therapy program. The length of the therapy program varies depending on the severity and duration of the diagnosed conditions and the initial etiology. It can range from several months to longer periods of time. Activities paralleling in-office techniques are typically taught to the patient to be performed at home, reinforcing the development and rehabilitation of visual skills in the office.

Research has demonstrated OVT can be an effective treatment option for

- Ocular motility dysfunctions (eye tracking disorders) (91–93)
- Nonstrabismic binocular disorders (inefficient eye teaming) (94–103)
- Accommodative disorders (focusing problems) (104–107)
- Strabismus (misalignment of the eyes) (108–114)
- Amblyopia (poorly developed vision) (115–120)
- Visual information processing disorders, including visual–motor integration and integration with other sensory modalities (121)
- Visual sequelae of ABI (122–131)

Individualized programming by developmental optometrists[‡] can consist of orthoptics (aligning of the eyes), OVT and neuro-optometric rehabilitation (NOR). Orthoptics has traditionally been defined as the aligning of the eyes. Optometric vision therapy is the integration of vision and visually guided activities with the patient's specific goals and needs. This includes basic principles of orthoptics and extends further into a more comprehensive model of vision and visual information processing. Neuro-optometric rehabilitation addresses not only those conditions found in the general population, but also the visual sequelae of ABI[§] (122–131). Optometric vision therapy and NOR are complementary in their nature, with the distinction that NOR specifically addresses patients with ABI.

Optometric Vision Therapy—Establishing A Plan Of Care What are the goals for the patient when conducting an OVT program? It is important to acknowledge that the eye care practitioner's goals may differ from the patient's (or parent/guardian's) goals. It is important that all individuals' goals, both short-term and long-term, be considered. The short-term goals should have a timeline that includes the initial few weeks/months, and the long-term goals can extend over years or even for a patient's lifetime.

Over the course of therapy, the goals for a patient with special needs change and evolve as some skills plateau and as other expectations are exceeded. Where physical limitations exist, compensatory strategies are guided. With continuous appraisal of the patient's progress and emerging needs, the therapist can modify the program so that the patient continues to make progress to meet the challenges encountered.

Practitioners should consider a life-span approach in the evaluation and treatment of patients with special needs so that specific concerns associated with aging can be anticipated. For example, a patient with Down syndrome and infantile esotropia should be managed initially for the infantile esotropia, but the parents should also be educated regarding the possibility of accommodative esotropia occurring as the child develops.

When developing an OVT program for a patient, the practitioner should begin by assessing the patient's abilities and potential. Goals should be tailored not only for the patient but also with the patient's active participation. Ideally, the practitioner should seek to gain the maximum potential function available from vision and visual processing.

Depending on the nature of the case, different activities are used and may be performed at different levels of difficulty. However, there are certain principles or models that can be applied to assist in organizing the therapy program. Ciuffreda and Ludlam offer a conceptual model for approaching mild TBI cases, which may be applied for patients with special needs. They suggest approaching the case using four tiers: Tier 1 is a basic optometric examination, Tier 2 addresses oculomotor-based vision problems, Tier 3 addresses non–oculomotor-based vision problems, and Tier 4 addresses non–vision-based problems (132). For some patients with special needs, the non–vision-based problems take priority. Part of the treatment plan includes integrating treatment with other professionals such as occupational therapists, physical therapists, and speech-language pathologists.

Once a treatment plan is established, the practitioner may benefit from keeping the principles of learning in mind for every activity attempted. Pepper (133) recommends guiding progress along the following five steps listed in Table 25.3. When employing this approach to a specific activity, such as the ability to fixate upon a target, skills can be improved using the Pepper Principles of Learning as follows: (a) "Can I fixate the target?" Yes. (b) "How well?" Observe how easily the patient can

TABLE 25.3 Pepper Principles of Learning

Step 1	Can I do it?
Step 2	How well can I do it?
Step 3	How long can I do it?
Step 4	Can I accept change?
Step 5	Can I problem solve?

[‡]Currently, there is no official designation for this subgroup of optometrists. They are often referred to as: Behavioral, Developmental, Neurocognitive, Neurodevelopmental, Neuro-Optometric, or Neurorehabilitative, depending on personal orientation and/or geographic predilection of the practitioner. For purposes of brevity, they will be referred to as "developmental optometrists" within this chapter.

[§]ABI includes but is not limited to traumatic brain injury (TBI), cerebrovascular accident (CVA—"stroke"), neurological disorders (e.g., multiple sclerosis, Meniere disease, Parkinson disease, Guillain-Barre, etc.) and developmental conditions (cerebral palsy, Down syndrome, etc.).

localize the target. Does it require excessive effort? (c) "How long?" Observe the patient's ability to sustain the activity. If, for example, the target is a Lang stereo test, the patient will need to maintain fixation long enough to realize depth. (d) "Can I accept change?" This offers the practitioner the opportunity to modify the environment to promote further learning. Thus, a child may be able to sustain target fixation from a sitting position, but not be able to do so while standing. (e) "Can I problem solve?" How well can a patient recover if the demands of the task are too great? If the patient's balance is interfering with his ability to sustain fixation, can he recognize the problem and attempt to recenter himself before attempting fixation again?

The problem-solving principle can be used at any cognitive level. Consider the task of reading. Can the patient read the text? How well? How long? Can the patient accept change, whether it is a change in font size or type, vocabulary, or grade level concepts? Can the patient problem solve? In this case, comprehension and language skills play a role. If the patient were to skip two lines of print, does the child realize this quickly because the context of the story no longer makes sense? Alternatively, does the child not realize he missed anything and continues to read on a word-by-word basis? Within any OVT activity, the learning principles outlined here can be applied for all patients to help them achieve their maximum potential.

Research over the last two decades has shown that cortical plasticity is active throughout an individual's life span and can be used to improve vision function even in adults (134). In spite of this, there are still some practitioners suggesting that amblyopia cannot be improved after a certain age. This misconception is attributed to a misinterpretation of Hubel and Wiesel's work which identified a so-called critical period in cases of deprivation amblyopia in cats (135). Rather than consider a critical period of development after which improvements in function cannot be made, it is better to consider the presence of a neurologically sensitive period during which changes in function become more deeply rooted (135–144). The prognosis for treatment of amblyopia, for instance, is influenced by time of onset and duration of any maladaptations present (145).

Visual skills necessary for effective visual processing have been shown to improve with vision therapy. Levi (137) published a paper that demonstrates that patients with amblyopia can achieve improvement via the same perceptual learning mechanisms that operate in the normal visual system. It is hypothesized that these mechanisms account for some of the improvement that occurs in the treatment of adults with amblyopia. Optometric vision therapy is an effective treatment throughout the life span of a patient. An OVT program is designed to support development, decreasing unwanted developmental adaptations such as strabismus and amblyopia or visual sequelae secondary to near-point stress. Optometric vision therapy is also effective for conditions often found in the geriatric populations (such as neurologic disorders and cerebrovascular accidents), in which the goal is to recover optimal function.

THE NEUROLOGIC BASIS FOR OPTOMETRIC VISION THERAPY

If you stand on one foot with your eyes open and then with them closed, you will immediately realize the importance of vision to balance. Recent fMRI studies have documented that vision is reciprocally interwoven with the other sensory modalities of the body (146). With a large portion of the visual system connected with other sensory systems, how can we understand the visual process except to observe how it interacts with the rest of what we do? Vision is not an isolated sensory system. It is an intricate sensorimotor system with neural connections through all lobes of the brain, even in blind individuals! (147–149).

The visual system is involved in most brain processes via reciprocal interweaving and multisensory integration (150,151). Over 1 million nerve fibers exit each eye. This represents about 70% of the sensory nerve fibers in the entire body. Of those nerve fibers, 10% do not go directly to the visual cortex (152), but travel to other parts of the brain including the brainstem. At the brainstem, the superior colliculus integrates with other sensory systems including tactile, proprioceptive, auditory, and vestibular. These connections provide important visual information for the integration of movement, balance, posture, and the orienting and localizing of objects of regard. Figure 25-17 illustrates the integration of sensory inputs involved in the visual process.

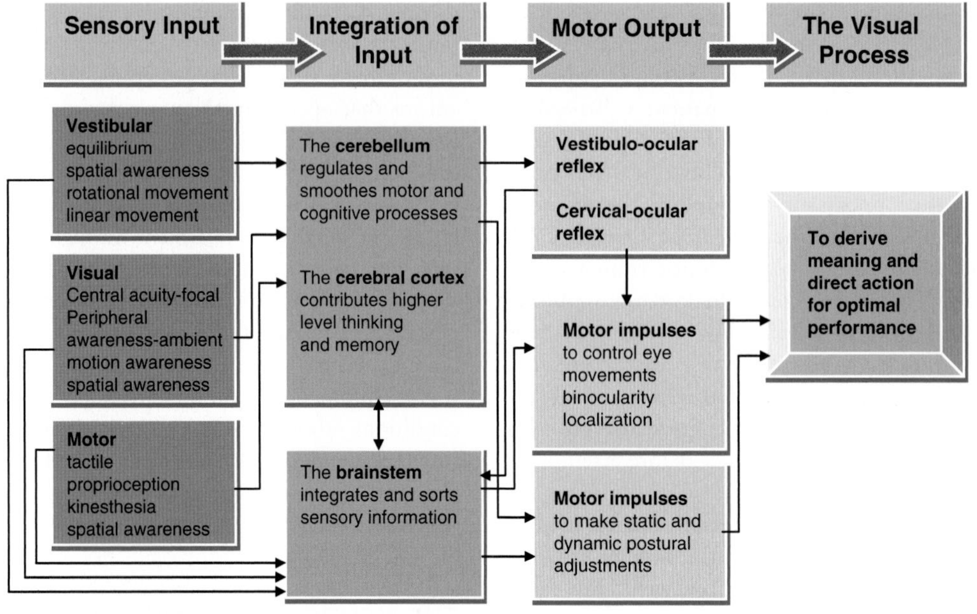

FIGURE 25-17. Integration of sensory input to the visual process. Artwork courtesy of Marc B. Taub, OD, MS

With this integration of systems in mind, developmental optometrists frequently work in coordination with other professionals such as occupational therapists, physical therapists, speech therapists, chiropractors, physiatrists, and other members of the rehabilitation team. Multidisciplinary cooperation provides the basis for appropriate and effective treatment and the opportunity for individual patients to reach their maximum potential. (For an illustration of the intricate circuitry of vision in the brain, see Felleman and vanEssen's depiction of 32 visual cortical areas, connected by 187 linkages, most of which are reciprocal pathways.) (153)

Subcortical And Cortical Pathways In Optometric Vision Therapy and Neuro-Optometric Rehabilitation Many pathways in the brain are required for functional vision. When we look at the reciprocal interweaving of the sensory systems, we quickly realize the complexity of the visual process and pathways (155). Many of these pathways are well known but not always evaluated in regards to the effects of vision therapy. The understanding of these pathways can lead to a better understanding of the development of vision, child development, and the wide array of visual disorders.

The brain can be divided up into cortical areas (the "gray matter") and subcortical areas (which include the brainstem, cerebellum, and midbrain). The cerebral cortex is highly developed in humans, and it is directly responsible for cognitive processing. The subcortical areas are evident in varying stages of development throughout the animal kingdom. Generally, the subcortical processes encompass body regulatory functions, reflexes, and basic sensory and motor processing.

Figure. 25-18 illustrates how subcortical skills form a foundation that must be integrated for higher level, cortical learning to take place. It also indicates how vision is integrated with other forms of sensory input in the development of complex behavior, performance, and interaction skills. The multitude of complex behaviors we use in daily life are the result of the integration of sensory inputs for subcortical and cortical learning (154).

Some patients with special needs are unable to cortically drive eye movements. This may be a result of cortical defects such as hydrocephalus or CVA. For example, patients with gaze palsy are unable to voluntarily move their eyes either to the right or left of midline. Over time, these patients often find abnormal ways to compensate and move their eyes. For example, if the patient is unable to move his eyes directly to a target to his right, he may *move his head in the opposite direction*, to the left. This produces an eye movement to the right within the

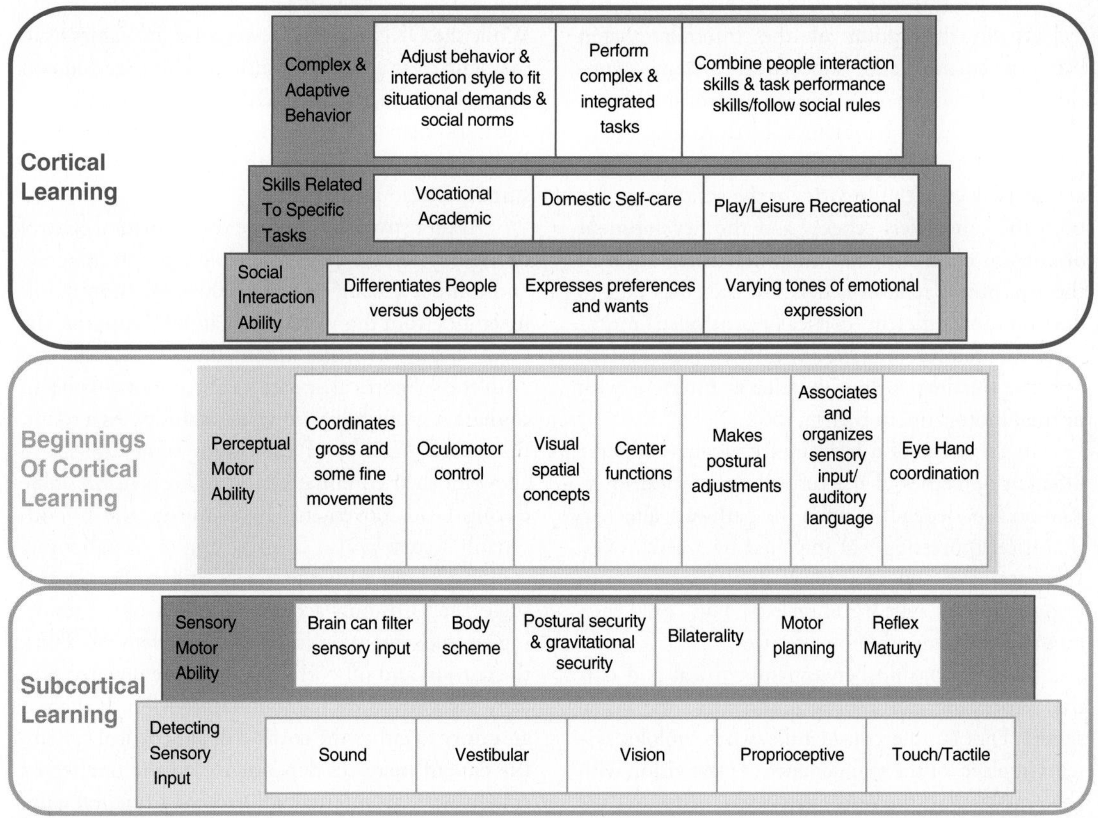

FIGURE 25-18. Interrelationship of cortical and subcortical learning, Adapted from the works of Laura Barker and Bonnie Hanschu by Heidi Clopton. Used with permission.

orbit (opposite the head rotation), taking advantage of the subcortical VOR. The patient may then make a *second* head movement *back* toward the target on his right, this time with the eyes prepositioned for the object of regard. This combines the subcortical eye movement within the orbit with a cortical head movement back toward the object of regard. This complex string of actions circumvents the need for the voluntary (cortical) initiation of a saccade, which has been rendered dysfunctional due to the gaze palsy.

In addition to apparent delays and limitations in visual processing, neurologic limitations, motor limitations, and cognitive limitations must all be taken into consideration when designing a vision therapy program for a patient with special needs.

The subcortical system is fairly well established at birth, whereas many of the cortical pathways emerge *after* birth. There is a reciprocal relationship in which the subcortical pathways initially establish behavioral patterns. These patterns are integrated with sensory processing and are then established into cortical pathways of behavior. If interference occurs early in subcortical development, such as with cerebral palsy or Down syndrome, the cortex may have difficulty in integrating and overriding the subcortical system. These systems may be thought of on a continuum as they are involved in ocular motor and body control. If either the cortical or subcortical system is dysfunctional for any reason, the other system may take precedence. However, due to the reciprocal nature of these two systems, any limitation in one is likely to create limitations in the other system. Ideally the two systems work in harmony with each other.

As an illustration of the interrelationship between cortical and subcortical systems, consider the development of motor control in infants: Primitive reflexes are present at birth to help establish early motor patterns in the infant. These reflexes are interwoven with the cortex as the child integrates both the subcortical reflexes and the development of cortical control of movement. If integration of these primitive reflexes is delayed, the child fails to develop more efficient (cortically controlled) motor patterns, reinforcing the primitive (subcortical) reflexes. Retained primitive reflexes interfere with normal motor function (155,156).

In the event of a head injury, we may observe different outcomes of the cortical–subcortical interrelationship, depending upon the pathways affected. If cortical processing was impaired by a cerebrovascular accident, this may result in the spontaneous reappearance of subcortical reflexes. This could then interfere with smooth motor control.

The relationship between subcortical and cortical processing can also be observed in the visual system. For example, consider the two neurologic systems in place for the maintenance of clear vision with head movement: the vestibular–ocular reflex (VOR) and optokinetic nystagmus (OKN). The VOR is based in the brainstem (subcortical), with a latency of about 16 ms. The OKN is based on both subcortical and cortical processing, with a longer latency of 140 ms. The VOR provides us with the ability to respond to head movement *immediately*, but it cannot be sustained with an extended period of head movement. While the OKN is slower to respond, it enables us to maintain clear vision with sustained head movement. The subcortical system (VOR) and the cortical–subcortical system (OKN) work in concert (reciprocally) to maintain clear vision both immediately and with sustained head movement.

As these two systems develop, the neural control of these systems evolves to enable them to integrate and work as a team. At birth, 100% of vision stability comes from the VOR. After about 3 months, the OKN begins to make a contribution as well, and both the subcortical and cortical components begin to share responsibility for visual stability. As a result, the neural "gain"* of each subsystem adjusts to allow for their combined effect to keep vision stable during head movement. By maturity, the smooth pursuit system is also contributing to overall visual stability, along with the OKN and VOR. At this stage, the VOR only accounts for 60% of the resulting eye movement on initial head movement. Thus, the cortical and subcortical systems are now reciprocally interwoven to maintain clear vision. If there is an injury to either the cortical or subcortical system, the patient increases dependence on the unaffected system with an internal adjustment in neural gain. However, if the damage is substantial such that one cannot sufficiently adjust the performance of the complementary system, blur or disequilibrium may be experienced (as illustrated above in Case 5, Occlusion section). In this instance, saccadic and pursuit eye movement therapy can be provided to improve gaze stability (157,158).

Vision Development: Orientation And Localization The foundation of any OVT program should include a consideration of the orientation and localization ability of the patient. This is consistent with Ciuffreda and Ludlam's recommendation to address oculomotor-based vision problems early in the treatment plan (132). Goodale suggests that the brain did not develop to think, but rather to *act* (159). In order to interact with anything around us, we must first have a sense of where *we* are, and then we can negotiate ways to interact with the world around us. Accordingly, the first step in an OVT program is often to help the patient develop a sense of his or her body in space. This provides a reference point from which one can respond to all sensory inputs from within one's peripersonal space (160).

The postural control of a patient should be observed, taking into account overall body tone and the presence of body and/or head tilt. There are two primary reasons why a patient may adapt an abnormal head posture. One is to compensate for an eye muscle limitation (such as with a superior oblique palsy) or eye movement abnormality (such as with gaze-dependent nystagmus). A patient may also display an abnormal head posture secondary to variations in neck muscle tone. Rigidity or contracture of a neck muscle may result in torticollis with a particular direction of turn and/or tilt. Hypotonic neck muscles result in reduced control of head posture, where the head may fall forward, backward, or sideways. This is a common concern in patients with cerebral palsy but may also occur to a milder extent in children with general hypotonicity. The inability to hold the head straight is likely to have a negative impact on binocular fusion and coordination. Thus, postural control can have an enormous impact on visual control, due in large part to the fact that the visual system is most efficient when the two eyes are on the same horizontal plane. In the absence of a paretic vertical extraocular muscle, binocular coordination is under the lowest amount of strain when the eyes are free to converge and diverge in the horizontal plane without a vertical component.

If a patient has not been assessed for orientation and postural control, a referral may be considered for occupational and/or physical therapy. Alternative motor-enhancing therapies, such as the Feldenkrais method (161) and Alexander technique (162), may also be considered (163). In addition, chiropractic adjustments may help train the patient to maintain better overall body and head alignment (164). The patient may also need support via equipment such as a wheelchair with headrests and/or side rests. Optometric vision therapy may also be considered while comanaging the patient with his or her occupational or physical therapist. This multidisciplinary approach provides the most efficient way for the patient to make progress. Often, the goals each provider has for the patient are met more rapidly with a team approach. For a comprehensive review of the use of complementary and alternative medical therapies, see Chapter 26, Complementary and Alternative Approaches.

In the development of spatial organization, the extraocular muscles (EOMs) provide important proprioceptive and somatosensory cues for visual localization (165). As many patients with special needs have visual deficits, they have not learned to depend upon vision to inform their sense of space and spatial organization. By developing body organization, they can learn to appreciate space, and later integrate this skill with their visual perception of space. Thus, proprioceptive and somatosensory cues often make a critical contribution to an OVT program.

There has also been a considerable amount of research confirming the importance of proprioception in the EOMs (166–169). During therapy, this may play an important role in the ability of patients to feel where they are aiming their eyes and to tie this into their sense of space. More recently, muscle fibers in EOMs have been identified that demonstrate a 1:1 relationship between nerve and muscle fiber. These Feldenstruktur fibers may provide eye muscle positional and directional information, including feedback to and from the vestibular system, to maintain alignment (170,171). In patients who have had EOM surgery, some of these fibers have been severed, which may result in the loss and/or diminution of proprioceptive feedback via these fibers. This may be an additional impediment to visual performance, as proprioceptive feedback mechanisms that normally support visual function have been compromised.

Spatial localization is supported by a combination of visual and motor input, including proprioceptive feedback via the EOMs. Once visual information reaches the primary visual cortex, it is processed along one of two major pathways: the ventral stream and the dorsal stream (Fig. 25-19). The ventral stream is often referred to as the *what* pathway, and the dorsal stream refers to the *where* and *how* pathway (172). When an individual reaches for an object, one needs to know where it is, relative to oneself. Recent studies have helped neuroscientists understand that the information considered in the dorsal stream is not simply where the target is, but how we act upon objects (159,173). This provides a comprehensive understanding of the visual process and our ability to anticipate and *act* within our world. This also further supports the need to go beyond the basic refraction of our patients when addressing the visual needs of a patient with special needs.

Optometric vision therapy procedures that offer the patient the opportunity to integrate a tactile or motor-based understanding of space with what they see will translate into a visual understanding of space. For example, if a patient reports on the Worth 4-Dot as having 2, 3 or 5 dots, indicating suppression or inadequate localization, it is recommended that the patient be directed to reach and touch the target,

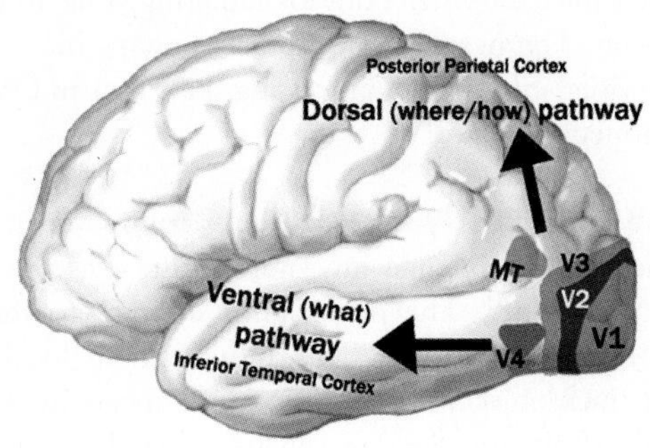

FIGURE 25-19. Visual processing divides into a dorsal ("where?") stream and a ventral ("what?") stream. Artwork courtesy of Kelin Kushin

which provides somatosensory input to localization. This is often a starting point for therapy. Emphasis in therapy should be directed toward accurate proprioceptive experiences with real objects in space, rather than using virtual targets on a computer. Treatment is expanded outward from arms' reach and peripersonal space through the use of therapeutic procedures such as the Brock string (174,175). In this way, the Brock string extends from the patient's hand across the room, creating a tangible extension from oneself into the surrounding space. This allows the patient to observe a distance target as single because vision and proprioception (of the EOMs) are both involved in localization. Over time, the patient learns to localize accurately without needing to use tools or physically touch the object to confirm where it is.

TABLE 25.4 Versional Eye Movements

Subsystem	Stimulus	Function
Fixational	Stationary target	To stabilize a target onto the fovea
Saccadic	Step of target displacement	To acquire an eccentric target onto the fovea
Pursuit	Target velocity	To match eye velocity with target velocity to stabilize the retinal image
Optokinetic	Target or field velocity	To maintain a stable image during sustained head movement
Vestibular	Head acceleration	To maintain a stable image with the target on the fovea during transient head movement.

Ciuffreda KJ, Tannen B. Eye movement basics for the clinician. In: Introduction to eye movements. St. Louis: Mosby; 1995. p. 1–9.

OVERVIEW OF VISUAL SKILLS AND CONDITIONS

Visual skills are the basic requirements for gathering information. They include oculomotor control, accommodation, and binocular function. Ideally, patients should be able to point their eyes at any distance and coordinate the two eyes with little conscious thought or effort. Visual skills work in conjunction with all of our senses so that we can function effectively. Because these skills are reciprocally interwoven with the other senses, their development needs more than just an orthoptic intervention. The visual system does not work in isolation but rather is integrated with the total human experience. Effective treatment of visual skill dysfunction requires an integrated approach. In addition, an evaluation of visual information processing is often an important step before embarking on an OVT program. This section covers the basic visual skills for gathering visual information. The next section explores how to incorporate visual information processing skills into an OVT treatment program.

Oculomotor Dysfunction Oculomotor dysfunction can include any nonspecific eye movement disorder. The oculomotor system provides information that allows the individual to localize and track objects in space, to derive meaning, and to direct action. Since it can be affected by many different inputs, one must evaluate this system by more than simply observing the eyes tracking a target (smooth pursuit) and jumping between targets (saccade). Versional eye movements may be fixational, saccadic, pursuit, optokinetic, or vestibular in origin. The neurologic pathways can be modified by both involuntary and voluntary inputs. Table 25.4 reviews the purpose of each versional eye movement subsystem (176).

Oculomotor dysfunction can result from an actual neurologic deficit, which is the case in some patients with special needs. But, it is just as likely that oculomotor dysfunction is a result of a deficit in the ability to exert cortical functional neuromuscular control over the EOMs. The origin of the problem may be perceptual, rather than motor. This is seen when a lack of proprioceptive awareness results in a deficit of where the body is in space. After strabismus surgery, a patient can struggle with an inability to use proprioceptive information from the EOMs to keep the eyes aligned. Treatment of oculomotor dysfunction should include gaining feedback and control over each of these five subsystems, with the added support of tactile feedback and elevating one's level of consciousness for proprioception of the EOMs (177). For a more comprehensive review, please see Chapter 18, Diagnosis and Treatment of Oculomotor Dysfunction.

Accommodative And Nonstrabismic Binocular Disorders Accommodative disorders refer to deficits in the ability to sustain focus and to easily shift focus between far and near. Nonstrabismic binocular disorders are difficulties in eye teaming that include over/underconvergence or problems in maintaining coordination. The possible clinical diagnoses include accommodative insufficiency, accommodative infacility, spasm of accommodation, convergence insufficiency, convergence excess, divergence insufficiency, divergence excess, binocular instability, basic esophoria, and basic exophoria.

In contrast to oculomotor dysfunction, which is primarily involved with directing the eyes along the *x*- and *y*-axes (horizontal and vertical directions), both accommodative and binocular functions have a correlation with localization along the *z*-axis. Since these two processes are neurologically cross-linked, they cannot be fully isolated from one another. When one increases accommodative effort, there is a neurologic input to converge the eyes; when one increases convergence, there is a neurologic input to accommodate.

In OVT, one of the goals in the management of accommodative and binocular conditions is to increase the flexibility between these two interconnected systems. This refers to the ability to maintain a constant amount of accommodation over a range of vergence demands and being able to maintain a constant degree of vergence or fusion over a range of accommodative demands. This results in greater comfort, flexibility, and efficiency when reading, when attending to information presented at near, and when functioning in a dynamic visual environment.

Lenses, prisms, filters, and occlusion can be used to help patients achieve their highest potential. They may be applied therapeutically, as in a spectacle lens, or they may be used as interventions in an active OVT program. An in-office OVT program helps the patient understand accommodation and vergence control along the *z*-axis, introducing spatial localization into accommodative and binocular activities. Opportunities are presented for biofeedback (visual, tactile, even auditory) and for integration of accommodative and binocular skills across the senses (including visual–motor, visual–vestibular, visual–proprioceptive, and visual–auditory sense integration). Biofeedback and integration help to solidify the learning experience so that the changes incorporated in one's perception of the world have a long-lasting effect. When an individual learns to use accommodation and binocularity for gathering information about the world in relation to himself or herself, these skills are integrated and supportive of the person as a whole.

For a more comprehensive review of these conditions, please see Chapter 19, Diagnosis and Treatment of Binocular Vision and Accommodative Dysfunction.

Strabismus And Amblyopia Strabismus, often referred to as squint, is the nonalignment of the visual axes of the two eyes. There are over 70 different types of strabismus (178). Diagnostic codes classify strabismus into general categories that include amblyopic, paralytic, mechanical, neuromuscular, intermittent, and vertical. There are many different approaches used in the treatment of strabismus. Some doctors tell the parents of young patients with strabismus that they will "grow out of it." While there is limited research available that supports the preceding statement, it is generally not supported by those who actively treat strabismus (179). The concern here is that many patients do not simply grow out of the strabismus, and each should be evaluated with regard to development and the need for possible intervention. By guiding young patients to have experiences that reinforce binocular vision, an OVT program can provide the best opportunity for the child to gain functional vision without surgery. Many of the principles regarding localization and orientation (addressed early in this chapter) are critical in providing young patients with strabismus with a framework for understanding space. Because patients with strabismus are not aiming both eyes at the object of interest, their ability to localize objects based on visual input may not be the most reliable mode of gathering spatial information. These patients may learn to rely on other sensory systems, such as touch and hearing, to build an understanding of space. These senses can be integrated with the visual system by first providing a way to understand space via available systems and subsequently integrating this understanding with visual input.

The same principles apply with older patients whose strabismus has persisted. When working with patients who are self-motivated to address their strabismus (e.g., adolescents, adults, or even precocious children), the therapist may tap into top-down visual processing techniques. So in addition to the bottom-up (i.e., experience-driven) activities, mature patients may use cognitive processing as a tool toward gaining oculomotor control and enhancing binocular function.

When the eye turn is large, the clinician can assist a patient in experiencing binocular vision on a sensory level with the use of prisms and filters (either colored or polarized). Once patients learn how to process visual information simultaneously at one binocular posture, they can start to expand their sensorimotor fusion, learning to converge and diverge the eyes in tandem around this point. Sensory fusion is a strong prognostic indicator that the patient will be able to reduce the degree of the turn. More importantly, the sensory experience of binocular vision greatly enhances quality of life (180); lenses and prisms may simply provide a means toward achieving this end.

It is indeed possible to change the degree of the deviation in strabismus (181–184). This is done through the slow and fast fusional vergence responses (185). Clinically, this has been documented in esotropia cases occurring in a patient with Guillain-Barre syndrome (186) and one with Arnold-Chiari malformation (187). These two cases were treated differently: The first case applied traditional orthoptics, and the second used compensatory prism and vestibular therapy. Both were successful in changing the underlying deviation.

If the patient is unable to gain motor control over the strabismus, a surgical approach can also be considered in conjunction with OVT. In such cases, OVT supports the sensory development of binocular vision before and after surgery. The surgery serves to reduce the motor fusion requirements for the patient.

Strabismus may correlate with other visual processing deficits. Often there are oculomotor and fixational dysfunctions, especially among patients with strabismic amblyopia. Infantile esotropia usually develops because of a visual motion processing disorder, rather than a muscle dysfunction (188,189). Since many patients with strabismus have multiple factors that contributed to the condition (190), it is helpful for the clinician to take a broad approach in treatment. A multifaceted program can help the patient develop sensory input skills, motor output skills, and visual information processing skills (such as spatial localization and organization) over the same time frame.

Amblyopia is an impairment of vision in one or both eyes in which the best corrected visual acuity is poorer than 20/20 in the absence of any obvious structural anomalies or disease (191). There are three primary reasons that an eye does not develop good vision. These are referred to as amblyogenic factors:

- Constant unilateral strabismus, which results in different images projecting onto the two foveae, requiring suppression of the input from one eye to avoid visual confusion.
- High uncorrected refractive error, which results in a defocused image projecting onto the fovea of one or both eyes.
- Deprivation, resulting from any obstruction that prevents information from reaching the fovea of one or both eyes (i.e., ptosis, cataract) (192).

Amblyopia is a diagnosis of exclusion. Before initiating treatment of amblyopia, it is important that the clinician identify one or more amblyogenic factors and rule out any pathology or disease that may be present. If no amblyogenic factor is identified, it may be necessary to refer the patient for imaging studies to rule out an organic cause of the vision loss.

Amblyopia is not a problem of the eye itself but rather a problem of the brain interpreting the information it receives. Particularly when there are unequal inputs between the two eyes, binocular development is affected (193). Especially in the case of strabismic amblyopia, the patient has great difficulty localizing objects with the amblyopic eye. In addition, visual information processing is negatively impacted.

The Amblyopia Treatment Studies (ATS) from the Pediatric Eye Disease Investigator Group (PEDIG) (194) have been undertaken to explore the many variables in the passive and active treatment of amblyopia. These include severity, age, patching time, spectacle correction, use of atropine compared to patching, active versus passive treatment while patching, and binocular function via the use of Bangerter filters (195).

With the understanding of the development of the visual system, OVT treats amblyopia with a multi-tiered approach, designed to provide a clear image on the amblyopic eye, and develop the ability to use this visual information. Amblyopia treatment during OVT integrates movement tasks, accommodative and binocular therapy, bilateral integration tasks, and visual information processing (perceptual) activities (196). Visual–perceptual therapy alone has been demonstrated to improve amblyopia in juveniles and adults (197,198).

A comprehensive overview of amblyopia and strabismus is found in Chapter 20, Diagnosis and Treatment of Strabismus and Amblyopia.

ORTHOPTICS AND NEURO-OPTOMETRIC REHABILITATION

Orthoptics has its roots as far back as the late 1700s and has been used to treat patients with strabismus with relative success (199). This form of therapy is generally accepted by ophthalmology as a valid treatment modality for strabismus and amblyopia (200) and was the only available treatment for eye alignment disorders until strabismus surgery was developed in the early 1900s. Even though it is accepted as a valid treatment, it is rarely practiced by ophthalmology. This may be because the emphasis of training is placed upon the surgical techniques for alignment and not nonsurgical treatment.

Traditionally, orthoptics as a procedure views the visual system in isolation of all other sensory systems. Because of this narrow view and limited approach, there has been limited success with orthoptic treatment for many of the other visual problems. This modality can help certain cases, but it does not directly treat some of the underlying cause(s) of oculomotor deficits, amblyopia and strabismus (201). Optometric vision therapy/neuro-optometric rehabilitation consider the visual system, the brain, and other sensory systems as operating in concert, rather than as isolated parts (202). This expanded view of visual processing provides the foundation for the treatment of a number of different visual conditions and also provides a better understanding of the etiology of strabismus and amblyopia. This is particularly important when treating someone with developmental disability.

Neuro-Optometric Rehabilitation

Neuro-optometric rehabilitation uses our understanding of the neurologic mechanisms underlying various visual skills and carefully directs treatment to address any deficits identified. Neuro-optometric rehabilitation activities are used in coordination with an OVT program, not independent from it.

Developmentally, we learn to maintain orientation to our surroundings during movement. The integration of eye movements with vestibular input is a critical aspect of this development. Many patients with strabismus and other eye-movement deficits have underlying neurologic deficits, such as a paretic muscle or deficiencies in saccadic and/or smooth pursuit eye movements in a particular direction. Neuro-optometric rehabilitation is the identification and remediation of these specific deficits. Here, we consider OKN and postrotary nystagmus (PRN) as part of an NOR program.

Optokinetic Nystagmus Optokinetic nystagmus eye movements stabilize the eyes during sustained tracking of a large moving visual scene. This causes an illusory sensation of self-rotation in the opposite direction (203). At birth there is a subcortical pathway that drives each eye to move in the *temporal-to-nasal* direction, in response to movement of the visual field in that direction. That is, when the visual field is progressing from one's right to one's left, the right eye receives a signal to move from right to left. *The left eye receives no such signal until after 3 months of age*, when the monocular *nasal-to-temporal* OKN develops. This is concurrent with the cortical development of motion processing and stereopsis (204). Clinicians can test for the presence of OKN monocularly, assessing the symmetry of response in the temporal-to-nasal and nasal-to-temporal directions. In many patients with infantile onset strabismus, nasal-to-temporal OKN fails to develop. Thus, the OKN can be used to differentiate between infantile onset strabismus and acquired strabismus (205,206). Accordingly, patients with infantile esotropia benefit from lateral tracking activities in an effort to establish nasal-to-temporal tracking in both OKN and smooth pursuits. Binasal occlusion may also support these patients in disrupting a cross fixational pattern in esotropia (see Occlusion section, above).

Postrotary Nystagmus Postrotary nystagmus occurs in response to the sudden cessation of rotational movement. Rotation provides the vestibular system with a large angular acceleration stimulus. This triggers the VOR to move the eyes opposite the direction of rotation. The sudden stop (postrotation) provides a large *deceleration* stimulus to the VOR. Visual stability is regained as the subcortical response (VOR) is integrated with the cortical visual response of motion processing and fixation. When the two responses are effectively working together, the duration of the PRN is around 7 to 12 seconds, depending on patient's age and cortical status (207). If the patient suppresses the PRN (with a shorter duration), they are visually (cortically) overriding the vestibular system (subcortical) response. This may result from a hyporegistration of the vestibular system (i.e., input from the vestibular system has a lower-than-normal impact upon oculomotor response). If the PRN lingers beyond 12 seconds, the patient is generally unable to cortically override the vestibular system. This may result from a hyperregistration of the vestibular system (i.e., input from the vestibular system has a greater-than-normal impact upon oculomotor response). Either form of response may be observed in those patients with special needs, depending on the nature of the condition.

In NOR, the clinician may make use of the PRN response in patients with esotropia. The patient should be rotated in the direction of the eye that deviates inward (i.e., left eye in, rotate to the left) with the speed of one rotation per second. When the patient is stopped, a left-beating PRN response is stimulated, which drives the esotropic eye outward and thus lessens the angle of strabismus. When performed with eyes open, the OKN serves to enhance the left-beating PRN response. This is particularly powerful in many esotropes, because their temporal-to-nasal OKN is often stronger than the nasal-to-temporal OKN. Additional cortically driven eye movement activities (smooth pursuits and saccades) help the patient to integrate and stabilize the PRN response.

Postrotary nystagmus may be applied during OVT/NOR. During this therapy, you would vary the number of turns, frequency of therapy throughout the day, and whether the patient should perform the technique with eyes closed or open. Patients can practice PRN at home with the assistance of a caretaker. As PRN engages several different neurologically driven oculomotor control mechanisms, it is an excellent activity with which to begin an in-office therapy session. As the patient dampens the PRN, they are engaging fixation while heightening awareness to peripheral areas of the retina. This automatic central–peripheral integration helps to prepare the patient for other forms of OVT. While in the general population, up to 10 rotations are used, in the special needs population, much less is required to stimulate a powerful response.

Caution should be taken when first introducing this activity, as the patient might be hypersensitive and develop a visceral response to this type of intervention. The literature also suggests that there is some concern for the possibility of inducing a seizure response with rotary stimulation (208). However, it may not actually be the rotation but rather periodic photic simulation from either an open window or the patient gazing upward at lighting that can trigger a seizure. Because of these risks, rotational techniques should be used with clinical discretion. Patients with a compromised neurologic system may not be able to efficiently dampen the subcortical input from the vestibular system and could find the experience disruptive.

VISION AND LEARNING

Visual skills are critical to development and learning (209). This suggests that vision may be an even more important consideration in the ability of patients with special needs to learn. Visual testing should include ocular health, far/near visual acuity, and the refractive status. Basic testing should also assess the visual information acquisition skills: ocular motility, accommodation, and binocularity. These skills are essential for all students, in particular, special needs students, to perform well in the classroom.

It is important to rule out the presence of a visual skills deficit, which may interfere in a child's ability to learn efficiently and effectively in a classroom setting. Likewise, a patient with an ABI should have an evaluation for visual efficiency and processing skills if undergoing a neuropsychological battery. This will help the treatment team better understand how the ABI and the visual skills are interfering with the patient's ability to perform higher-level information processing tasks.

In school, a student might be able to obtain 20/20 visual acuity at far and near, but performance may suffer because of other visual skill deficits. Some of the common vision-related educational and visual complaints are reading delays, avoidance of close work, headaches, tired eyes, strain, poor attention, rubbing eyes, covering an eye, skipping lines, and negative behaviors (i.e., attention deficit hyperactivity disorder). All of these may result from poor visual functioning at near. While in the classroom, students require at least 17 visual skills to be able to keep pace with the demands of school (Fig. 25-20).

There has been some confusion in the media regarding the role of vision in learning. The American Association for Pediatric Ophthalmology and Strabismus has suggested that vision therapy does not help in cases of learning disabilities and dyslexia (210). This misleading paper suggests that optometrists are attempting to directly treat learning disabilities and dyslexia, as opposed to treating visual skills that support one's ability to learn and to read. Several well-documented papers rebut the

Classroom Task	Eye Movement Control	Simultaneous Focus at Far	Sustaining Focus at Far	Simultaneous Focus at Near	Sustaining Focus at Near	Simultaneous Alignment at Far	Sustaining Alignment at Far	Simultaneous Alignment at Near	Sustaining Alignment at Near	Central Vision	Peripheral Vision	Depth Awareness	Color Perception	Gross Visual-Motor	Fine Visual-Motor	Visual Perception	Visual Integration
Reading	XX			XX	XX			XX	XX	XX	XX		XX	XX		XX	XX
Writing	XX			XX	XX			XX	XX	XX	XX			XX	XX	XX	XX
Copying (Chalkboard to desk)	XX	XX		XX		XX		XX		XX	XX			XX	XX	XX	XX
Copying (At desk)	XX			XX	XX			XX	XX	XX	XX			XX	XX	XX	XX
Taking Notes	XX	XX		XX		XX		XX		XX	XX			XX	XX	XX	XX
Classroom discussion		XX				XX				XX	XX			XX		XX	XX
Classroom demonstration		XX	XX			XX	XX			XX	XX	XX	XX	XX		XX	XX
Movies and T.V.		XX	XX			XX	XX			XX	XX		XX	XX		XX	XX
Dancing and physical Ed.	XX	XX		XX		XX		XX		XX	XX	XX		XX		XX	XX
Craft Activities	XX	XX	XX	XX	XX	XX	XX	XX	XX	XX	XX	XX	XX	XX	XX	XX	XX
Play	XX	XX	XX	XX	XX	XX	XX	XX	XX	XX	XX	XX	XX	XX	XX	XX	XX

FIGURE 25-20. An accounting of tasks in the classroom and the visual skills they require.

position statement (211,212). Visual skills can influence how well children learn and should be diagnosed and treated. This is true particularly for children who have been identified with learning disabilities or dyslexia (213).

Difficulty in any single or combination of the skills referenced above may be the result of compromised sensorimotor systems. When vision is inefficient, it can interfere with the learning process. This can lead to avoidance of task, negative behaviors, reduced performance, and challenges with sustained attention. The student may have to work harder than necessary to organize thinking and to complete homework assignments. These visual inefficiencies can also lead to behaviors resulting in misdiagnosis and inappropriate labels. The behaviors can be mistaken for attention deficit disorder, sensory integration dysfunction, and even food allergies. Visual deficits may not be clearly observable to the parent or caretaker of special needs patients, as many special needs patients do not understand or report their symptoms. Unlike visual dysfunctions, most other sensorimotor processing dysfunctions have readily observable motor dysfunctions, such as speech impediments that result from a hearing deficit or a gustatory–motor dysfunction.

One common concern in the area of learning is reading. Deficient visual skills can influence both learning to read and reading to learn. If a patient with special needs has deficient visual acquisition skills, he or she may not be able to attend to instruction and learn how to read. If these deficiencies are adequately addressed, they would otherwise be visually prepared to respond to reading instruction. Once the visual skills are addressed, these patients may no longer require supplementary time and instruction for reading remediation. In this way, by addressing the visual skills deficits, OVT can indirectly support reading, without directly addressing the educational process of reading. Likewise, children who start out as good readers in the early grades (when the print is large), but develop poor visual skills, may suffer an apparent loss in reading ability when the print gets smaller. Once these students improve their visual skills, reading should become more comfortable and efficient. Following visual skills therapy, such students may appear to become instantaneous readers, because they had already learned to read, but were suffering interference from inefficient visual skills.

Visual Information Processing Once visual information has successfully been transferred to the cortex via the visual pathway, the information is available for processing. There are several visual information processing skills through which data is managed and organized, instantaneously, over time, and over space. Visual information is both processed independently of and related to all other sensory inputs, allowing one to derive meaning from one's surroundings and to direct action. John Streff (214)* described the process of visual integration of new information with one's existing understanding of the world as follows:

> *Every time the visual system receives a stimulus, it analyzes and matches it against the memory banks of cumulative experience of the whole body/mind system. Accordingly, the way it integrates ("sees") that stimulus or image is conditioned by the previous experience of the whole organism. At the same time the new stimulus is added to and synthesized with the old experience, becoming a part of the analyzing, matching mechanism that is applied to the next stimulus.*

Visual information processing skills include visual discrimination, visual closure, form perception, visual form constancy, visual figure ground, visual–spatial relations, tachistoscopic visual memory, visual sequential memory, visual spatial memory, and the integrative skills of visual motor integration, tactile–visual integration, and auditory-visual integration.

Deficits may occur in any of the visual processing skills. They can be developmental in origin or can be acquired, as in brain injury. Several of these skills directly impact the reading process, along with the visual acquisition skills. Specifically, reading may suffer with deficits in visual discrimination, visual closure, form perception, visual figure ground, tachistoscopic visual memory (via visual span), and visual sequential memory.

The literature identifies many different factors that may contribute to reading deficits. Phonologic processing deficits have been demonstrated to affect reading ability (215,216). Various visual components may also have an impact on reading and fluency Magnocellular processing deficits have been demonstrated in students with a reading disability (217–219). The visual span, which refers to the number of letters (horizontally arranged) that can be processed in a single glance, has a direct impact on reading speed (220). Visual-spatial attention deficits may impair visual processing of words, affecting their translation into phonemes (221,222). At the intersection of visual and auditory processing of information is the underlying temporal processing. Disabled readers have been demonstrated to require a longer amount of time to integrate visual processing of words, as well as other word-like stimuli (219,223). Even cerebellar morphology has been shown to correlate with the presence of dyslexia, suggesting differences in neurologic organization (224). Since both visual and nonvisual factors may negatively affect reading ability, a careful evaluation of visual skills and visual information processing is indicated in any patient with a reading disability, even if phonologic deficits have been identified (225,226).

For a more comprehensive view of this topic, please see Chapter 21, Diagnosis and Treatment of Vision Information Processing Disorders.

Visual Sequelae Of Acquired Brain Injury

There are many visual conditions that are associated with ABI (227). These include anomalies of accommodation, vergence, version, photosensitivity, and the field of vision. They are amenable to noninvasive rehabilitative interventions including OVT and the application of lenses, prisms, selective occlusion, and tints (228). Often, the visual impact arises as part of a syndrome of conditions associated with acquired brain injury, such as visual midline shift syndrome (VMSS) or PTVS (229).

Visual midline shift syndrome occurs in response to an alteration in neurologic processing from one side of the body. To help the body re-establish a sense of balance, patients with ABI may perceive a distortion in their perception of visual space in the horizontal, vertical, and even anteroposterior dimension. Visual midline shift syndrome can be treated with low power yoked prism lenses. These lenses can provide a stimulus for change, modifying the patient's perception of their visual midline. This midline misalignment may stem from a change in processing or feedback from the proprioceptive, tactile, vestibular, and visual worlds (229,230).

Posttrauma vision syndrome is a much more inclusive diagnosis that may encompass such characteristics as exotropia or high exophoria, accommodative dysfunction, convergence insufficiency, low blink rate,

*This quote is attributed to John Streff and was originally found in his lecture notes given while teaching at the Southern College of Optometry in 1971.

spatial disorientation, poor fixation, impaired smooth pursuit, and unstable ambient vision. Symptoms include diplopia, objects appearing to move, staring behavior, poor visual memory, photophobia, asthenopia, and associated neuromotor difficulties (229). Stress results from a mismatch between one's internal sense of space and one's external reality. Through OVT and NOR, opportunities are presented to interact with space and reestablish an internal representation of one's visual world that is consistent with external reality (229,230).

COMPREHENSIVE TREATMENT OF A PATIENT WITH SPECIAL NEEDS

A 13-year-old boy with cerebral palsy is a wheelchair user who has been in the care of three different developmental optometrists since the age of 5 years. He has been involved in an active in-office OVT program for approximately 6 years, working with two practitioners, 4 years with one, 2 with the second.

His visual needs have evolved tremendously since the age of 8. When he presented, he had a constant alternating exotropia of about 50 to 55$^{\Delta}$. Visual acuities were reduced, about 20/80 in each eye. Eye contact was poor, but the child was highly engaged verbally. He also showed a knack for computational skills.

The first practitioner worked on foundational concerns, with the goal of helping this child localize and interact with space and visual information. Spatial awareness is of great importance for any wheelchair user, as they must learn to "drive" and navigate their wheelchair safely.

Foundational Activities Included

- Maintaining fixation
- Visually tracking a Marsden ball while lying on the floor (removing "gravity" from the equation)
- Developing visual memory (so that he could absorb more information in a glance)
- Increasing visual-spatial awareness with the use of yoked prisms during in-office activities

The managing optometrist also participated in in-service visits to the school in order to provide the following supportive recommendations for necessary visual adaptations:

- In the classroom
- On handouts
- On appropriately sized/spaced printed materials

At the age of 11, this patient was transferred into the care of the second optometrist, with the hopes that she would be able to assist him in making progress on binocular skills. Up to this point, the exotropia had not been addressed directly.

Diagnostic testing revealed a potential for combining right-eye and left-eye information with the use of compensatory base-in prism. Approximately 30$^{\Delta}$base-in was required to enable this patient to converge only 20 to 25$^{\Delta}$ of the 50 to 55$^{\Delta}$ turn. Cover testing revealed a tendency for the eyes to default to upgaze, with greater difficulty maintaining fixation into downgaze.

Glasses were designed to improve visual acuity (with corrective Rx), facilitate binocular alignment (with the use of corrective prisms), and allow the patient to hold his eyes in a more natural posture (with the use of yoked prisms).

Spectacle Hardware Figure 25-21 shows this patient wearing frames from Specs4Us, secured with a mini-Croakies adjustable strap. Fresnel prisms were applied in combination with ground-in prism to facilitate alignment and minimize spectacle weight. Trivex material was selected to offer impact resistance and to reduce the dispersion which is inherent in prisms.

Spectacle Software This prescription is corrective, approximately emmetropic but with about 1.5D of oblique cylinder OU:

OD + 0.75 − 1.00 × 030;
OS + 0.75 − 1.50 × 160.

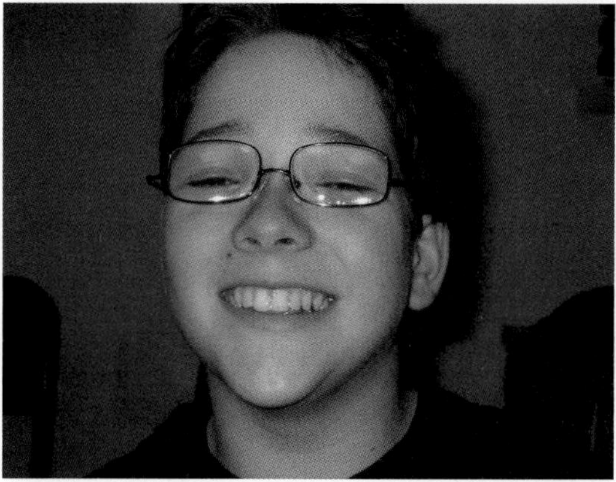

FIGURE 25-21. A patient with large-angle XT, wearing Specs4Us frame for low bridge, secured with mini-Croakies adjustable strap. Lenses in Trivex with antireflective coating. Prescription incorporates a combination of Fresnel prism and ground-in prism, base-in OU, as well as yoked prism base-up OU.

His initial Rx incorporated 3^base-down ground-in OU (yoked for spatial shifts that facilitate comfort and stability, particularly with his eyes defaulting into upgaze) with 7$^{\Delta}$base-in ground-in OU, and 8$^{\Delta}$base-in Fresnel prism OU for a compensatory prism total of 30$^{\Delta}$base-in.

Optometric Vision Therapy Program When this patient entered therapy with the second optometrist, at age 11, he still had not developed his sense of laterality on himself, let alone others. He was using large print on all classroom handouts, with limited information presented on a page. He did not undertake to write anything by hand, nor did he type on a computer keyboard. All testing responses were given via dictation to an aide. He could not read independently for more than a page or two before fatiguing. He would take about an hour to read three printed pages.

The fact that this patient had strabismus was significant, because the large-angle turn denied him the potential to learn to appreciate spatial organization from a binocular perspective. Being a wheelchair user, his motor interactions with the 3-D world were also somewhat limited. In this case, the development of spatial organization in the space of the mind can help the patient learn to appreciate the world he must navigate, even before he learns to see it as such. Spatial organization and visualization provide the scaffolding for developing the binocular experience of stereopsis. And once the patient learns to see and use stereoscopic vision, he may continue to reinforce his spatial organization and navigation skills.

The therapy program was designed to

- Develop visually-guided motor skills
  - improve fixation accuracy and duration of fixation on near-point activities at a desk
  - improve convergence and spatial organization, hitting Marsden ball
  - improve motor control: timing and strategy to catch Marsden ball
  - improve fine motor skills, beginning with finger placement (e.g., on a Visual Motor Form C)
  - attempt fine motor control of a writing utensil, rudimentary writing activities (visually guided control of starting/stopping, reducing spasticity after each mark, see Fig. 25-22)
- Develop oculomotor skills and rhythm
  - implement metronome for timing in saccadic eye movement activities

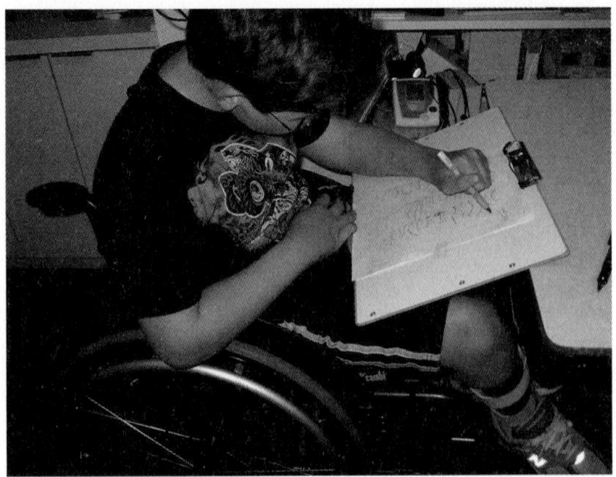

FIGURE 25-22. Writing activity adapted for working in a wheelchair, supporting a slant desk between the physical desk and his lap. The patient is using thick three-sided pencil, bracing the pencil against index finger in two places to stabilize. Fine-motor control is limited in the left hand, but better with the right. Gross motor control is very limited on the right side. The patient is practicing starting/stopping horizontal lines with visually guided placement of pencil on start/stop points. The challenge remains to control stopping without spastic jerk.

  - develop ability to process visual information monocularly while eye is held in adduction (using base-out prism)
- Build laterality and directionality skills
  - provide mechanisms for embedding his own laterality
  - develop projection of laterality onto others
  - develop directionality: laterality of objects relative to one another
  - develop directional language
- Build visual memory
  - develop visual–spatial memory in particular, to assist with spatial planning
- Build visualization
  - develop the ability to create pictures in the mind
  - develop the ability to manipulate the pictures in his mind
  - develop the ability to keep the pictures/objects still and adjust his perspective or vantage point in his mind
  - develop ability to "pre-plan a navigation course" in his mind when driving the wheelchair
- Build spatial organization
  - understand space conceptually
  - use directional language in a practical way
  - represent 3-dimensional constructions (block towers) in 2-dimensional space from a single perspective or vantage point

    - create 3-dimensional structures (block towers) from 2-dimensional "floor plans"
    - relate spatial language and experience to binocular activities in both free space and with vectograms (see Fig. 25-23)
- Develop head and neck postural control
    - reinforce proprioception for primary head posture
    - use VOR to isolate and reinforce effects of specific head movements—turning, tilting, tipping
    - reinforce advantages of proper head posture in binocular perception activities
- Develop stereopsis
    - relate stereo perception to motor activities
    - build 3-dimensional point-localization skills in space
    - develop motor control of pressure applied when interacting with visual–motor targets

With a considerable amount of fixational work, and with the glasses, visual acuities gradually improved to about 20/40 OD and 20/50 OS in the first year of therapy.

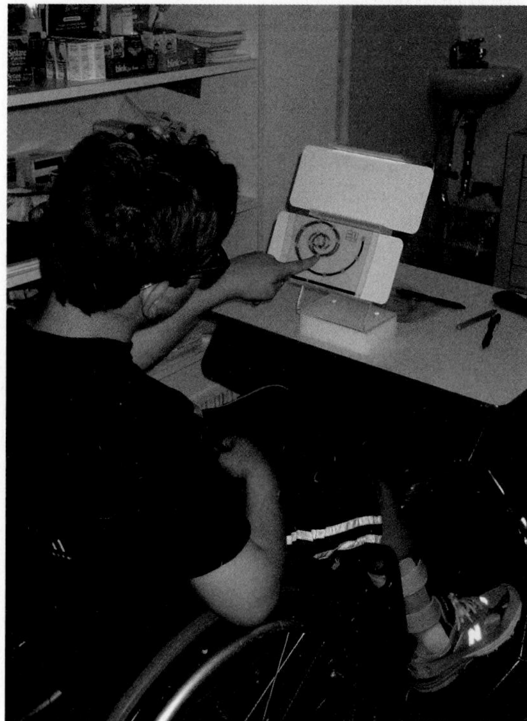

FIGURE 25-23. Patient with large angle XT describing appearance of 3-D Vortex vectogram and localizing in space.

With the spectacle correction and OVT, this patient developed the ability to hold his eyes in binocular alignment when visually attending. He consistently appreciated 400″ stereoacuity. He accurately reported size changes and localization on Quoits vectograms, and developed the ability to describe relative spatial locations with simultaneously presented vectograms.

Occlusion

During a period of therapy, this patient had misplaced his glasses for a period of about 2 months. When new glasses were made, he showed difficulty keeping his eyes in binocular alignment, having become reaccustomed to alternately suppressing vision. Binasal occlusion was applied for a brief period to draw greater attention to his peripheral awareness, supporting his gross appreciation of stereopsis. Greater attention was taken, in-office, to reinforce binocular processing activities during this period. After approximately 3 weeks, the binasal occlusion was removed and was no longer necessary.

Change in Spectacle Prescription

Reevaluation at age 12 revealed a greater range of binocular function and flexibility, as well as oculomotor range. A trial of yoked prism revealed much greater head and neck stability with the application of base-up prism at this juncture (Fig. 25-21).

The spectacle Rx was updated with mild adjustments to refractive correction.

$$OD + 0.50 - 1.50 \times 030;$$
$$OS + 0.75 - 1.75 \times 015.$$

Yoked prism was reoriented to 2^{Δ} base-up OU. Corrective prism was reduced to 5^{Δ}base-in ground-in OU, maintaining the 8^{Δ}base-in Fresnel OU, for a total of 26^{Δ}base-in. This also served to reduce the spectacle weight and lens thickness.

Continuing Progress in an Active Optometric Vision Therapy Program With consistent binocular function and performance, this patient holds his eyes in alignment a majority of the time, not only when visually attending. His visual acuities have also improved in his second year of therapy, achieving 20/25 OD, 20/30 OS, and now 20/20 OU.

Many of the classroom adaptations have been altered accordingly, as he is now able to manage a greater amount of material on a page, and can view a smaller font comfortably. He still prefers larger spacing between lines of text, to help him keep his place across a line. He now reads with much greater speed and less effort, reporting that he can read about 15 to 20 pages in an hour now, at 18 pt and double-spaced at a 24″ working distance.

Rather than design a finite course of treatment with an expected goal or conclusion, goals for this patient have been established, met, and reset as a constantly evolving treatment plan. In addition, the patient voices his concerns or challenges as they present, and a plan is created to help achieve each new goal. In this regard, OVT has become an adjunct to an overall educational plan, supporting this child in any challenges that arise.

CONCLUSION

Optometric vision therapy and neuro-optometric rehabilitation are two modalities that can provide the optometrist with the tools to treat patients with special needs. When combined with lenses, prisms, selective occlusion and tints, patients have the opportunity to develop and/or recover those visual skills that can allow them to reach their maximum potential. This can improve their performance in school, open up opportunities for employment, and improve their overall quality of life.

REFERENCES

1. Akinci A, Oner O, Bozkurt OH, Guven A, et al. Refractive errors and ocular findings in children with intellectual disability: a controlled study. J AAPOS. 2008;12:477–81.
2. Donati RJ, Maino DM, Bartell H, Kieffer M. Polypharmacy and the lack of oculo-visual complaints from those with mental illness and dual diagnosis. Optometry. 2009;80:249–54.
3. Woodhouse JM, Griffiths C, Gedling A. The prevalence of ocular defects and the provision of eye care in adults with learning disabilities living in the community. Ophthalmic Physiol Opt. 2000;20:79–89.
4. North RV, Kelly ME. A review of the uses and adverse effects of topical administration of atropine. Ophthalmic Physiol Opt. 1987;7:109–14.
5. Twelker JD, Mutti DO. Retinoscopy in infants using a near noncycloplegic technique, cycloplegia with tropicamide 1%, and cycloplegia with cyclopentolate 1%. Optom Vis Sci. 2001;78:215–22.
6. Manny RE, Fern KD, Zervas HJ, Cline GE, et al. 1% Cyclopentolate hydrochloride: another look at the time course of cycloplegia using an objective measure of the accommodative response. Optom Vis Sci. 1993;70:651–65.
7. West D, Somers WW. Binocular balance validity: a comparison of five common subjective techniques. Ophthalmic Physiol Opt. 1984;4:155–9.
8. Gallop S. Viewpoint: reconfiguring lens power for improved function. J Behav Optom. 2011;22:99–104.
9. Smith K, Weissberg E, Travison TG. Alternative methods of refraction: a comparison of three techniques. Optom Vis Sci. 2010; 87:E176–82.
10. Cotter SA. Management of childhood hyperopia: a pediatric optometrist's perspective. Optom Vis Sci. 2007;84:103–9.
11. O'Leary CI, Evans BJ. Criteria for prescribing optometric interventions: literature review and practitioner survey. Ophthalmic Physiol Opt. 2003;23:429–39.
12. Lyons SA, Jones LA, Walline JJ, Bartolone AG, et al. A survey of clinical prescribing philosophies for hyperopia. Optom Vis Sci. 2004;81:233–7.
13. Farbrother JE. Spectacle prescribing in childhood: a survey of hospital optometrists. Br J Ophthalmol. 2008;92:392–5.
14. Reiter C, Leising D, Madsen EM. Survey of German clinical prescribing philosophies for hyperopia. Optom Vis Sci. 2007;84:131–6.
15. Harvey EM, Miller JM, Dobson V, Clifford CE. Prescribing eyeglass correction for astigmatism in infancy and early childhood: a survey of AAPOS members. J AAPOS. 2005;9:189–91.
16. Miller JM, Harvey EM. Spectacle prescribing recommendations of AAPOS members. J Pediatr Ophthalmol Strabismus. 1998;35:51–2.
17. Moore B. Refractive error in young children. In: Moore B. Eye care for infants and young children. Boston: Butterworth-Heinemann; 1997.
18. Tassinari JT. Monocular estimate method retinoscopy: central tendency measures and relationship to refractive status and heterophoria. Optom Vis Sci. 2002;79:708–14.
19. Koslowe KC. The dynamic retinoscopies. J Behav Optom. 2010;21:63–7.
20. Marran L, Schor CM. Lens induced aniso-accommodation. Vis Res. 1998;38:3601–19.
21. Tassinari JT. Change in accommodative response and posture induced by nearpoint plus lenses per monocular estimate method retinoscopy. J Behav Optom. 2005;16:87–93.
22. Goss DA, Groppel P, Dominguez L. Comparison of MEM retinoscopy and Nott retinoscopy, and their interexaminer repeatabilities. J Behav Optom. 2005;16:149–55.
23. Suemaru J, Hasebe S, Ohtsuki H. Visual symptoms and compliance with spectacle wear in myopic children: double-masked comparison between progressive addition lenses and single vision lenses. Acta Med Okayama. 2008;62:109–17.
24. Gwiazda J, Hyman L, Hussein M, Everett D, et al. A randomized clinical trial of progressive addition lenses versus single vision lenses on the progression of myopia in children. Invest Ophthalmol Vis Sci. 2003;44:1492–500.
25. Rainey BB, Brooks CW. The use of low powered progressive addition lenses for non-presbyopic patients. J Behav Optom. 1997;8:65–9.
26. Nandakumar K, Leat SJ. Bifocals in Down Syndrome Study (BiDS): design and baseline visual function. Optom Vis Sci. 2009;86:196–207.
27. Nandakumar K, Leat SJ. Bifocals in children with Down syndrome (BiDS): visual acuity, accommodation and early literacy skills. Acta Ophthalmol. 2010;88:e196–e204.
28. Woodhouse JM, Cregg M, Gunter HL, Sanders DP, et al. The effect of age, size of target, and cognitive factors on accommodative responses of children with Down syndrome. Invest Ophthalmol Vis Sci. 2000;41:2479–85.

29. Cregg M, Woodhouse JM, Pakeman VH, Saunders KJ, et al. Accommodation and refractive error in children with Down syndrome: cross-sectional and longitudinal studies. Invest Ophthalmol Vis Sci. 2001;42:55–63.
30. Three Rivers Optical. Available from: www.threeriversoptical.com. Last Accessed October 14, 2010.
31. Signet Armorlite. Available from: www.signetarmorlite.com/professional/index.asp?page_id=211. Last Accessed October 14, 2010.
32. Essilor. Available from: http://www.essilor.com/Essilor-Anti-Fatigue,190. Last Accessed October 14, 2010.
33. Birnbaum, M. Optometric management of nearpoint vision disorders. Santa Ana: Optometric Extension Program Foundation; 2008.
34. Bixenman WW. Vertical prisms: Why avoid them? Surv Ophthalmol. 1984;29:70–8.
35. Karania R, Evans BJW. The mallett fixation disparity test: influence of test instructions and relationship with symptoms. Ophthalmic Physiol Opt. 2006;26:507–22.
36. Kommerell G, Gerling J, Ball M, de Paz H, Bach M. Heterophoria and fixation disparity: a review. Strabismus. 2000;8:127–34.
37. Hock DR, Coffey B. Effects of yoked prism on spatial localization and stereolocalization. J Behav Optom. 2000;11:143–8.
38. Cook DL. Optometric management of patients with incomitant strabismus. J Beh Optom. 2004;15:10–6.
39. Averbuch-Heller L, Dell'Osso LF, Jacobs JB, Remler BF. Latent and congenital nystagmus in Down syndrome. J Neuroophthalmol. 1999;19:166–72.
40. Ciuffreda MA, McCann AL, Gruning CF, Ciuffreda KJ. Multimodal treatment of congenital nystagmus: a case study. J Behav Optom. 2003;14:143–8.
41. Abel LA. Infantile nystagmus: current concepts in diagnosis and management. Clin Exp Optom. 2006;89:57–65.
42. Ordonez XP, Ciuffreda KJ. Reading eye movements in patients with nystagmus and proposed therapeutic paradigms. J Behav Optom. 1997;8:99–103.
43. Margolis NW, Suter PS. Visual field defects and unilateral spatial inattention: diagnosis and treatment. J Behav Optom. 2006;17:31–7.
44. Prisms restore lost peripheral vision. First Report: Englander Communications, May, 2001. Available from: www.eri.harvard.edu/faculty/peli/driving/index.htm. Last Accessed August 18, 2011.
45. Houston KE. Measuring visual midline shift syndrome and disorders of spatial localization: a literature review and report of a new clinical protocol. J Behav Optom. 2010;21:87–93.
46. Massucci ME. Prism adaptation in the rehabilitation of patients with unilateral spatial inattention. J Behav Optom. 2009;20:101–5.
47. Lazarus SM. The use of yoked base-up and base-in prism for reducing eye strain at the computer. J Am Optom Assoc. 1996;67:204–8.
48. Horner SH. The use of lenses and prisms to enhance visual training. Santa Ana: Optometric Extension Program Foundation. 1973. p. 45.
49. Birnbaum MH. Alternative approaches to lens prescribing. In: Optometric management of nearpoint vision disorders. Santa Ana: Optometric Extension Program Foundation, Inc.; 2008. p. 161–92.
50. Medic8 Glasses for infants and children. Available from: www.medic8.com/healthguide/articles/glasses4kids.html. Last Accessed October 14, 2010.
51. How to ensure your glasses fit correctly. Available from: www.stingyspecs.com.au/fit-your-glasses-correctly.html. Last Accessed October 14, 2010.
52. Walsh G. The weight of spectacle frames and the area of their nose pads. Ophthalmic Physiol Opt. 2010;30:402–4.
53. Eng H, Chiu RS. Spectacle fitting with ear, nose and face deformities or abnormalities. Clin Exp Optom. 2002;85:389–91.
54. Steel SE, Mackie SW, Walsh G. Visual field defects due to spectacle frames: their prediction and relationship to UK driving standards. Ophthalmic Physiol Opt. 1996;16:95–100.
55. Dille JR, Marano JA. The effects of spectacle frames on field of vision. Aviat Space Environ Med. 1984;55:957–9.
56. Superior Precision Eyewear for Children who are Special. Available from: www.specs4us.com. Last Accessed October 14, 2010.
57. Miraflex Children's Eyewear. Available from: http://miraflex.info. Last Accessed May 23, 2011.
58. Classé JG. Ophthalmic lenses. University of Alabama at Birmingham's Clinico-legal Aspects of Optometry. 2010.
59. Prevent Blindness America Impact Protection and Polycarbonate Lenses. Available from: www.preventblindness.org/resources/fact sheets/ImpactPoly_FS94.PDF. Last Accessed October 15, 2010.
60. Mattison-Shupnick M. Trivex material- unique attributes make it more than a niche material. Available from: www.2020mag.com/CE/TabViewTest/tabid/92/LessonId/106793/Default.aspx. Last Accessed October 19, 2010.
61. Jalie M. Materials for spectacle lenses: optical and mechanical performance. Optometry Today. 2005;25(2):26–32.
62. Aasuri MK, Venkata N, Preetam P, Rao NT. Management of pediatric aphakia with silsoft contact lenses. CLAO J. 1999;25:209–12.
63. Sclafani LA. Kids and contacts: pediatric aphakia contact lens fitting. Rev Optom. 2002;139:3 Available from: http://cms.revoptom.com/index.asp?page=2_463.htm. Last Accessed September 27, 2011.
64. Tychsen L. Refractive surgery for special needs children. Arch Ophthalmol. 2009;127:810–3.
65. Mojon-Azzi SM, Kunz A, Mojon DS. Strabismus and discrimination in children: are children with strabismus invited to fewer birthday parties? Br J Ophthalmol. 2011; 95:473–6.
66. Lukman H, Kiat JE, Ganesan A, Chua WL, et al. Strabismus-related prejudice in 5–6-year-old children. Br J Ophthalmol. 2010;94:1348–51.
67. Durnian JM, Owen ME, Baddon AC, Noonan CP, et al. The psychosocial effects of strabismus: effect of patient demographics on the AS-20 score. J Am Assoc Pediatr Ophthalmol Strabismus. 2010;14:469–71.
68. Bez Y, Coşkun E, Erol K, Cingu AK, et al. Adult strabismus and social phobia: a case-controlled study. J Am Assoc Pediatr Ophthalmol Strabismus. 2009;13:249–52.
69. Mojon-Azzi SM, Mojon DS. Strabismus and employment: the opinion of headhunters. Acta Ophthalmol. 2009;87:784–8.
70. Mojon-Azzi SM, Potnik W, Mojon DS. Opinions of dating agents about strabismic subjects' ability to find a partner. Br J Ophthalmol. 2008;92:765–9.

71. Maples WC, Bither M. Treating the trinity of infantile vision development: infantile esotropia, amblyopia and anisometropia. Optom Vis Dev. 2006;37:123–30.
72. Jackson J, Castleberry C, Galli M, Arnoldi KA. Cerebral palsy for the pediatric eye care team part II: diagnosis and treatment of ocular motor deficits. Am Orthopt J. 2006;56: 86–96.
73. Maino D. The number of placebo controlled, double blind, prospective, and randomized strabismus surgery outcome clinical trials: none. Optom Vis Dev. 2011;42: 135–8.
74. London R. Passive treatments for early onset strabismus. Probl Optom. 1990;2:480–95.
75. Padula WV, Argyris S, Ray J. Visual evoked potentials (VEP) evaluating treatment for post-trauma vision syndrome (PTVS) in patients with traumatic brain injuries (TBI). Brain Inj. 1994;8:125–33.
76. Tassinari JD. Binasal occlusion. J Behav Optom. 1990;1:16–21.
77. Gallop S. A variation on the use of binasal occlusion-a case study. J Behav Optom. 1998:9:31–5.
78. Sarniguet-Badoche, JM. Early medical treatment of strabismus before the age of 18 months. In: Strabismus II. Proceedings of the 4th Meeting of the International Strabismological Association; October 25–29, 1982, Asilomar, California (Pt. 2). Orlando: Grune and Stratton; 1984. p. 83–9.
79. Wittenberg S. Pinhole eyewear systems: a special report. J Am Optom Assoc. 1993;64:112–6.
80. Rutstein RP. Use of bangerter filters with adults having intractable diplopia. Optometry. 2010;81:387–93.
81. Proctor A. Traumatic brain injury and binasal occlusion. Optom Vis Dev. 2009;40:45–50.
82. Arai T, Ohi H, Sasaki H, Nobuto H, et al. Hemispatial sunglasses: effect on unilateral spatial neglect. Arch Phys Med Rehabil. 1997;78;230–2.
83. Beis JM, Andre JM, Baumgarten A, Challier B. Eye patching in unilateral spatial neglect:efficacy of two methods. Arch Phys Med Rehabil. 1999;80:71–6.
84. Rethy S and Rethy-Gal S. Decreasing behavioral flexibility (of adjustment to strabismus) as the cause of resistance against treatment during the first year of life. In: Strabismus II. Proceedings of the 4th Meeting of the International Strabismological Association; October 25–29, 1982: Asilomar, California (Pt. 2) Orlando: Grune and Stratton; 1984. p. 91–9.
85. West RW. Differences in the perception of monocular and binocular gaze. Optom Vis Sci. 2010;87:112–9.
86. Press L. (June 1, 2011). Photodocumentation of Non-Surgical Treatment of Strabismus. Available from: http://visionhelp.wordpress.com/2011/06/01/4802/. Last Accessed June 2, 2011.
87. London R, Scott SH. Sensory fusion disruption syndrome. J Am Optom Assoc. 1987;58:544–6.
88. Pratt-Johnson MB and Tillson G. The loss of fusion in adults with intractable diplopia. Aust N Z J Ophthalmol. 1988;16:81–5.
89. American Optometric Association. Position statement on vision therapy. J Am Optom Assoc. 1985;56:782–3.
90. Vision Therapy: information for health care and other allied professionals. Optom Vis Sci. 1999;76(11):739–40.
91. Gur S, Ron S. Training in oculomotor tracking: occupational health aspects. Isr J Med Sci. 1992;28:622–8.
92. Ciuffreda KJ, Suchoff IB, Marrone MA, Ahmann E. Oculomotor rehabilitation in traumatic brain-injured patients. J Behav Opt. 1996;7:31–8.
93. Ron S. Plastic changes in eye movements of patients with traumatic brain injury. In: Fuchs A Beckett W, Editors. Progress in oculomotor research. Amsterdam: Elsevier; 1981. p. 233–40.
94. Birnbaum MH, Soden R, Cohen AH. Efficacy of vision therapy for convergence insufficiency in an adult population. J Am Optom Assoc. 1999;70;225–32.
95. Ciuffreda KJ. The scientific basis for efficacy of optometric vision therapy in nonstrabismic accommodative and vergence disorders. Optometry. 2002;73:735–62.
96. Cohen A, Soden R. Effectiveness of visual therapy for convergence insufficiencies for an adult population. J Am Optom Assoc. 1984;55:491–4.
97. Cooper J, Duckman R. Convergence insufficiency: incidence, diagnosis and treatment. J Am Optom Assoc. 1978;49: 673–80.
98. Cooper J, Selenow A, Ciuffreda KJ, Feldman J, et al. Reduction of asthenopia in patients with convergence insufficiency after fusional vergence training. Am J Optom physiol Opt. 1983;60:982–9.
99. Gallaway M, Scheiman M. The efficacy of vision therapy for convergence excess. J Am Optom Assoc. 1997;68:81–6.
100. Grisham JD, Bowman MC, OWyang LA, Chan CL. Vergence orthoptics: validity and persistence of the training effect. Optom Vis Sci. 1991;68:441–51.
101. Scheiman M, Cotter S, Cotter S, Cooper J, et.al. Randomized clinical trial of treatments for symptomatic convergence insufficiency in children. Arch Ophthalmol. 2008;126:1336–49.
102. Scheiman M, Mitchell GL, Cotter S, Cooper J, et al. A randomized clinical trial of treatments for convergence insufficiency in children. Arch Ophthalmol. 2005;123:14–24.
103. Scheiman M, Mitchell GL, Cotter S, Kulp MT, et al. A randomized clinical trial of vision therapy/orthoptics versus pencil push-ups for the treatment of convergence insufficiency in young adults. Optom Vis Sci. 2005;82:583–93.
104. Bobier WR, Sivak JG. Orthoptic treatment of subjects showing slow accommodative responses. Am J Optom Physiol Opt. 1983;60:678–87.
105. Cooper J, Feldman K, Selenow A, Fair R, et al. Reduction of asthenopia after accommodative facility training. Am J Optom Physiol Opt. 1987;64:430–6.
106. Goss DA, Strand K, Poloncak J. Effect of vision therapy on clinical test results in accommodative dysfunction. J Optom Vis Dev. 2003:34:61–3.
107. Russell GE, Wick B. A prospective study of treatment of accommodative insufficiency. Optom Vis Sci. 1993;70:131–5.
108. Altizer LB. The nonsurgical treatment of exotropia. Am Orthopt J. 1972;22:71–6.
109. Chryssanthou G. Orthoptic management of intermittent exotropia. Am Orthopt J. 1974;24:69–72.
110. Coffey B, Wick B, Cotter S, Sharre J, et al. Treatment options for intermittent exotropia: a critical appraisal. Optom Vis Sci. 1992;69:386–404.
111. Cooper J, Medow N. Major review: intermittent exotropia-basic and divergence excess type. Bin Vis Eye Muscle Surg. 1993;8:185–216.

112. Etting GL. Strabismus therapy in private practice: cure rates after three months of therapy. J Am Optom Assoc. 1978;49:1367–73.
113. Flax N, Duckman RH. Orthoptic treatment of strabismus. J Am Optom Assoc. 1978;49:1353–61.
114. Ziegler D, Huff D, Rouse MW. Success in strabismus therapy: a literature review. J Am Optom Assoc. 1982;53:979–83.
115. Birnbaum MH, Koslowe K, Sanet R. Success in amblyopia therapy as a function of age: a literature review. Am J Physiol Opt. 1977;54:269–75.
116. Fitzgerald D, Krumholtz I. Maintenance of improvement gains in refractive amblopia: a comparison of treatment modalities. Optometry. 2002;73:153–9.
117. Garzia RP. Efficacy of vision therapy in amblyopia: a literature review. Am J Optom Physiol Opt. 1987;64:393–404.
118. Krumholtz I, Fitzgerald D. Efficacy of treatment modalities in refractive amblyopia. J Am Optom Assoc. 1999;70: 399–404.
119. Rutstein RP, Fuhr PS. Efficacy and stability of amblyopia therapy. Optom Vis Sci. 1992;69:747–54.
120. Wick B, Wingard M, Cotter S, Scheiman M. Anisometropic amblyopia: is the patient ever too old to treat? Optom Vis Sci. 1992;69:866–78.
121. Seiderman A. Optometric vision therapy results of a demonstration project with a learning disabled population. J Am Opt Assoc. 1980;51:489–93.
122. Zelinsky D. Neuro-optometric diagnosis, treatment and rehabilitation following traumatic brain injuries: a brief review. Phys Med Rehabil Clin N Am. 2007;18:87–107.
123. Ciuffreda KJ, Ludlam DP, Kapoor N. Clinical oculomotor training in traumatic brain injury. Optom Vis Dev. 2009;40:16–23.
124. Cohen AH. The role of optometry in the management of vestibular disorders. Brain Inj Prof. 2005;2:8–11.
125. Fox RS. The rehabilitation of vergence and accommodative dysfunctions in traumatic brain injury. Brain Inj Prof. 2005;2:12–5.
126. Ciuffreda KJ, Kapoor N, Han Y. Reading-related ocular motor deficits in traumatic brian injury. Brain Inj Prof. 2005;2:16–21.
127. Suchoff IB. The diagnosis of visual unilateral spatial inattention. Brain Inj Prof. 2005;2:22–5.
128. Suter PS, Margolis N. Managing visual field defects following acquired brain injury. Brain Inj Prof. 2005;2:26–9.
129. Hillier CG. Vision rehabilitation following acquired brain injury: a case series. Brain Inj Prof. 2005;2:30–2.
130. Padula WV, Argyris S. Post trauma vision syndrome and visual midline shift syndrome. NeuroRehabilitation. 1996 6:165–71.
131. Padula WV, Wu L, Vicci V, Thomas J, et al. Evaluating and treating visual dysfunction. In: Zasler N. Brain injury medicine: principles and practice. New York: Demos Med Pub; 2007.
132. Ciuffreda KJ, Ludlam DP. Conceptual model of optometric vision care in mild traumatic brain injury. J Behav Optom. 2011;22:10–2.
133. Pepper RC, Nordgren MJ. Stress-point learning-A multisensory approach to processing information. Santa Ana: Optometric Extension Program Foundation; 2006.
134. Maino D. Neuroplasticity-teaching an old brain new tricks. Rev Optom. 2009;146:62–70.
135. Constantine-Paton M. Pioneers of cortical plasticity: six classic papers by Wiesel and Hubel. J Neurophysiol. 2008, 99:2741–4.
136. Knudsen EI. Sensitive periods in the development of the brain and behavior. J Cogn Neurosci. 2004;16:1412–25.
137. Levi DM. Perceptual learning in adults with amblyopia: a reevaluation of critical periods in human vision. Dev Psychobiol. 2005;46:222–32.
138. Heimel JA, Hermans JM, Sommeijer JP. Neuro-Bsik Mouse Phenomics consortium, et al. Genetic control of experience-dependent plasticity in the visual cortex. Genes Brain Behav. 2008;7:915–23.
139. Harvey EM, Dobson V, Clifford-Donaldson CE, Miller JM. Optical treatment of amblyopia in astigmatic children: the sensitive period for successful treatment. Ophthalmology. 2007;114:2293–301.
140. Caleo M, Restani L, Gianfranceschi L, Costantin L. Transient synaptic silencing of developing striate cortex has persistent effects on visual function and plasticity. J Neurosci. 200725;27:4530–40.
141. Lewis TL, Maurer D. Multiple sensitive periods in human visual development: evidence from visually deprived children. Dev Psychobiol. 2005;46:163–83.
142. Duffy KR, Livingstone MS. Loss of neurofilament labeling in the primary visual cortex of monocularly deprived monkeys. Cereb Cortex. 2005;15:1146–54.
143. Bottjer SW. Neural strategies for learning during sensitive periods of development. J Comp Physiol. A. 2002;188:917–28.
144. Domenici L, Cellerino A, Berardi N, Cattaneo A, et al. Antibodies to nerve growth factor (NGF) prolong the sensitive period for monocular deprivation in the rat. Neuroreport. 199427;5:2041–4.
145. Matta NS, Singman EL, Silbert DI. Evidenced-based medicine: treatment for amblyopia. Am Orthopt J. 2010;60:17–22.
146. Alvarez TL, Vicci VR, Alkan Y, Kim EH, et al. Vision therapy in adults with convergence insufficiency: clinical and functional magnetic resonance imaging measures. Optom Vis Sci. 2010;87:985–1002.
147. Cattaneo Z, Vecchi T. The neuroscience of visual impairment. Boston: MIT Press; 2011. p. 75–112.
148. Cattaneo Z, Vecchi T. Spatial cognition in the blind. In: Blind vision: the neuroscience of visual impairment. Massachusetts: MIT Press; 2011. p. 113–36.
149. Alesterlund L, Maino D. That the blind may see: a review. Blindsight and its implications for optometrists. J Optom Vis Dev. 1999;30:86–93.
150. Maravita A, Spence C, Driver J. Multisensory integration and the body schema: close to hand and within reach. Curr Biol. 2003;13:R531–9.
151. Ladavas E. Functional and dynamic properties of visual peripersonal space. Trends Cogn Sci. 2002;6:17–22.
152. Snell RS, Lemp MA. The visual pathway. In: Clinical anatomy of the eye. 2nd ed. Malden: Blackwell Science, Inc.; 1998. p. 379–412.
153. Felleman DJ, VanEssen DC. Distributed hierarchical processing in the primate cerebral cortex. Cereb Cortex. 1991;1:1–47.

154. Barker L. Evaluation and treatment of sensory processing disorder. Chattanooga: Ready Approach Lecture Series; July 2010.
155. Goddard-Blythe S. The well balanced child-movement and early learning. London: Hawthorn Press; 2004.
156. Goddard S. A teacher's window into the child's mind. Eugene: Fern Ridge Press; 1996.
157. Kasai T and Zee DS. Eye-head coorination in labyrinthine-defective human beings. Brain Res. 1978;144:123–41.
158. Herdman SJ. Vestibular rehabilitation. 3rd ed. Philadelphia: FA Davis Company; 2000.
159. Goodale MA. Action insight: the role of the dorsal stream in the perception of grasping. Neuron. 2005;47:328–9.
160. Holmes NP, Spence C. The body schema and multisensory representation(s) of peripersonal space. Cogn Process. 2004;5:94–105.
161. The Feldenkrais Method of Somatic Education. Available from: www.feldenkrais.com. Last Accessed August 8, 2011.
162. The Complete Guide to the Alexander Technique. Available from: www.alexandertechnique.com. Last Accessed August 8, 2011.
163. Sanders H, Davis MF, Duncan B, Meaney FJ, et al. Use of complementary and alternative medical therapies among children with special health care needs in southern Arizona. Pediatrics. 2003;111:584–7.
164. Troyanovich SJ, Harrison DE, Harrison DD. Structural rehabilitation of the spine and posture: rationale for treatment beyond the resolution of symptoms. J Manipulative Physiol Ther. 1998;21:37–50.
165. Jackson R. Action binding: dynamic interactions between vision and touch. Trends Cogn Sci. 2001;5:505–6.
166. Buisseret P, Gary-Bobo E. Development of visual cortical orientation specificity after dark rearing: role of extraocular proprioception. Neurosci Lett. 1979;13:259–63.
167. Buisseret P, Singer W. Proprioceptive signals from extraocular muscles gate experience dependent modifications of receptive fields in the kitten visual cortex. Exp Brain Res. 1983;51;443–50.
168. Gauthier GM, Nommay D, Vercher JL. Ocular muscle proprioception and visual localization of targets in man. Brain. 1990;1113:1857–71.
169. Gauthier GM, Nommay D, Vercher JL. The role of ocular muscle proprioception in visual localization of targets. Science. 1990;249:58–61.
170. Brunech R, Ruskell GL. Myotendinous nerve endings in human infant and adult extraocular muscles. Anat Rec. 2000;260:132–40.
171. Brunech JR, Ruskell GL. Muscle spindles in extraocular muscles of human infants. Cells Tissues Organs. 2001;169:388–94.
172. Goodale MA, Milner AD. Sight Unseen-an exploration of consciousness and unconscious vision. Oxford, England: Oxford University Press; 2004.
173. Nassi JJ, Callaway EM. Multiple circuits relaying primate parallel visual pathways to the middle temporal area. J Neurosci. 2006;26:12789–98.
174. Maravita A, Iriki A. Tools for the body (schema). Trends Cogn Sci. 2004;8:79–86.
175. Berti A, Frassinetti F. When far becomes near: remapping of space by tool use. J Cogn Neurosci. 2000;12:415–20.
176. Ciuffreda KJ, Tannen B. Eye movement basics for the clinician. In: Introduction to eye movements. St. Louis: Mosby; 1995. p. 1–9.
177. Schaaf RC, Lane SJ. Neuroscience foundations of vestibular, proprioceptive and tactile sensory strategies. OT Practice. 2009;14:CE1–8.
178. Hertle RW. Classification of eye movement abnormalities and strabismus (CEMAS). Washington: Workshop, National Eye Institute; 2008.
179. Clarke VN, Noel LP. Vanishing infantile esotropia. Can J Ophthalmol. 1982;17:100–2.
180. Barry S. Fixing my gaze. New York: Basic Books; 2009.
181. Schor CM. Neuromuscular plasticity and rehabilitation of the ocular near response. Optom Vis Sci. 2009;86:788–802.
182. Munoz P, Semmlow JL, Yuan W, Alvarez RL. Short term modification of disparity vergence eye movements. Vis Res. 1999;39:1695–1705.
183. Thiagarajan P, Lakshminarayanan V, Bobier WR. Effect of Vergence adaptation and positive fusional vergence training on oculomotor parameters. Optom Vis Sci. 2010;87:487–93.
184. Sreenivasan V, Bobier W, Irving E, Lakshminarayanan V. Effect of vergence adapatation on convergence-accommodation: model simulations. Trans Biomed Eng. 2009;56:2389–95.
185. Schor CM, Ciuffreda KJ. Vergence eye movements-basic and clinical aspects. Boston: Butterworth- Heinemann; 1983.
186. Cooper J, Ciuffreda KJ, Carniglia PE, Zinn KM, et al. Orthoptic treatment and eye movement recordings in Guillain-Barre syndrome. 1995;15:249–56.
187. Baxstrom CR. Nonsurgical treatment for esotropia secondary to Arnold-Chiari I malformation: a case report. Optometry. 2009;80:472–8.
188. Valmaggia C, Proudlock F, Gottlob I. Optokinetic nystagmus in strabismus: are asymmetries related to binocularity? Invest Ophthalmol Vis Sci. 2003;44:5142–50.
189. Gerth C, Mirabella G, Li X, Wright T, et al. Timing of surgery for infantile esotropia in humans: effects on cortical motion visual evoked responses. Invest Ophthalmol Vis Sci. 2008;49:3432–27.
190. Tychsen L. Motion sensitivity and the origins of infantile strabismus. In: Simons K, editor. Early visual development-normal and abnormal. New York: Oxford University Press; 1993. p 364–90.
191. Optometric clinical practice guideline: care of the patient with amblyopia. St. Louis: Am Optom Assoc; 2004:http://www.aoa.org/documents/CPG-4.pdf.
192. Swartout-Corbeil DM, Steefel L, Gale T. "Amblyopia." Gale encyclopedia of children's health. Gale Encyclopedia of Public Health; 2006.
193. Hess RF, Mansouri B, Thompson B. A binocular approach to treating amblyopia: antisuppression therapy. Optom Vis Sci. 2010;87:697–704.
194. Amblyopia. National Eye Institute National Institutes of Health. Available from: www.nei.nih.gov/health/amblyopia/factsaboutamblyopia.pdf. Last Accessed August 11, 2011.
195. Amblyopia Treatment Studies. Available from: www.abcd-vision.org/amblyopia/ats-pedig.html. Last Accessed August 11, 2011.

196. Levi DM, Li RW. Perceptual learning as a potential treatment for amblyopia: a mini-review. Vis Res. 2009;49:2535–49.
197. Li RW, Young KG, Hoenig P, Levi DM. Perceptual learning improves visual performance in juvenile amblyopia. Invest Ophthalmol Vis Sci. 2005;46:3161–8.
198. Polat U, Ma-Naim T, Belkin M, Sagi D, et al. Improving vision in adult amblyopia by perceptual learning. Proc Natl Acad Sci. 2004;101:6692–7.
199. Revell MJ. Strabismus-A history of orthoptic techniques. London, England: Barrie and Jenkins Ltd;1971.
200. Bredemeyer HG, Bullock K. Orthoptics-theory and practice. St. Louis: CV Mosby Co.; 1968.
201. Pediatric eye disease investigator group. The clinical spectrum of early-onset esotropia: experience of the congenital esotropia observational study. Am J Ophthalmol. 2002;133;102–8.
202. AOA and COVD joint policy on "The Distinction between Vision Therapy and Orthoptics." Available from: www.aoa.org/documents/DefinitionsOptometricVisionTherapy.pdf. Last Accessed August 17, 2011.
203. Wong AMF. Eye movement disorders. New York: Oxford University Press; 2008. p. 22.
204. Bosworth RG, Birch EE. Direction-of-motion detection and motion VEP asymmetries in normal children and children with infantile esotropia. Invest Ophthalmol Vis Sci. 2007;48:5523–31.
205. Aiello A, Wright KW, Borchert M. Independence of optokinetic nystagmus asymmetry and binocularity in infantile esotropia. Arch Ophthalmol. 1994;112:1580–3.
206. Tychsen L. Motion sensitivity and the origins of infantile Esotropia. In: Simons K, editor. Early visual development: normal and abnormal. New York: Oxford University Press; 1993. p. 364–90.
207. Ottenbacher K. Patterns of postrotary nystagmus in three learning-disabled children. Am J Occup Ther. 1982;36: 657–63.
208. Winkler PA, Ciuffreda KJ. Ocular fixation, vestibular dysfunction, and visual motion hypersensitivity. Optometry. 2009;80:502–12.
209. Scheiman M, Rouse M. Optometric management of learning-related vision problems. St. Louis: Mosby-Year Book; 1994.
210. American Academy of Pediatrics, Section on Ophthalmology, Council on Children with Disabilities American Academy of Ophthalmology, American Association for Pediatric Ophthalmology and Strabismus and American Association of Certified Orthoptists: learning disabilities, dyslexia and vision. Pediatrics. 2009;124:837–44.
211. Bowan MD. Learning disabilities, dyslexia, and vision: a subject review-A rebuttal, literature review and commentary. Optometry. 2002;73:553–75.
212. Lack D. Another joint statement regarding learning disabilities, dyslexia, and vision—a rebuttal. Optometry. 2010; 81:533–43.
213. Li A. (Alicia) Classroom strategies for improving and enhancing visual skills in students with disabilities. Except Child. 2004;36:38–46.
214. Titcomb R, Okoye R, Schiff S. Introduction to the Dynamic Process of Vision. In: Gentile M. Functional visual behavior. Bethesda: American Occupational Therapy Association. 1997. p. 27.
215. Shaywitz SE, Fletcher JM, Holahan JM, Shneider AE, et al. Persistence of dyslexia: the connecticut longitudinal study at adolescence. Pediatrics. 1999;104:1351–9.
216. Schulte-Korne G, Deimel W, Barling J, Remschmidt H. Speech perception deficit in dyslexic adults as measured by mismatch negativity. Int J Psychophysiol. 2001:40: 77–87.
217. Stein J, Walsh V. To see but not to read: the magnocellular theory of dyslexia. Trends Neurosci. 1997;20:147–52.
218. Solan HA, Hansen PC, Shelley-Tremblay J, Ficarra A. Coherent motion threshold measurements for M-cell deficit differ for above and below average readers. Optometry. 2003;74:727–33.
219. Talcott JB, Hansen PC, Assoku EL, Stein JF. Visual motion sensitivity in dyslexia: evidence for temporal and energy integration deficits. Neuropsychologia. 2000;38:935–43.
220. Legge GE, Cheung SH, Yu D, Chung STL, et al. The case for the visual span as a sensory bottleneck in reading. J Vis. 2007;7:1–15.
221. Vidyasagar TR, Pammer K. Dyslexia: a deficit in visuo-spatial attention, not in phonological processing. Trends Cogn Sci. 2009;14:57–64.
222. Vidyasagar TR. Neural underpinnings of dyslexia as a disorder of visuo-spatial attention. Clin Exp Optom. 2004;87:4–10.
223. Williams MC, Lecluyse K. Perceptual consequences of a temporal processing deficit in reading disabled children. J Am Optom Assoc. 1990;61:111–21.
224. Rae C, Harasty JA, Dzendrowskyj TE, Talcott JB, et al. Cerebellar morphology in developmental dyslexia. Neuropsychologia. 2002;40:1285–92.
225. Lane KA. Vision processing and reading. OEP Clin Curr. 1985;1(1–3):1–20.
226. Birnbaum MH. Vision disorders frequently interfere with reading and learning: they should be diagnosed and treated. J Behav Optom. 1993;4:66–71.
227. Kapoor N, Ciuffreda KJ. Vision disturbances following traumatic brain injury. Curr Treat Options Neurol. 2002;4:271–80.
228. Suter PS, Harvey LH. Vision rehabilitation-multidisciplinary care of the patient following brain injury. New York: CRC Press; 2011.
229. Padula WV. Neuro-optometric rehabilitation. Santa Ana: Optometric Extension Program Foundation; 1988.
230. Padula WV, Argyris S. Post Trauma Vision Syndrome and Visual Midline Shift Syndrome. Available from: www.padulainstitute.com/post_trauma_vision_syndrome.htm#vmss. Last Accessed August 12, 2011.
231. Croakies Available from: http://croakies.com/kidsmicrosuiter.aspx. Last Accessed June 15, 2011.

CHAPTER 26

Patricia S. Lemer, MEd, NCC

Complementary and Alternative Approaches

INTRODUCTION

A variety of well-documented interventions for individuals with special needs are presented in earlier chapters of this book. Several traditional treatments, including the use of medications, placing a child in special education, and providing counseling, all are efficacious. Information on these and other conventional alternatives is readily available and will not be included in this chapter. Many less well-known options fall under the umbrella of "*complementary and alternative medicine*" or CAM, because they are used together with (complementary) or in place of (alternative) conventional medicine.

WHAT IS CAM?

The National Center for Complementary and Alternative Medicine (NCCAM) defines CAM as "a group of diverse medical and health care systems, practices, and products that are not generally considered part of conventional medicine. The boundaries between CAM and conventional medicine are not absolute, and specific CAM practices may, over time, become widely accepted" (1).

Whatever the treatment methods, the ultimate goal for individuals with special needs is to eliminate undesirable behaviors, as well as mitigate underlying dysfunction in one or more of the body's systems that might be causing such behaviors. Negative behaviors such as hyperactivity, poor attention, perseveration, and impulsivity are generally unacceptable, while positive behaviors such as relatedness, eye contact, self-control, heightened attention, and increased independence, self-confidence, speech, and language are desirable.

Because individuals with different diagnoses have varying etiologies, pinpointing single causes is often very difficult. Many early medical and environmental conditions are now considered risk factors for developmental delays, leading to special needs. Risk factors include, but are not limited to, the following:

- Prenatal and birth complications, such as gestational diabetes, oxygen deprivation, or breech presentation
- Skin eruptions, such as eczema, acne, and rashes
- Self-limited diets often consisting primarily of wheat and dairy products
- Digestive problems including chronic constipation, diarrhea, and/or reflux
- Allergy symptoms such as colic, ear infections, red ears and cheeks, black circles under the eyes, and puffy faces
- Respiratory reactions, such as asthma and allergies
- Sleep problems
- Hyperactivity
- Hypotonia

Sometimes, when treatments focus on and ameliorate physiologic problems, even partially, negative behaviors often decrease, and desired behaviors increase spontaneously (2).

Physicians deliver primary care for individuals with special needs; however, other health care and educational professionals provide important adjunct interventions. Today's well-educated parents learn about new treatments quickly by using computers and smart phones or flocking to conferences with hundreds of vendors selling thousands of products promising to improve behavior, language, learning, social skills, and almost everything else. Which alternative and complementary approaches are sound, which will work for their child, and which are risky, not worth the expense, or outright bogus, can be difficult to determine.

In this chapter, the goal is to offer professionals and parents alternatives, so that they can make educated choices. Informed decisions allow limited resources to be allocated with care.

TOTAL LOAD THEORY

While diagnoses differ, children with special needs have an important commonality: a huge total load. Total load theory is a multifactorial approach describing the cumulative effect of the individual assaults on the body as a whole (3). The cluster of symptoms that eventually leads to a diagnosis involves many organ, muscle, and sensory systems of the body being stressed to their limits. Each individual has a personal load limit, as does a bridge. When that limit is exceeded, skin, respiratory, digestive, immunologic, language, motor, and attention problems occur. These coexist with the developmental, cognitive, and sensory issues, and their relationship is very complex.

Timing of the assaults is crucial. Pregnancy and the first two years of life, especially the end of the second year, are particularly vulnerable periods, when neuronal growth is rapid.

Components of the total load include, but are not limited to, the following:

- ***Structural problems*** resulting from traumatic birth or other injury
- ***Biomedical dysfunction*** such as allergies, eczema, rhinitis, sinusitis; bacterial, viral, and yeast infections; digestive and respiratory problems
- ***Environmental assaults*** from chemicals, pesticides, food additives, pollen and heavy metals, including aluminum, antimony, arsenic, cadmium, lead and mercury, and possibly from electromagnetic fields (4)

The idea of total load brings together a coherent theory of etiology and also offers possible solutions. Each therapy or intervention that removes load factors is part of a larger whole and therefore may be partially, but not necessarily completely, effective. The sum is greater than the individual parts.

Before practitioners prescribe CAM treatments, they must take an exhaustive history. Oral and written questions can take hours and pages to uncover all prenatal, natal, environmental, and social factors, including toxic exposures to pesticides, chemicals, or tobacco or building materials; medications, vaccine reactions; pet products; travel; changes in environment and water; family strife; lack of sensory stimulation; and more. Some factors may be obvious, such as moving into an older house with lead paint, but others may be subtler, such as toxic lawn treatments that are tracked daily into the home.

APPROACHES TO REDUCE THE TOTAL LOAD

Alternative and complementary treatments focusing on physiologic relationships occurring in the body neurologically, metabolically, and psychologically can be categorized as follows:

- **Structural therapies** including chiropractic, chiropractic neurology, craniosacral therapy, osteopathy
- **Reflex integration** of approximately 100 primitive reflexes, involuntary, stereotyped movements, which babies are born with and account for most of the movement patterns during the first few months of life
- **Biomedical interventions** that boost the depressed immune system, remove pathogens from and heal the damaged gastrointestinal system, enhance neurologic and metabolic function, and remove the toxins from the body including dietary modification, nutritional supplementation, and homeopathy
- **Sensory therapies that complement vision therapy**, including occupational therapy, listening therapies, educational kinesiology, music therapy, neurofeedback and animal therapies
- **Therapies focusing on developing communication and social skills**, including Son-Rise, Developmental Individual, Relationship-Based (DIR) Model, and Relationship Development Intervention (RDI) Program
- **Energy therapies** that modify or manipulate underlying intangible impediments, many of which are based on ancient eastern healing techniques that are thousands of years old

Structural Therapies Chiropractors, chiropractic neurologists, osteopaths, and craniosacral therapists evaluate cranial, upper cervical, and pelvic alignment as well as possible defects in facial development or dental occlusion. Structural stressors, in any of these areas, derived from birth and other trauma, can affect bodily systems profoundly, by disrupting blood flow and lymphatic drainage. They also can weaken the brain's defenses, making the body susceptible to invasion by lead, aluminum, and mercury and the microorganisms that feed on them, as well as set the body up for ear and other infections (5).

Professionals then design a variety of treatment procedures focusing on the two-way interaction between the sensory systems, including vision, and the central nervous system. The goal of structural therapy is to realign the body's internal parts and bring the body into balance. Treatment, which could include manipulation or use of cold lasers or other tools, enhances the nervous system's ability to handle sensory stimulation. Some treatments look similar to optometric vision therapy, including ocular–motor activities and computer-based techniques. (Chapter 25, Optometric Management of Functional Vision Disorders). After structural treatment, increased proprioceptive feedback to the peripheral and central nervous systems can improve brain integration and facilitate improved responses to other therapies (6).

Reflex Integration Most individuals with special needs still retain some primitive reflexes. Visually, they help infants to focus on and identify what they see, to coordinate the eyes to work together, and to develop accommodation and depth perception. Neurologically, primitive reflexes provide infants with learning experiences that build the foundation for all motor and cognitive skills. The interference of reflexes with the development of complex motor skills most probably accounts for some babies' odd movement and behavior patterns (7).

When babies, for whatever reason, fail to gain full control over one or more primitive reflexes, the reflexes remain present and voluntary movement patterns cannot develop. These children eventually may be diagnosed as dyspraxic or apraxic, learning disabled, having an attention deficit, or on the autism spectrum (8,9).

Some developmental optometrists, occupational and physical therapists, and others are now including reflex integration programs into their therapy protocols. Intervention programs focus on several reflexes that are thought to most affect development. These include the Moro, tonic labyrinthine, spinal Galant, asymmetrical, and symmetrical tonic neck reflexes (10,11).

Biomedical Interventions Treatments for immune system, gastrointestinal, metabolic, and other medical problems are crucial to the care of individuals with special needs, as many encounter health problems from almost the first day of life. These treatments are extremely complex and must be individualized. A well-known program for using biomedical interventions for autism and related disorders is available from the Autism Research Institute (ARI) at www.autism.com. For further information on autism, please refer to Chapter 8, Autism.

Although history taking alone is sometimes adequate to determine an appropriate beginning treatment plan, laboratory testing is frequently necessary to investigate gut flora, specific nutritional deficiencies, or the presence of toxic agents. Fortunately, some very sophisticated blood, urine, and stool tests are available to pinpoint exactly what has gone awry with the immune, digestive, and respiratory systems and the body's ability to detoxify. These tests measure the following factors:

- Strength of immediate and delayed reactions to various common foods, including gluten and casein peptides
- The presence of abnormal organic acids associated with yeast, fungal, and clostridia metabolism
- Undesirable invaders such as intestinal parasites, viruses, yeast, and bad bacteria
- Amino acid and fatty acids
- Unusually high antibody titers resulting from markedly abnormal responses to childhood vaccinations and to various pathogens, such as Lyme, strep, and herpes
- Environmental toxin and blood ammonia levels
- Excessive levels of toxic metals and deficiencies of essential minerals
- Total immunoglobulins and lymphocyte levels

The two most common treatment protocols to address immune system dysfunction include identifying and stopping all possible problematic exposures, along with increasing function with nutritional supplementation.

Dietary Modification Changing the diet can be crucial in improving the behavior of children with special needs (12). Studies show that removal of gluten (the protein in many grains, including wheat), casein (the protein in dairy products), soy, sugar, and yeast can make a marked and often immediate difference in approximately one-third of children with special needs. Some improve dramatically; another third show improvement in secondary symptoms, such as poor sleep and preservative behavior, although their diagnosis remains (13). Children on dairy-free diets and others with calcium (Ca) deficiency may be irritable, hyperactive, sleep-disturbed and inattentive, and have stomach and muscle cramps and tingling in arms and legs. These symptoms often disappear with properly balanced supplements of calcium and magnesium.

As early as the 1950s, pioneers in this field, Drs. William Crook (14), Benjamin Feingold (15), and Doris Rapp (16) showed that unprocessed foods are less likely to cause problems than those with additives, and that a consistent assault of single food products, such as milk and wheat products cannot be tolerated by some children. Crook and Rapp developed rotation diets that alternate grains, meats, fruits, nuts, seeds, and legumes. Feingold removed artificial colors, flavors, and foods containing salicylates. The gluten- and casein-free (GF/CF) diet is particularly common in treating children with autism spectrum disorders and helpful in those with other special needs as well (17). Two other popular diets for individuals with special needs are the Specific Carbohydrate Diet (SCD) (18) and Body Ecology Diet (BED) (19). Both are quite restrictive but show marked changes in behavior and reduction of symptoms in some of the most difficult cases.

Nutritional Supplementation What comprises appropriate nutrition is a matter of great controversy; both deficiencies and toxic levels can be at fault. While biomedical treatments can be extremely helpful for many with special needs, patients' tendency towards picky eating can often interfere with success. Their self-restricted diets, poor absorption, inherited nutrient deficiencies, and/or impaired ability to detoxify environmental chemicals and pollutants combine to make them needier nutritionally than typical children. A logical step is the therapeutic use of nutritional supplements to close the gap between what is eaten and what the body requires.

Vitamins and minerals can often enhance cognition, improve speech and language, help sleeping patterns, lessen irritability, and decrease self-injurious and self-stimulatory behavior, without side effects (17). A special case is Down syndrome. Kent MacLeod, a Canadian pharmacist, has had success with vitamin and mineral supplementation that corrects what he believes is a metabolic defect caused by the chromosomal abnormality (20).

Minerals are perhaps the most important of the body's nutrients, as vitamins, proteins, enzymes, amino acids, fats, and carbohydrates all require minerals for activity. Mineral deficiencies are very common in children who eat high-carbohydrate and processed foods. Key vitamins include the antioxidants A, C, and E, vitamin D, and vitamins B_6 and B_{12}, especially when combined with magnesium, the fourth most abundant mineral in the body. It is essential for over 300 biochemical bodily reactions and the single most important mineral for maintaining proper electrical balance and facilitating smooth metabolism in the cells (21). Vitamins and minerals most often used therapeutically are noted in Table 26.1.

Other supplements used for those with special needs include the following:

- **Essential Fatty Acids (EFAs)** are crucial to maintaining a healthy immune system. Omega 3 and omega 6 fatty acids must be ingested, because the body cannot produce them. Fortunately, both are found in a variety of foods, including nuts and seeds, fish, and oils, including flaxseed, borage, and cod-liver.
- **Amino acids** are subunits of protein molecules that result from completed digestion. When absorbed into the bloodstream, they aid in ridding the body of toxins that are by-products of normal metabolism, as well as those that come from bowel germs, impure waste, and food.
- **Probiotics and Antifungals** In order to reestablish intestinal integrity and to mend the leaky gut, over-the-counter and prescribed supplements are often recommended. These fall into two categories: *pro*biotics, meaning "in support of life," and *anti*fungals, drugs that kill the yeasts and fungi. Probiotics, including acidophilus and lactobacillus, replace the good bacteria in the gut, and are available over the counter. Antifungals, needed to wipe out the yeasts, require a doctor's prescription. These products are often used together and in conjunction with the elimination of all sugars, including fruits, from the diet.
- **Miscellaneous supplements** Herbs, digestive enzymes, and plant extracts, including algae, can also be taken in combination with vitamins, minerals, antifungals, amino acids, and probiotics in the treatment of undesirable behaviors,

TABLE 26.1 Vitamin and Mineral Supplements for Individuals with Special Needs

Supplement and Purpose

Vitamins

Vitamin A

- Metabolites from vitamin A are involved in the normal function of retinoid receptors in the eye. Critical for vision, sensory perception, language processing, and attention (22,23).

B vitamins

- Enhance health of nerves, hair, skin, eyes, liver, mouth. Increase muscle tone in gastrointestinal tract (24)

  Vitamin B6

  - Used with magnesium to increase social engagement, language, and appropriate facial expressions. Decreases obsessive behavior and tactile sensitivity (25).

  Vitamin B12

  - Deficiency causes early regression in infants. In children, slow thinking, confusion, memory issues, depression, and psychotic states. Supplementation enhances cognition and awareness (26).

Vitamin C

- Potent antioxidant. Enhances selenium utilization.

Vitamin D

- Regulates calcium status. Regulates immune function. Essential for brain development during gestation and early years of life.

Vitamin E

- Potent antioxidant. Promotes proper metabolism and reception of Vitamin D and calcium.

Minerals

Calcium

- Most abundant mineral in the body. Neutralizes excess aluminum. Must be supplemented in dairy-free diets.

Magnesium

- Improves digestion, hypersensitivity to sound, irritability, muscle cramps, cold hands and feet, insomnia, carbohydrate cravings, numbness and tingling, and the inability to inhale deeply. Used frequently with vitamin B_6 (27)

Selenium

- Important for immune function. Often deficient in low-protein diets (28).

Zinc

- Protects against adverse effects from heavy metals. Essential to health of ocular tissue. Cofactor for vitamin A (29).

including hyperactivity. Creatine use has shown an increase in muscle strength in muscular dystrophies with activities of daily living improving as well (30). Ginseng appears to have beneficial effects on cognition, behavior, and one's quality of life (31). The use of melatonin can be effective for dementia-related psychopathologic behavior problems (32).

Homeopathy Homeopathy is a 200-year-old approach that provides substances to stimulate and harness the body's own ability to heal itself. Homeopathic practitioners can be traditional MDs, naturopaths, osteopathic physicians, or lay persons. Many physicians combine traditional and homeopathic treatments, depending upon the patient's symptoms and history. The healer evaluates and treats physical, mental, and emotional symptoms (33).

Homeopathy, like other treatments in this chapter, focuses on the individual, not the diagnosis. Thus, people with similar diagnoses may be given very different treatments or "remedies," depending on what characteristics cluster together, with the ultimate goal to bring the body into balance. Homeopathy is hugely popular in Europe and is being used more widely in North America today.

Detoxification Living in a toxic world bombards the body with substances that cause damage to its tissues and thus weaken health by contributing to its body burden and total load (34). Health care practitioners use a combination of laboratory tests to identify toxins and determine an appropriate detoxification treatment plan. Foods, supplements, prescriptive medications, homeopathy, and other means are part of ever-changing protocols. The ultimate goal is to find where toxic metals and other substances are hiding in the body, and to force excretion through the skin, urine, bowels or hair, without overburdening vital organs (35).

Treatments That Affect Sensory Processing The senses allow us to process, organize, and give meaning to our world. The bodies of many children with special needs do not process touch, movement, balance, smell, sound, or vision efficiently. A variety of approaches are designed to improve all types of sensory processing.

Occupational Therapy Please refer to Chapter 28, The Multidisciplinary Approach, for a comprehensive discussion.

Listening Therapies Good listening requires that the various components of the ear and the two ears work together. The coordination of sounds allows the ear to send messages to the brain to be interpreted and stored. The vestibular system is also key to efficient processing of sound. These auditory difficulties could very well be related to the repeated inner ear infections many children diagnosed with special needs experienced as babies (36).

Several types of auditory training have been developed to normalize the way individuals with special needs process sound, and they all require specialized electronic equipment. Digitally modified music stimulates the vestibular system, located in the inner ear, which, in turn, activates the language centers of the brain, eye movements, and the digestive system. Thus, far more than hearing may be influenced (37).

The most common approaches are Berard AIT, designed to reduce hypersensitivity to sound and equalize the perception of all frequencies (38) and the Tomatis method designed specifically to improve listening and communication skills directly (39).

Research is ongoing to evaluate the effectiveness of listening therapies for individuals with special needs. Parents report a reduction in temper tantrums, sound and tactile sensitivity, hyperactivity, impulsivity, and distractibility. Increased eye contact, as well as the ability to follow directions, pay attention, remember, speak, socialize, move, draw, and play independently is reported. Sometimes sleep and other activities are disturbed temporarily, but a return to normality is usually seen in a short time (40).

Educational Kinesiology Also known as Brain Gym, educational kinesiology (EK) is a therapy that purportedly improves sensory function by enhancing neuropathways. Developed in the 1970s by Dr. Paul Dennison, an educator who was trying to understand his own learning and visual problems, it is based on an understanding of the interdependence of physical development, language acquisition, and academic achievement. Central to EK is the relationship between dysfunctional behavior and stress. Dennison synthesized the pioneering work of optometrists, chiropractors, and learning specialists to integrate a series of movements that together reduce an individual's stress (41).

Brain Gym movements can be incorporated into the school program several times a day for a few minutes to wake up the body to learn (42). Starting with a readiness routine called PACE, for **P**ositive, **A**ctive, **C**lear and **E**nergetic, it includes drinking ample water (to nourish the neuropathways), and then a number of techniques with catchy names such as Brain Buttons, Cross Crawls, and Hook-Ups. Carla Hannaford has written an understandable discussion of this interesting technique (43), and Cecilia Freeman has shown how to use it with children with various types of special needs (44).

Sensory learning is a unique program founded in 1997 by Mary Bolles, a mother who was seeking help for her son. She discovered that combining visual, auditory, and vestibular into one multisensory experience resulted in improved perception, understanding, and the ability to learn. The visual component uses syntonics: colored lights that pulse on and off about six times per minute. The vestibular stimulation is delivered on a motion table that rotates in various planes. The auditory part uses headphones that contain modulated music. Sensory Learning Program centers are nationwide.

HANDLE, an acronym for the **H**olistic **A**pproach to **N**euro**D**evelopment and **L**earning **E**fficiency, is another multisensory program that also targets nutritional and digestive problems. This approach was developed by the late Judith Bluestone. Since 1994, the HANDLE organization has trained many therapists who have treated thousands of individuals worldwide for learning disabilities, attention deficits, autism, Pervasive developmental disorder (PDD), dyspraxia, language disorders, Tourette syndrome, and a plethora of perceptual and behavioral disorders.

Strengthening the vestibular system, enhancing muscle tone, and increasing differentiation are the goals of HANDLE. These are all accomplished through deceptively simplistic activities that are sensitive to the client's physical and social–emotional needs. Small, measured doses of specific activities are incorporated daily at home or in a day care/school setting.

Music/Rhythm Therapy Interactive metronome (IM) is a computerized program that challenges the participant to precisely match the computer's rhythm by tapping hand and/or foot sensors. Feedback tells whether the response was early, late, or just right. During a full training, over 35,000 responses are possible. More than 2,000 clinics in North America offer this training.

In a study concerning music therapy, pain was reduced by up to 50% in some patients and decreased the need for morphine-like analgesics (45). Music therapy also appears to improve walking skills of those with acquired brain injury, was superior to placebo therapy for improving verbal and gestural communicative skills of those with autism, and may be of use for the treatment of depression (46–48).

Neurofeedback Neurofeedback has emerged as a powerful tool for those with special needs. Individuals from a number of disciplines have embraced it because it complements biomedical and sensory methods so well. Neurofeedback takes the form of a visual display with auditory signals and occasionally tactile feedback. The visual display serves the dual purpose of entertaining the subject and training the brain. The dual nature of this process makes it possible for the training to proceed even with nonverbal individuals with autism.

The brain continuously does its best, primarily at an unconscious level, to adjust to the demands of its environment, regardless of the cognitive level of the patient. Individuals often appear calmer after just the first few minutes of training. As sessions continue, many demonstrate the ability to focus and concentrate for longer periods of time, exhibit less or no self-stimulatory behaviors, and respond with appropriate reactions (49).

Animal Therapies This type of technique is now available using our feathered and furry friends to enhance behavior and learning. Dogs, cats, rabbits, birds, dolphins, and other creatures serve to enhance sensory processing, increase relatedness, and help individuals with special needs develop better language skills (50).

Treatments That Enhance Communication and Social Skills Poor, unusual, and absent communication skills and interpersonal relationships are hallmarks of individuals with special needs. Many "relationship-based" copyrighted programs are now on the market for those with specific diagnoses. Some that are worthy of further investigation are the following:

- **Son-Rise**, developed by psychologist Barry Kaufman and his wife, the founders of The Option Institute, whose unique feature is the commitment to happiness. Parents of children with special needs are encouraged to explore their own belief systems and to question judgments that are limiting them (51).
- **Developmental, Individual, Relationship-Based (DIR) Model,** developed by late psychiatrist, Stanley Greenspan, MD, which combines sensory, motor, language, and play techniques through a system called FloorTime (52).
- **Relationship Development Intervention (RDI) Program,** developed by psychologist Steven Gutstein, PhD, which is similar to DIR, but more structured (53).

Energy Therapies Therapists in all disciplines are adding tools to their tool chest whose main purpose is to move energy around and thus enhance healing. These include various types of massage, Reiki, and work with family constellations. The latter, which grew out of the family systems movement in the 1950s, is especially popular in Germany, where it was developed by psychoanalyst Bert Hellinger. Instead of focusing on an individual's history from birth, it addresses dysfunction and suffering related to painful events in the family's past (54).

CONCLUSION

Some exciting new treatment options for individuals with special needs address causes, in addition to treating symptoms, by removing individual stressors leading to the total load that eventually result in one or more diagnoses. In addition to social, academic, and language benefits, many times, long-standing health problems are also alleviated. Eye care professionals and others working with children who have special needs have an ethical obligation to become aware of and conversant about these new programs. They can then access them in their communities in order to educate parents and help them sift through the many options for intervention for their children.

REFERENCES

1. United States Department Health and Human Services. CAM basics: what is complementary and alternative medicine? Handout D347. Available from: http://nccam.nih.gov/health/whatiscam. Last Accessed August 13, 2011.
2. Autism Research Institute. 2009 Parent ratings of behavioral effects of biomedical interventions: Publication 34. Available from: www.autism.com/fam_ratingsbehaviorbiomedical.asp. Last Accessed August 13, 2011.
3. Lemer P. Total load theory: how the cumulative effect of many factors causes developmental delays. New developments 2007, Summer, 12:4. Available from: www.oepf.org/ICBOFlash/Handouts/Lemer%20375-total-load-theory.pdf. Last Accessed August 13, 2011.
4. Gilbert SG. Scientific consensus statement on environmental agents associated with neurodevelopmental disorders. The Collaborative on Health and the Environment's Learning and Developmental Disabilities Initiative; [July 2008]. Available from: http://www.ldanys.org/images/uploads/misc/1218746794_LDDIStatement.pdf. Last Accessed August 13, 2011.
5. Frymann VM. Birth trauma: the most common cause of developmental delays. New Developments; 1996, Summer 1:4.
6. Melillo R, Leisman G. Neurobehavioral disorders of childhood: an evolutionary perspective. New York: Springer; 2009.
7. Goddard S. Reflexes, learning and behavior: a window into the child's mind. Eugene: Fern Ridge Press; 2005.
8. Berne SA. Without Ritalin. New York: McGraw Hill; 2006.
9. Berne SA. The primitive reflexes: treatment considerations in the infant. Optom Vis Dev. 2006:37(3):139–45.
10. Gonzales SR, Ciuffreda K, Hernandez LC, Escalante JB. The correlation between primitive reflexes and saccadic eye movements in 5th grade children with teacher-reported reading problems. Optom Vis Dev. 2008:39:140–5.
11. Mowbray L. The primitive reflex training program. Bloomington: Visual Dynamix; 2009.
12. Converse J. Special-needs kids eat right. New York: Perigee Press; 2009.
13. Shattock P, Whiteley P. How dietary intervention could ameliorate the symptoms of autism. Pharm J. 2001;7:7155–8.
14. Crook WG. Solving the puzzle of your hard-to-raise child. Jackson: Professional Books; 1987.
15. Feingold B. Why your child is hyperactive. New York: Random House; 1985.
16. Rapp D. Is this your child? New York: Quill Books; 1991.
17. Silberberg B. The autism and ADHD diet. Naperville: Sourcebooks; 2009.
18. Gottschall E. Breaking the vicious cycle. Ontario: Kirkton Press; 1994.
19. Gates D. The body ecology diet: Recovering your health and rebuilding your immunity. Atlanta: Body Ecology; 2006.
20. Macleod K. Down syndrome and vitamin therapy. Toronto: Kemanso Publishing Ltd; 2003.
21. Dean C. The magnesium miracle. New York: Ballantine Books; 2006.
22. Kirschmann J. Nutrition almanac. New York: McGraw Hill; 2006. p. 23–56.
23. Megson, M. Is autism a G-alpha protein defect reversible with natural vitamin A? Med Hypotheses. 2000;54:979–83.
24. Rimland, B. High dosage levels of certain vitamins in the treatment of children with severe mental disorders. In: Hawkins D, Pauling L, editors. Orthomolecular psychiatry. New York: Freeman; 1973. p. 512–38.
25. Mousain-Bosc M, Roche M, Polge A, Pradal-Prat D, et al. Improvement of neurobehavioral disorders in children supplemented with magnesium-vitam in B_6. Magnes Res. 2006;1: 53–62.
26. James SJ, Cutler P, Melnyk S, Jerrigan S, et al. Metabolic biomarkers of increased oxidative stress and impaired methylation capacity in children with autism. Am J Clin Nutr. 2004;80(6):1611–7.
27. Rimland B, Baker SM. Brief report: alternative approaches to the development of effective treatments of autism. J Autism Dev Disord. 1996;26(2):237–41.
28. Litov RE, Combs GF Jr. Selenium in pediatric nutrition. Pediatrics. 1991;87:339–51.
29. Grahn BH, Paterson PG, Gottschall-Pass KT, Zhang Z. Zinc and the eye. J Am Coll Nutr. 2001;20:106–18.
30. Kley RA, Tarnopolsky MA, Vorgerd M. Creatine for treating muscle disorders. Cochrane Database Syst Rev. 2011;Issue 2. Art. No.:CD004760. DOI: 10.1002/14651858.CD004760.pub3.
31. Geng J, Dong J, Ni H, Lee MS, Wu T, Jiang K, et al. Ginseng for cognition. Cochrane Database Syst Rev 2010;Issue 12. Art. No.: CD007769. DOI: 10.1002/14651858.CD007769.pub2.
32. Jansen SL, Forbes D, Duncan V, Morgan DG, Malouf R. Melatonin for the treatment of dementia. Cochrane Database Syst Rev. 2006;Issue 1. Art. No.: CD003802. DOI: 10.1002/14651858.CD003802.pub3.
33. Lansky A. Impossible cure: the promise of homeopathy. Portola Valley: RL Ranch Press; 2003.
34. The Environmental Working Group. EWG tests find high BPA loads on receipts. Available from: www.ewg.org/featured/15. Last Accessed August 8, 2011.
35. Baker SM. Detoxification and healing. New York: McGraw Hill; 2003.
36. Schmidt MA. Childhood ear infections. Berkeley: North Atlantic Books; 2004.
37. Davis DS. Sound bodies through sound therapy. Budd Lake: Kalco Publishing; 2004.
38. Berard G. Hearing equals behavior. New Canaan: Keats Publishing; 2000.
39. Sollier P. Listening for wellness: an introduction to the Tomatis method. Toronto: The Mozart Center Press; 2006.
40. Davis D. Every day a miracle: success stories with sound therapy. Landing: Kalco Publishing; 2006.
41. Dennison PE, Dennison GE. Brain gym teachers edition, revised. Ventura: Edu-Kinesthetics; 2010.
42. Cohen I. Hands on: how to use brain gym in the classroom. Ventura: Edu-Kinesthetics; 2002.
43. Hannaford C. Smart moves: why learning is not all in your head. Arlington: Great Ocean Publishers; 1995.

44. Freeman C. I am the Child. Ventura: Edu-Kinesthetics, Inc.; 1998.
45. Cepeda MS, Carr DB, Lau J, Alvarez H. Music for pain relief. Cochrane Database of Systematic Reviews 2006, Issue 2. Art. No.: CD004843. DOI: 10.1002/14651858.CD004843. pub2.
46. Bradt J, Magee WL, Dileo C, Wheeler BL, McGilloway E. Music therapy for acquired brain injury. Cochrane Database of Systematic Reviews 2010, Issue 7. Art. No.: CD006787. DOI: 10.1002/14651858.CD006787.pub2.
47. Gold C, Wigram T, Elefant C. Music therapy for autistic spectrum disorder. Cochrane Database of Systematic Reviews 2006, Issue 2. Art. No.: CD004381. DOI: 10.1002/14651858. CD004381.pub2.
48. Maratos A, Gold C, Wang X, Crawford M. Music therapy for depression. Cochrane Database of Systematic Reviews 2008, Issue 1. Art. No.: CD004517. DOI: 10.1002/14651858. CD004517.pub2.
49. Hill RW, Castro E. Healing young brains: the neurofeedback solution. Charlottesville: Hampton Roads Publishing; 2009.
50. Lemer PS. Envisioning a bright future: interventions that work for children and adults with autism spectrum disorders. Santa Ana: OEPF; 2008.
51. Kaufman BN. Son rise: the miracle continues. Tiburon: HJ Kramer; 1994.
52. Greenspan SL, Wieder, S. The child with special needs: encouraging intellectual and emotional growth. New York: Perseus Books; 1998.
53. Gutstein S. The RDI book. Houston: Connections Center; 2009.
54. Ulsmer R. The healing power of the past: systemic therapy of Bert Hellinger. Nevada City: Underwood Books; 2005.

CHAPTER 27

Sidney Groffman, OD, MA, FAAO, FCOVD
Jeffrey Cooper, MS, OD, FAAO
Paul Harris, OD, FCOVD, FACBO, FAAO
Marc B. Taub, OD, MS, FAAO, FCOVD

Technology for Rehabilitation, Treatment, and Enhancement

Traditional optometric vision therapy (OVT) requires the use of an optometrist and/or therapist who has sufficient knowledge and experience to administer treatment using various devices such as stereoscopes, vectograms, and anaglyphs. It also requires the patient to be sophisticated enough to provide reliable and accurate responses. The child with special needs is more likely to have communication or attention problems resulting in a greater need for instrumentation to objectively determine appropriate responding. Even with the best therapist, the changing of targets or stimuli during traditional OVT is often slow, arduous, and maybe unreliable at times. Further, there has been little standardization of instructional sets, rate and amount of stimulus changes, and means to apply positive and negative reinforcements. These factors can result in variability of treatment and its results.

According to Duckman (1), "the most compelling device for use in a visual therapy program that deals with persons who have handicaps is the computer. Computers have the capability of drawing out and maintaining a child's attention better than any other device..." Individual differences in patient characteristics present a pervasive problem to optometrists. At the onset of OVT, patients of any age will differ from one another in various intellectual and perceptuomotor abilities and skills, in interest and motivation, in family and cultural background, and in personal styles of work and thought. These differences, in turn, appear directly related to differences in the patient's progress, and must be considered in planning learning strategies for an OVT regimen (2). This is particularly true in patients with special needs whose differences in characteristics may be exaggerated. The following is a list of the many useful features that help us work with patients with special needs:

1) *Patient Acceptance*: This is stimulated by the ubiquity of computers and their offspring in all areas of society and the belief that computers help us to perform more efficiently and rapidly. Patients expect to use and benefit from complex electronic devices. Therapy is more motivating (3) and effective when patients believe in the mystique of the modality.
2) *Flexibility*: Computers are not limited to one function or level of difficulty. With appropriate software, it is possible to use computers for a large number of OVT procedures. Almost all visual skills and visual information processing abilities can be enhanced, remediated, and/or improved using a computer. Computer programs are available for both office and home therapy (4).
3) *Proven Learning Principles*: Optometric vision therapy is a learning process, and is subject to the principles of educational therapy (5) and the laws of learning. The general procedure in OVT is to improve the individual processes, abilities, and components to higher levels of performance. This requires a thorough and well-structured protocol consisting of a sequence of programmed steps. This type of protocol is important for patients with special needs. Operant conditioning is a valuable structured motivational technique for OVT (6,7). Computers are particularly well suited to provide programs of this nature (8).
4) *Adaptable Programming*: Computers are uniquely adaptable to the OVT needs of special populations because:

- Programs are user friendly and self-instructional
- The primary interaction can be between the patient and the program, rather than the patient and the therapist

- Stimuli are divided into small, discrete units
- Computer programs provide a large number of stimuli for many activities and an infinite number for others
- The stimuli can be programmed in sequences ranging from simple to complex
- Each stimulus requires an overt response from the patient
- Each response is recorded by the computer and immediate feedback can be provided
- A computer stores information during each session and can furnish a visual, auditory, or printed summary of the patient's activities
- Some programs permanently store results and/or are connected to the Internet

EVIDENCE-BASED STUDIES USING COMPUTERIZED VT

Cooper and Feldman (7,9) were the first to demonstrate the effectiveness of computerization in OVT by using random dot stereograms (RDSs) in an operant conditioning paradigm. Random dot stereograms, which are devoid of monocular cues, create stereoscopic demands that can only be appreciated during binocular fusion. Since bifoveal fixation is required, stereopsis on an RDS cannot be appreciated by patients with constant strabismus, including microtropia, regardless of the size of the disparity of the targets (9). When the RDSs are presented in an operant conditioning paradigm, the patient makes a response to the stereoscopic stimulus; correct responses are positively reinforced, while incorrect responses are negatively reinforced (7,10,11).

In a subsequent study, Cooper and Feldman (10) used an operant conditioning paradigm to determine if computer-based RDS vergence therapy improved vergence amplitudes. The experimental group received vergence therapy while the control group did not. The stimuli presentation other than vergence was identical in both groups. Both groups received identical stimuli and reinforcement. This study clearly demonstrated that automated computerized OVT resulted in a rapid increase of fusional amplitudes with concurrent transference of this ability to other vergence tasks such as vectograms.

Cooper (12) later reported that patients with clinically diagnosed vergence anomalies, who failed to respond to traditional methods using an experienced therapist, could be successfully treated with automated vergence therapy. Daum et al. (13) demonstrated that automated therapy produced more effective results than those obtained with traditional use of prisms, stereoscopes, and vectograms. Additionally, he showed that shorter, more frequent sessions were preferable to longer, spaced-out therapeutic sessions. From Daum's results, one may infer that once or twice a week in-office therapy should be augmented with effective home therapy to improve results.

Cooper et al. (14) performed the first prospective controlled study that evaluated the ability of OVT to eliminate the signs and symptoms associated with convergence insufficiency (CI). Again, one group received vergence therapy (experimental) while the other group did not (control). Both groups received identical RDS stimuli with appropriate reinforcement. They used a scaled questionnaire before and after treatment. Patients were treated in an A-B-A crossover design to control for experimental bias, placebo, and order effects. It was found that therapy improved convergence amplitudes, reduced asthenopia as measured on their scaled questionnaire, and flattened fixation disparity curves. Similar results were found in a study with automated accommodative therapy (15).

Kertesz and Kertesz (16,17) treated a group of CI patients who had failed traditional orthoptic treatment regimens. They used automated large stimuli vergence targets. The researchers reported that 23 of 29 patients studied (80%) showed significantly increased fusional ranges with a concurrent reduction of symptoms. Feldman et al. (18), in a subsequent study, found that the size of fusional amplitudes was directly related to the size of the stimuli, that is, the larger the target the larger the amplitude. Neither detail nor disparity influenced fusional amplitudes. From this research, they suggested that therapy should begin with large stimuli, progressing to smaller stimuli.

Sommers et al. (19) used computerized vision therapy techniques and compared them to traditional techniques. Patients treated with computerized techniques showed more rapid and complete improvement of their binocular anomalies. Similar findings have been reported by Griffin (20). These studies suggest that computerized vision therapy, using RDSs in an operant conditioning paradigm, is more effective than traditional therapy. In addition, it decreases the need for an experienced therapist and shortens therapy by improving motivation and reliability. This is especially important in the child with special needs. The Convergence Insufficiency Clinical Trial (21) compared in-office with supplemental home therapy to placebo therapy, and pencil push-ups. The Computer Orthoptics and Home Therapy System (HTS) programs were used in conjunction with vectograms, Brock string, lifesaver cards, etc. In-office therapy, which consisted of the Computer Orthoptics program, was controlled by the therapist, and the automated HTS was used in both studies. The results demonstrated that OVT with the use of HTS at home was the most effective treatment, when compared to base-in prism, placebo therapy, or pencil push-ups, in reducing asthenopia in symptomatic children with CI.

Goss et al. (22) performed a study to determine the effect of normalization of accommodation, vergence, and eye movements according to specific criteria on reading scores. The subjects were third graders who were randomized into one of two groups. One group ($n = 63$) served as a control receiving no treatment, and the other group performed active therapy using the HTS program. The group that completed the HTS program improved their reading scores on the STAR reading achievement test by 1.8 years as compared to the control group's improvement of 0.9 years. This study provides further support for the inclusion of OVT in a program to improve reading scores.

Cooper (23) conducted a retrospective study of prepresbyopic patients who completed the HTS program for a variety of nonstrabismic vergence anomalies. Prior to and immediately after treatment, all patients in this study took a 15-question symptom questionnaire, the Convergence Insufficiency Symptom Survey (24). Treatment consisted of various accommodative and vergence activities. Pre- and posttreatment symptoms were 32.8 (sd = 8.1) and 20.6 (sd = 11.5), respectively. These changes were both clinically and statistically significant. Forty percent eliminated their symptoms, and 55% improved. Improvement in both convergence and divergence amplitude was clinically significant. Most of the patients finished the program by 40 sessions (equivalent to 8 weeks). They concluded that the HTS system should be used in those patients demonstrating symptoms associated with an accommodative/vergence anomaly when in-office vision therapy was not practical.

OFFICE-CENTERED PROGRAMS

Computer Orthoptics Computer Orthoptics is a group of in-office therapy programs that was first introduced in 1982. The original system used anaglyphs to diagnose and treat various oculomotor, accommodative, and vergence disorders. In 1988, a more advanced computerized therapy program was introduced that used liquid crystal glasses to present binocular stimuli. Liquid crystals allow for the presentation of full-color, realistic stimuli. More recent versions, The Computer Orthopter (VTS3 and VTS4) were developed and produced by HTS Inc. in 2005 and 2011, respectively (Fig. 27-1). This instrument simulates the performance of a vectogram, stereoscope, troposcope, and Brock stereo motivator in a single unit. Changing stimuli is easily and rapidly performed.

This comprehensive unit has a diagnostic program that includes testing of phorias, fusional amplitudes, fixation disparity, suppression, motor fields, pursuits, and saccades. The therapeutic program includes techniques for ocular motility, accommodation, and vergence. Stimuli consist of a variety of targets: first-degree (simultaneous perception), second-degree (flat fusion), and third-degree targets (stereopsis). These targets vary in size and suppression control features (Fig. 27-2). They can be presented at the objective angle to treat strabismus or in an operant conditioning paradigm, to improve both fast and slow disparity vergence. Targets may be presented at near or projected at distance. Stimuli can either be monocularly flashed or alternatively flashed at various frequencies to break suppression. Vergence targets can be presented manually (examiner controls the targets) or automatically (program controls changes in vergence and/or movement of targets). One of the most important features is that stimuli can be presented at both distance and near. Distance projection is stereoscopically compelling.

The real power of the Computer Orthopter (VTS3) is the combination of first-, second-, and third-degree targets (Fig. 27-3) in an operant conditioning paradigm. Therapy is automatically altered based upon previous responses. Thus, successful viewing of an RDS results in positive reinforcement and a concurrent increase in vergence, while an incorrect response results in delivery of negative reinforcement with concurrent decrease in vergence. The Computer Orthopter allows the use of line or traditional stereograms, which have subtle monocular cues. However, they have been camouflaged to make it difficult to use monocular cues. These stimuli should be used with strabismic patients who cannot appreciate an RDS or for those patients in whom smaller targets are necessary. Accommodative stimuli are employed using a similar operant conditioning

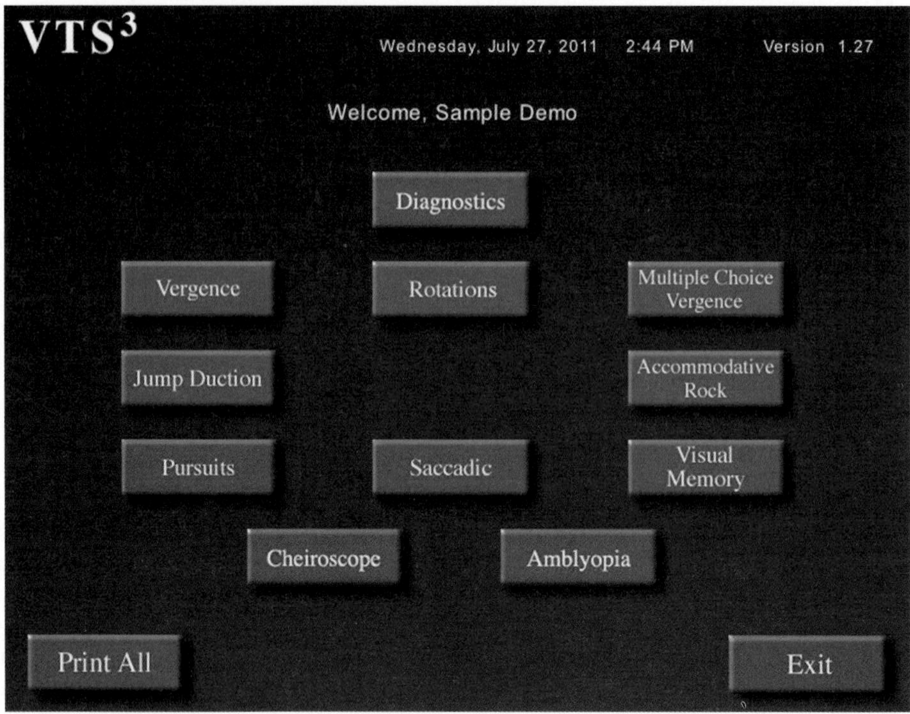

FIGURE 27-1. Computer Orthoptics VTS3 vergence main menu. (Image courtesy of HTS Inc.)

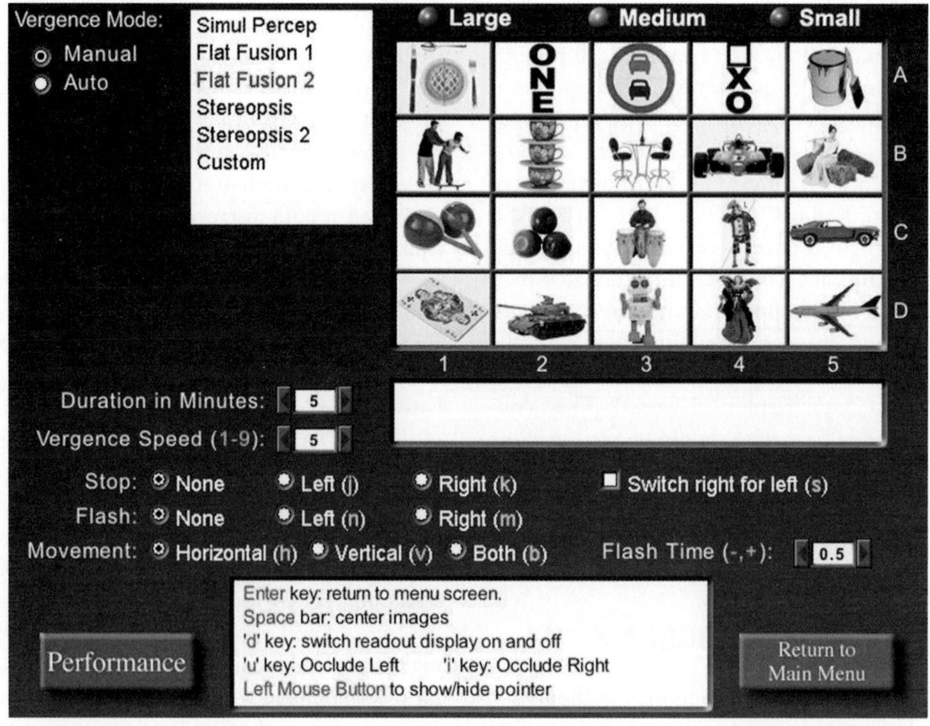

FIGURE 27-2. Computer Orthoptics VTS3 vergence parameters menu. (Image courtesy of HTS Inc.) (See also Color Section.)

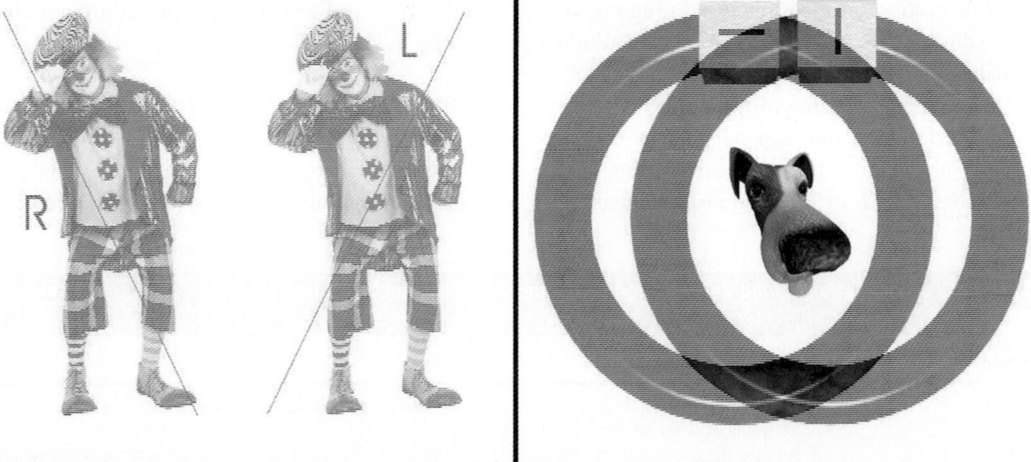

FIGURE 27-3. Depicts computer Orthoptics VTS3 two different targets for improving either fusional amplitudes or stereoscopic appreciation. The target on the left consists of two different dichoptic stimuli that are viewed using liquid crystal glasses to separate the right and left views. The clown on the left is seen by the right eye, while the clown on the right is seen by the left eye. The R and L serve as suppression controls. The eyes are required to converge to see a single, binocular image. Manipulation of the targets is used to train fusion. The target on the right is made up of a central fixation target seen by both eyes (dog) and peripheral rings, which can be separated to created either crossed or uncrossed retinal disparity. Alteration in the separation of the rings results in a change in retinal disparity or stereopsis. (Image courtesy of HTS Inc.) (See also Color Section.)

paradigm. This regimen has been scientifically tested to show its validity (22).

VisionBuilder The VisionBuilder program, written by Jan Erik Haraldseth, a Norwegian optometrist, is designed to be an adjunct tool used as part of a comprehensive OVT program. The first versions of the software were made expressly for use in the office under the direct supervision of the optometrist or a vision therapist. Very soon after the program came into use, the optometrists and therapists demanded a version of the software that could be used at home

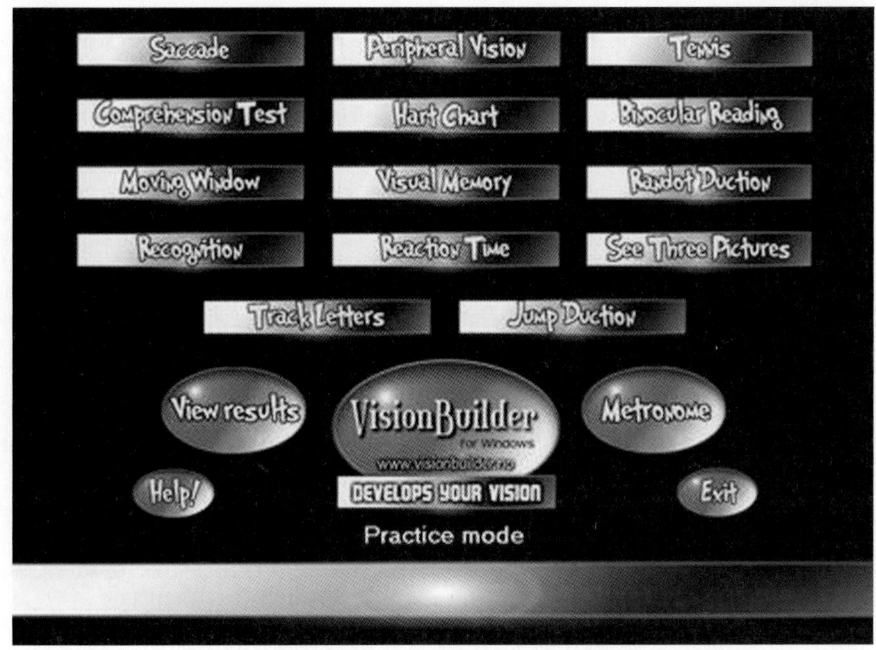

FIGURE 27-4. VisionBuilder main menu.

by patients to continue their practice during the week between their OVT sessions. As a result, VisionBuilder is available in both a home and office version.

The program includes 14 main modules plus a metronome function that can be used in conjunction with other vision therapy activities (Fig. 27-4). The purpose of each of the modules is explained in Table 27.1, and several of the procedures are shown visually in Figures 27-5–27-7.

Computerized Perceptual Therapy

Individuals with special needs may exhibit significant deficits in both visual skills and visual information processing abilities. They require complete

TABLE 27.1 Descriptions of the Various Modules of the VisionBuilder Program

Module	Description of Module
Saccade	Arrows come on in random locations on the screen, and the patient has to hit the arrow on the keypad that corresponds to the arrow on the screen. The size of the arrows can be changed to alter the difficulty of the activity, which also reports back the average response time as well as percentage correct. For work with amblyopes or to do monocular work in a binocular field, a red lens can be used over one eye.
Peripheral vision	The purpose of the peripheral vision module is to learn to parallel process a central task while expanding the volume of space attended to. They are to keep their eyes focused in the center of the screen, and read the numbers out loud as they appear. At varied intervals, an arrow will appear on the screen somewhere in the periphery. Whenever an arrow appears, the patient is to hit the correct left or right arrow key that matches the direction the arrow is pointing.
Tennis	The Tennis module is very similar to the old game "Pong". The value of it in a vision therapy program is tremendous. It helps the patient learn to predict when and where the moving object will hit the side wall and to direct the paddle to intercept it. This helps with most tasks where they have to interact with moving objects and predict their paths.
Comprehension test	This section of VisionBuilder is used by the patient to self-evaluate his or her current reading speed level under conditions of comprehension. The figures attained here will be used in setting the Moving Windows section. So the main purpose will be to get a baseline level of reading speed with comprehension. This can also be done periodically to assess progress made with the mechanics of reading.
Hart chart	This module of VisionBuilder allows you to make your own Hart charts with a nearly unlimited variation of font sizes, upper case only, mixed upper and lower case letters and even to add numbers into the mix. A key feature is the ability to print the chart with fewer columns or rows to help the developmentally challenged child accomplish this task more easily.
Binocular reading	Using the red/blue glasses can provide you with a reading sample with some letters in blue, some in red, and some in a middle color, pink, that is seen by both eyes.
Moving window	The moving window exposes only a portion of the reading material and covers up the previously read section, so that it is not possible to go back and re-read. This helps in stopping regressive eye movements (backward movements that tend to slow down reading speed). It promotes a smooth left-to-right, top-to-bottom reading pattern and by slowly increasing the speed of the window, allows you to improve your reading speed.
Visual memory	The objects presented are rectangles with different markings. Some are shaded, some have lines going in one direction, some have lines in multiple directions, and there are various combinations. Because these objects are more difficult to "name" than traditional symbols, the idea is to encourage remembering based on what they look like, rather than remembering your verbal descriptions.
Randot duction	This module is excellent for building the quality of binocularity by using the popular RDS training paradigm.
Recognition	Here words or phrases are flashed for varying periods of time, based on your selection, and then selected from lists which mostly consist of very similar distracters.
Reaction time	Here you can drill with purely visual stimuli, purely auditory stimuli, or a combination of both visual and sound stimuli. The patient is asked, in each instance, to react as soon as he or she perceives the event you are waiting for, by depressing the spacebar. The program reports back their score in milliseconds.
See three pictures	A classic part of many vision therapy programs involves using physiological diplopia techniques and well-drawn pictures to observe multiple images with more visual information than is present in either of the two original targets.
Letter tracking	Allows the optometrist or therapist to generate new, randomly generated letter tracking paragraphs as needed for working with patients of all levels of skill.
Tachistoscope	You can do traditional tach work where you show something for a brief period of time, and the patients have to simply recall what it was they saw. Board tach: Here a shape is projected onto the writing surface via a data projector connected to the computer's second video output channel. The patient then is asked to go to the board and draw the object that was flashed in the same place and the same size that it appeared.

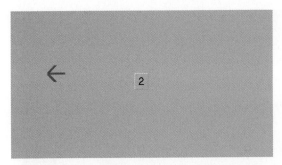

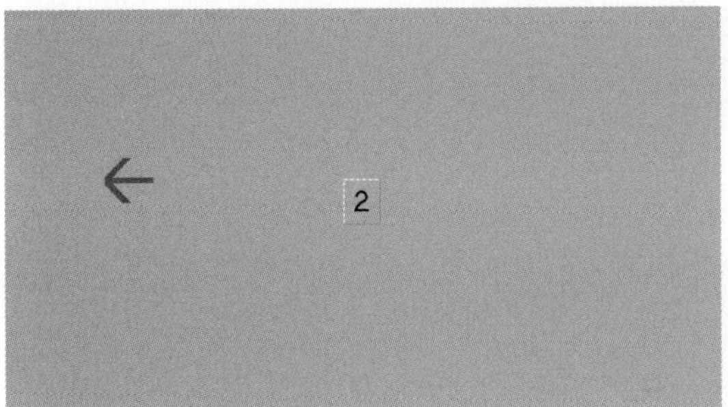

FIGURE 27-5. The peripheral vision module is depicted. This is an example of what the screen might look like at one point in time. At this moment, the patient should say the number "2" out loud while tapping the left arrow button. The numbers continually change in the center, while the arrow disappears as soon as the key stroke is completed and reappears in a new random position on the screen and in a new random orientation. Average response time and percentage of correct responses is returned upon completion of the task.

optometric assessments in both of these areas (25). Some of the conditions that should be evaluated include attention deficit/hyperactivity deficit (26–28), autism (29–32), traumatic brain injury (33,34), cerebral palsy (35–37), Down syndrome (38–40), dyslexia (41–43), dyscalculia (44,45), emotional disorders (46), epilepsy (47), multiple sclerosis (48), and Williams syndrome (49,50). There have been a number of articles regarding the value of computers in the treatment of patients with special needs including those with cerebral palsy and dyslexia (51–54).

Computerized perceptual therapy (CPT) is an office-centered program designed by Sidney Groffman OD, and distributed by Home Therapy Services Inc. It consists of 18 individual programs based on the perceptuocognitive simultaneous–sequential theory of Luria (55) and Das (56) (Fig. 27-8). This theory states that information is processed either simultaneously or sequentially, with both being essential for learning. The individual programs as well as the areas they stimulate can be found in Table 27.2, and several of the procedures are shown visually in Figures 27-9 and 27-10.

FIGURE 27-6. This shows sample text for use with the binocular accommodative rock procedure in VisionBuilder. Unlike the conventional Polaroid or Red/Green strips, this random pattern helps deal with suppression better. (See also Color Section.)

Sanet Vision Integrator Using a 46 inch touch screen monitor, the Sanet Vision Integrator (SVI) is designed to improve visual abilities for a wide range of patients with visually related learning problems, strabismus, amblyopia, and traumatic brain injury (Fig. 27-11). It is also effective for sports vision enhancement work with athletes. The key features that make this "all in one" instrument so useful are the variety of programs and ways that visual abilities can be enhanced. The programmable instrument incorporates features of a saccadic trainer, virtual rotator, tachistoscope, and programmable metronome. The SVI instrument actually "speaks," instructing the patient to respond to verbal commands, improving auditory–visual integration and memory. In addition, it has an adjustable stand that accommodates patients of different heights and also allows those with disability or who are not ambulatory patients access to the unit (Fig. 27-12).

The SVI can be used to enhance pursuits, saccades, fixation stability, eye–hand coordination, and visual reaction time, as well as speed and span of recognition, automaticity, and contrast sensitivity, visual and auditory sequencing, and memory. This program should be quite effective when working to improve visual acuity and eliminate suppression in patients with amblyopia. In addition, it can be used in patients with acquired brain injury to help them adapt to visual field loss, visual–spatial neglect and visual–vestibular integration problems, and, in patients with rhythm, reading, and math problems.

Neuro-Vision Rehabilitator The neuro-vision rehabilitator (NVR) is a state-of-the-art vision therapy system (software program) that uses an interactive interface and bluetooth software that integrates a remote, an interactive balance board, and infrared head sensor (Fig. 27-13). The therapy procedures and sequences were developed by Allen H. Cohen, OD. The NVR represents the only interactive, integrative, real space vision therapy system specifically designed to address visual processing problems commonly experienced by patients with neurologic insult, acquired brain injury, posttrauma vision syndrome, and stroke. The NVR can also be used in children with visually related learning problems.

The NVR system provides five specialized therapy modules which are based on the concept

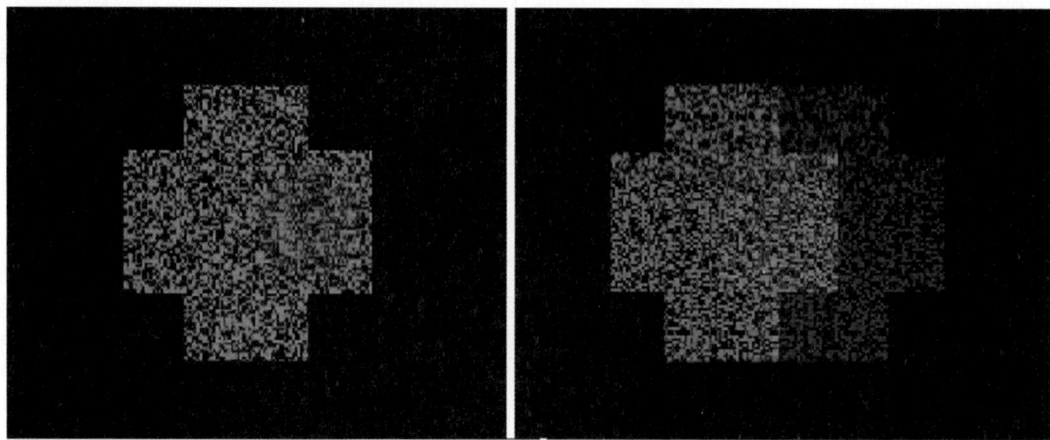

FIGURE 27-7. A (left): shows the standard RDS pattern used in VisionBuilder with a cross pattern. Here the circle is shown in the right branch of the cross. **B (right):** shows the RDS displaced with significant base-out demand for glasses with the red lens in front of the right eye. (See also Color Section.)

of top-down processing. It is designed to enhance ocular motor control, visuomotor and binocular performance while integrating vision, auditory, proprioception, balance, and visuomotor control. Using the remote, integrative balance board and infrared head sensor, an interactive interface is created that provides uniquely powerful procedures designed to significantly enhance deficits in visual processing skills in real space. Neuroscience has demonstrated that repetition, multisensory feedback, and active participation in sensory motor tasks are essential for affecting synaptic and neuroplastic changes. These are the changes that translate into increased speed of information processing and performance.

HOME-CENTERED PROGRAMS

HTS iNet Some patients are not able to participate in therapy within a traditional office setting.

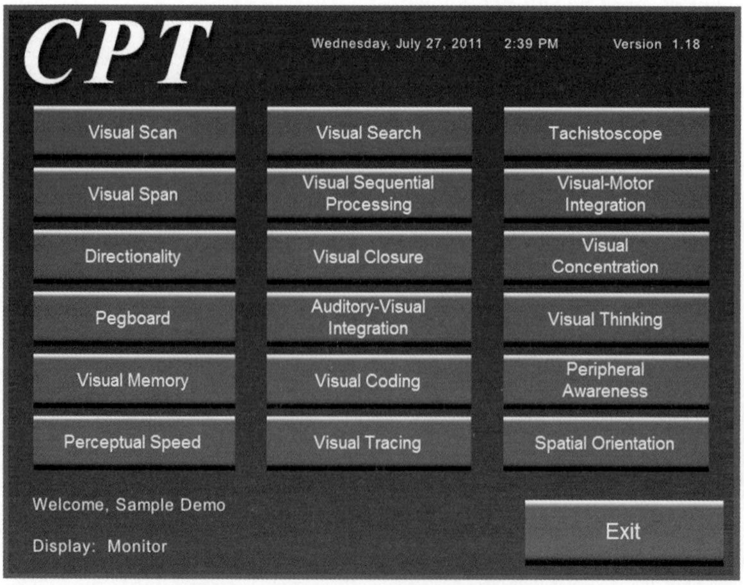

FIGURE 27-8. Main menu of CPT. (Image courtesy of HTS Inc.)

TABLE 27.2 Descriptions of the Various Modules of the CPT Program

Skill	Patient Requirements	Areas Stimulated
Visual–motor integration	To accurately hit a moving ball with a bat as many times as possible. The speeds of the ball, the size of the bat, the distraction elements, are all selectable.	Fine motor control Ocular motor control Hand–eye coordination Visual planning Ocular pursuit A high level of visual attention.
Tachistoscope	To identify a stimulus displayed simultaneously for various brief exposure times.	Perceptual speed Visual memory Perceptual integration Temporal visual processing Visual attention
Visual concentration	To remember the location of hidden pairs of stimuli that are located on various sized grids.	Visual spatial memory Spatial visualization Visual planning Visual attention
Visual search	To locate a designated stimulus that is hidden in an array on the screen. The array is organized in columns of rows and a variable number of stimuli will be found at random locations.	Visual planning Perceptual speed Figure–ground perception Visual memory Temporal visual processing Visual attention Ocular motility directionality
Visual closure	To identify incomplete stimuli that are presented on the screen in an increasing degree of completeness starting at 1% and finishing at 100%.	Visual closure Visual figure–ground Visual discrimination Perceptual speed Visualization Visual attention Perceptual organization
Visual sequential processing	There are two components; 1) A multistimuli one that requires the patient to identify multiple stimuli that are repeated in a sequence presented in a designated pattern at a specified speed 2) A single stimulus component that requires the patient to identify and count the number of times a designated stimulus appears in a sequence of varied stimuli presented at a designated speed and pattern.	Sequential processing Temporal visual processing Visual attention Speed of processing Visual sequential memory saccadic fixation.
Visual thinking	To fill in various sized grids with stimuli that differ from one another in one, two, or three attributes. The stimuli may be geometric forms, numbers, colors, or pictures. When using geometric forms as the stimuli: The attributes are four shapes, two sizes, and four colors. The patient places the forms adjacent to each other on the grid but the forms must differ from each other by one, two, or three differences.	Visual discrimination Spatial relations Visual attention Visualization Visual planning Visual conceptualization.
Visual memory	There are two components 1) Visual Sequential Memory requires patients to identify, recall, and motorically indicate the correct order of a sequence of colored stimuli that are displayed in the cells of a matrix grid. 2) Visual Spatial Memory requires patients to identify, recall, and motorically indicate the spatial location of an array of colored stimuli that are briefly displayed in the cells of a matrix grid.	Visual spatial memory Visual sequential memory Visual processing speed Eye–hand coordination Visual attention Spatial visualization
Visual span	To identify a sequence of stimuli displayed one at a time at various speeds of presentation. The patient must remember the exact order of the sequence and type in or vocalize the response.	Visual sequential memory Auditory sequential memory Temporal visual processing Perceptual speed Visual attention.

(*Continued*)

TABLE 27.2 Descriptions of the Various Modules of the CPT Program (*Continued*)

Skill	Patient Requirements	Areas Stimulated
Spatial orientation	To react quickly to a target that is moving through a map-like grid As the target makes turns, either to the right or left, the patient responds indicating right or left on the mouse.	Direction sense Spatial visualization Visual attention Ocular pursuit Eye–hand coordination.
Peripheral awareness	To maintain attention on a central target while increasing awareness of peripheral targets or activities.	Peripheral awareness Form recognition fields Temporal visual processing Visual attention
Computer pegboard	To reproduce a stimulus presented on a 9 × 9 grid on one side of the screen, in a blank grid on the other side of the grid. The stimuli designs range from simple to complex, have one to three colors, and the patient may be asked to reproduce a direct copy of the stimulus or in one of four spatial directions.	Spatial relations Spatial visualization directionality Eye–hand coordination figure-ground perception Visual attention Visual planning.
Visual coding visual	To quickly identify a symbol/digit, or other code, displayed in a key, and then to complete a task in which only the symbols or other objects are displayed.	Perceptual speed Visual memory Working memory directionality Figure-ground perception visual attention Saccadic fixation.
Directionality–spatial visualization	To visualize specified directional movements of a visual form. There are four directional moves: 1) Right requires that the form be moved 90 degrees to the right; 2) Left requires that the form be moved 90 degrees to the left; 3) Upside down requires that the form be inverted vertically; 4) Side to Side requires that the form be flipped laterally. There can be 1–5 transformations required for each individual stimulus.	directionality Spatial visualization Visual spatial memory Spatial working memory Visual attention.
Visual scan	To locate designated stimuli that are embedded in a large scattered array of distracter stimuli.	Visual planning Perceptual speed Figure–ground perception Directionality Temporal visual Processing ocular motility
Auditory–visual integration	To remember an auditory or visual stimulus consisting of dots, dashes, or dot/dashes. The computer will then sequentially present 3–8 possible response choices that are either visual or auditory.	Visual/auditory attention Auditory sequential memory Visual sequential memory Working memory Visual/auditory integration Auditory/visual integration Auditory/auditory integration Visual/visual integration Temporal visual processing
Visual perceptual speed	To discriminate stimuli composed of letters, numbers, codes, pictures, symbols, shapes, or colors as rapidly as possible. The patients may be required to match a model stimulus, find two stimuli that are alike, or locate the one stimulus that is different from all the other stimuli. The program may be used by patients of all ages and can be very helpful for special needs patients.	Perceptual speed Visual attention Visual planning Visual scanning Ocular motility
Visual tracing	To accurately and rapidly trace a number of tangled lines, visually or motorically, from their starting point on the left side of the screen to their end point on the right side of the screen. If the lines are traced visually, a response is made by selecting a number on the keyboard. If the lines are traced motorically with the mouse, the computer will respond automatically.	Self-generated ocular pursuits Figure–ground perception Visual attention Spatial visualization Perceptual speed Visual planning Eye–hand coordination.

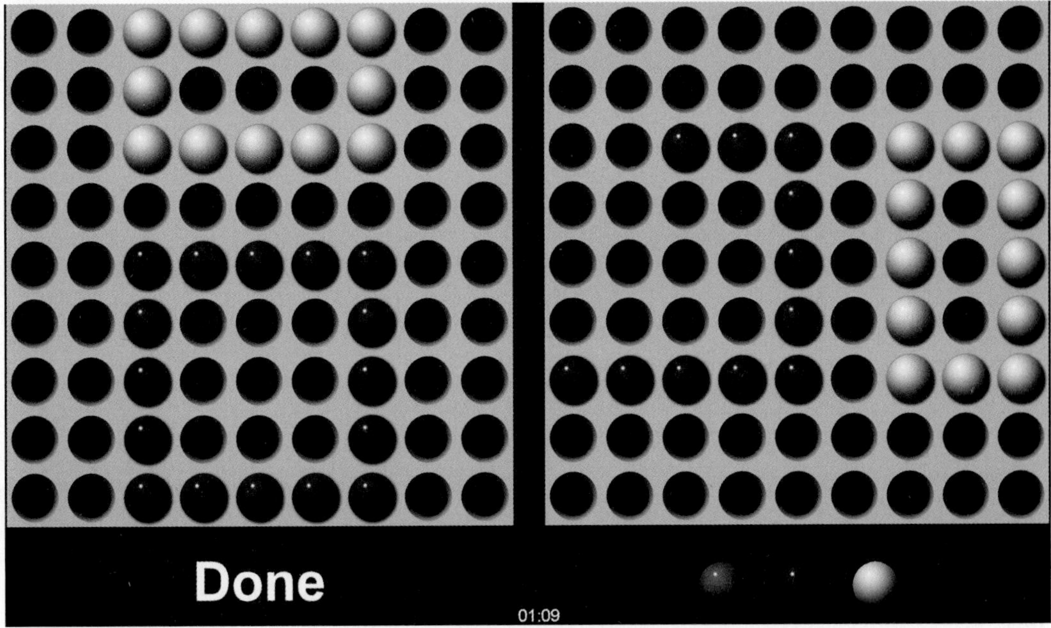

FIGURE 27-9. Pegboard module of the CPT. (Image courtesy of HTS Inc.) (See also Color Section.)

They may not have the time, may live too far from an office that provides in-office vision therapy, or cannot afford in-office therapy. Though office-based therapy is considered the standard, stand-alone home therapy has its place in the treatment regimen. In addition, office therapy, augmented by home therapy, dramatically enhances the effectiveness of in-office therapy by reinforcing office-based learned skills (57).

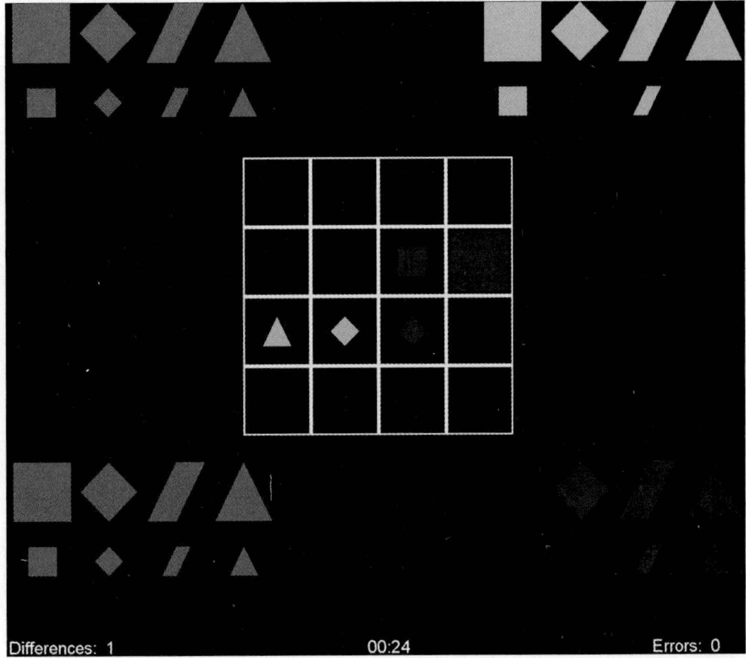

FIGURE 27-10. Visual thinking module of the Computerized Perceptual Therapy (CPT). (Image courtesy of HTS Inc.) (See also Color Section.)

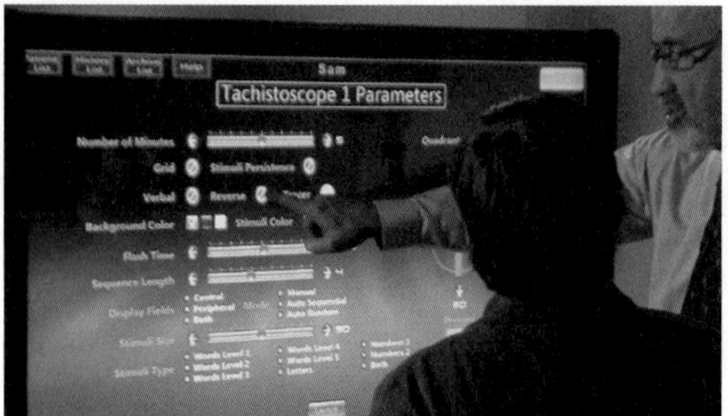

FIGURE 27-11. The SVI is a 46 inch touch screen, programmable instrument that incorporates features of a saccadic trainer, virtual rotator, tachistoscope, and metronome. Image courtesy of HTS Inc.

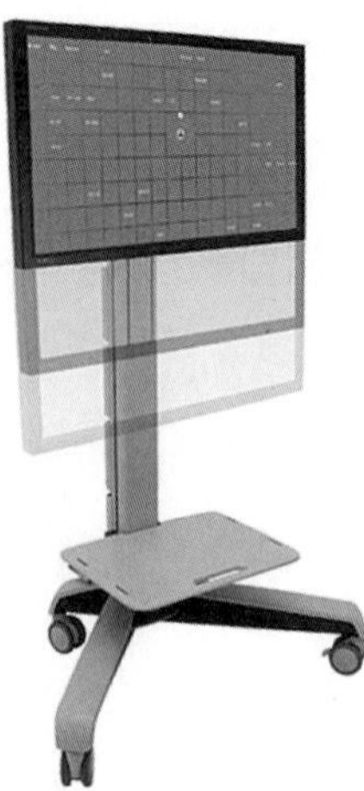

FIGURE 27-12. The open design and adjustable screen height allows for the use of this instrument in patients with special needs. Image courtesy of HTS Inc.

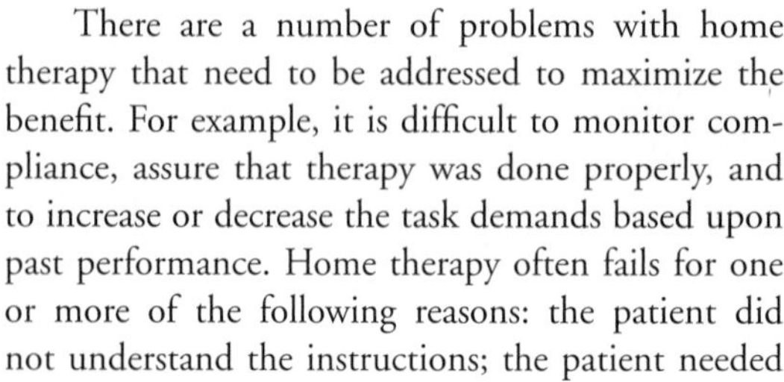

There are a number of problems with home therapy that need to be addressed to maximize the benefit. For example, it is difficult to monitor compliance, assure that therapy was done properly, and to increase or decrease the task demands based upon past performance. Home therapy often fails for one or more of the following reasons: the patient did not understand the instructions; the patient needed more than one technique to alter vergence behavior; the parent could not work with the child, so that the therapy was not performed or was carried out incorrectly.

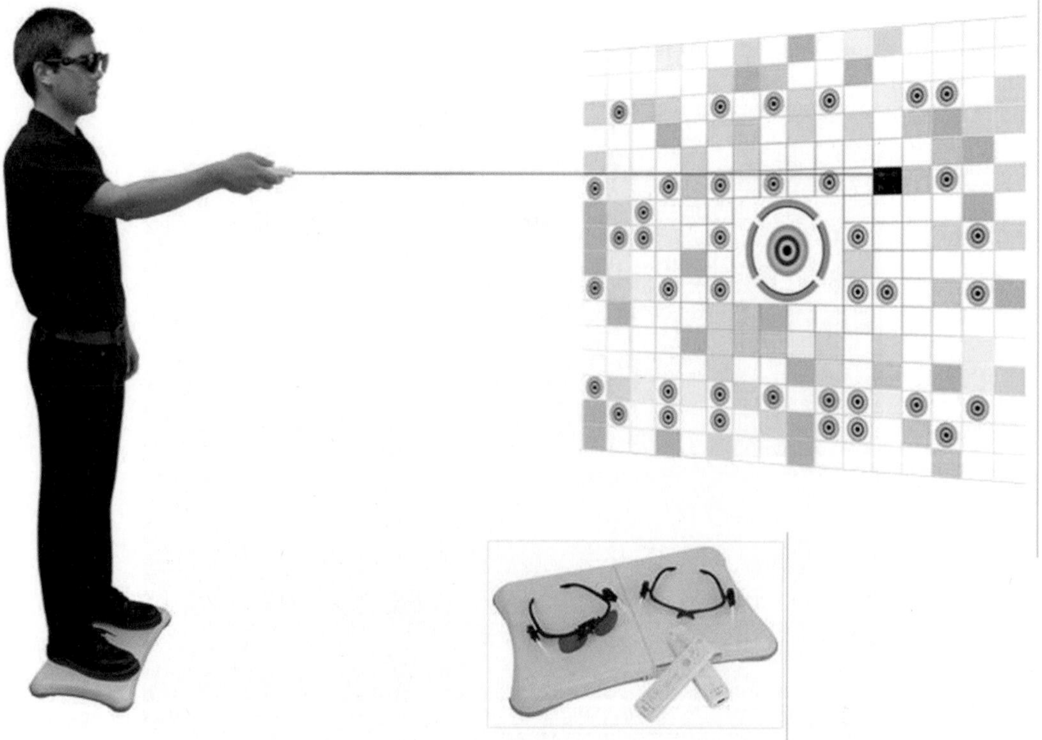

FIGURE 27-13. The NVR employs the use of a remote, balance board, and head sensor in free space. (Image courtesy of HTS Inc.) (See also Color Section.)

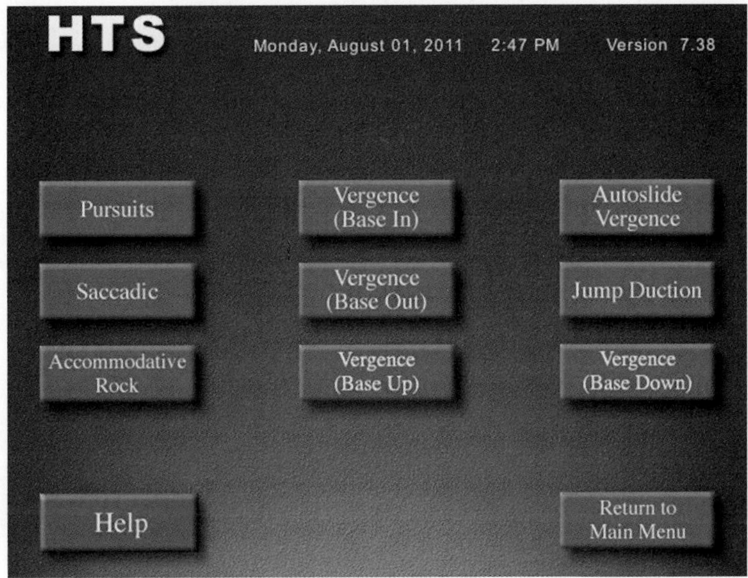

FIGURE 27-14. The HTS iNet main menu. (Image courtesy of HTS Inc.)

Recently, HTS revamped its previous home-based computerized program to address some of these shortcomings (Fig. 27-14). The newer version improves compliance by providing detailed instructions for performing various techniques and provides Internet access to allow the doctor/technician to remotely monitor, control, and reinforce therapy (Fig. 27-15). The use of a disc allows the patient to perform therapy with or without Internet capabilities.

Therapy can be prescribed in either an "auto mode" or "manual mode." In the auto mode, therapy is predetermined with alterations based upon previous progress. The doctor/therapist can

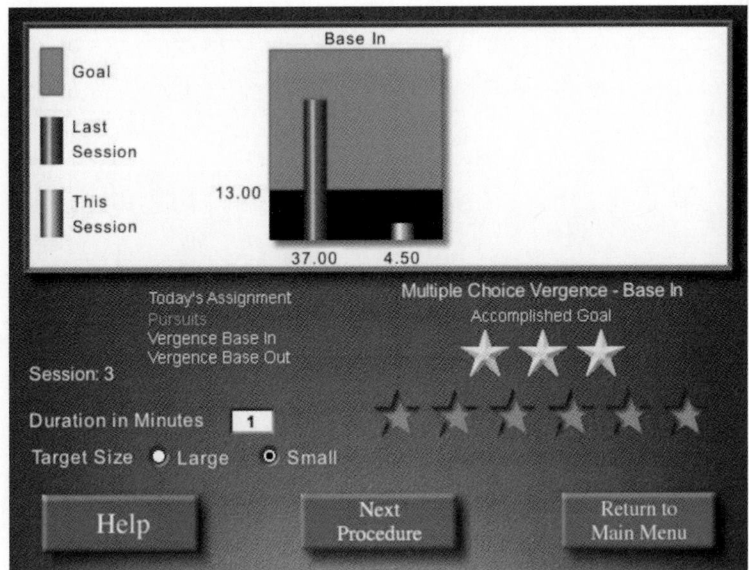

FIGURE 27-15. This screen on the HTS program is shown to the patient as motivation as a signal of the progress made. (Image courtesy of HTS Inc.)

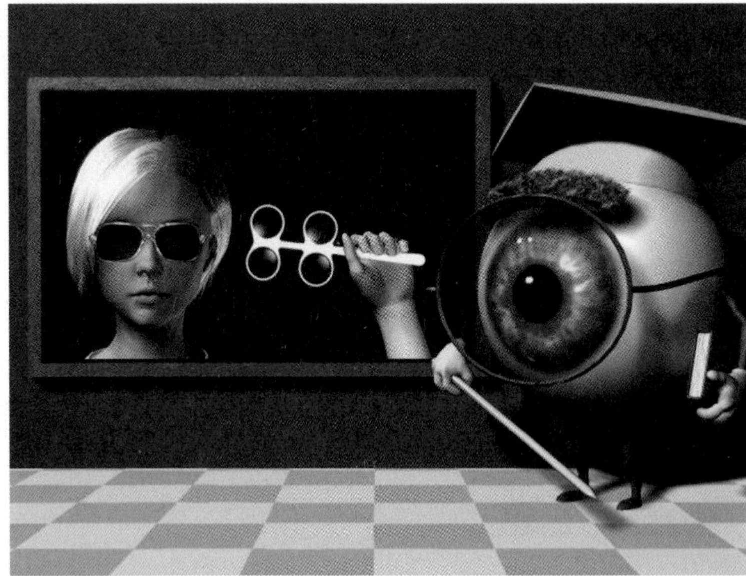

FIGURE 27-16. The HTS program uses this "instructor" to lead the patient through the procedures. (Image courtesy of HTS Inc.)

modify the "Auto Program," for example, eliminating accommodative rock in presbyopic patients. It begins therapy with help screens using a "video man" to describe each therapeutic regimen in detail (Fig. 27-16). After the patient understands the directions, the program automatically begins therapy. Ocular motilities, accommodation, and vergence therapy in an operant conditioning paradigm are incorporated. Correct responses are positively reinforced with a concurrent increase in the difficulty of the task, while incorrect responses are negatively reinforced with concurrent reduction in the difficulty.

The purpose of therapy is to systematically develop the appropriate reflex. The computer automatically

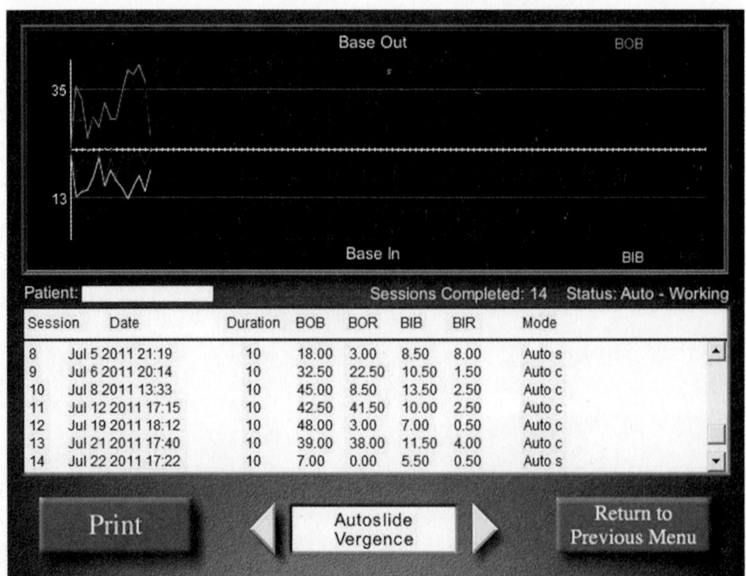

Session	Date	Duration	BOB	BOR	BIB	BIR	Mode
8	Jul 5 2011 21:19	10	18.00	3.00	8.50	8.00	Auto s
9	Jul 6 2011 20:14	10	32.50	22.50	10.50	1.50	Auto c
10	Jul 8 2011 13:33	10	45.00	8.50	13.50	2.50	Auto c
11	Jul 12 2011 17:15	10	42.50	41.50	10.00	2.50	Auto c
12	Jul 19 2011 18:12	10	48.00	3.00	7.00	0.50	Auto c
13	Jul 21 2011 17:40	10	39.00	38.00	11.50	4.00	Auto c
14	Jul 22 2011 17:22	10	7.00	0.00	5.50	0.50	Auto s

FIGURE 27-17. This HTS screen allows for the tracking of patient progress by the clinician from a remote location. (Image courtesy of HTS Inc.)

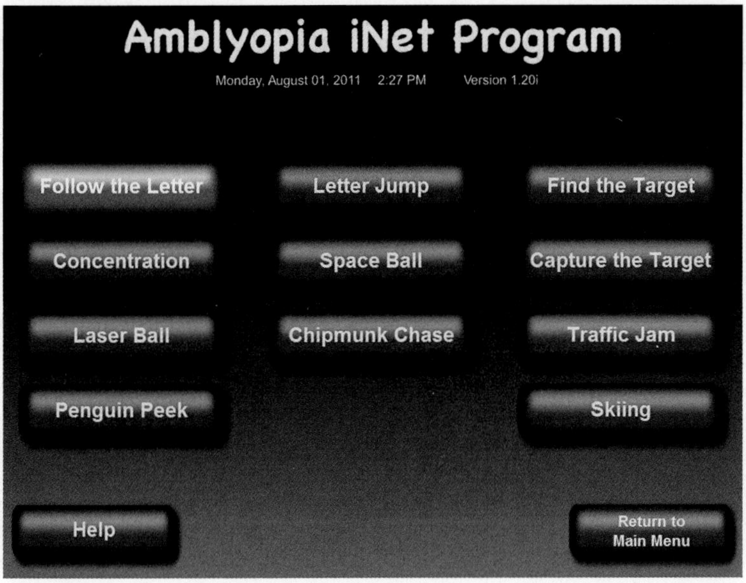

FIGURE 27-18. The main menu of the Amblyopia iNet program. (Image courtesy of HTS Inc.)

assigns the patient three tasks a day; the computer determines time and order. The patient follows the simple instructions. At the end of each session, there is an automatic recording of each task. The performance screen allows the doctor, parent, and patient to view previous performance two ways. The first provides tabular data of each session that includes the date, time, task performed, level achieved, and the level of performance. The second is a graph of all the sessions, so that one can quickly determine the cumulative effects of therapy (Fig. 27-17). Therapy is manipulated based upon previous performance, that is, success leads to harder tasks.

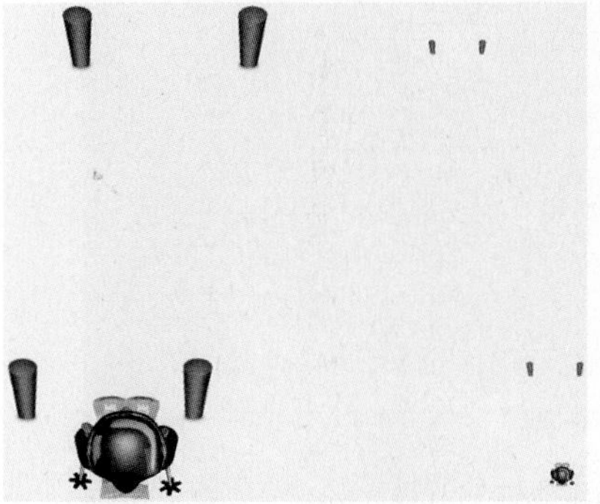

FIGURE 27-19. Typical amblyopia therapy task found in the Amblyopia iNet program. In this task the skiing penguin is guided through the gates. As the visual acuity improves, the penguin and gates become smaller. On the left, the targets are 20/200 and on the right they are 20/30.

Amblyopia iNet Home Therapy Systems has released a new home therapy amblyopia program designed to systematically improve hand–eye coordination, visual acuity, crowding effect, and visual memory (Fig. 27-18). The doctor inputs the visual acuity and the side of the amblyopic eye. Then the patient is instructed to use the program five days a week. Six of the 12 activities in the amblyopia program are randomly assigned each day; thus, at the end of two days, each task has been performed one time. Success results in decreasing the size of the target so that it is harder to resolve. Additionally, in tasks where the targets are moving, the speed is systematically made faster with success. The doctor has the option of eliminating the patch and performing the tasks monocularly in a binocular field. This feature is double-password protected to make sure the doctor wants to prescribe therapy in this manner to decrease the possibility of inducing intractable diplopia. Figure 27-19 shows a typical procedure found on this program.

Perceptual Therapy System II Perceptual Therapy System II (PTSII) is based on the same principles of the CPT office program. Like the office-centered program, PTSII is equally effective regardless of the perceptuocognitive domain preferred. Perceptual Therapy System II contains 11 therapy programs

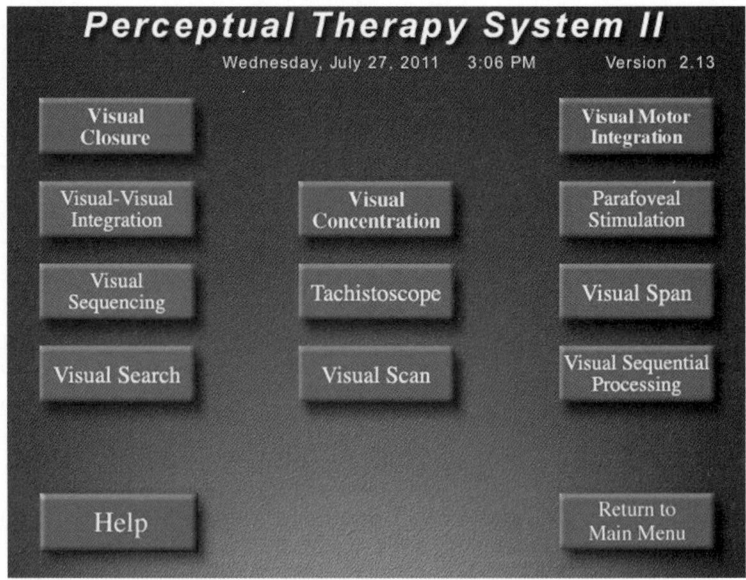

FIGURE 27-20. Main menu of the PTSII. (Image courtesy of HTS Inc.)

(Fig. 27-20), of which nine are similar to CPT programs. They are Visual Closure (Fig. 27-21), Visual Sequencing, Visual Search, Visual Concentration, Tachistoscope, Visual Scan, Visual Motor Integration, Visual Span, and Visual Sequential Processing. The other two are Visual–Visual Integration, which differs from Auditory–Visual Integration in that no auditory stimuli are used, and Parafoveal Stimulation, which is uniquely designed to actively stimulate the area of the retina that is served by the magnocellular (M) system

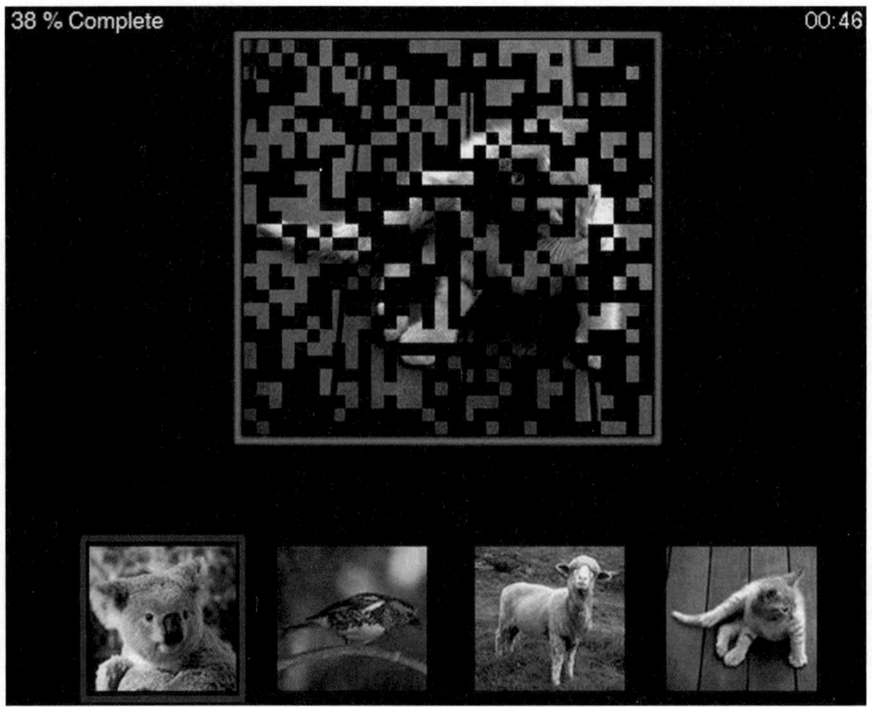

FIGURE 27-21. Visual closure module of the PTSII procedure. (Image courtesy of HTS Inc.)

during reading. The M system controls the ability to change visual fixation from word to word as we read. Magnocells are large neurons in the lateral geniculate body that are responsible for timing visual events not identifying their form. An efficient M system enables us to read smoothly, rapidly, and fluently. The Parafoveal Stimulation program also involves temporal vision processing. Temporal vision processing is a complex process by which an individual processes brief components and rapid sequences of information. It involves a hierarchy of temporal information processing functions ranging from the perception and identification of stimuli to individualizing and perceiving multiple stimuli presented in sequence. Deficits in temporal vision information processing are often associated with reading disability. Many of the other programs in CPT and PTS II address temporal processing.

Dynamic Reader Program Reading fluency is the ability to read connected text rapidly, accurately, effortlessly, and automatically with little conscious attention to the mechanics of reading (58). It is the bridge between word recognition and comprehension. Reading fluency, in essence is a measure of the cumulative reading skills at a particular reading level (59). Dysfluent readers read less text than their peers and have less time to remember, review, or comprehend the text. They expend more cognitive energy than their peers, have poor attention skills, and are less able to integrate segments with other parts of the text. Reading fluency is a critical component for all aspects of learning. The problem is widespread with nearly half of American fourth graders not achieving a minimal level of fluency in their reading (59). Dynamic Reader is a reading fluency program that has three distinct steps listed in Table 27.3. Figure 27-22 provides a visual representation of the program.

Perceptual Visual Tracking Perceptual visual tracking (PVT) is a unique computer program that is specifically designed to improve academically relevant visual tracking skills for patients with learning-related visual disability. Many special needs patients fall into this category. The patient is required to track stimuli that move from left to right and top to bottom, with various speeds and sizes. Identification of specific stimuli is required, and the tasks become progressively more difficult. Patients will develop better perceptual tracking, increased visual attention, faster speed of information processing, improved visual reaction time, orthographic processing, rapid automatized processing, and more efficient ocular motor skill (Fig. 27-23).

ADDITIONAL PROGRAMS

There are several other computer programs and online resources that should be considered for use with patients with special needs. Due to space limitations, they are not fully discussed here, but can be found in Table 27.4.

CONCLUSION

The use of computers for OVT has been discussed in the optometric literature for decades (60,61) and

TABLE 27.3 Descriptions of the Distinct Steps of the Dynamic Reader Reading Fluency Program

Dynamic Reading Steps	Description of Process
Moving test dynamic reading	The material to be read remains in the center of the screen and does not move down the page from top to bottom; therefore, saccadic eye movements are not required. This prevents the loss of place and visual attention that may occur when the print moves down to the next line. This step introduces the concept of dynamic reading with its emphasis on fluency. This step is valuable because it is easier to achieve success.
Standard dynamic reading	The print moves left to right and top to bottom. The reading rate starts at a level that should be comfortable for the patient. It increases as the patient progresses. This step continues the emphasis on fluency and reduction of fixations and regresses. It introduces the added complexity of top-to-bottom reading.
Whole line dynamic reading	The text to be read does not move left to right but is presented an entire line at a time. The patient must self-generate left-to-right eye movements while processing the information. The reading material moves down the page one line at a time to the end of the passage. The speed is determined by the patient's reading rate and comprehension level. This is a critical bridge to normal reading.

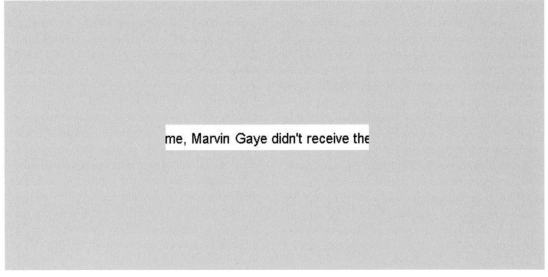

FIGURE 27-22. Depicts the Dynamic Reader Program, standard dynamic reading procedure (Moving Window). (Image courtesy of HTS Inc.)

should be considered a standard for optometric care in this area. Computer-aided OVT can be successfully implemented either in-office in conjunction with traditional techniques, as a stand-alone therapy, or home-based concurrently with office-based treatment. Computerization improves patient motivation, eliminates experimental bias, simplifies therapy goals, provides immediate reinforcement to encourage

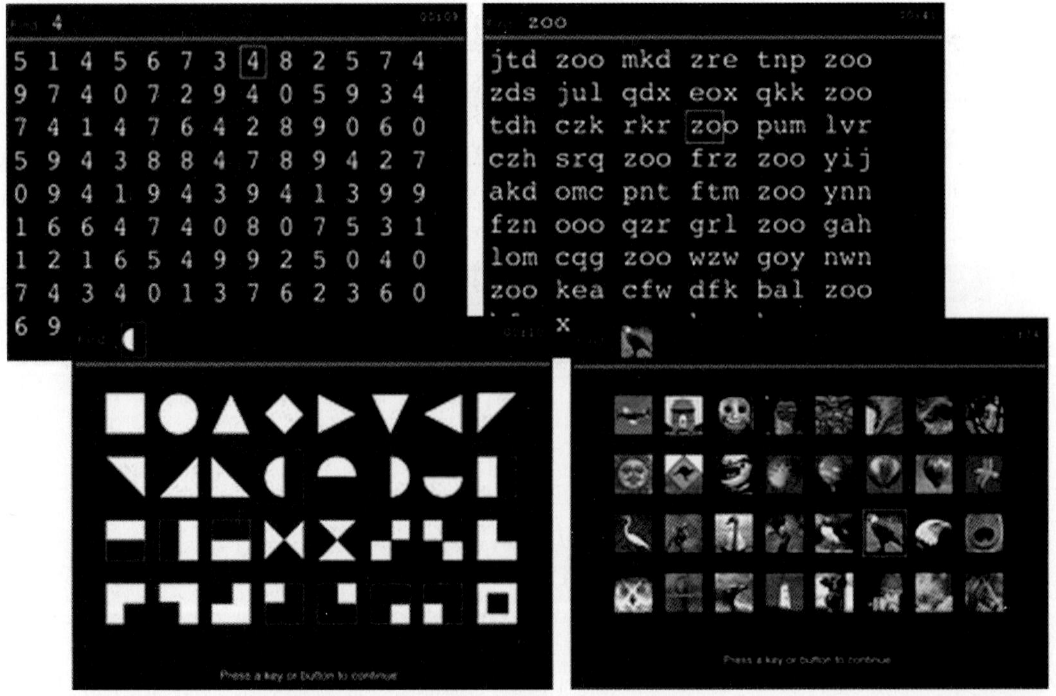

FIGURE 27-23. PVT program, various procedures. (Image courtesy of HTS Inc.)

TABLE 27.4 Additional Programs and Online Resources

Program/Online Resource	Additional Information and Associated Research Support
Brainware safari:	www.brainwareforyou.com (Helms D, Sawtelle SM. A study of the effectiveness of cognitive therapy delivered in a video game format. Optom Vis Dev. 2007;38:19–26.)
PATH to reading:	www.pathtoreading.com/home.htm (Lawton T. Training Direction-Discrimination sensitivity remediates aWide spectrum of reading skills. OptomVis Dev. 2007:38:33–47; Lawton T. Filtered text and direction discrimination training improved reading fluency for both dyslexic and normal readers. Optom Vis Dev. 2008;39:114; Lawton T. Stephey D. Field of view, figure/ground discrimination, sequential memory, and navigation skills improve following training on motion discrimination in older adults. Optom Vis Dev. 2009:40:82–93.)
Computer aided vision therapy	http://cavt.net
Subitizing	(Math programs) (45,54) (Fischer B, Köngeter A, Hartnegg K. Effects of daily practice on subitizing, visual counting, and basic arithmetic skills. Optom Vis Dev. 2008:39:30–34.)
Sub iNet	www.visiontherapysolutions.net/subinet.php
FixTrain+	www.lookingforlearning.com/train/school/index.htm
Eye can learn	www.eyecanlearn.com
Funschool	www.funschool.kaboose.com
The Kidz page	www.thekidzpage.com/learninggames/index.htm
Brain games	www.sheppardsoftware.com/braingames/braingames.htm
Brain injury	www.psychological-software.com

correct responding, and provides meaningful data to evaluate progress. In patients with special needs, OVT must take into account their demands, and potentially, the use of computer-based techniques may allow for the maximum benefit to be achieved.

REFERENCES

1. Duckman RH. Management of functional and perceptual disorders in patients with developmental disabilities. In: Maino DM, editor. Diagnosis and management of special populations. St Louis: Mosby; 1995. p. 256.
2. Groffman S. Consideration of individual characteristics and learning theory. In: Press LJ, editor. Applied concepts in vision therapy. St Louis: Mosby; 1997. p. 43.
3. Groffman S. Motivational factors in visual therapy: comparison of computerized vs. manipulative techniques. J Am Optom Assoc. 1993;67:344–9.
4. Groffman S, Press LJ. Computerized perceptual therapy programs, part 1 and 2. In: Press LJ, editor. Computers and visual therapy programs. Santa Ana: OEP Foundation; 1992.
5. Woolf D. Education psychology as applied in vision training. Am J Optom Arch Am Acad Optom. 1948;25:561–78.
6. Groffman S. Operant conditioning and vision training. Am J Optom Arch Am Acad Optom. 1969;46:583–94.
7. Cooper J, Feldman. Operant conditioning and the assessment of stereopsis in young children. Am J Optom Physiol Opt. 1978;55:532–42.
8. Groffman S. Slot machines and vision therapy. J Optom Vis Dev. 2004;35:134–8.
9. Cooper J, Feldman J. Random-dot-stereogram performance by strabismic, amblyopic, and ocular-pathology patients in an operant-discrimination task. Am J Optom Physiol Opt. 1978;55:599–609.
10. Cooper J, Feldman J. Operant conditioning of fusional convergence ranges using random dot stereograms. Am J Optom Physiol Opt. 1980;57:205.
11. Feldman J, Cooper J. Rapid assessment of stereopsis in preverbal children using operant techniques: a preliminary study. J Am Optom Assoc. 1980;51:767–71.
12. Cooper J. Review of computerized orthoptics with specific regard to convergence insufficiency. Am J Optom Physiol Opt. 1988;65:455–63.
13. Daum KM, Rutstein RP, Eskridge JB. Efficacy of computerized vergence therapy. Am J Optom Physiol Opt. 1987;64:83–9.
14. Cooper J, Selenow A, Ciuffreda KJ, et al. Reduction of asthenopia in patients with convergence insufficiency after fusional vergence training. Am J Optom Physiol Opt. 1983;60:982–89.
15. Cooper J, Feldman J, Selenow A, et al. Reduction of asthenopia after accommodative facility training. Am J Optom Physiol Opt. 1987;64:430–36.
16. Kertesz AE. The effectiveness of wide-angle fusional stimulation in the treatment of convergence insufficiency. Invest Ophthalmol Vis Sci. 1982;22:690–93.
17. Kertesz AE, Kertesz J. Wide-field fusional stimulation in strabismus. Am J Optom Physiol Opt. 1986;63:217–22.
18. Feldman J, Cooper J, Eichler R. Effect of various stimulus parameters on fusional horizontal amplitudes in normal humans. Bin Vis Eye Mus Surg Qtly. 1993;8:23–32.
19. Sommers W, Happel A, Phillips J. Use of personal microcomputer for orthoptic therapy. J Am Optom Assoc. 1984;55:217–22.

20. Griffin JR. Efficacy of vision therapy for nonstrabismic vergence anomalies. Am J Optom Physiol Opt. 1987;64:411–14.
21. Scheiman M, Mitchell GL, Cotter S, et al. A randomized clinical trial of vision therapy/orthoptics versus pencil pushups for the treatment of convergence insufficiency in young adults. Optom Vis Sci. 2005;82:583–95.
22. Goss DA, Downing B, Lowther A, et al. The effect of HTS Vision Therapy conducted in a school setting on reading skills in third and fourth grade students. Optom Vis Dev. 2007;38:27–32.
23. Cooper J. Diagnosis and treatment of accommodative and vergence anomalies using computerized vision therapy. Pract Optom. 1998;9:6–10.
24. Borsting EJ, Rouse MW, Mitchell GL, et al. Validity and reliability of the revised convergence insufficiency symptom survey in children aged 9 to 18 years. Optom Vis Sci. 2003;80:832–8.
25. Das M, Spowart K, Crossley S, et al. Evidence that children with special needs all require visual assessment. Arch Dis Child. 2010;95:888–92.
26. Rommelse NNJ, Stighcel S, Witlox J, et al. Deficits in visuo-spatial working memory, inhibition and oculomotor control in boys with ADHD and their non-affected brothers. J Neural Transm. 2008;115:249–60.
27. Mayes SD, Calnoun SI. Learning, attention, writing, and processing speed in typical children and children with ADHD, autism, anxiety, depression, and oppositional-defiant disorder. Child Neuropsychol. 2007;13:469–93.
28. Granet BD, Gomi CF, Ventura R, et al. The relationship between convergence insufficiency and ADHD. Strabismus. 2005;13(4):163–8.
29. Simmons DR, Robertson AE, McKay LS, et al. Vision in autism spectrum disorder. Vis Res. 2009;49:2705–38.
30. Dakin S, Frith U. Vagaries of visual perception in autism. Neuron. 2005;48:497–507.
31. Pellicano E, Gibson l, Mayberry M, et al. Abnormal global processing along the dorsal visual pathway in autism; a possible mechanism for weak visuospatial coherence. Neuropsychologia. 2005;43:1044–53.
32. Coulter R. Understanding the visual symptoms of individuals with autism spectrum disorder (ASD). Optom Vis Dev. 2009;40:164–75.
33. Kapoor N, Ciuffreda KJ. Vision disturbance following traumatic brain injury. Curr Treat Options Neurol. 2002;4:271–80.
34. Gianutsos R, Suchoff IB. Neuropsychological consequences of mild brain injury and optometric implications. J Behav Optom. 1998;9:3–6.
35. Koeda T, Inque M, Taheshita K. Constructional dyspraxia in preterm diplegia: Isolation from visual and visual perceptual inpairments. Acta Paediatr. 1997;86:1068–73.
36. Pagliano E, Fedrizzi E, Erbetta A. Cognitive profiled and visuoperceptual abilities in preterm and term spastic diplegic children with periventricular leukomalacia. J Child neurol. 2007;22:282–8.
37. Kozeis N, Anogelanaki A, Mitova DT, et al. Visual function and visual perception in cerebral palsied children. Ophthalmic Physiol Opt. 2007;27:44–53.
38. Woodhouse JM, Pakeman VF, Saunders JM, et al. Visual acuity and accommodation in infants and young children with Down's syndrome. J Intellect Disabil Res. 1996;40:49–55.
39. Visu-Petra L, Benga O, Tingas I, et al. Visual-spatial processing in children and adolescents with Down's syndrome: a computerized assessment of memory skills. J Intellect Disabil Res. 2007;51:942–52.
40. Lanfranchi S, Carretti B, Spano G, et al. A specific deficit in visuospatial simultaneous working memory in Down syndrome. J Intellect Disabil Res. 2009;53:474–83.
41. Sireteanu R, Goebel C, Goertz R, et al. Do children with developmental dyslexia show a selective visual attention deficit? Strabismus. 2006;14:85–93.
42. Vidyasagar TR, Pammer K. Dyslexia: a deficit in visuo-spatial attention, not in phonological processing. Trends Cogn Sci. 2009;14:57–63.
43. Palomo A, Puell MC. Binocular function in school children with reading difficulties. Graefes Arch Clin Exp Ophthalmol. 2010;248:885–92.
44. Ansari D, DonlanC, Thomas MSC, et al. What makes counting count? Verbal and visuo-spatial contributions to typical and atypical number development. J Exp Child Psychol. 2003:60–63.
45. Groffman S. Subitizing: Vision therapy for math deficits. Optom Vis Dev. 2009;40:229–38.
46. Dickstein DP, Treland JE, Snow J, et al. Neuropsychological performance in pediatric bipolar disorder. Biol Psychiatry. 2004;55:32–9.
47. Dow C, Seidenberg M, Hermann B. Relationship between information processing speed in temporal lobe epilepsy and white matter volume. Epilepsy Behav. 2004;5:916–25.
48. Drew MA, Starkey NJ, Isler RB. Examining the link between information processing speed and executive functioning in multiple sclerosis. Arch Clin Neuropsychol. 2008;24:47–68.
49. Olitsky SE, Sadler LS, Reynolds JD. Subnormal binocular vision in the Williams syndrome. J Pediatr Ophthalmol Strabismus. 1997;34:58–60.
50. Nakamura M, Watabane K, Matsumoto A, et al. Williams syndrome and deficiency in visuospatial recognition. Dev Med Child Neurol. 2001;43:617–21.
51. Lorusso ML, Facoetti A, Toraldo A, et al. Tachistoscopic treatment of dyslexia changes the distribution of visual-spatial attention. Brain Cogn. 2005;57:132–42.
52. Berry AS, ZantoTP, Clapp WC et al. The influence of perceptual training on working memory in older adults. Available from: www.plosone.org. 2010;5:1-8. e11537.
53. Akhutina T, Foreman N, Krichevets A, et al. Improving spatial functioning in children with cerebral palsy using computerized and traditional game tasks. Disabil Rehabil. 2003;25:1361–71.
54. Fischer B, Gebhardt C, Hartnegg K. Subitizing and visual counting in children with problems in acquiring basic counting skills. Optom Vis Dev. 2008;39:24–9.
55. Miller DC. Luria's theory of brain functioning. Educ Psychol. 1992;27:493–512.
56. Das JP, Kirby JR, Jannan RF. Simultaneous and successive cognitive processes. New York: Academic Press; 1979.
57. Daum K. Double-blind placebo-controlled examination of timing effects in the training of positive vergences. Am J Optom Physiol Opt. 1986;63:807–12.
58. Solan HA, Shelley-Tremblay S, Larson S, Mounts J. Silent word reading, fluency, and temporal vision processing: difference between good and poor readers. J Behav Optom. 2006;17:1–9.

59. Rasinski TV. Assessing reading fluency. Available from: www.prel.org/products/re_/assessing fluency.po.2005. Last accessed March 1, 2011.
60. Maino D. The process approach, microcomputers, and therapy. In: Press L, editor. Computers and Vision Therapy Programs. Santa Ana: Optometric Extension Program; 1992. p. 51–7.
61. Maino D. Computer saccadic and accommodative rock visual therapy program. Pediatr Optom Vis Ther. 1992;2:3.

CONFLICT OF INTEREST *Dr. Cooper is a developer of the Computer OrthoptorTM and HTSTM and has a financial interest in these systems. This chapter was adapted from* Cooper J. Computerized Vision Therapy for Home and Office Treatment of Accommodative and Vergence Disorders, and Amblyopia. J Behav Optom. 2007:88–93.

Dr. Harris has no financial interest in any of the products discussed in this chapter.

Dr. Groffman is a developer of CPT, PTSII, Dynamic Reader, PVT, and Subitizing and has a financial interest in these programs.

CHAPTER 28

Danielle L. Hinton, MD
Deborah S. Hoffnung, PhD, ABPP-CN
Elizabeth Bishop, MSSW
F. Fred Hidaji, MD
Glenda Brooks, LCSW
Julie S. Marshall, MA, CCC-SLP, BRFS
Marc B. Taub, OD, MS, FAAO, FCOVD
Monika Kolwaite, PT, NCS
Orli Weisser-Pike, OTR/L, CLVT, SCLV
Pamela J. Compart, MD
Robin D. Lewis, OD, FCOVD
Robert Hohendorf, OD

The Multidisciplinary Approach

The idea of a multidisciplinary or a team approach is crucial in the care of patients with special needs. The question is not *if* a multidisciplinary team is to be used but rather, *"Who is to be on that team?"* In addition to optometrists and patients, occupational therapists, speech and language pathologists, physical therapists, psychologists, physicians, educators, friends, and parents must all be a vital part of that team. Every member of the team can potentially help develop, improve, and integrate the learning process of each special needs individual. Each brings potential benefits as well as fiscal costs. The core issue is, "What are the best possible uses of the patient's resources to meet their goals?"

A care-giving team, whether the team has multiple members or as few as two, ideally derives its advantages from a coordinated and collaborative effort to provide care. At its best, multidisciplinary cooperation can provide a greater-than-linear addition of efficiency and improved access to care from a wider variety of professionals. When misapplied, the team can misuse the patient's resources, increasing the time, energy, and financial burdens borne by the patient with little benefit in meeting the individual's goals.

When we talk about multidisciplinary teamwork, it is useful to think about what this implies. Multidisciplinary means that we have all taken different paths to learning that will uniquely affect the way we see and understand our patients' wants and needs. How team members respond to the patients we work with depends heavily on our frame of reference. Our frames of reference provide the contexts within which we understand our patients. We form individual frames of reference based on the variation of our individual life experiences that include the influences placed upon us by the educational environments in which we participated. The result is that each of us, even within the same profession, will have some surprising differences in how we come to understand what we do. In the right circumstances, the disparity provided by our differing frames of reference can provide improved context, increase depth of understanding, provide synergistic outcomes, and improve the efficacy of actions taken on behalf of our patients. Some of the potential members of the multidisciplinary team related to the care of patients with special needs are introduced in this chapter. The goal in doing this is that we may all understand the backgrounds and roles of the various professionals involved.

BEHAVIORAL–DEVELOPMENTAL PEDIATRICS

Behavioral–developmental pediatrics is a subspecialty of pediatrics. Pediatricians complete 3 years of general pediatric residency training, but those in this subspecialty obtain 3 years of additional specialty training in pediatric behavioral and developmental disorders. Behavioral–developmental pediatricians are trained in a broad variety of areas, allowing them to view a child in his/her entirety. Specialty areas typically covered in training include genetics, neurology, and psychiatry. Physicians also work with and learn from educational specialists, speech pathologists, occupational and physical therapists, psychologists, and social workers.

Training programs vary in the scope of topics covered and which areas receive emphasis. Similarly, behavioral-developmental pediatricians (BDPs) can choose to practice more broadly or focus on more specific areas within their training. For example, some choose a more behavioral emphasis, while others focus more on neurodevelopmental disorders. Those with a more behavioral emphasis might focus increasingly on the diagnosis and treatment of disorders such as attention deficit hyperactivity disorder (ADHD), depression, and anxiety and bipolar disorders. Those with a neurodevelopmental emphasis might focus more on disorders such as autism, learning or intellectual disability, cerebral palsy, and complications of prematurity.

There is much overlap between these two areas, and many behavioral–developmental pediatricians work with children with a variety of disorders and delays. In addition, numerous children have a combination of disorders that require a broader view and approach. For example, many children with ADHD also have learning disabilities.

Behavioral–developmental pediatricians play an important role in the overall management of children with special needs. These pediatricians, secondary to the breadth of their training, are able to identify a broad range of dysfunctions or needs and can then either treat the child or refer to the appropriate services. In an era in which children often have a doctor for each individual body part or system, a BDP can look at the whole person and place the relevant symptoms in a larger context.

As with other areas of medicine, the best test for diagnosing behavioral or developmental disorders is the individual's history. Behavioral–developmental pediatricians take an in-depth history that covers a variety of areas (Table 28.1). This history provides information that can guide further diagnostic workup and therapeutic interventions. For example, a history that reveals that a child lives in an older home might result in further investigation for lead exposure, while a child with constipation, fatigue, weight gain, and cognitive delays might be hypothyroid.

A complete general physical and neurologic examination is performed by the BDP. This is done with an eye toward clues to a variety of diagnoses. For example, certain findings on the skin may indicate the potential for abnormal brain development as skin and brain originate from the same embryonic source (ectoderm). An early insult to the fetus might then affect both of these organ systems. A child's head circumference can also provide helpful information. If too small, it might indicate poor brain growth or malformation, but if too large, it might indicate hydrocephalus. Any dysmorphic features such as unusual facial features, large ears, etc., are noted as possible clues for genetic syndromes. Close attention is also paid to the neurologic examination (reflexes, strength, tone). Lastly, there are physical examination findings that might indicate nutritional deficiencies that can affect brain function. For example, eczema or keratosis pilaris ("chicken skin") can be seen with essential fatty acid deficiencies. Essential fatty acids are needed for optimal brain health and function.

TABLE 28.1 Areas Covered during the History Component of an Examination with Behavioral–Developmental Pediatrician

Category	Important Points
Pregnancy history	Mother's health during pregnancy; cigarette, alcohol, or drug use; results of amniocentesis or ultrasounds
Birth and neonatal history	Full-term or premature birth; complications at delivery; postdelivery complications (e.g., jaundice, infections, etc.)
Past medical history	Injuries (especially significant head injuries), hospitalizations, surgeries, illnesses, environmental exposures (e.g., lead), hearing and vision, medications, "review of systems" (e.g., allergies, illnesses, GI health, sleep, weight/growth, etc.)
Diet	Variety of food intake; adequacy of calcium and protein intake; risk factors for nutritional deficiencies that can affect brain function (e.g., iron deficiency anemia, vitamin D deficiency, zinc deficiency)
Developmental milestones	History regarding speech/language, gross and fine motor, social/adaptive skills. Looking for delays and/or atypical qualities to development
Behavioral symptoms	Inattention, hyperactivity, impulsivity, depression, anxiety, mood swings, irritability, aggression, autism symptoms, sensory sensitivities, or sensory processing issues
Social history	Peer and family relationships; family stressors
Family history	Genetic predispositions to physical, neurologic, or mental health disorders

Additional data are obtained through questionnaires completed by parents or teachers and direct examination in the office. Testing varies depending on the child's age and the diagnoses in question. Testing can be performed to obtain information concerning cognitive and language levels, as well as gross, fine, and visual motor function. The child's mental health can be assessed through direct questioning and observation or through questionnaires which the child completes. Questionnaires can also be completed by the parents to obtain further information regarding a child's adaptive skills (such as feeding, dressing, etc.), as well as by the child's teacher or other therapists to provide information on the child's functioning in settings other than the home.

Based on the history, physical examination, and other data obtained, medical testing is then done to confirm diagnoses (such as genetic syndromes) or provide a basis for treatment. Testing might include blood and urine testing for genetic, metabolic, or nutritional issues. An electroencephalogram (EEG) may be ordered if there is a question or history of seizures. Imaging of the brain (such as computed tomography [CT] or magnetic resonance imaging [MRI] scans) may also be indicated.

A treatment plan is then devised based on all of the above factors. Some of these treatments may be carried out directly by the BDP. Other interventions may require referrals to other specialists for further diagnostic workup or to other practitioners for therapies. Potential treatments or interventions include the following:

- Referral for treatment of identified or suspected hearing or vision impairments
- Treatment of nutritional deficiencies
- Advice regarding school placement and the need for educational/special educational supports—such as a Section 504 plan or Individualized Educational Plan
- Recommendations for specific therapies—such as vision, speech/language, occupational, and physical therapy
- Referrals for counseling, psychotherapy, or family therapy
- Prescription of medications
- Referrals to other specialists—for example, neurologists, psychiatrists, physiatrists, optometrists

A case example might be helpful in better understanding the above process. Johnny is an 8-year-old child who presented to a BDP because of school's concern that he might have ADHD. He was inattentive at school, often daydreamed, and had trouble completing tasks. He particularly had problems when asked to do math, at school or as part of his homework. A detailed history revealed that he had frequent ear infections and that the fluid in his ears took a long time to resolve. He was a picky eater and often would not eat anything for breakfast other than dry cereal or a doughnut. At school, he was a generally happy child but had turned into the class clown and was more frequently being sent to the principal's office for disrupting the class. His physical examination in the office was normal except for fluid in his ears. He was referred to an ENT specialist and found to have decreased hearing. This resulted in the placement of tubes in his ears. Referral was also made to an optometrist who ruled out the need for glasses as well as a visual efficiency issue related to fusion, accommodation, or eye movements.

Blood testing revealed that Johnny was iron and zinc deficient, both of which can affect brain functioning. Studies have shown that iron deficiency can result in worsened ADHD symptoms (1,2). Zinc deficiency was likely contributing to his picky eating. Zinc and iron supplements were initiated. In addition, lack of protein intake in the morning was likely leading to low blood sugar in the midmorning, which can result in inattention. Adding protein to breakfast and lunch was recommended. Johnny was referred for educational testing and was found to have a math learning disability. His acting out in class served a helpful function for him. It helped him get sent to the principal's office during math lessons and thus allowed him to avoid work. Addressing his math disability and providing additional educational support decreased his disruptive behaviors and allowed him to feel more successful at school. The above interventions resulted in significant improvement. However, Johnny continued to have some residual difficulty focusing in class and completing his assignments, so a low dose of a stimulant medication was added which improved his attention. This type of comprehensive approach allows the BDP to view a child's symptoms within the context of his/her entire medical, educational, social, and family system in order to make the most accurate diagnoses and to formulate the most appropriate treatment plans.

NEUROPSYCHOLOGY

In neuropsychology, it is quite common to encounter individuals with special needs, particularly those with physical disabilities and limitations in sight or hearing. Conducting assessments with these individuals poses numerous challenges for the neuropsychologist.

Clinical neuropsychology is a specialty field of psychology that examines brain functions including attention, learning, and memory, as well as language, visuospatial abilities, and reasoning. Other areas evaluated often include motor and sensory operations, mood, and behavior. Neuropsychologists work in a variety of settings, including schools, medical centers, brain and spinal cord injury rehabilitation programs, and private practice groups. Subspecialization includes, but is not limited to, learning disabilities, ADHD, epilepsy, memory disorders, dementia, brain tumor, and stroke.

A number of clinical and functional questions may prompt referral for a neuropsychological evaluation. These include issues of diagnosis, treatment suitability and response, and learning disability. Other issues of concern are decision-making capacity and questions of a forensic nature related to incarceration, disability claims, and other legal proceedings. The most common referral sources include neurologists, neurosurgeons, pediatricians, psychiatrists, primary care physicians, attorneys, and the court system, as well as patients and their families.

A typical evaluation includes a review of the medical record, ancillary testing results (e.g., MRI, EEG), an interview with the patient and the family, observation of behavior, administration of statistically validated assessment measures, and analysis and interpretation of test data. All of this information, combined with the results of testing, is then summarized into a written clinical report, which includes diagnoses and recommendations. Findings can be communicated to the client and the referral source in writing, by phone, and/or in a feedback session, as desired. The cognitive domains that are typically assessed and examples of the tests that are used to measure these functions are listed in Table 28.2.

Neuropsychologists work in a variety of settings and a diverse patient population with the recommendations being as unique as the patients they serve. These include suggestions for further assessment and treatment of physical, mood, and sleep disorders, as well as proposed accommodations for school and/or the workplace.

Standardized tests have been developed and selected based on statistical reliability and validity. Validity generally refers to a test's ability to measure the construct or brain function that it purports to measure, such as memory. Reliability refers to the consistency with which a test generates the same score under similar retest conditions.

For the most part, the development of neuropsychological measures also includes the collection of performance scores within a defined group. Commercially developed tests aim to collect scores from a sample based on the United States census, while more specialized tests may use a sample of convenience or a sample from the population of interest. "Norms" are then developed that represent the average or median performance on the test earned by the group to which it was administered. For many cognitive functions, variables that are found to affect test performance, such as age, education, and gender, are also taken into account to define expectations about normal performance on the task. In clinical practice, individual patients' scores are then compared to these norms, and the degree of deviation from the median score is used to indicate the presence (or absence) and degree of dysfunction demonstrated. The legitimacy of basing interpretations on these deviation scores requires the administration of tests in the same (standardized) manner as the test was administered when the norm scores were collected. Otherwise, deviations in a patient's score from the mean of the norm group cannot be interpreted in a reliable and valid manner because of the number of other factors that may have been introduced by the modifications in administration.

Evaluating the patient with special needs often requires that modifications be made to standardized testing procedures. The goal of adaptation is to preserve, as much as possible, a test's ability to measure a construct of interest (e.g., fluid intelligence, reasoning ability, etc.) while minimizing the impact of confounding variables that are unrelated to that construct. For example, it is not surprising that low vision has been shown to affect performance on measures of visual processing, yet it is important to recognize that low vision would likely also impact an individual's performance on a test of memory that requires the learning and retention of visually presented designs. Modifications to testing can be negligible to extensive and may include any of the following changes: how a response is given (pointing versus a verbal response), alteration of the testing stimuli (magnification of a picture for those with low vision), use of an amplification system, writing out and/or repetition of instructions for those with

TABLE 28.2 Domains Assessed and Measures Commonly Used in the Neuropsychological Evaluation

Cognitive Domain Assessed	Examples of Tests within That Domain
General intellectual and cognitive abilities	• Weschler Adult Intelligence Scale • Wechsler Intelligence Scale for Children • Repeatable Battery for the Assessment of Neuropsychological Status
Academic functioning	• Wechsler Test of Adult Reading • Woodcock Johnson Tests of Achievement • Wide Range Achievement Test
Attention	• Continuous Performance Test • Digit span tasks • Stroop test • Trail Making test • Paced Auditory Serial Addition Test
Language	• Boston Naming Test • Controlled Oral Word Association Test • Token tests • Sentence repetition tasks
Visuospatial functioning	• Hooper Visual Organization Test • Block design tasks • Judgment of line orientation tasks • Rey Complex Figure Test
Memory	• Wechsler Memory Scale • California Verbal Learning Test • Rey Auditory Verbal Learning Test • Brief Visuospatial Memory Test • Test of Memory and Learning • Children's Memory Scale
Reasoning	• Wisconsin Card Sorting Test • Verbal similarities tests • Matrix reasoning tasks • Tower of London
Sensory and motor functioning	• Finger tapping • Grip strength • Grooved pegboard • Reitan-Klove Sensory–Perceptual test
Mood and personality	• Beck Sepression Inventory • Beck Anxiety Inventory • Minnesota Multiphasic Personality Inventory

poor hearing, additional time for completion of the task or avoidance of timed tasks for those with motor slowing, and the use of a sign-language interpreter trained to translate examiner instructions and patient responses verbatim.

However, as described above, changes to testing procedures generally invalidate existing norms because these norms were developed based on testing done in a standardized manner in a population without disabilities. As noted by Hill-Briggs et al. (3), little research has been conducted to validate the accommodation and modification practices that deviate from standard test administration or to develop interpretive guidelines specifically for persons with physical or sensory disabilities. Thus, the effects of disability and modification-related factors on performance are, for the most part, unknown. For example, verbal fluency tasks are commonly used to evaluate an individual's ability to quickly generate words within a given category or beginning with a given letter in a minute's time. Performance on these tasks is used as an indicator of mental speed and verbal generation abilities. On this measure, the hearing-impaired and/or mute individual using sign language may have an advantage, as some words seemingly have a sign that is faster to communicate than stating the word aloud.

Alternatively, they may also be at a disadvantage, as other words must be spelled out because there is no corresponding single sign for the word. It is clearly inappropriate to compare the score of an individual who has signed a list of words to that of a group of individuals with intact speech and hearing who have spoken these words.

Nevertheless, testing of individuals with disability using appropriate accommodations *does* allow for inferences to be made regarding performance and abilities. Reluctance to assess individuals with physical and sensory disabilities because of the limitations in available tests and norms would be, in and of itself, unethical. Any accommodations and modifications should be clearly noted on the test protocols as well as stated in the report. Any conclusions (including limitations in measuring the construct of interest) should be qualified appropriately. Given the increasing cultural diversity and the advancing age (decreased hearing, vision, and physical ability) of the population, the standardization of modifications to testing procedures and the collection of normative data derived from special needs populations using these modifications is essential. Similarly important is the education of specialists in complementary fields, such as optometry, ophthalmology, audiology, and speech-language pathology, regarding the services available from the neuropsychologist, and the considerations taken, in assessing the cognitive functions of individuals with visual, auditory, and hearing impairments.

OCCUPATIONAL THERAPY

Occupational therapy (OT) promotes engagement and participation in everyday activities in a manner that supports health, well-being, and life satisfaction (4). The profession is underpinned by the notion that engagement in meaningful and purposeful occupations facilitates well-being. This emphasis on well-being is also supported by the World Health Organization, which defines health as "not merely the absence of disease or infirmity" but rather "a state of complete physical, mental and social well-being" (5). Furthermore, the International Classification of Functioning, Disability and Health (ICF) (6) measures a person's well-being by his/her ability to participate in life situations (7). Drawing on the language of the ICF, the profession of OT describes its domain and process in the Occupational Therapy Practice Framework, a document that includes within it the language and concepts relevant to the profession (8). In this document, the term occupation is used "to capture the breadth and meaning of everyday activity." Recognition of the inherent therapeutic value contained within everyday activities is a central tenet of the profession's philosophy. Engagement and participation in life activities is both the means by which well-being is achieved and the desired outcome.

Since OT is concerned with the promotion of health, it is only natural that therapists are typically found in the health care workforce. Occupational therapy practitioners may have a bachelor's, master's, or doctoral level degree, while OT assistants have an associate degree. OTs are responsible for evaluating the client and creating an intervention and discharge plan. They are also accountable for all aspects of OT service delivered, while their assistants provide intervention. Occupational therapy practitioners offer care in hospitals, nursing homes, private clinics, early intervention centers, schools, and many other settings, including clients' homes and workplaces. The natural environments in which occupations occur are part and parcel of the dynamic therapeutic process, whereby the OT practitioner may engineer the environment to enable access or remove barriers to participation in desired activities. In all circumstances, OT practitioners use knowledge and apply skilled methods to facilitate the goals of the client.

In the health care system, OT commonly falls under the umbrella of physical medicine and rehabilitation. Clients are referred by order of physicians who deem the therapy medically necessary in order to promote, restore, and remediate, as well as preserve, adapt, modify, or compensate for the client's inability to participate in life activities. In the educational system, the school team may request an OT evaluation for a student, which also requires a physician's order. Direct access to OT is also available, but clients do not have the benefit of accessing health care insurance reimbursement for these services.

Clients referred to OT may have an acute condition, such as a bone fracture, that prevents the individual from dressing while adhering to certain medical precautions. Acute conditions are expected to heal in time after which the client may not require OT intervention. On the other hand, individuals with chronic conditions may require periodic OT for a longer period of time or over the course of the client's lifetime. Typically these clients are considered as having "special needs." For example, a child born with Down syndrome may have difficulty sucking from a bottle, sensitivity to sounds, and hand weakness. These difficulties will negatively affect the child's ability to achieve developmental milestones, such as eating and drinking, tolerating noisy environments with unexpected sounds, and manipulating toys. Using skilled interventions, OT practitioners work to remove barriers to participation and promote development and engagement in everyday routines. Table 28.3 shows several examples of OT areas of intervention.

How Did Low Vision Become a Rehabilitation Area in Occupational Therapy? In the United States, several important changes were made in the health care environment in the late 1990s. Recognizing the growing needs of seniors with permanent vision loss from age-related eye diseases and the lack of services available to this segment of the population, the government-run health care insurance, known as the Centers for Medicare and Medicaid Services, conceded that despite being a sensory impairment, low vision interfered with one's ability to participate in necessary and desired activities of daily living in the same way that other medical conditions resulted in reduced physical functioning (9). This recognition enabled physicians, including ophthalmologists and optometrists, to prescribe to their clients with low vision, rehabilitation services delivered via OT. Likewise, it enabled a large segment of the population to receive therapy as a benefit of their health insurance coverage.

The American Occupational Therapy Association (AOTA) was the first OT membership organization to realize the importance of certification for practitioners working with adults with low vision. The Occupational Therapy Code of Ethics (10) requires OT practitioners to achieve high standards of competency. To facilitate professional development in low vision, in 2006, the AOTA began offering its members a specialty certification in low vision based on a peer-reviewed reflective portfolio. The AOTA delineated four competencies composed of 27 criteria that reflect the specialized OT practice in the field of low vision. The criteria encompass the standards of knowledge, performance, critical reasoning, ethical reasoning, and interpersonal skills. To apply for certification, OT practitioners must meet specific eligibility requirements, including a minimum of 600 hours delivering low vision rehabilitation. The portfolio is an assemblage of evidence of professional development activities for each criterion with narrative self-assessments on how these activities helped the applicant achieve the overarching competencies. Applications are peer reviewed and scored according to AOTA guidelines. Occupational therapists who achieve specialty certification receive the designation specialty certification low vision, while OT assistants receive the designation specialty certification low vision assistant (11).

What Are Examples of Occupational Therapy Interventions for Clients with Low Vision? Occupational therapy for clients with low vision includes a variety of skilled techniques to promote functioning and remove barriers to participation. For example, an OT practitioner may work with the client to maximize his or her remaining vision by the facilitation of scotoma awareness, identification of the preferred retinal locus (PRL) and training in efficient PRL placement for reading and writing. Occupational therapists may design pen-on-paper exercises to practice and achieve the skill of PRL-hand coordination in preparation for writing checks. When using a prescribed optical device, such as a stand magnifier for reading one's mail, the OT practitioner may recommend and position a table easel to promote good posture, reduce neck strain, and insure the client is viewing from the appropriate distance for the device. The OT practitioner might recommend a lamp in a closet to

TABLE 28.3 Examples of OT Interventions for Clients with Special Needs

Interventions	Goal
Cognitive skills	Problem solving and adaptation to novel or unexpected situations
Gross- and fine-motor skills	Proximal stability of the trunk and shoulders and distal control of the hands for the development of age-appropriate grasp, release, and prehension
Self-care skills	Participation in eating, dressing, toileting, and bathing using alternative techniques and/or adaptive equipment
Sensory integration skills	Regulation of overactive or underactive sensory systems, particularly proprioceptive, tactual, and vestibular systems

improve the client's ability to identify and match clothing, may train the client in nonvisual methods to dial phone numbers, and program the client's telephone with frequently called numbers to facilitate efficient and safe communication in cases of emergency. Other common areas for OT intervention in clients with low vision are medication, home, and financial management, shopping, and access to community resources.

Service gaps continue to remain with regard to access to OT services for young clients with low vision. While it is common for OT practitioners to treat young clients through educational systems, these clients typically receive OT to address deficits relating to sensory integration dysfunction, autism, cerebral palsy, intellectual disabilities, and other developmental delays. While it remains uncommon for OT practitioners to treat young clients with low vision, the earlier intervention occurs, the greater the impact and easier the adaptation process will be for the patient and his or her family.

OPHTHALMOLOGY

As most aspects of the oculovisual diagnosis and management of the special needs patient are covered elsewhere in this text, this section will focus on the role that the ophthalmologist plays in treatment of such patients. The goal of this section is to describe the subspecialties of ophthalmology, with particular attention to the role each may play in low vision treatment. Of course, there are many more similarities than differences between the fields of optometry and ophthalmology. Traditionally, the distinctions have centered on surgical scope of practice, but other differences exist, allowing optometry and ophthalmology to be complementary. This can then allow each profession to best serve the mutual goal of improving the lives of patients with special needs and reduced vision. Familiarity with ophthalmology and its various subspecialties is essential in the management of patients with special needs to facilitate appropriate comanagement.

After 4 years of medical school, the ophthalmologist in training completes 1 year of internship (either surgical or medical) and a general ophthalmology residency of 3 to 4 years. Following completion of the residency, some choose to undergo a 1- or 2-year fellowship in one or more of these areas: Cornea/Anterior Segment, Retina/Posterior Segment, Pediatrics/Strabismus, Oculoplastics, Glaucoma, Neuro-ophthalmology

General ophthalmologists have, in years past, been the gatekeepers of the ophthalmic world, dealing with optometric referrals directly and deciding on the need for referral to an ophthalmic subspecialist. But as the optometric scope of practice has expanded in the past few decades, optometrists have become more adept at direct subspecialty referrals. Comprehensive treatment of the special needs patient will often require the intervention of one or more of these subspecialties.

Cornea/Anterior Segment This field deals with diseases involving the ocular surface (cornea, conjunctiva, tear insufficiency). In addition, corneal surgeons are trained to perform the more complicated anterior segment surgeries, such as corneal transplantation, endothelial grafts, keratoprosthesis implantation, conjunctival grafting, and corneal refractive surgery. They also are skilled at managing corneal disease such as herpetic eye disease, autoimmune sclerokeratopathies, and chronic corneal degenerations.

Retina/Posterior Segment Retinal specialists have at their disposal several diagnostic and surgical techniques not generally used by nonspecialist ophthalmologists. Retinal detachment repair, macular surgery, and pars plana vitrectomy are among the surgeries usually only performed by retinal surgeons. Retinal specialists also make frequent use of fluorescein angiography, indocyanine green angiography, and optical coherence tomography (OCT) to make diagnostic and therapeutic decisions. To allow for mastery of these techniques, retinal fellowships are 2 years in length.

Some retinal disorders that the optometrist may encounter in the special needs patient are

1. Age-related macular degeneration (AMD)
2. Diabetic retinopathy
3. Retinopathy of prematurity (ROP)
4. Retinal detachment
5. Cystoid macular edema
6. Autoimmune retinopathies
7. Hereditary retinal degenerations
8. Albinism

In years past, AMD came with a dismal prognosis and poor treatment options. Treatment of AMD has, in recent years, taken a leap forward following the release of the Age-Related Eye Disease Study study advocating the use of nutritional supplements (vita min C, vitamin E, beta-carotene and zinc) (12) as well as the advent of vascular endothelial growth factor inhibitors (anti-VEGF). Retinal surgeons are now able to effectively stabilize devastating disorders, like wet AMD, with these drugs (13,14).

Likewise, treatment of proliferative diabetic retinopathy has advanced significantly in the past decade. Though panretinal and focal laser remains a mainstay of treatment, retinal surgeons have learned to modulate the disease using anti-VEGF agents synergistically with laser treatment to minimize the amount of laser needed and reduce laser-related side effects.

With the emergence of excellent neonatal care, more severely premature babies are surviving, making retinopathy of prematurity an increasingly common cause of low vision. The Early Treatment for Retinopathy of Prematurity Study has led to more aggressive early laser treatment for so-called prethreshold ROP (15). Preserving vision in this class of special needs patients is particularly important, because their visual limitations often coexist with cerebral palsy and other systemic conditions. The use of anti-VEGF agents for the treatment of ROP appears very promising, but is presently in the research realm.

Pediatrics/Strabismus Depending on their training, pediatric ophthalmologists may be specialized to treat childhood and adult strabismus (i.e., strabismologists) or may practice a more comprehensive scope of care that also includes lacrimal disorders, pediatric cataracts, and congenital glaucoma or ptosis. Optometric vision therapy (OVT) and orthoptics are very unlikely to have been a part of the pediatric ophthalmologist's education, in either residency or fellowship. Most pediatric ophthalmologists' training focuses on the optical and surgical correction of strabismus, as well as occlusion therapy for amblyopia.

Strabismus in the special needs patient is often sensory in nature; that is, the misalignment is a result of the poor vision, not the converse. These patients are more likely to have reduced fusional ability. As such, correction of the strabismus may not result in improved visual function, but the benefits of improving a sensory strabismus can easily be underestimated. Strabismus is a cosmetically disfiguring condition similar to a cleft lip, which any physician would not hesitate to correct.

Diplopia in adults is a most difficult problem to correct. Adults with new-onset strabismus and diplopia can often have a very difficult time coping and functioning. Prisms can help, but are not always the best solution. Consequently, some of the most gratifying interventions a pediatric ophthalmologist provides are corrective surgery in such patients. Adjustable suture techniques in strabismus surgery, in which the surgeon fine-tunes the amount of surgery after the patient is awakened from anesthesia, provides increased success in alleviating diplopia in complicated strabismus.

Oculoplastics Disorders involving the lids, lacrimal system, and orbit are the purview of the oculoplastic surgeon. Blepharoplasty is a mainstay of the practice of most oculoplastic surgeons, but they also treat pediatric and adult-onset ptosis, cancers of the lids and ocular adnexa, and eyelid trauma. The specialist will also use surgical intervention for orbital fracture, congenital eyelid abnormality, orbital tumor, and lacrimal duct obstruction. Patients with special needs who are born with genetic defects may have coexisting craniofacial defects. The oculoplastic surgeon, working with the craniofacial surgeon, is typically involved in such cases.

Ocular Oncology A fairly recent addition to the subspecialties of ophthalmology is that of ocular oncology. As the treatment of ocular cancer becomes more complex, a multidisciplinary approach is necessary. For example, the treatment of retinoblastoma has evolved from simple enucleation to using a much more powerful array of tools including I^{131} plaque therapy and chemoreduction (16). The ocular oncologist provides a bridge between the worlds of ophthalmology and oncology, allowing for the latest therapies to be available to the patient. Training as an ocular oncologist usually includes completion of an oculoplastics fellowship followed by a year or more of a specialized ocular oncology exposure.

Glaucoma Fortunately, the arsenal of medical and surgical interventions available for treating glaucoma has expanded dramatically over the past several decades. Modern perimetry and OCT have improved diagnostic accuracy and the ability of the specialist to monitor glaucoma progression. Medical glaucoma management has improved through the shift towards prostaglandin analogs and topical carbonic anhydrase inhibitors.

The role of the glaucoma specialist is most prominent in the arena of surgery. Glaucoma specialists are fellowship trained to deal with failures of medical management and have many techniques at their disposal. Laser trabeculoplasty has been a valuable adjunct to topical medications, while glaucoma unresponsive to medical therapy can now be adequately controlled with modern surgical therapies, such as trabeculectomy and tube shunts, using antimetabolites (e.g., mitomycin and 5-fluoruracil). Endocyclophotocoagulation and cyclocryotherapy are treatments used if conventional medical and surgical therapy fails.

Neuro-ophthalmology The neuro-ophthalmologist deals with problems involving the optic nerve and brain. Even when the ocular diagnosis may already be clear, the neuro-ophthalmologist can work to rule out a systemic cause for vision loss and determine if it is stable or worsening. This intervention can clarify the exact nature of a neurologic disorder involving the eyes, thus preventing further visual loss and progression of a system-wide disease, such as myasthenia gravis or multiple sclerosis.

Conclusion A wonderful synergy between the fields of optometry and ophthalmology has arisen over the past two decades. With our mutual goal of delivering efficient, effective, compassionate care, cooperation is becoming more and more common. The result is excellent eye care for a greater number of people than ever before. With continued expansion of knowledge about what each of our fields is capable of, we can look forward to even more improvement in the delivery of care of patients with special needs.

OPTOMETRY

Optometry is an international profession. The World Council of Optometry represents 250,000 optometrists from 94 member organizations in 45 countries (17). Doctors of optometry are the largest eye care profession in the United States with 35,000 optometrists serving patients in nearly 6,500 communities (18).

Prior to admittance into optometry school, optometrists typically complete 4 years of undergraduate study, culminating in a bachelor's degree. Required undergraduate coursework is extensive and covers a wide variety of advanced health, science, and mathematics courses. Because a strong background in science is important, many applicants major in the sciences, such as biology, physics, engineering, or chemistry, as undergraduates.

Optometry school in the United States consists of 4 years of postgraduate, doctoral-level study concentrating on the health and structure of the eye, the visual process, and systemic disease. In addition to vision-specific courses, optometrists take systemic health courses that focus on a patient's overall medical condition as it relates to the health of the eyes and visual process. Optometric coursework includes classroom and laboratory study of pharmacology, optics, vision science, and biochemistry, as well as extensive clinical training in the diagnosis and treatment of visual disorders. During optometry school, besides successfully completing a rigorous academic and clinical program, each student must pass a state and national board examination before he or she can practice.

Upon graduation, approximately 20% of all students are accepted into residency programs. These residency programs may be based within universities/colleges, hospitals, and even within multipractitioner/discipline practices. They are usually 1 year in duration and concentrate on specific areas such as eye disease, contact lenses/cornea, and vision rehabilitation/low vision, as well as pediatrics, binocular vision, and optometric vision therapy. Additional programs feature the diagnosis and management of patients with traumatic/acquired brain injury and other areas of specialty.

Although several certification programs are either being developed or currently exist for optometry, the oldest and most respected program is that of the College of Optometrists in Vision Development (COVD). College of Optometrists in Vision Development certifies, through a rigorous program of academic and clinical skills verification, that optometrists are qualified to use optometric vision therapy as a treatment modality. The American Board of Optometry and the American Board of Clinical Optometry are both currently devising certification venues for primary care optometrists, while the American Board of Certification in Medical Optometry certifies doctors in medical optometry.

Optometrists are experts at understanding the role of lenses and the impact lenses can have on human performance. Lenses can include contact lenses, glasses, magnifiers, and telescopes. The optimal design, prescription, and use of lenses can be of enormous significance in improving balance and mobility, attention, and visual awareness.

Optometrists have a distinctive understanding of the role of overall health and the visual process.

Not only do optometrists diagnose and treat diseases of the eyes and related structures, they understand the relationships present between systemic illness or disability and visual performance. Many optometrists encourage preventative measures by promoting nutrition and hygiene education to their patients to minimize the impact or risk of systemic and eye disease. The optometric perspective allows the development of an optimal integrated treatment program including all facets of eye and vision care. He/she is responsible for providing the multidisciplinary team with as complete assessment of visual function and health as possible, including potential strategies for the remediation of visual inadequacies that hinder the performance of daily living skills and academic performance.

Optometric vision therapy, which includes the use of lenses, is a uniquely optometric treatment program. Optometric vision therapy is a program of doctor-supervised therapeutic procedures directed at the development, remediation, or enhancement of various visual skills and vision information processing outcomes. Visual skill development achieved through OVT is important in patients with developmental or learning delay where various aspects of visual performance have not advanced as expected. Neurorehabilitative optometry, which includes OVT, focuses on the restoration of functional visual and vision information processing/perceptual skills and competence following illness or injury affecting performance and an individual's quality of life.

The role of the optometrist will vary depending upon the needs of the patient. The visual process is complex and nearly invisible in its mechanics and influences on human behavior, yet is often in need of attention when developmental or behavioral problems are noted. An eye examination or screening that is based only on visual acuity and refractive error assessment is frequently inadequate to diagnose the majority of performance-based functional visual problems usually seen in the patients with special needs. This is because visual inadequacies contributing to developmental/behavioral problems are only rarely based on how clearly one sees. For example, the inability to consistently direct the eyes at lines of print or to maintain steady focus for reading is not often evaluated in many visual acuity–based assessments. This is even more evident when considering vision screenings. It may be necessary to seek the participation of an optometrist with special interest or additional expertise when dealing with special needs populations. In most cases, those optometrists will be those who provide OVT directly or will have an established referral relationship with an OVT provider.

It is up to the multidisciplinary team, including the optometrist, to design an overall treatment plan, taking into consideration the potential resources the patient has at his/her disposal. It is impossible for all therapies to be provided at one time; therefore, the treatment plan must account for the individual patients' needs and abilities. For example, while a patient hospitalized after a stroke or head injury must be medically stable before much visual intervention is possible, the use of a well-designed pair of glasses relatively early in the process may make occupational, physical, psychoeducational, speech, and language therapies much more effective. Optometric vision therapy may need to wait until more basic life skills are restored, or may be used as an integral part of the restoration process, depending on the patient's needs, environment, and resources.

When a patient has reading and learning problems, the immediate use of appropriate lenses and OVT will usually make academic therapies more effective and should be given a high priority. Optometric vision therapy, which includes the use of standard lenses, prism, and varifocal lens designs, should be provided ahead of or concurrent with academic therapies, as it is designed to develop the visual skills needed for best success with academics.

All doctors and therapists want to help and are deeply committed to the therapies they provide. Potential problems develop when the focus moves away from solving patient problems to professional turf battles. It takes insight, confidence, and discipline to keep our focus on the needs of the patient.

It will often confuse the patient and his or her family when various professions that may be similar in what they do, recommend differing approaches to patient care. Many OVT activities may appear similar to OT activities and even use very comparable equipment. The line separating the two professions is not always clear. The difference is that neurorehabilitative optometrists have a significantly different frame of reference from other therapists. When an optometrist or vision therapist provides OVT, the therapy is being done somewhat differently from the therapy any other profession offers.

The secret of success when involved in a multidisciplinary team is working together and keeping the patient as the number one priority. The secret of teamwork is developing strong trusting relationships within and among team members. In the end, it is not as much about what initials caregivers have in terms of training and professional degrees, as it is the ability of the individual members of the team to provide what the patient needs in the most efficient manner, providing the right tools and experiences for the patient at the right time.

PHYSICAL THERAPY

A physical therapist's primary role is to help regain physical ability after disease or injury. The profession began in the United States when returning veterans from World War I and II required a higher level of intervention to succeed in rehabilitation. Due to medical advances, these veterans survived unheard of trauma, but there was a lack of any medical service to help them recover physical skills. Initially, surgeons treating WWI veterans began hiring women (often nurses) to administer exercise, massage, and physical education. This practice increased with WWII veterans and then exploded with the polio epidemic in 1952 (19). For such a short history, physical therapy (PT) has evolved well beyond administering basic exercise and physical education. Today's physical therapist has a broad scope of practice that includes regaining movement lost from injury or disease, specializing in deep tissue wound care, or even consulting on ergonomics in various industrial settings. The PTs education originally required "on the job" training, but today's graduates earn a Doctorate in Physical Therapy. (They are assisted by PT assistants, "PTAs," who require an Associate degree.) Up until the late 1990s, PT could only be accessed through the referral of a physician, but 45 states now allow some provision for PT services to be available without a direct referral.

Physical therapists are governed and licensed by individual states, but are organized nationally by the American Physical Therapy Association (APTA). In 2008, the Department of Labor Statistics estimated there were 185,500 therapists working in the United States in a wide variety of settings (20). Physical therapy was initially only offered in hospital settings, but is now routinely provided in schools, fitness gyms, industrial settings, nursing facilities, private homes, sports training facilities and outpatient clinics. The APTA has eight specialty certifications including Cardiovascular & Pulmonary, Clinical Electrophysiology, Orthopedics, Geriatrics, Sports, Women's Health, Pediatrics, and Neurology (21). While few therapists obtain these credentials, most concentrate experience in one of these fields of care.

Cardiovascular and Pulmonary This concentration manages the delicate balance between cardiac and respiratory functioning after injury, surgery, or disease. Examples of this population would be those recovering from heart transplant, cardiac bypass, and heart attack, as well as managing those with emphysema or pulmonary fibrosis. During rehabilitation, physical conditioning needs to be closely monitored to gauge the body's reaction to exercise and pharmaceuticals. While the physical therapist has very little to do with which medications are prescribed, he or she must have a working knowledge of the mode of action and side effects of the particular medication to recognize contraindications to care.

Clinical Electrophysiology and Wound Care Clinical electrophysiology and wound care are separate areas of practice, but the two are grouped together when discussing areas of concentration because they comprise the smallest divisions of PT. Electrophysiology involves the evaluation of the neuromuscular system. Surface or needle electrodes are used to measure the intensity of muscle contraction or the quality of nerve conduction. This field requires specific credentialing to conduct these evaluations, but all physical therapists are able to interpret and explain findings. Electrophysiology is used to differentiate diagnoses between central and peripheral nerve impairments or to determine difference between muscular and neurological breakdown. Examples include differentiating between multiple sclerosis and Guillain-Barré syndrome or between myasthenia gravis and amyotrophic lateral sclerosis.

Wound care is common in an acute care setting. Wounds seen are often the result of immobility ("pressure sores") and are referred for debridement, vacuum care, dressing recommendation, and medication application. Since the majority of these wounds are the result of immobility, the therapist must create a healing environment to reduce shearing or maceration and recommend appropriate seating. The plan of care would also include increasing mobility to prevent future wounds.

Geriatrics The ability to move changes as we age. While some of these changes are the result of personal choices (exercise, diet, lifestyle), other changes are the result of cellular breakdown. Examples include changes in cardiovascular responses to physical activity, metabolic processing of medications, and changes in posture and muscle force generation. Often, the primary diagnosis for referral must be differentiated from secondary diagnoses resulting from the aging process. The clinician tailors the plan of care to address all the systemic changes experienced during aging such as muscle atrophy, skin thinning, diminished sensation, and decreased collagen elasticity.

Sports This specialized division of PT revolves around preventing and recuperating from sports injuries, as well as enhancing sport-specific functions. Examples of treatment include changing movement patterns to avoid chronic overuse of susceptible muscle groups, recovering from surgical repair, or improving timing and accuracy of movements. While a sports PT works in the clinic to achieve these results, they also work closely with athletic trainers who are on the field.

Women's Health The primary area of concentration in women's health is pelvic floor dysfunction. Examples of pelvic floor dysfunction could be due to urinary or bowel incontinence and painful scar tissue buildup from episiotomies, or painful intercourse. Physical therapy treatment focuses on strengthening the muscles of the pelvic floor to resolve these issues since they often occur because of skeletal muscle weakness. Common methods of treatment use Kegel exercises, electrical stimulation, or biofeedback devices. Also included in this specialty is the treatment of osteoporosis and lymphedema. Osteoporosis is most commonly seen in aging females, and lymphedema is most frequently seen after breast cancer treatment.

Pediatrics The vast majority of pediatric patients are referred because of a congenital deficit or developmental delay. Often, these patients are learning to move for the first time rather than "relearning" motion like an adult. Children learn about their environment by exploring the world around them. Children with limited mobility may be limiting their intellectual (including visual), emotional, and physical development. The focus is to teach physical developmental abilities, prevent deformities during the growth process, and assess the child's environment. PT is often performed at school or home, so direct recommendations can be made concerning what might be needed in that particular setting, as well as find ways to help that child interact with peers.

Neurology This field focuses on primary impairments of the neurological system. Common diagnoses for this category are traumatic brain injury (TBI), cerebral vascular accident, Parkinson's, multiple sclerosis, Guillain-Barré, peripheral neuropathy, spinal cord injuries, and encephalopathy. The focus of therapy is either on regaining lost function or teaching compensation techniques to most efficiently use remaining abilities. This often relies on finding the most effective teaching method to relearn movement and control. New technologies, such as body weight–supported treadmills, functional electrical stimulation devices, or balance training machines are often incorporated to provide many avenues for the brain to relearn mobility.

Orthopedics Orthopedics focuses on muscle and skeletal disorders. This includes recovering from total joint surgeries, disorders causing back pain, amputation, and even occupational health consulting. Orthopedic PTs often rely on manual techniques to administer care, such as joint mobilizations, soft tissue stretching, or guided exercise. Many practitioners in this setting concentrate even further into specific areas of dysfunction, such as ankle and foot, spine, and temporomandibular joint disorders. This type of care is predominately found in outpatient settings.

No matter if the deficit is from a sports injury or brain injury, regaining physical ability is a coordinating process between neurologic and muscular systems. While all these fields of care focus on different aspects of neuromuscular dysfunction, they all incorporate motor learning as part of the treatment process. The brain assembles a plan for movement by gathering sensory information that tells where the body is in space and where it is going. Proprioceptive systems, tactile sensation, and auditory cues are all important in gathering reference information for the brain. The most efficient and reliable sensory information the brain receives, however, is through the visual system. Therefore, the vision professional is paramount in helping to achieve optimal physical functioning. If the athlete has a deficit in depth perception, muscle force generation, timing, and accuracy are all off. If the child with cerebral palsy cannot see her environment, she will not be motivated to explore and learn. For complex injuries like TBI, the individual needs to be able to accurately see his surroundings before he can begin to comprehend what he needs to do in order to sit, stand, walk, or talk. Too often, vision care is provided at the end of rehabilitative care, when it is often most beneficial at the very beginning of the therapeutic intervention.

PHYSIATRY

Physical Medicine and Rehabilitation (PM&R), also known as physiatry (derived from the Greek words "physikos" meaning physical and "iatreia" meaning art of healing), was established by the American Board of Medical Specialties in 1947. The development of the specialty began during World War I and progressed after World War II, when rehabilitation needs increased for injured veterans. Medical residency training involves one year of general medicine to develop fundamental skills, followed by 3 years of training focused on the PM&R specialty. Fellowships for subspecialization are available in pediatric rehabilitation medicine, spinal cord injury medicine, neuromuscular medicine, hospice and palliative medicine, pain medicine, and sports medicine.

The purpose of PM&R is to address impairments and disabilities through prevention, diagnosis, and nonsurgical treatment of nerve, muscle, and bone disorders. The primary focus is to develop a comprehensive program of recovery after injury for the entire body through medical, social, emotional, and vocational means. Emphasis is placed on restoration of function and improving quality of life. The scope of PM&R is broad and involves an array of simple to complex diagnoses affecting all ages (Table 28.4). For example, in the pediatric population, a physiatrist may treat an individual with cerebral palsy, Down syndrome, or muscular dystrophy. When working with the geriatric population, the physiatrist may encounter an individual with a cerebrovascular disease or Parkinson disease.

The cornerstone of PM&R training and practice is the multidisciplinary approach, using a team of medical specialists. This team is led by a physiatrist who provides medical care and coordinates the treatment plan. These plans are individualized to address the specific needs of each patient. The role of the team is to apply the components of the treatment plan that are unique to one's area of expertise. The multidisciplinary team may include, but is not limited to, physical therapists, occupational therapists, speech–language pathologists, optometrists, social workers, nurses, case managers, and other physicians (Table 28.5).

TABLE 28.4 Common Physical Medicine and Rehabilitation Patient Diagnoses

Medical Category	Examples
Amputation	Transfemoral (above knee), transtibial (below knee)
Brain injury	Traumatic, acquired
Nerve pain	Diabetic neuropathy, carpal tunnel syndrome
Sports-related injury	Rotator cuff tear, tendinitis, ankle sprain
Spinal cord injury	Traumatic, nontraumatic
Back pain	Lumbar herniated disk, facet arthropathy
Work-related injury	Cumulative trauma disorders
Stroke	Hemorrhagic, thrombotic
Neck pain	Cervical herniated disk, myofascial pain
Movement disorder	Huntington disease, Parkinson disease
Myopathy	Duchenne muscular dystrophy

The individualized plan for a stroke patient, for example, may include medical management from the physiatrist, emphasizing recurrent stroke prevention, treatment of comorbid conditions, such as diabetes mellitus or hypertension, and specific recommendations to the team regarding the patient's motor, cognitive, visual, or linguistic impairment. The physical therapist may enforce gait training with a rolling walker, perform neuromuscular reeducation, and teach techniques for transfer training with loss of leg function. The occupational therapist can address issues with dressing, grooming, and bathing techniques, while leading exercises for strengthening of a weak arm. The speech therapist may enforce mouth and lip exercises or use special devices for improving slurred speech and swallowing dysfunction. The optometrist ensures the maximum visual function including treatment of visual field loss (e.g., homonymous hemianopia) and diplopia. The nurse often administers medications, monitors medical status, and reenforces the overall stroke therapy program. Another physician, such as a neurosurgeon, may be consulted for specialized management of injury caused by the stroke, especially if it involves a hemorrhage requiring surgical intervention. Case managers and social workers often communicate with families, caregivers, and outside resources to enhance the transition to the home or another facility where the patient may complete his or her recovery.

In the patient population treated by physiatrists, a significant number of disorders often associated with

TABLE 28.5 The Physical Medicine and Rehabilitation Multidisciplinary Team

Specialty	Brief Summary of Collaborative Role with Physiatrist
Physical therapy	Execute gait training Wheelchair mobility Functional electrical stimulation of the lower extremity Transfers Equipment evaluation
Occupational therapy	Provide ADL and self-care training Functional electrical stimulation of the upper extremity Recommendation of assistive devices
Speech therapy	Enhance communication and cognitive skills Evaluate swallowing deficits
Optometry	Ensure maximal visual function at distance and near Treat any learning-related vision problems Reduce or eliminate visual field loss and/or diplopia
Nursing	Perform bladder and bowel training Wound care Medication administration
Case management	Communication between family and team
Social work	Utilization of community resources
Physicians	Consultants such as neurologists and surgeons

visual impairments, in addition to neuromuscular or cognitive deficits, are found. Some of the age-related diagnoses in the elderly population include cataracts, macular degeneration, glaucoma, and diabetic retinopathy. In the younger populations, a physiatrist may encounter patients with retinopathy of prematurity, congenital cataracts, rubella syndrome, and retinitis pigmentosa. The young and middle-aged populations may have visual impairments linked to cerebral palsy, acquired immunodeficiency syndrome (AIDS), or other central nervous system infections, such as cryptococcal meningitis. Diabetic retinopathy also affects this age group and, with progression, may lead to proliferative retinopathy. Additionally, those with stroke, TBI, and multiple sclerosis are among the high-risk population for vision problems.

The physiatrist should routinely evaluate all rehabilitation medicine patients for visual problems. Obtaining a history focused on functionally related vision problems is pertinent. Questions may address mobility and activities of daily living problems associated with visual impairment. Components of the neurologic examination, such as visual acuity, extraocular movements, and visual field testing, are useful in identifying deficits that should be referred to a vision specialist.

It is common for a rehabilitation medicine patient to have more than one impairment contributing to a disability. A stroke patient may not only have a motor deficit (e.g., hemiplegia) but may also have a visual field deficit. This combination limits functional mobility and self-care, while increasing the safety risk. A patient with TBI may have a cognitive impairment in addition to a visual disturbance. Examination of this type of patient may be difficult if TBI sequelae, such as agitation and impulsiveness, are present. The patient with multiple sclerosis can have vision problems such as optic neuritis and a neurogenic bladder. These can limit independence with a resultant decreased ability to care for oneself. An amputee with a gait disturbance is at greater risk for falls when a concomitant visual impairment is present. Those with polyneuropathy often have problems with proprioception and sensory feedback during ambulation. If a vision problem is also present, a loss of balance due to decreased visual input could occur.

Physiatrists are trained to perform diagnostic and therapeutic procedures along with other interventions to address the impairments of those affected by nerve, bone, or muscle disease leading to injury or disability. Since diskitis or facet arthropathy often causes back pain, an intervention often used is fluoroscopically guided steroid injections. Intra-articular (joint) injections may be used for pain related to degenerative changes caused by osteoarthritis. Myofascial pain syndrome will frequently require localized intramuscular injections to resolve symptoms. Chemodenervation injections (i.e., botulinum toxin or phenol) are performed for treatment of spasticity and dystonia to both relieve pain and prevent muscle contracture. Electrodiagnostic techniques, such as electromyography, nerve conduction studies, and somatosensory evoked potentials, are used to determine neuromuscular injury that causes pain, weakness, and numbness. Other interventions include the formulation of exercise programs for tetraplegia, paraplegia, and other neuromuscular impairment. Exercise programs can also be designed to increase bone mass and decrease loss of bone mineral density. Physiatrists are trained to recommend the most appropriate prosthetics for amputees and orthotics for conditions requiring bracing. Additionally, wheelchair evaluation and design are skills employed by the physiatrist to enhance mobility as well.

SOCIAL WORK

Historical Reference for Social Work Multidisciplinary Practice Social work as a profession is relatively young with just over 100 years of recognition and training in United States; however, the impact on society has been tremendous. Social work pioneers were not highly educated health care workers or political powerhouses. They were, however, individuals who saw problems in society and appreciated the interconnectedness of those problems with the rest of the world. Poverty and sickness were not linked to social status but occurred anytime to anyone. What did divide people were the options available. While wealth and privilege were connected, so were poverty and lack of choice. Social workers sought to change this unfair system first with volunteer work and later as great facilitators linking charitable organizations. Early social workers were primarily women with a collaborative spirit to maximize the limited resources and shine light on the problems of society. As recognition of the needs of people living in poverty grew, more individuals and organizations and the government took notice. These quintessential multidisciplinary leaders breached the divide among health care and government services, Christian charity, and public/community responsibility. They were both organizers of people as well as innovative problem solvers. This role and flexibility has not changed in 100 years of practice.

Early social workers were leaders and innovators in the social services movement. The brief timeline in Figure 28-1, including the recognition of the profession in 1898, depicts the emergence of social work as a profession alongside the growing response to health care issues in the United States. Hull House, organized by Jane Addams in the late 19th century, was the first settlement house in the country and was the embodiment of creative problem solving and multidisciplinary practice. It incorporated social and civic clubs for children, a public kitchen, an art gallery, and coffeehouse. It also included a gym, bathhouse, bookbinder, music school, drama group, library, and an employment agency. All of the elements of that program sought to blend the fabric of social work practice to address the whole person, family, and community at the most immediate level and need. Today, multidisciplinary practice follows the same model, involving numerous health and social service disciplines to address the complex needs of people with disabilities and their families. After the Great Depression, the country sought to rebuild the infrastructure of its people with government assistance programs, such as The New Deal (1935–1940). At the same time, the foundations of social work practice also expanded, as government was incorporated into the social services plan. An explosion of programs, geared at addressing health and social ills of women, minorities, children, and the poor, emerged through the late 20th century and continue to serve at-risk groups. These early efforts began the tradition of improving the lives of the "underserved population."

How Does Social Work Interact with Other Members of the Team? Social work practice continues to be a profession that sees people and society as an interconnected system. Compton and Galaway (22) state, "*Systems theory serves social work well in that it offers a conceptual framework that supports the purpose of the profession by shifting our attention from either the person or the environment to problems in the interaction.*" Because of this perspective, those in the field are aptly positioned to address the individual needs of clients with an understanding that environment, politics, health care systems, and other professions are interconnected and not isolated pieces in the overall treatment plan.

The role of the professional social worker is quite fluid, as they are not confined to one theory or prescribed treatment. Most importantly, insight is provided into the construct of a family system that will highlight strengths and weaknesses of any treatment or intervention path for a client. Moreover, a social worker is a valuable resource to a multidisciplinary team as he/she has the knowledge and skill to recommend additional supports and services that might be necessary for intervention success.

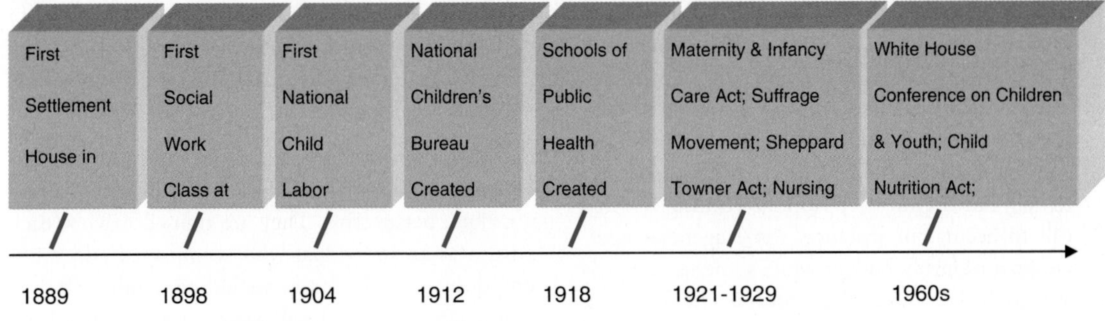

FIGURE 28-1. A timeline concerning the development of social work as a profession.

Social workers have two main areas of focus identified as the micro and macro level. Micro level practice focuses on the individual or family system; macro level focuses on the larger influences of the environmental and societal systems. The micro and macro levels are seen as having a direct affect on the person, family, and support services they require.

Social workers interact on the multidisciplinary team a little differently than other professions. While tests or screening tools are not used, a very specific set of criteria, by which the team can make an efficacious decision, can be provided. Social workers conduct need assessments based upon interviewing clients and investigating deeper into the stressors and strengths of the individual and family. The biopsychosocial framework that addresses the amount of risk and resiliency to stress that an individual may possess is one such framework. The affect that environment has on natural resources and protective factors will have consequences on any intervention or treatment plan. For example, a person living in poverty choosing to ration expenses might not seek medical treatment for a minor issue, however, that if left untreated could develop into a major health problem.

Social work practice follows the Person in Environment (PIE) approach that stipulates working within the limits of a person's current situation instead of against it. The PIE approach takes into account all the factors and stressors that might affect the person's ability to recover. This assessment looks at the person's inclination towards resiliency based upon the amount of factors that place them at risk. The scope of the assessment makes the social worker vital to the success of the multidisciplinary team.

Who Are Social Workers? What Do they Do? A professional social worker receives a degree from a program approved by the Council on Social Work Education. The degrees offered are at the bachelor's, master's, and doctoral level of proficiency. Job expectations can vary significantly based on the agency and population served, but there are similarities among social work jobs, and it is realistic to have certain expectations as follows.

- **Social workers are problem solvers.** They can help define and resolve problems. They are trained in listening and communication skills to detect what is not being said. A good listener can discover a lot about a situation. Soliciting information by statements such as, "Tell me more about that" can be a relief to the family and patient rather than being considered "nosey." Many times, the social worker is the primary team member who is there to listen and assist them with the "rest of the problem." They are there not to pry but to partner with the patient and family to determine what obstacle(s) prevents the treatment plan from being followed.

  The patient and family are often embarrassed to tell their doctor about their obstacles. It may be humiliating to admit that they cannot afford their medication, that the medication causes them difficulty with sexual performance, or that their living conditions are less than ideal. Conversations should be affirming, should be empathic, and should validate the concerns of each patient. It can be quite therapeutic for someone to normalize the patient's problems. A simple statement such as, "We help many patients to apply for drug assistance" can be reassuring.
- **Social workers are trained to provide support groups**. Expertise in listening and communicating allows for the facilitation of groups that aid those involved. Setting up and facilitating groups, whether psychoeducational or therapeutic, is often the role of the social worker.

- **Social workers are knowledgeable about community resources.** In the current climate of health care, we all must do more with less. Many, if not most of our resources are shrinking. Often, social workers will develop networks with their community resource providers; they know who to call and the most appropriate timing for that call to occur. For instance, some agencies operate on a monthly budget while some use a yearly approach. The end of the month or the fiscal year is often when the money gets very tight around agencies. It is important to be familiar with the requirements of each resource agency so the family does not waste time applying for assistance if they will not meet the guidelines for that particular program.
- **Social workers will advocate for their clients.** A good social worker will "go to bat" when needed, contacting others on behalf of their client. Whether it is approaching an agency or an estranged relative, it is sometimes possible to create resources specifically for that client. Social workers must respect confidentiality, observe The Health Insurance Portability and Accountability Act (HIPPA) policies, and be mindful of personal boundaries. Many times, however, an agency, church, or relative is glad to help once they are made aware of a need. A skillful social worker may be able to assist their client process a situation so that they may see alternatives that were previously ignored.
- **Social workers usually work with the families of patients.** The social worker is often the liaison between the medical team and the patient's family. They can gather needed information and provide it to the family. Families want to hear medical information from the doctor and other personnel; however, details about the clinic, office hours, services offered, etc. can be provided by the social worker. Families will often contact the social worker in confidence, to ensure that the clinic knows pertinent details of their loved one's situation.
- **Social workers are trained to provide counseling.** This is subject to the level of education and expertise of the social worker. If the appropriate counseling cannot be provided, the social worker should be able to identify a counselor in the area who can help.
- **A social worker should be able to make a home visit if needed.** In the TV series, *House,* Dr. House usually has his medical team to visit the patient's home to investigate for disease pathogens. A home visit can reveal a lot that is missed in the sterile office environment.

Social workers can be an excellent addition and valuable asset to the multidisciplinary team as they bring a unique perspective. They are trained to view each person as an individual who is impacted and influenced by outside forces including family, church, work, and existing local, state, and national laws. Furthermore, the interaction among all of these forces is not static but constantly changing. A good social worker should be respectful, caring, and nonjudgmental of each client and his or her world. Most importantly, they should serve as advocates for their clients when interacting with the public and the multidisciplinary team.

SPEECH–LANGUAGE PATHOLOGY

The field of Speech–language pathology developed from the early "speech elocutionists" who, in the 1800s, became popular with people wishing to improve their speaking ability. Eventually, elocutionists organized themselves and formed the National Association of Speech Elocutionists. Over the next two decades, universities began to train elocutionists, and by 1925, "Speech Correction" was a new profession. The American Academy of Speech Correction eventually became the American Speech Language Hearing Association (ASHA). American Speech Language Hearing Association is the certifying agency for speech-language pathologists (SLPs) in the United States. There are similar credentialing agencies throughout the world as well (23).

Early on, the focus was on the nonverbal child, stuttering, voice disorders, articulation disorders, and children with cleft lip and palate. The field of speech-language pathology has expanded so greatly that ASHA now has 16 Special Interest Divisions, and many SLPs specialize in one or two specific areas within the scope of the profession.

In general, SLPs who are ASHA certified are able to evaluate, diagnose, and treat disorders of speech, language, cognitive communication, and swallowing/oral motor disorders in individuals of all ages (24). As of 2009, there were nearly 120,000 ASHA certified SLPs (25).

Once certified, the SLP is required to maintain continuing education to remain certified (26). In addition, many states have licensure laws, and ASHA has a written Code of Ethics to which certified SLPs must abide (27).

A description of the areas within the scope of clinical practice follows, including the related Special Interest Division where applicable. Not all the Special Interest Divisions are mentioned, as some are related to research, administration, or audiology only.

Language Learning and Education (Special Interest Division 1) Language Learning and Education covers the areas of learning disability, specific language impairment, and preliteracy/literacy issues (28). As of 2009, about 50% of certified SLPs were employed in educational settings with 22% working in elementary schools (25).

These professionals encounter the language and literacy problems that can prevent children from achieving academic success. They assist in the planning and implementing of remediation of any deficits present. Early intervention with the preschool population has seen a tremendous increase in the past two to three decades with an emphasis on identifying risk factors so that academic failure can be prevented. Many SLPs serve as part of early intervention teams.

Neurogenic Speech and Language Disorders (Special Interest Division 2) Speech–language pathologists also work with people having speech and language disorders secondary to stroke, TBI, Parkinson disease, and other neurological events (29). Forty percent of certified SLPs work in heath care settings, such as hospitals, skilled nursing facilities, home health agencies, and rehabilitation centers (25).

Problems after a neurological event, which would fall under the scope of speech-language pathology, include difficulty speaking, problems with comprehending speech, impaired problem-solving and organizational abilities, and difficulty swallowing.

Voice and Voice Disorders (Special Interest Division 3) Problems with the sound quality or the production of the human voice also fall under the purview of the SLP. Speech-language pathologists in this specialty area work closely with otolaryngologists to treat people with overuse problems, such as edema, polyps and nodules, vocal fold paralysis, or other malfunction and resonance disorders. A few SLPs may have special training and experience to work with the professional speaker and singer (30).

Stuttering and Other Disorders of Fluency Special Interest Division 4, Fluency and Fluency Disorders, includes stuttering, cluttering, and neurogenic stuttering. Stuttering is a disrupted flow of speech, which can sound like repetitions of sounds, prolonged sounds, or no sound at all (blocked sound). It may also be characterized by excessive use of interjections such as "um," abandonment of speech attempts, avoidance of speaking situations, or circumlocution. Cluttering is a rare disorder characterized by unfinished words, rapid and irregular speech rate and excessive use of interjections, somewhat unclear articulation, and some lack of organization of the speech output. Neurogenic stuttering, or stuttering that occurs in a previously fluent person after a neurologic event, is rare. Early referral to SLP is recommended for young children who are thought to be stuttering, especially those who have a family history of chronic stuttering, are male, or have any other areas of speech or language development that also appear delayed or disordered (31).

Cleft Lip and Palate and Other Craniofacial Anomalies Orofacial disorders are considered a part of Special Interest Division 5. Children and adults with craniofacial anomalies are typically managed by a team of specialists, including an SLP, audiologist, pediatrician, ENT physician, surgeon, and related professionals. Craniofacial anomalies often result in speech and resonance disorders. Some of the causes of these anomalies are cleft lip and palate, Apert Syndrome, Treacher Collins Syndrome, and Crouzon Syndrome. Several of these conditions are discussed in greater detail in Chapter 7, Oculo-Visual Abnormalities Associated with Rare Neurodevelopmental Disorders. Hearing loss and/or structural defects in the ear are also common (32).

Hearing Loss and Deafness Many SLPs work with children and adults with hearing loss in the area of Aural Rehabilitation (Special Interest Division 7). Aural rehabilitation is delivered as part of a team which includes speech pathology and audiology, a physician or surgeon, and other related practitioners. Family members are always important members of the team. Aural rehabilitation is sometimes referred to as aural *habilitation* for those patients who have never been able to hear (as opposed to someone who was able to hear in childhood and lost the hearing later). Aural rehabilitation typically is recommended after a person has been fitted with a hearing aid or AIDS or has had unilateral or bilateral cochlear implant. Techniques for improving the ability to listen, hear, perceive, and interpret sound are part of aural rehabilitation, as is improving expressive and receptive communication. The use of technology to improve safety, quality of life, and ability to function in school or workplace are also part of this process (33).

Some SLPs teach sign language to those children whose families wish for their child to use sign language. Some families have several members of the family who are deaf and use sign language and wish for their child to learn sign as well. Others determine that sign language is the best mode of communication for their child. Hearing-impaired or deaf speakers also require extensive speech therapy to learn not only the phonemes of speech, but also the features of speech, such as loudness, intonation, and prosody.

Augmentative and Alternative Communication (Special Interest Division 12) SLPs also serve those who need a form of communication other than speech. A person who is cognitively able to comprehend and formulate language, but physically unable to speak in a commensurate manner, may be a candidate for augmentative or alternative communication (AAC) (34). An AAC system can be as simple as a set of photos or pictures (low tech) or highly advanced computer-generated communication. Sign language is considered an alternative communication system. Most systems rely on vision; therefore, any AAC user should be evaluated visually in conjunction with system selection and implementation. Augmentative or alternative communication systems use objects, photographs, drawings, black and white line drawings, words, and letters. Visual acuity, visual fields, and visual scanning are important to maximize using this technology. A team of professionals may be needed in order to assess a person's ability to access AAC, including the vision specialist, occupational therapist, physical therapist, cognitive specialist, and SLP.

Feeding and Swallowing The ability to eat and drink is vital to one's quality of life. There are many illnesses and conditions that can result in an impaired ability to eat and drink. These conditions include stroke, TBI, head and neck cancer, cerebral palsy, and prematurity. In the 1980s, the diagnosis and treatment of Swallowing Disorders (Special Interest Division 13) became a specialty area for SLPs, partly because of their in-depth understanding of oral structure and function. Today, SLPs with special training are able to evaluate the oral, pharyngeal, and esophageal phases of chewing and swallowing in children and adults. A full case history, observation of eating and drinking, and administration of specialized tests help the SLP determine what deficits exist. The safety of oral feeding following a stroke or other neurologic insult may be in question and the SLP's expertise assists in determining when and if a patient may safely eat or drink by mouth. Strategies and techniques to assist with safe, successful eating and drinking are developed for the individual patient. The SLP is involved in training the patient, family, and caretakers to follow all appropriate intervention plans (35).

Articulation and Phonology One of the original areas of expertise for speech-language pathology is phonologic development and disorders. This was referred to as the area of *articulation* by earlier practitioners. Many people think of the "kid who does not pronounce 'r' correctly" as the typical client of the SLP. It is true that most SLP's have worked with someone who needed to improve their "r" sound or correct a lisp. There are children who have difficulty developing the full repertoire of sounds and skills required to produce clear connected speech. Some children appear to have a motor planning problem (developmental apraxia) or have a muscle weakness (dysarthria) due to an underlying neurological issue. They may also have delayed speech development or exhibit a slower acquisition of speech sounds because of a chronic middle ear infection and resultant inner ear fluid retention.

Some adults require remediation of speech sounds or may wish to improve their speech sound production if they speak with a foreign accent. SLPs create treatment plans to assist children (and possibly adults) in accurate speech sound production. Auditory, visual, and tactile methods are utilized depending on the type of problem and underlying etiology.

Interface of the Vision Professional with the Speech-Language Pathologist There are many occasions for a SLP to refer a patient for a vision evaluation. In early intervention, children with history of prematurity, fetal exposure to detrimental substances, or other health problems often have vision problems. So much of how we work with young children is through visual means, so an SLP will be interested in what access, visually, a child has to their visual world, as well as what size and type of stimuli might be best to use depending upon the recommended treatment program.

The use of visual communication systems for the AAC user is another occasion where the input of the vision professional is valuable. A communication system that relies on vision will not be useful if it is set up in a manner not visually accessible to the user. The vision professional should help in the determination of size and placement of icons, whether color or black and white is to be used, and what the overall size of the system should be.

In rehabilitation settings, patients with neurologic deficits often experience vision changes. The SLP uses many items that depend upon the visual system when evaluating patients, including objects, drawings, photographs, and written material. An accurate assessment of the patient's skills with these items requires an underlying knowledge of their visual function. Finally, children and adults who are deaf and blind represent another population in which understanding and collaboration between disciplines becomes crucial.

CONCLUSION

Treating patients with special needs requires a multidisciplinary approach in which all members of the team are working toward common goals. Communication is the key; there are often many different treatments and therapies recommended by the various professionals. While written reports are helpful, simply picking up the phone can be the best approach. As an individual client's needs, strengths, and weaknesses differ, the order of importance of treatments needs to be considered, keeping in mind the available resources. Whether the patient's first interaction is with the developmental pediatrician, physiatrist, or optometrist, building a trusted network of professionals is crucial. The goal is to enhance patient care.

REFERENCES

1. Juneja M, Jain R, Singh V, et al. Iron deficiency in Indian children with attention deficit hyperactive disorder. Indian Pediatr. 2010;47(11):955–8.
2. Jonofal E, Lecendreux M, Arnulf I, et al. Iron deficiency in children with attention-deficit/hyperactivity disorder. Arch Pediatr Adolesc Med. 2004;158(12):1113–5.
3. Hill-Briggs F, Dial JG, Morere DA, et al. Neuropsychological assessment of persons with physical disability, visual impairment or blindness, and hearing impairment or deafness. Arch Clin Neuropsychol. 2007;22:389–404.
4. Policy Manual. American Occupational Therapy Association. Available from: http://www.aota.org/Governance/40517.aspx. Last Accessed October, 2010.
5. Preamble to the constitution of the World Health Organization. World Health Organization. Available from: http://whqlibdoc.who.int/hist/official_records/2e.pdf. Last Accessed October, 2010.
6. International classification of functioning, disability, and health (ICF). World Health Organization. Available from: http://www.who.int/classifications/icf/wha-en.pdf. Last Accessed October, 2010.
7. ICF Checklist. World Health Organization. Available from: http://www.who.int/classifications/icf/training/icfchecklist.pdf. Last Accessed October, 2010.
8. American Occupational Therapy Association. Occupational therapy practice framework: Domain and process. 2nd ed. Bethesda: American Occupational Therapy Association; 2008. p. 62.
9. Program Memorandum Transmittal AB-02-078. Centers for Medicare and Medicaid Services. Available from: http://www.cms.gov/transmittals/downloads/AB02078.pdf. Last Accessed October, 2010.
10. American Occupational Therapy Association. Occupational therapy code of ethics. Am J Occup Ther. 2005;59:639–42.
11. AOTA Low Vision Specialty Certification Handbook (OT). American Occupational Therapy Association. Available from: http://www.aota.org/Practitioners/ProfDev/Certification.aspx#areas. Last Accessed October 2010.
12. Age-Related Eye Disease Study Research Group. A randomized, placebo-controlled, clinical trial of high-dose supplementation with vitamins C and E, beta carotene, and zinc for age-related macular degeneration and vision loss: AREDS report no. 8. Arch Ophthalmol. 2001;119:1417–36.
13. Rosenfeld PJ, Brown DM, Heier JS, et al. Ranibizumab for neovascular age related macular degeneration. N Engl J Med. 2006;355:1419–31.
14. Andreoli CM, Miller JW. Anti-vascular endothelial growth factors for neovascular disease. Curr Opin Ophthalmol. 2007;18(6):502–8.
15. Good VW. Early treatment for retinopathy of prematurity cooperative group. The early treatment for retinopathy of prematurity study: structural findings at age 2 years. Br J Ophthalmol. 2006;90(11):1378–82.
16. Houston SK, Murray TG, Wolfe SQ, et al. Current update on retinoblastoma. Int Ophthalmol Clin. 2011;51(1):77–91.
17. World Council of Optometry. Available from: http://www.worldoptometry.org/. Last Accessed January, 2011.
18. American Optometric Association. Available from: http://www.aoa.org/x5879.xml. Last Accessed December, 2010.
19. Murphy W. Healing the generations: a history of physical therapy and the American physical therapy association. Alexandria: APTA; 1995.
20. United States Department of Labor, Bureau of Labor Statistics. Available from: http://www.bls.gov/oco/ocos080.htm#emply. Last Accessed December, 2010

21. Professional Development. American Physical Therapy Association. Available from: http://www.apta.org/AM/Template.cfm?Section=Certification2&Template//TaggedPage/TaggedPageDisplay.cfm&TPLID=206&ContentID=60265. Last Accessed December, 2010
22. Compton BR, Galaway B. Social work processes. 4th ed. Belmont: Wadsworth Publishing Company; 1989.
23. Cornett B.S, Chabon S.S. The clinical practice of speech-language pathology. Columbus: Merrill; 1988.
24. American Speech Language Hearing Association: Information for the Public: Speech, Language and Swallowing. Available from: http://www.asha.org/public/speech. Last Accessed January, 2011.
25. American Speech Language Hearing Association 2009 ASHA Member Counts. Available from: http://www.asha.org/uploadedFiles/2009MemberCounts.pdf. Last Accessed October, 2010.
26. American Speech Language Hearing Association: Information for Students-Certification Available from: http://www.asha.org/certification/slp_standards.htm#Std_IImpl. Last Accessed January, 2011.
27. American Speech Language Hearing Association: Code of Ethics Available from: http://www.asha.org/docs/html/ET2010-00309.html. Last Accessed January, 2011.
28. American Speech Language Hearing Association Special Interest Division 1: Language Learning and Education. Available from: http://www.asha.org/Members/divs/div_1.htm. Last Accessed October, 2010.
29. American Speech Language Hearing Association Special Interest Division 2: Neurophysiology and Neurogenic Speech and Language Disorders. Available from: http://www.asha.org/Members/divs/div_2.htm. Last Accessed October, 2010.
30. American Speech Language Hearing Association Special Interest Division 3: Voice and Voice Disorders. Available from: http://www.asha.org/Members/divs/div_3.htm. Last Accessed October, 2010.
31. American Speech Language Hearing Association Special Interest Division 4: Fluency and fluency Disorders. Available from: http://www.asha.org/Members/divs/div_4.htm. Last Accessed October, 2010.
32. American Speech Language Hearing Association Special Interest Division 5: Speech Science and Orofacial Disorders. Available from: http://www.asha.org/Members/divs/div_5.htm. Last Accessed October, 2010.
33. American Speech Language Hearing Association Special Interest Division 7: Aural Rehabilitation and Its Instrumentation. Available from: http://www.asha.org/Members/divs/div_7.htm. Last Accessed October, 2010.
34. American Speech Language Hearing Association Special Interest Division 7: Augmentative and Alternative Communication. Available from: http://www.asha.org/Members/divs/div_12.htm. Last Accessed October, 2010.
35. American Speech Language Hearing Association Special Interest Division 13: Swallowing and Swallowing Disorders (Dysphagia). Available from: http://www.asha.org/Members/divs/div_13.htm. Last Accessed October, 2010.

CHAPTER 29

David A. Damari, OD, FCOVD, FAAO

Disabilities and the Education System

"In 2008, President George W. Bush signed the Americans with Disabilities Act Amendments Act (ADA), which was intended as an amplification of the original ADA signed by his father in 1990." These two acts have bookended an era of remarkable change in the way disabilities are viewed by the American public and its legal system. The ADA as amended (hereafter simply referred to as the ADA) was the response of Congress to several key decisions by the Supreme Court that, in the view of several key congressmen and senators, placed unintended restrictions on the way the original ADA was applied in the workplace. As providers of vision care, it is important that we understand not just the old, almost mathematical standard of visual disability that was developed for the Social Security Act (SSA) in the 1930s, but the new standards of the ADA, the ADAAA, the Individuals with Disabilities Education Act (IDEA), and Section 504 of the Rehabilitation Act (§504) (Table 29.1). All these laws are driven far more by the individual's quality of life and day-to-day functioning and not by some arbitrary mathematical standard. As such, these laws require evaluations that are functional or developmental in nature and certainly evaluations of the individual's visual functioning in the context of the quotidian demands of the individual's academic or occupational life.

Although this chapter is largely about how individuals with disabilities navigate the educational system in the United States, it may provide valuable context pertaining to two early laws that largely, though not exclusively, pertained to adults.

THE BEGINNINGS: THE SOCIAL SECURITY ACT

One of the major initiatives of the New Deal, the SSA was signed into law by Franklin Delano Roosevelt in 1935. It was designed as a "safety net" to protect the finances of Americans who had retired or had severe disabilities and, therefore, could not work. As a consequence, the definition of disability created by this law was an attempt, largely by representatives of the American Medical Association, to codify the ability to work.

The visual disability aspects of this law are fairly well known to eye care professionals. Visual disability is referred to as "blindness," and for decades since the colloquial shorthand for visual disability has been "legal blindness." Blindness, under the SSA, is defined simply as a visual acuity in the better-seeing eye of 20/200 or worse. There is also a provision for visual field loss, but, interestingly, the way the provision is phrased is that "[a]n eye which is accompanied by a limitation in the fields of vision such that the widest diameter of the visual field subtends an angle no >20 degrees *shall be considered for purposes of this paragraph* as having a central visual acuity of 20/200 or less" (emphasis mine). (1) It is apparent that the only important visual disability to those pioneers in disability assessment was loss of central vision resolution, that visual field loss was an afterthought, and that no other visual disorders warranted any attention.

As simplistic as this model of visual disability is (for it remains the SSA definition, with some minor modifications), the only eye care professional who was allowed to make the assessment of disability was "a physician skilled in the diseases of the eye," and until 2007, the Social Security Administration interpreted that rule to mean only those with a medical degree were so skilled. This interpretation was finally and formally changed in 2007, so that now optometrists can also document disability for the purposes of the SSA.

TABLE 29.1 Disability Laws in the United States

Summary of Major Components of Various Disability Laws in the United States

Law	Coverage	Major Points
Social Security Act (SSA)	• >65 y • Permanently disabled	• Disability determined by formulae • Entitlement law (tax breaks or federal funds)
Rehabilitation Act Section 504	Disabled individuals using public institutions that receive federal funds	• Civil rights law (equal access) • Mostly affects K-12 education • Those institutions must provide services that allow equal access to disabled individuals
Individuals with Disabilities Education Act (IDEA)	Children with disabilities in the K-12 educational system	• Entitlement law for the most part (children with disability are entitled to accessible public education) • Most commonly covers learning disabilities (LD) and attention deficit/hyperactivity disorder (ADHD) • Created the system of special education services in the United States
Americans with Disabilities Act as amended or ADA Amendments Act	All individuals with disabilities in the United States using public (although not federal) buildings All individuals with disabilities employed by firms with ≥15 employees All individuals with disabilities using public facilities or services of privately or publicly held corporations	• Civil rights law (equal access) • Mostly affects those not covered by IDEA or §504 • Disability determined by substantial impairment in major life activities • Covered institutions must provide services that allow equal access to disabled individuals • Includes institutions that offer testing services under Title III

This model of visual disability was exclusive until the 1970s. At that point, veterans of the Vietnam War were returning with various disabilities that clearly impacted their quality of life and their access to many aspects of public life but did not necessarily impair their ability to work or fall under the neat, quantitative formulae of the SSA. Clearly, an entitlement act like the SSA did not address all the needs of individuals with disabilities. A new model was needed.

THE BEGINNINGS OF CHANGE: THE REHABILITATION ACT

The SSA is an **entitlement law**; that is, an individual who falls under the qualifications of that law is entitled to money from the federal government, to a significant deduction on his taxes, or both. However, the SSA is silent on access. There are no provisions to ensure that an individual with a disability can get into a public building without being carried, or can take an examination that is intended to test a skill or knowledge base completely unrelated to his or her area of challenge, or can get a job for which he or she is otherwise completely qualified to do.

The need for a **civil rights law** for the disabled became more apparent to legislators as the veterans of the Vietnam War were coming home with various injuries and the civil rights movements for blacks and women were changing the national psyche about equal access. Therefore, in 1973, Congress passed and President Richard Nixon signed the Rehabilitation Act. Its stated purpose was to "empower individuals with disabilities to maximize employment, economic self-sufficiency, independence, and inclusion and integration into society...[and] to ensure that the Federal Government plays a leadership role in promoting the employment of individuals with disabilities..., and in assisting States and providers of services in fulfilling the aspirations of such individuals with disabilities for meaningful and gainful employment and independent living" (2). This act, in addition to funding vocational rehabilitation services, research, and independent living services, created a National Council on Disability, appointed by the President, to promote these services and opportunities.

Title V of the Rehabilitation Act is the portion that deals with enforcement of rights and advocacy for individuals with disabilities. Section 504 of Title V provides for "[n]ondiscrimination under Federal grants and programs." Because almost all educational programs in the United States, and certainly all primary and secondary (K-12) public educational programs, receive federal funds, this section of the act applies to more individuals with disabilities in the educational system than any other law.

Whereas the Rehabilitation Act does fund some programs, as listed above, §504 is an unfunded mandate. State education budgets and local school districts must fund the programs that will provide equal access to the individuals who qualify under §504. Therefore, the funds available may often have a direct and inverse relationship to how much documentation the school district requires in order to classify a student under §504. In other words, in tight budgetary times, the clinician should understand that the school district will create several, perhaps even dozens, of documentation obstacles for arriving at a classification of the child as disabled under the Rehabilitation Act. The law is typically interpreted to cover those schoolchildren with physical or mental disorders, while those with learning disabilities most commonly get their services under the IDEA (see below).

A note of caution is in order here. Visual disorders that have been shown to have a deleterious effect on classroom performance (such as eye movement, accommodative, or binocular vision disorders or visual information processing delays) require specific and sometimes extensive data for proper documentation. Unfortunately, these claims are often plagued by poor documentation or, even when the documentation is of high quality, misinterpretation by educational and medical professionals who have little understanding of any visual disability that doesn't meet the standard of the SSA—poor visual acuity. Therefore, it is critical that the eye care professional documenting a visual condition for an individual who needs classroom accommodations be very forthcoming in providing data and explanations of how the diagnosed condition has a direct impact on the child's access to normal classroom materials.

For example, a child with a convergence insufficiency will probably have visual functioning deficits that cause significant difficulties when doing most classroom desk work and reading assignments. However, the condition rarely has any effect on distance visual acuity. This requires the eye care professional to supply the school with the data that demonstrate how the diagnosis was made. I usually do this by using Morgan's normative values, which have been revalidated in several subsequent studies and have an advantage for this purpose over the Optometric Extension Program (OEP) Analytical Expecteds in that they have a mean and standard deviation. Therefore, they can be reported as standard scores or percentile scores, which are easily interpreted by educational professionals and psychologists.

THE ADOLESCENCE OF DISABILITY LAW: THE INDIVIDUALS WITH DISABILITIES EDUCATION ACT

The IDEA is, like the SSA, an entitlement law. It entitles each child (and the definition of child is quite loose, as shown in the next paragraph) with disabilities access to the education system. It was initially known as PL94-142 or the Education for All Handicapped Children Act when it was first passed and signed by President Gerald Ford in 1975 and made provisions for Committees on Special Education (CSE) in the public school system, as well as other school district–based initiatives to help the education of learning disabled students. In its latest permutation, signed by George W. Bush in 2004, it became the Individuals with Disabilities Education Improvement Act, but it is still largely known by the acronym IDEA.

The IDEA has four parts. Part A lays out the legislative details and provisions of the act. Part B deals with the education of children and young adults from ages 3 to 21 years. Part C details programs and entitlements for children younger than three who are identified as being "at risk." Part D gives support for grants and other initiatives to improve the education of disabled children nationally (3).

The presence of a learning disability under the IDEA must be determined by a CSE, and the basic makeup of that CSE is mandated by the law. At minimum, the committee must include the individual's parents, his "regular teacher," and an evaluator. As defined on the Department of Education's Web site, a "qualified evaluator" is often a school psychologist, speech/language pathologist, or remedial reading teacher (4), although in today's health care climate, licensed social workers and other specialists with master's degrees are often used to run the psychoeducational testing that sets the stage for the determination of a disability. It is of interest that optometrists are also specifically listed as qualified evaluators in the amended act.

There are generally three criteria used to determine the presence of a learning disability, although this can vary somewhat from state to state. These criteria are as follows:

- A significant demonstrated difference is found between the child's achievement and his or her grade level or chronological age (the discrepancy definition).

- The child does not make significant progress over the course of 1 or 2 years.
- The child exhibits a pattern of strengths and weaknesses relative to his or her age.

The last two definitions of disability are a significant departure from the older versions of the law, and are a result of the increasing criticism of the discrepancy model by educational professionals, members of the academe, and child advocates. In fact, the new law specifically states that jurisdictions "shall not be required to take into consideration whether a child has a severe discrepancy between achievement and intellectual ability in oral expression, listening comprehension, written expression, basic reading skill, reading comprehension, mathematical calculation, or mathematical reasoning" (5). The major criticism has been that the discrepancy model allows a school district to wait for up to 2 years while the child is failing to learn basic skills before he or she can possibly qualify for services under the IDEA. However, being able to wait for 2 years before paying for an evaluation or remedial services has obvious budget implications for school districts that provide a short-term incentive for them to keep using the discrepancy model in their analysis of learning disabilities.

Because of the definitions of learning disability included in this law, those individuals with significant cognitive or developmental challenges are often covered under §504, and the academic interventions get additional funding under the state's IDEA budget.

DISABILITY LAW MATURES: THE AMERICANS WITH DISABILITIES ACT

The Americans with Disability Act as amended has three large areas of coverage, or "titles." Title I covers every type of employer, with the exception of organizations with <15 employees, the United States Government, and "bona fide private membership club[s]." Title II covers access to the services and facilities of state and local governments, including public transportation. It also specifically covers Amtrak. However, it implicitly does **not** include the services or facilities of the federal government, other than Amtrak. Title III covers public access to services and facilities of privately held corporations with 15 or more employees and nonprofit organizations (6).

While the ADA is, first and foremost, intended as an employment civil rights law, and most of the direction of the 2008 version was meant to close loopholes by employers to avoid employment of workers with disabilities, higher education is clearly covered under titles II (for public universities) and III (for private institutions of higher education).

The definition of disability in the ADA as amended has far more in common with §504 than it does with the SSA. The definition has three aspects:

- "A physical or mental impairment that substantially limits one or more major life activities...
- a record of such impairment; or
- being regarded as having such an impairment...." (7)

This is the same language as the original ADA of 1990. It is still up to the courts to decide the meaning of the two major descriptors in the definition: "substantially limits" and "major life activities." However, Congress went further in their description of major life activities in the 2008 law. Major life activities are now expanded to include "major bodily functions" and activities including, but "not limited to, caring for oneself, performing manual tasks, seeing, hearing, eating, sleeping, walking, standing, lifting, bending, speaking, breathing, learning, reading, concentrating, thinking, communicating, and working" (8). This last element of the list is clearly intended as a slap at the Supreme Court, who had decided in one major ADA case that "working" included too broad a range of activities to be interpreted as a major life activity (9).

It is beyond the scope of this paper to describe the landmark cases in modern (i.e., post-SSA) disability law, but suffice it to say that some of the major controversies are:

- To what cohort should a person who claims to be disabled be compared?
- What documentation can be requested in the institution's quest to determine if an individual's claim of disability is legitimate, and what constitutes a "qualified evaluator"?
- How many years, under how many different laws, and how many times does a person have to be defined as disabled before he or she can be considered disabled without further review?
- Who gets to decide what constitutes a reasonable accommodation?

Often, the Rehnquist court answered these questions, only to have the answers made ambiguous again by the passage of the amended act in 2008 and the subsequent guidelines handed down by the Obama administration's Department of Justice. The Roberts court has, to date, not heard any major ADA cases.

It is important to note that it is not only doctors of optometry who are identifying vergence, accommodative, and other eye movement disorders as disabling under the ADA —eye surgeons are claiming these conditions are disabling to their patients, as well. In fact, in a review of the rate of claims filed with certain testing organizations for accommodations under the ADA for both traditional (acuity loss and field loss) and nontraditional (ocular motor issues) visual disabilities in 1998, it was found that the rate of claims for nontraditional visual disabilities from ophthalmology was slightly higher than that from optometry, at 60% versus 54% (10).

One interesting case involved a contact lens–wearing patient of a surgical clinic who had been diagnosed with dry eye for years. When no clinical findings supported the diagnosis, and the patient requested a letter from her ophthalmologist for test accommodations for a national licensing examination, he submitted the records of examinations showing the symptoms he had interpreted as dry eye: headaches when reading and using the computer, fatigue and sleepiness with reading, and difficulty attending to near point visual tasks. When the documentation was reviewed and the request denied on the grounds that the documentation did not support the diagnosis, the surgeon finally did some binocular testing. It revealed that his contact lens patient had a significant convergence insufficiency, and she was then granted accommodations on that basis.

NAVIGATING THE STORM: OPTOMETRY'S ROLE IN ADVOCATING FOR THE VISUALLY DISABLED

The AMA and the federal government initially mandated that under the SSA only an ophthalmologist could determine what constituted a visual disability. Under the more modern disability laws, the determination of disability is made by reviewing the patient's functional limitations in the context of his or her day-to-day living activities. In other words, this is a task tailor-made for the clinical training and visual science expertise of the optometrist. Patients are often seeking our aid in seeing if they qualify as disabled under §504 if they are in K12 education or under the ADA if they are in higher education or about to take a standardized examination. Here are some basic guidelines to help you help your patients through the process.

The diagnosis is not the disability. This is nearly a direct quote from Sandra Day O'Connor in one of the most formative of the ADA Supreme Court decisions. Even though Congress has largely invalidated most of the tenets of that decision, this one still stands. What it means for you is that the determination of disability must be made not by looking at the patient's diagnosis, but by determining if the functional limitations placed on that individual by his visual impairment are substantial enough to impede major life activities. This cannot be done by fiat or mathematical formulae. It can only be done by a thoughtful clinician who asks the right questions and can make a clear-eyed, disinterested judgment. However, you should also know that if there is no well-accepted, International Classification of Diseases (ICD)-9 or -10 listed diagnosis, there will be no respect for your determination either. For example, Irlen syndrome (also known as Scotopic Sensitivity Syndrome or Meares-Irlen syndrome) is not a diagnosis under the ICD and, therefore, it is not a disability—it is merely a collection of symptoms.

Documentation is everything. Schools or testing organizations rely on your judgment to determine if your patient is indeed disabled and what accommodations are most appropriate. However, in the majority of cases, they are not going to just accept your word for it because you say it is so. You must back up your judgments with data and a solid, clearly explained rationale. I have seen many claims of convergence insufficiency with absolutely no binocular testing data given, and at least once the diagnosis of accommodative insufficiency claimed after the evaluator did the entire examination after the application of mydriatics. These claims will not stand.

While you should be your patient's advocate, you should not compromise professional ethics. If you firmly believe your patient is disabled because of a complete history, solid evidentiary data, and a data-driven diagnosis, then by all means you should strongly advocate for accommodations and programs to allow equal access for her. However, if you are tempted to write a letter simply because the patient's parents paid a lot of money for your professional evaluation and she is really a sweet kid, do not do it.

Navigating the ins and outs of the public schools' special education system often requires patience, documentation, and the force of will.

Because schools are run by humans, and teachers are humans, and parents are strongly biased humans, and schools are funded by taxpayers' money at the federal, state, and local levels, the determination of who gets special education services is often much more complicated than you might think it should be. If you firmly believe that a patient deserves services under the law, then you should supply the patience and documentation, and you should count on the parent for the force of will.

Though a diagnosis lasts forever, a disability does not. If you have a patient with an eye movement, vergence, or accommodative dysfunction who has been through a program of optometric vision therapy, you probably still use the original diagnosis code to bill for the progress evaluations. This is standard procedure and well accepted by third-party payers because the condition needs to be actively monitored, even after all symptoms may be resolved. However, in the world of disability analysis, the determination is made by looking at functional limitations, not old diagnoses. Therefore, the school or testing organization is well within its rights to ask for *current* data and symptoms in the documentation supplied to support a claim of disability.

Often, this situation leads to the most difficult discussions with patients or their parents. As an example, you have a patient who successfully completed a program of optometric vision therapy, and you like the patient and her family. Now, she is taking the LSAT and would like extended time. She asks you to write the letter for test accommodations based on her convergence excess. It is certainly ethical to write that she still has convergence excess. However, you are obligated to supply the current data and symptoms in your documentation, even though you suspect that these data do not support any claim of a *current* disability. You might have a frank discussion with your patient about the very strong possibility that accommodations will be denied because her visual functioning is much improved.

Extended time is not the only available accommodation. By far, the most popular test accommodation is extended time on testing. There may be a good reason for this popularity among test takers: there are some pilot studies indicating that extended time gives an unfair advantage to all test takers, no matter their disability status, although the data are still somewhat limited to pilot studies at this point. However, there are many visual conditions—convergence insufficiency, accommodative disorders, etc.—for which extended time on the near point task *exacerbates* the symptoms and thus the impairment. It does not serve your patient well to request extended time for a condition that gets worse with time. Other options available from most testing organizations are occlusion of one eye, extra breaks, enlarged print or ZoomText (on computer-based tests). It is highly advisable to work with your patient to determine the accommodation that would best provide equal access to the examination, not unfair advantages.

CONCLUSION

Optometry has much to offer to patients with visual disabilities at all educational levels today. The IDEA, ADAAA, and Section 504 of the Rehabilitation Act are a solid troika of laws that allow individuals with disabilities to participate fully in our educational system, so that they can maximally contribute to society without being held back because of accessibility problems.

REFERENCES

1. Social Security Act Sec. 216. [42 U.S.C. 416] "Other Definitions". Available from: http://www.ssa.gov/OP_Home/ssact/title02/0216.htm#act-216-i-1. Last Accessed January 17, 2011.
2. Rehabilitation Act Amendments of 1973 at Available from: http://www.access-board.gov/enforcement/Rehab-Act-text/intro.htm. Last Accessed January 17, 2011.
3. United States Department of Education IDEA. Available from: http://idea.ed.gov/download/statute.html. Last Accessed January 17, 2011.
4. IDEA statute, Section 632 (Definitions), 4(F).
5. IDEA statute, Section 614 (b)(6)(A).
6. ADA Amendments Act statute. Available from: www.access-board.gov/about/laws/ada-amendments.htm. Last Accessed March 18, 2011.
7. ADA Amendments Act Section (4), "Disability Defined and Rules of Construction."
8. ADA Amendments Act Section (4)(a)(2)(A).
9. O'Connor, Sandra Day. Sutton v. United Air Lines, Inc.; (1990). Paragraph (c).
10. Damari DA. Visual disability claims of medical students under the Americans with Disabilities Act (abstract). Annual Meeting of the College of Optometrists in Vision Development 1999.

CHAPTER 30

Jason Clopton, OD, FCOVD
Dan Fortenbacher, OD, FCOVD
Bradley Habermehl, OD, FCOVD

The Optometric Practice

Optometrists need to know not only the neurology, genetics, and other systemic and oculovisual anomalies associated with the patient with special needs but also the business aspects of running a medical office to serve those with disabilities. Having a professionally successful and monetarily profitable office ensures the ability to care for those most in need of the services unique to optometry. This chapter discusses office layout, equipment, staffing, billing/coding, and marketing.

PHYSICAL STRUCTURE, EQUIPMENT, STAFFING

The treatment of visual problems associated with special populations requires the application of sound methods of practice to ensure that the patient has the best opportunity for improvement. Evidence-based studies have shown that office-based optometric vision therapy (OVT), in conjunction with home-oriented activities, is the most effective method of treatment (1).

In addition to the judicious application of lenses, and prisms to improve visual function, the optometric practitioner who works with special populations must have an organized system of management for delivering office-based OVT. This section discusses the important elements (physical structure, equipment, and staffing) within the optometric practice required for implementing the delivery of the best diagnostic and therapeutic care.

Physical Structure While it is possible to provide OVT services in nearly any space that contains a floor, four walls, and a ceiling, the most effective delivery requires allocated and often separate space within the optometric practice. In this section, we discuss the core components of space including the reception/waiting, testing, conference, treatment, and administrative rooms and equipment.

Reception/Waiting Room A patient's first physical experience with any optometric practice will occur in the reception room. While most optometric practices are designed to handle the flow of the primary care patient, any reception room might receive a diverse group of patients, from young children to seniors. In an OVT practice that provides care for patients with special needs, the reception room should be designed to cater to the needs of parents or guardians waiting for the patient. In addition, when families have one person in treatment, it is common for additional young children to tag along. Given the diverse needs of patients and their caretakers or families, the reception room must have adequate space and provisions.

For example, a successfully designed reception room should cater to the needs of young children by providing toys, a variety of children's books, and related age-appropriate materials (Fig. 30-1). Other important amenities include coffee, tea, water, free WiFi, and an assortment of the usual reception room reading material (Fig. 30-2). It also is a good idea for the reception room to convey the type of optometric care that is being provided. Effective messaging materials include posters, brochures, special books, success stories, etc., all of which emphasize the role of vision in learning and life skills (Fig. 30-3). While these items might seem insignificant to the effective delivery of care, it actually plays a significant role in the patient experience because other family members who are waiting as long as 45 to 60 minutes will need space to accommodate their needs during that time.

Testing Room The diagnostic evaluation of a patient with special needs requires the use of space beyond the confines of the optometric examination

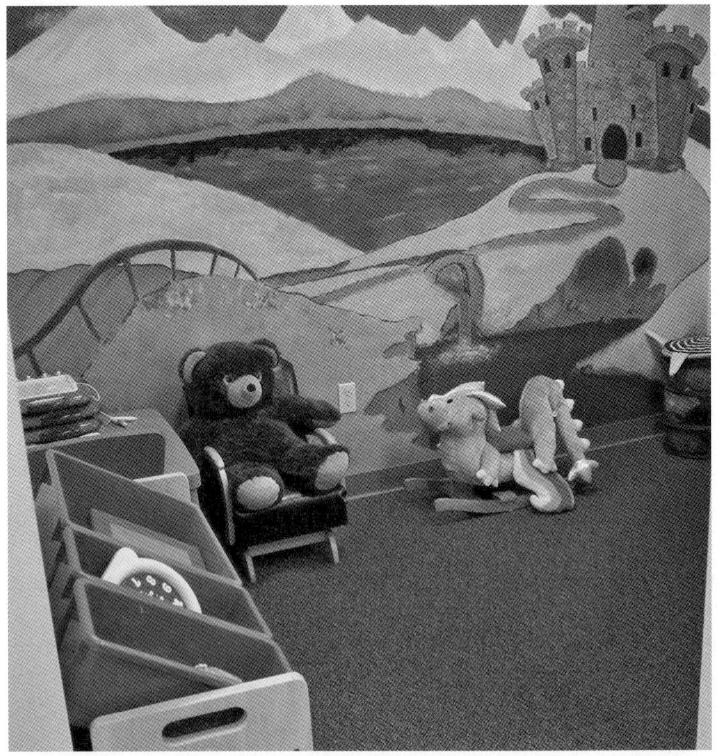

FIGURE 30-1. A "kid's zone" can help patient anxiety while waiting for their appointment.

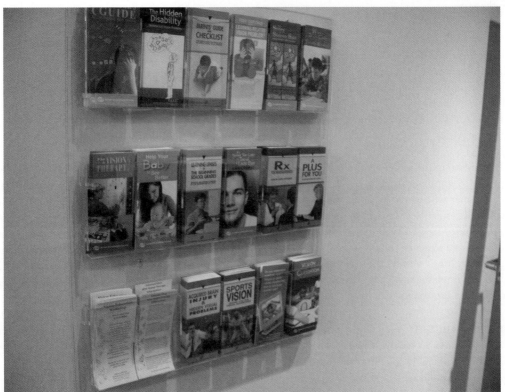

FIGURE 30-2. Reading material can provide education on various topics.

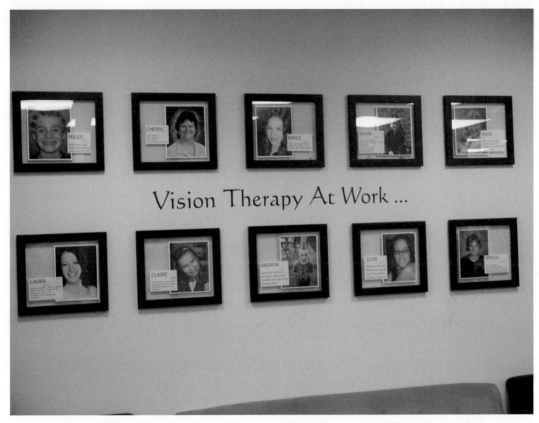

FIGURE 30-3. Success stories can demonstrate the power of vision therapy and provide waiting room decor.

room. Whether it is to observe the application of yoked prism or to watch the response to tests of visual information processing, visually directed gross motor skills or visual–vestibular integration procedures, the allocation of space for effective and discreet testing is essential.

Conference Room After diagnostic evaluations are complete, a practitioner must take the time to compile the test results and present the information to the patient, parent/guardian, and/or responsible family member. In some offices, the practitioner conducts this conference in the examination room, but in other practices, a specifically appointed conference room is preferred. This should be furnished with comfortable chairs and a conference table with related handouts and communication materials nearby.

Treatment Room Providing office-based OVT begins by having the space to allow interaction between the doctor and/or vision therapist and the patient (Fig. 30-4). Because the delivery of care requires the use of specialized equipment, there must be enough room to store and use the equipment. The allocation of adequate space for treatment is a critical component in the delivery of therapy. While not every office has the flexibility to add more square footage, often, existing rooms can be modified by the use of walls for specialized equipment, rollaway counters or tables, and closets designed with special storage compartments.

Administrative Room One important area that practitioners too often overlook is the space needed for administrative support staff. The administrative elements of a practice that uses vision therapy as a treatment modality involves record-keeping systems that are unique to rehabilitative medicine. Consequently, a well-organized practice should set aside space for charting of a patient's examination procedures, therapy programming, progress notes, and insurance-related documentation.

Equipment The delivery of OVT for patients with special needs requires the use of a wide variety

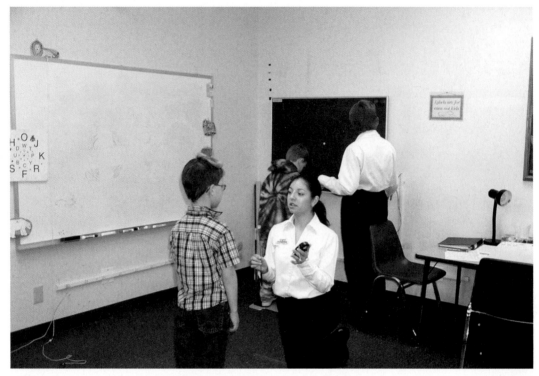

FIGURE 30-4. An example of a vision therapy room.

of essential equipment. One of the best resources for help in deciding which equipment to obtain is the Optometric Extension Program Foundation (OEPF). Their website lists OVT supplies and equipment in alphabetical order (2).

The instrumentation used in the delivery of OVT requires floor, wall, ceiling, and tabletop space. While optometric practices often have finite space, there are creative ways to acquire the space needed to accomplish the activities. For example, because lenses and prisms are so important during patient interaction, space must be allocated for their effective storage and ease of access for treatment (Fig. 30-5). In addition to storage drawers, a practitioner may use wall-mounted storage compartments and rollaway carts to keep these tools close at hand.

Staffing The key to the successful delivery of treatment is organized methodology of care. Whether it is an optometric practitioner providing individual care to a patient or a trained optometric vision therapist working under the supervision of an optometric practitioner, the interaction between the patient, doctor, and professional staff is a critical element needed for successful patient outcomes.

The team approach to care creates efficiencies and challenges. Effective use of trained paraprofessionals enables improved patient access to care because the doctor can provide care to more patients per unit time. To maximize efficiency and minimize challenges in a team atmosphere, training and organization are key to consistent delivery of OVT in the optometric practice. While there may be a variety of ways to organize a team, in general, the structure of the team can be divided into the following:

- Doctor(s)
- Optometric vision therapy assistants (OVTAs)
- Certified optometric vision therapists (COVTs)
- Administrative staff

Regardless of the recruitment method used, experience shows that successful candidates for employment in a practice that provides OVT, must enjoy working with children and exhibit a strong desire to help others. Other positive qualities include the ability to learn quickly and to work well within a team environment. Practitioners should understand that it is rare to recruit OVT staff that has all of the needed training and clinical skills to begin working with patients. Therefore, a practitioner should have

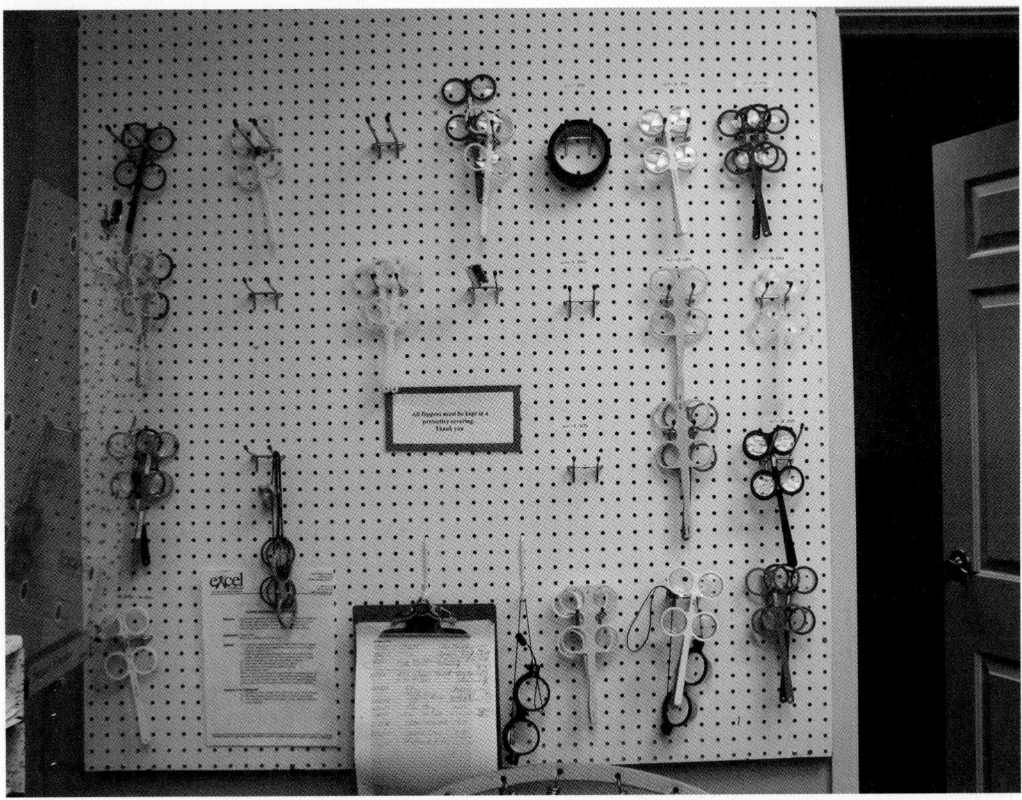

FIGURE 30-5. A space-saving method to store lenses.

an effective system for training and educating new staff and for continuing the education of existing staff. Three organizations can assist an optometric clinician: OEPF (3), the College of Optometrists in Vision Development (COVD) (4) and the Neuro-Optometric Vision Rehabilitation Association (5). All three organizations have as their mission to serve optometry and to provide continuing education and other vital programs. The American Optometric Association (AOA) (6) and the American Academy of Optometry (7) also provide political stability, intensive research support, and educational courses to improve primary and specialized care.

The Doctor In addition to staff education and training, practitioners who work with special needs patients must place a priority on their own continuing education in the area of pediatrics, developmental vision, and OVT. In addition to continuing education programs, COVD provides a board certification process in developmental vision and OVT for doctors and therapists. Information regarding the fellowship process can be found at www.covd.org (4). Once an optometrist becomes a fellow of COVD, therapists who are employed by the fellow may pursue board COVT. Attaining these prestigious designations is important to the development of a qualified team of professionals who work with the doctor to deliver OVT for those with special needs.

Optometric Vision Therapy Assistant The OVTA works with the patient by providing activities during the course of the session, under the supervision of the doctor. Activities are typically preprogrammed by the doctor and/or other experienced vision therapists on the team to meet the individual needs of the patient. The OVTA provides therapeutic activities that include the right amount of complexity and variety so that the patient can achieve success.

Certified Optometric Vision Therapist The OVTA who is employed by a Fellow of COVD may qualify for the COVD board certification process, upon documenting 2,000 hours of experience as an OVTA and completing the three-part examination process, which involves open book questions, closed book examination, and oral interview. The certification process is designed to enhance the knowledge and understanding of developmental vision and OVT and to show that the individual has met the criteria of advanced competency.

Administrative Staff Administrative staff plays an important role within the office structure. These individuals wear many hats that range from scheduling appointments to understanding and communicating effectively the multitude of issues that occur with third party health care plans and patient reimbursement. While it is possible to combine the administrative duties of primary care and OVT, experience shows that it is often better to have at least one administrative staffer who is dedicated to the OVT team. This promotes consistency across the variety of administrative duties. Through the effective use of space, organization, training, and administration, the delivery of effective rehabilitative/developmental vision care for those with special needs is assured of success.

CODING AND BILLING

The number one rule in coding and billing is that those that pay the bill make the rules. With that in mind, every provider should know that there are differing rules for each payer. Cash payers are convenient, require little paperwork or staff time, and provide immediate compensation. Managed care organizations are third party payers that require a great deal of paperwork and staff time and provide compensation in a less than immediate fashion. When providers accept assignment from a third party payer, they sign a contract with that third party and agree to follow the rules that have been set out in that contract.

On occasion, practitioners that examine special needs patients often code outside of routine practices. Because of this, knowledge of all the rules from each third party (managed care companies or the government programs such as Medicare/Medicaid) must be considered. Sometimes there are no rules established or associated with some of the codes that can and should be used by optometrists but are routinely used by other professions on a daily basis (see 96000 and 97000 series codes below). Coding and billing is used every day by all providers who contract with a third party payer. Different third parties (insurance companies) pay differing amounts for the same services. Some third parties (commercial insurance companies) will negotiate the fees paid to the provider and some do not (Medicare). Most commercial payers pay a percentage of what Medicare allows. Regarding coverage, in most cases, Medicare sets the rules for what is and is not covered.

When a patient comes to the office of a provider and the provider has a contract with the insurance company, the patient usually will pay the contracted amount (co-pay and/or deductible). The provider accepts whatever amount the third party payer agrees to pay in addition to the co-pay and/or deductible of that patient. After collecting the co-pay and/or deductible at the time of services rendered, the additional amount (if any) for the services that the patient has not paid is then billed to the third party payer as a courtesy to the patient. In most contracts, the provider may not bill a differing amount for the same service. However, since it can take considerable time to get reimbursement from any third party payer, you may allow for a prompt pay discount for patients paying cash.

Most states now have laws on how long the third party can take to reimburse the provider. Any reimbursement that goes beyond the date allowable should be paid with accrued interest. Each state has different laws regarding this issue, so providers should check with their own state on these regulations.

Coding and billing are thought of as the method of describing and paying for services and procedures that are provided to patients. In reality, they are two separate entities and a great deal more than that. Coding is a system of classifying procedures and services for systematic enumeration with the purposes of research, studies, and surgical and examination procedures. Billing is applying that systematic enumeration to what a provider does, enabling payment from a third party.

There are two forms of coding: diagnostic coding and procedural coding. The first, the International Classification of Disease (ICD) is a four- to five-digit system used by physicians and nonphysician providers to describe commonly accepted disease diagnoses. The current edition, ICD-9, is owned and copyrighted by the American Medical Association (AMA). There are other coding systems, but they are not widely used. ICD-9-CM does not include all diagnoses, but rather only the most of the common. Most of the rest of the world uses a much more inclusive system called ICD-10 (this is not owned or copyrighted by the AMA).

The other coding system is the Physicians' Current Procedural Terminology (CPT). It uses a standardized five-digit code with descriptive terms used to report the medical services and surgical procedures performed by physicians and other health care providers. The CPT coding system, which is proprietary, was developed and copyrighted by the AMA to provide enumeration of common procedures used by providers in the United States. Not all procedures fall under this code.

Current Procedural Terminology codes can be separated into service-based codes, surgical codes, and time-based codes. These types of codes are usually mutually exclusive, but can overlap in particular instances. Service codes are traditionally used for procedures done in the office or hospital. Time-based codes are used when varying procedures are done on a timed basis such as rehabilitation (97000 series) procedures. Service-based codes are not usually timed (but can be), do not require direct face-to-face time (unless timed) with the patient, and can only be billed one unit of each service-based code daily per discipline, per patient. There are rare exceptions where perhaps a provider could bill more than one unit on the same day, such as when a patient comes to the office with a specific problem, the problem was treated, and later that same day the patient returns with a different problem.

Current Procedural Terminology codes are also used to report the technical component (TC), the recording of the data, or professional component (PC), the interpreting of the data, of most outpatient services including procedures, laboratory, radiology, and same-day surgery. These two components can be done by different providers on different days with the appropriate modifiers. There are many dissimilar codes used in various professions, but for our purposes we will discuss those codes routinely used by eye care professionals: surgical (65000 series), general ophthalmic (92000 series), testing (96000 series), rehabilitation (97000), and evaluation and management (E&M) (99000 series) codes. There are criteria involved in each that must be satisfied to be able to correctly use any of these codes.

Optometry is legislated in each state by its own optometry practice act that describes what procedures an optometrist can perform under that state law. Many states allow optometrists to prescribe topical, ophthalmic, injectable, and oral medicines and perform surgery to practice to the highest level of their training. Since 1987, optometrists have been considered physicians by Medicare and the Centers for Medicare Services (CMS). In the CMS policy manual in Section 30.4—Optometrist's Services (Rev. 1, 10-01-03) B3-2020.25, it is stated that a "doctor of optometry is considered a physician with respect to all services the optometrist is authorized to perform under State law or regulation" (8). To be covered under Medicare, the services must be medically reasonable and necessary for the diagnosis or treatment of illness or injury, and must meet all applicable coverage requirements.

Surgical (65000 Series) Procedure Codes These codes can be used to describe the surgical procedure or the comanagement aspect of a procedure, such as cataract surgery. A modifier must be attached, describing what part of the procedure was performed by which provider. As these codes are not used in relation to vision rehabilitation, they will not be covered in greater detail.

General Ophthalmic (92000 Series) Procedure Codes General ophthalmic codes (CPT 92002/92012 and 92004/92014) are specific to optometry and ophthalmology. They represent a standard procedure for examination of a patient. There are specific criteria that must be met for a provider to bill these codes. 92002 is a *new* patient intermediate ophthalmic examination. 92012 is an *established* patient intermediate ophthalmic examination. 92004 is a *new* patient comprehensive ophthalmic examination. 92014 is an *established* patient comprehensive ophthalmic examination. Other codes in the 92000 series are performed outside of the routine codes and are usually more properly billed in conjunction with the 99000 series and a modifier when required. Typical procedures other than 92000 series pertinent to special needs patient care include the following:

Sensorimotor evaluation (CPT 92060) is a procedure for measuring the deviation of an eye in strabismus or other posturing diagnosis. This must have quantitative measurement in all major fields of gaze and be documented in at least nine different positions of gaze. This requires a separate interpretation and report.

Orthoptics/pleoptics (CPT 92065) is a procedure that is defined as orthoptic and/or pleoptic training under direct physician supervision. It was originally described as the aligning of the eyes using an orthoptor. The AMA has defined it as any procedure that includes aligning the eyes with lenses, prisms, or filters (patches). For this reason, this code has improperly come to include OVT.

Visual field examination (CPT 9208*x* [*x* = 1, 2, or 3]) is a bilateral procedure and billable for ICDs related to glaucoma, retinal and neurologic abnormalities, and visual field defects. It requires a separate interpretation and report. It is broken down into three different levels: 92081 is a limited evaluation and does not include measurement of isopters but is more than confrontation fields. 92082 is an intermediate evaluation that includes measurement of isopters but not threshold (campimetry). 92083 is the extended evaluation and includes measurement of isopters and threshold.

Prolonged physician service (99354/99355) is used if you spend more than the "normal" amount of time with a patient. The provider must document the amount of time spent with a patient, and the reason why (Table 30.1).

Testing (96000 Series) Timed Procedure Codes Testing codes include standardized testing that is performed outside of the 92000 or 99000 series. These codes have traditionally been used by providers like psychology and neurology but are allowed to be billed by any physician.

Developmental Testing: Limited (CPT 96110) is the use of developmental screening instruments of a limited nature. It is often reported when performed in the context of preventative medicine services. It is typically completed by a nonphysician provider.

Developmental Testing: Extended (CPT 96111) includes an assessment of motor, language, social, adaptive, and/or cognitive functioning by standardized instrumentation, with interpretation and report. It is billed in 1-hour units. Time spent interpreting and reporting may be other than when the patient is present. This service may be reported independently or in conjunction with another code describing a separate patient encounter on the same day as the testing. A physician or other trained professional typically performs this service. A specific example, given in the Medical Coding Companion series published by the AMA, is the Beery-Buktenika Test of Visual Motor Integration.

Neurobehavioral Status Exam (CPT 96116) is defined as the clinical assessment of thinking, reasoning, and judgment (e.g., acquired knowledge, attention, language, planning and problem solving, and visual spatial abilities). It is billed per hour of the physician's time, and includes both face-to-face and time interpreting results and preparing the report.

TABLE 30.1 Prolonged Physician Service Codes (99354/99355)

• <30 min	Not reported separately
• >30–74 min	99354 × 1 (2009 CMA allowable: $86.85)
• +30 min	99355 × 1 (2009 CMA allowable: $86.28)
• =75–104 min	99354 × 1 and 99355 × 1

Rehabilitation (97000 Series) Timed Procedure Codes The 97000 series codes are used to describe procedures performed in the rehabilitation and, since 2004, the habilitation setting. These codes have traditionally been used by physical medicine and occupational and physical therapy and are often mistakenly described as "OT/PT codes" by third party payers and other providers. These codes recently have been more properly used by any provider involved in the rehabilitation or habilitation process including occupational therapists, physical therapists, optometry, speech and language pathology, chiropractors, podiatry, and other physicians. 97000 series codes are time based due to the fact that a provider may use multiple techniques or procedures in a single therapy session to engage the patient in therapeutic activities and procedures.

Therapeutic Exercise (CPT 97110) incorporates rehabilitation principles related to increasing strength, endurance, flexibility, and range of motion to one or more areas of the body. This procedure code is billed in 15-minute increments. A therapeutic exercise is considered reasonable and necessary if the patient is having weakness, pain, contracture, stiffness (secondary to coordination deficits), abnormal posture, or muscle imbalance or the patient needs to improve mobility, stretching, strengthening, coordination, control of extremities, dexterity, and range of motion or endurance. At least one of these conditions must be present and documented in the medical record. Documentation for therapeutic exercise must show objective functional loss of joint motion, strength, mobility (e.g., degrees of motion, strength grades, and levels of assistance), or endurance and may be performed with a patient either actively, actively assisted, or passively participating.

Neuromuscular Reeducation (CPT 97112) is defined as a therapeutic procedure, in one or more areas that is 15 minutes in duration. These areas include reeducation of movement, balance, coordination, kinesthetic sense, posture, and proprioception. The patient must show functional limitations/deficits as a result of the neuromuscular impairment. Objective measurements/ratings of loss of balance, strength, coordination, and/or mobility must be indicated. The patient may need assistance for balance and mobility. As per the AMA, 97112 is intended to identify therapeutic exercise designed to retrain a body part to perform some task that the body part was previously able to do. This will usually be in the form of some commonly performed task for that body part.

Therapeutic Activity (CPT 97530) is considered reasonable and necessary for patients needing a broad range of rehabilitative techniques that involves movement. Movement activities can be for a specific body part or could involve the entire body. It is billed in 15-minute increments. This procedure involves the use of functional activities to improve functional performance in a progressive manner. The activities are usually directed at a loss or restriction of mobility, strength, balance, or coordination. They require the skills of a provider and are designed to address a specific functional need of the patient.

Development of Cognitive Skills (CPT 97532) is a therapeutic activity designed to improve attention, memory, and problem solving. It includes compensatory training and is provided through direct (one-on-one) patient contact by the provider in 15-minute blocks of time.

Sensory Integrative Therapy (CPT 97533) includes techniques to enhance sensory processing and promote adaptive responses to environmental demands. It is provided directly (one on one) by the provider in 15-minute increments.

In order for any of the therapeutic activities to be covered, all of the following requirements must be met: (a) the patient has a condition for which therapeutic activities can reasonably be expected to restore or improve functioning; (b) the patient's condition is such that he or she is unable to perform therapeutic activities except under the direct supervision of a physician or therapist; (c) there is a clear correlation between the type of exercise performed and the patient's underlying functional deficit(s) for which the therapeutic activities were prescribed. Therapeutic activities may be medically necessary when the professional skills of a provider are required, and the activity is designed to address the specific needs of the patient. These dynamic activities must be part of a documented treatment plan and intended to result in a specific outcome.

As can be seen by the definitions above, the rehabilitation/habilitation codes are a much better fit for the procedures that are performed in OVT. Orthoptics certainly fits into what optometrists do on occasion, but the 97000 series actually better describes what is actually happening in the modern OVT office. Orthoptics has its place when doing vectographic, orthoptic, or other stationary procedures, where the only system that is stimulated is the aligning of the oculomotor system. When other sensorimotor systems are being incorporated, orthoptics does not fit that description. A provider should use the code(s) that best describe what procedures are performed.

Evaluation and Management (99000 Series) Service Codes Evaluation and management codes are the 99000 series. They can only be used in a medical examination in which there is a medical diagnosis (generally anything other than myopia, hyperopia, astigmatism, and presbyopia). Evaluation and management codes have areas of documentation to determine the level of service provided. They must include at least some of the six documentation criteria for payment or time element. These seven areas of documentation include the (a) history; (b) examination; (c) level of medical decision making; (d) amount of counseling; (e) coordination of care; (f) nature of the presenting problem; and (g) time spent with the patient. Evaluation and management codes have guidelines for each of the previous areas of documentation that must include areas of history. Examples include whether the practitioner is seeing a new or established patient, the chief complaint, history of present illness, family history, past history, social history, and review of systems. Your documentation determines the level of coding used for a patient encounter. For instance, when determining the level of service, you must see what you have documented in the patient history. Levels for review of the patient history are divided into four categories, which are described along with their differences in Table 30.2.

The elements of the examination include visual acuity; gross visual field testing; ocular motility including primary gaze alignment and bulbar and palpebral conjunctivae inspection; ocular adnexa

TABLE 30.2 Requirements of Different Levels of History for the Evaluation and Management (99000) Series Codes

Level	Requirements
Problem focused history	• Chief complaint • 1–3 elements of the history of present illness
Extended problem focused history	• Chief complaint • one to three elements of the history of present illness • Ocular review of systems
Detailed history	• Chief complaint • One to three elements of the history of present illness • Ocular review of systems • Two-body review of systems • One of three problem focused—patient, family, or social history.
Comprehensive history	• The chief complaint • One to three elements of the history of present illness • Ocular review of systems • Two-body review of systems • Three of three problem focused—patient, family, or social history for a new patient • Two of three for an established patient

examination including lids, lacrimal glands, lacrimal drainage, orbits, and preauricular lymph nodes; and pupil and iris examination including shape, direct/consensual reaction, size, and morphology. The slit lamp examination of the corneas should include the epithelium, stroma, endothelium, and tear film. The anterior chamber structures assessed should note depth, the presence of cell and flare, and an evaluation of the lens (clarity, anterior and posterior capsule, cortex, and nucleus). Intraocular pressure measurements can include noncontact tonometry, Goldmann tonometry, and digital palpation, among others. Ophthalmoscopic examination through a dilated pupil of the optic discs should include the size, C/D ratio, appearance, and information about the nerve fiber layer. An assessment of the posterior segment notes information concerning the retina and blood vessels. The neurologic assessment should take into account the patient's orientation to time, place, and person, while the psychiatric assessment includes mood and affect (depression, anxiety, and agitation). Documentation of these different elements gives you the level of examination. A problem-focused (PF) examination is a limited evaluation and has one to five of the elements listed above. The expanded problem focused (EPF) is a limited examination and consists of six elements. A detailed examination is an extended examination and consists of nine elements. A comprehensive assessment is a complete single-system examination and includes all elements listed above.

There are various levels of medical decision making: straightforward (SF), low complexity (LC), moderate complexity (MC), and high complexity (HC). Straightforward takes into account that the number of diagnoses or management options should be minimal. The amount or complexity of data should be minimal or none, and risk of complications are also minimal. An LC level of decision making includes that the number of diagnoses or management options and amount or complexity of data are limited and the risk of complications is low. The next level is MC. In this category, the number of diagnoses or management options is multiple, and the amount or complexity of data and risk of complications are moderate. The HC level of decision making indicates that the number of diagnoses or management options and the amount or complexity of data are extensive, and the risk of complication is high. All of this will add up to which E&M code to properly use for the level of billing when examining a patient.

The practitioner has to determine the level of E&M by identifying the category of service. The extent of history taking, level of the examination, and the complexity of medical decision-making process should be assessed by reviewing the E&M descriptors. For example, on a new patient, you must have three of three for history, exam, decision making, or bill by time using documented face-to-face interaction with the patient. A new patient is defined as a patient who has not been seen in the office by anyone

TABLE 30.3 Evaluation and Management (99000) Code Series

Code	Level of History	Level of Exam	Level of Decision Making	Time
99201 =	PFH	PFE	SFDM	10
99202 =	EPFH	EPFE	SFDM	20
99203 =	DH	DE	LDM	30
99204 =	CH	CE	MDM	45
99205 =	CH	CE	HDM	60
99211 =	minimal			5
99212 =	PFH	PFE	SDM	10
99213 =	EPFH	EFE	LDM	15
99214 =	DH	DE	MDM	25
99215 =	CH	CE	HDM	40

PFH, problem focused history; EPFH, extended problem focused history; DH, detailed history; CH, comprehensive history; PFE, problem focused exam; EPFE, extended problem focused exam; DE, detailed exam; CE, comprehensive exam; SFDM, straightforward decision making; LDM, low-complexity decision making; MDM, moderate-complexity decision making; HDM, high-complexity decision making.

(including another similar practitioner) for a period of at least 3 years. The rules are similar for an established patient, but you only have to meet the level for two out of the three criteria (history, examination, or decision making). The information needed to properly and legally use the 99000 code series is listed in Table 30.3.

There are separate diagnostic codes that should be documented when performing procedures that are outside of the typical examination sequence. They must be separate from the examination and can be unilateral or bilateral and have a TC and PC. These separate diagnostic codes must be filed with corresponding ICD-9-CM codes. Examples include gonioscopy, visual fields, scanning laser, anterior or posterior photography, corneal topography, serial tonometry, and pachymetry.

Modifiers Modifiers are used for codifying in special circumstances such as performing multiple procedures, technical versus professional components, and differing providers performing postoperative procedures, on the same day. These modifiers are posted on the Health Insurance Claim Form with the code used for that procedure (e.g., 99213 with 92060-25 when performing a medical examination with a neuromuscular evaluation on the same day).

Modifier 25: Significant, separately identifiable E&M service by the same physician on the same day of a procedure or other service—E&M service or service by the same physician on the same day as the procedure or other service.

Modifier 51: Multiple procedures—When multiple procedures, other than E&M services, are performed on the same day or at the same session by the same provider, the primary procedure or service may be reported as listed. The additional procedure(s) or service(s) are identified by adding modifier 51.

Because optometrists who work with patients with special needs perform procedures that are not routine, we have historically had a more difficult time in the coding and billing arena. It means that when working with patients with special needs, a provider has to have a better overall understanding of coding and billing. It is imperative that coding and billing be done correctly. Audits can be costly, or they can be an affirmation that confirms the provider's ability to provide care and code and document properly.

MARKETING YOUR SPECIALTY 101

A practitioner may very well be the best doctor in his or her field in treating patients with special needs, but if no one knows who the practitioner is or how they can be helped by him or her, then the practitioner's knowledge and talents are of no use. As much as it is the responsibility of the practitioners to stay well educated in clinical advancements, it is also their responsibility to keep the practice and services well marketed for those who are seeking the care provided.

Getting Started The first step in marketing is choosing a brand that is identifiable with the practice. Some great examples of memorable brands would be the "swoosh" for Nike, the golden arches of McDonalds, and the light blue globe for AT&T. The brand may be colorful, abstract, or a simple metaphor for the specialty of the office. The goal is to make it a recognizable symbol of the practice. Once the brand has been designed, be sure to place it on everything that represents the practice including the Web site, business cards, stationery, handouts, informational pamphlets, literature, print ads, television commercials, and on the sign outside. Some practices have gone so far as putting their branding on the staff's uniforms, including shirts, jackets, and baseball caps.

Today, there are numerous sites online that will assist you in developing a logo so it is no longer necessary for a new or established practitioner to hire an expensive graphic designer to get an original, memorable logo. Some of the best do-it-yourself logo makers online include www.logoyes.com and www.logomaker.com. A useable logo with either of these sites can be designed for under $100.00.

It is not necessarily to spend a significant amount of money to market your services and practice, but time is required to make it happen. The key to being successful is to be consistent in the message and marketing. On average, a potential patient will see an advertisement seven times before calling to schedule an appointment. It is also important to remember that every opportunity to get your marketing and message in front of someone should be considered as an opportunity to plant seeds for future patients who might not need the services today but might seek them out in the future.

Marketing should ramp up around report card and back-to-school time to raise awareness, but the goal is to do something visible every week that brings attention to the practice. While the months of October and March tend to be the busiest times for marketing, the brand should be kept visible during quieter periods around the winter holidays and the middle of summer vacation.

Every marketing plan should include metrics that can measure if the return on investment is appropriate for the time and fiscal investment put into the program. These metrics should be easily measured and include increases in fiscal aspects of the practice but also patient satisfaction.

Social Networks Social networks like Facebook (www.facebook.com) and Twitter (www.twitter.com) can be an effective part of a marketing plan. Increasing numbers of people are drawn to social networks to find and share information. It is an inexpensive way to highlight the practice, where it is located, and the specialties provided. The use of social networking at least two to three times per week, sharing information and ideas, will keep people interested. The practitioners may want to take on this role themselves or hire a staff member to generate postings.

Facebook With over 800,000,000 users, Facebook is the largest of the social networking sites. Once thought to be a site just for college students, Facebook has now extended its reach to the business world and beyond. The practitioner may want to have both a personal page and one for his or her office so as to not mix business and personal relationships. A Facebook page is maintained to develop relationships, so the content should be meaningful and interesting to the followers. Always keep in mind that posts represent both the practice and practitioner at all times.

When creating a personal Facebook page, a representative picture is selected. It is thought that the best photos are those that show a doctor to be both knowledgeable and yet easy to approach. Searching for "friends" who are already on the network is the next task. This can be aided by searching a personal e-mail address book for contacts that may be on Facebook or providing the names of schools attended in the past, including high schools and colleges. Many Facebook users are excited to rekindle relationships that had slipped away due to the time constraints of modern life.

Facebook has done an excellent job updating their privacy settings so who is allowed to view the posts can be selected. For instance, lists can be created such as "high school," "sorority sisters," "golf buddies," and patients. A little bit of time organizing the lists can save a great deal of worry regarding who may be viewing personal posts.

When setting up a Facebook account for a practice, it is recommended to choose the "Facebook page" option. This setting will differentiate the practice's business page and entitle the account to certain benefits, such as weekly "insights" and demographic breakdowns of the page's followers. Once the page is published, e-mails will be sent from Facebook indicating how many fans joined the page that week, the number of wall posts, comments, and "likes" that were generated. Details regarding how many people visited the page that week as compared to the previous week will also be provided. For example, over the past several months, the Facebook page for The

Vision Therapy Group (the office of one of the coauthors) has consistently generated between 300 and 600 views per week. Not a bad return on investment for something that requires only minutes a day to maintain.

The practice page should display its logo as well as pictures and videos from the office. Consider posting content three to four times each week on topics ranging from news in the world of vision development and education to patient success stories and product recommendations. Facebook provides a great opportunity to be a resource for the page's followers and a positive reflection of the community. The Facebook page might draw attention not only to the practice but also to the field of OVT itself, by highlighting success stories in the media, even if they do not come from the office.

There are several pages on Facebook in which a link can be created to enhance the practice's message concerning the importance of yearly examinations and the benefits of OVT. In addition to COVD's Facebook pages "COVD" and "School screenings are not enough! Support comprehensive vision exams," there are also a number of patient-generated pages to which a referral should be made. One such page, "Vision Therapy Changed My Life," was started by a dedicated parent who was appalled by the fact that so many children were being labeled with learning disabilities, when they are often suffering from a difficulty in the way they process visual information. At the time of this writing, that particular fan page has over 425 members and continues to grow almost daily.

Twitter Another great social networking tool is Twitter. Twitter provides an opportunity for users to post status updates using 140 or fewer characters. It is possible to post articles and to "retweet" the posts of other users. Although many people who maintain Facebook pages also maintain Twitter accounts, many people use the sites for different purposes such as business or pleasure. Both Facebook and Twitter accounts can be linked so that status updates on one will be automatically published to the other. Because Twitter limits postings to 140 characters or less, longer Facebook status updates will become truncated.

It is important to maintain a Twitter account once it is set up. Many Twitter users start out making an account and then leave the account behind; abandoning an account is one of the biggest taboos in social media. It is akin to an empty dilapidated building with a giant sign boasting the practice's name and brand. It does not take a lot to maintain a Twitter account, but it does take some time.

The College of Optometrists in Vision Development maintains a Twitter account that currently has over 2,910 followers. The account is updated four to six times a week with important news, information, and inspirational stories about developmental optometry and OVT. The ultimate compliment on Twitter, undoubtedly, is what is referred to as the "retweet." It is when a post is reposted by another user so that it is available for his or her followers to read. There are many free programs available on the Internet that will allow the tracking of Twitter statistics. This will help in determining the effectiveness of postings.

Twitter is great in a number of ways, but one of the most important is the ability for users to search for key terms. For example, in setting a key term search for OVT, all relevant Twitter posts that include the words "optometric vision therapy" will be displayed. Be sure to list multiword terms within parentheses so that not every post that contains the words optometric, vision, or therapy is listed, unless of course, that is what is wanted. Posts go up daily on the topic of OVT and convergence insufficiency. Some posts are written by one of several OVT doctors or therapists who currently use Twitter, while other times, they are written by parents who just received a diagnosis and are looking for others who have had experience with OVT.

One of the most underused Twitter tools is the ability for users to create lists of their followers. Lists are helpful for a variety reasons. In the beginning, use lists generated by other users to build a network of followers. One of the biggest questions asked by Twitter followers is "How do I get more followers?" The answer is simple, "follow more people." In general, Twitter users will return the favor if they feel intentions are genuine (i.e., something is not trying to be sold). On COVD's Twitter page, a majority of COVD's followers are divided into lists. The College of Optometrists in Vision Development's list entitled "Eye Care" has over 500 members; the list for "Vision Therapy" has 348 members. That means there are 348 Twitter users on this list who are OVT doctors, therapists, parents, or patients, or have supported OVT by retweeting related posts.

Sovoto Connections within the OVT community are important for not only personal growth but also the improvement of the practice. Sovoto is a social networking site developed especially for doctors, therapists, and patients involved in OVT. Members connect with "friends," post on their walls, and share information about developmental optometry without all of the extras offered by Facebook and Twitter. At the time of this writing, active members regularly post topics for discussion as well as helpful videos and commentaries.

Blogging Many practitioners have decided to turn to blogging as a means of driving potential clients to their websites and other social media endeavors. Blogs are a means of communication that fosters an exchange between the reader and the author. Some blog topics are meant to be purely informative, while others serve to bring about discussion and even debate. Many doctors with a practice concentration of OVT currently host popular and dynamic blogs. This is important as Google now posts blogs in its search results. Perspective patients or parents who Google "vision therapy" or "special populations" are sure to come across a blog written by an optometrist interested in these areas. Table 30.4 lists several blogs.

It is important to remember that not all blog entries need to be lengthy in order to convey important messages. Some topics of interest may warrant a blog post that is several paragraphs in length, while others need only a few sentences that draw the reader's attention to a particular link. Time should be spent viewing blogs by other doctors before jumping into actual writing. Be sure to leave comments when a blog is interesting as this is another way to demonstrate that intentions are genuine.

Web Site A Web site should be a complete and well-planned representation of what services are available at the office. The Web site should be updated consistently with success stories and substantive information that will keep referral sources coming back. The news media and current patients might turn to the Web site to help them understand exactly what services are provided and the background of the practice including the practitioners and staff members. Pictures of all the members of the practice are always recommended as people are anxious to see those with whom they will be dealing. It is also advisable to post a biography of the lead practitioners and possibly key staff members. Remember to post the Web site address on every marketing piece produced. The Web site address should be short (the shorter the better) but also distinctive so that it can be easily remembered.

TABLE 30.4 Examples of Blogs Concerning Patients with Special Needs, OVT, and Other Topics of Interest

COVD Blog
http://covdblog.wordpress.com
MainosMemos
http://mainosmemos.blogspot.com
Eyes on the Brain
http:www.psychology.com/blog/eyes-the-brain
Adventures in Amblyopia
http://amblyopiakids.com
Autism Blogs
http://autism-hub.com/
Special Needs Blogs
http://specialchildren.about.com/od/blogs/Special_Needs_Blogs.htm
Traumatic Brain Injury
http://www.networkedblogs.com/search?q=traumatic+brain+injury
Dyslexia
http://www.networkedblogs.com/search?q=dyslexia
Bright Eyes News
BrightEyesNews.com
News From the AOA Blog
http://newsfromaoa.org
Little Four Eyes
http://littlefoureyes.com
Eye Can Too! Read
http:eyecantooread.blogspot.com
Down Syndrome Blogs
http://www.squidoo.com/downsyndromeblogs
Fragile X Blogs
http://www.networkedblogs.com/topic/fragile_x/
Learning Disabilities Blogs
http://www.networkedblogs.com/search?q=learning+disability
Edie Neurolearning
http://eideneurolearningblog.blogspot.com/
Gifted Children
http://giftedkids.about.com/

Newspaper Although fewer people subscribe than in the past, newspaper advertising is still a recommended tool primarily because of its affordability. Many offices have a great deal of success with infomercial news advertisements. They look like news articles with pictures and text on a specific topic but are actually advertisements that have been written either by someone in the office or by a service (Fig. 30-6). This type of advertisement appears to work well with grandparents who often clip out the articles in an effort to help a struggling grandchild. An educated grandparent can often be the best ally. It is estimated that as many as one-third of parents receive assistance of some sort from their child's grandparents.

Parents find Answers to their child's learning problems

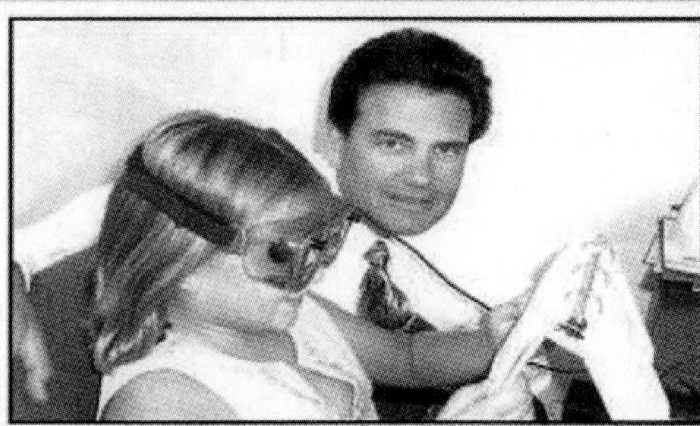

Dr. Habermehl uses computerized technology to help a student with reading problems

There's been a lot of attention lately on local schools, MEAP scores, and learning problems. Teachers are concerned about curriculum. Parents are asking about Ritalin. At the end of all this discussion is a child... a child who is struggling to read and write.

Many children are still waiting for answers to their dilemma. At the least, they are waiting for help with their homework. Or, in many cases, they quit trying and avoid schoolwork completely.

Many of these children may be diagnosed with a treatable vision-related learning problem. Vision is used for 80% of our learning process. Many children have not developed their visual system to be able to handle the demands of school.

The American Optometric Association (AOA) states that ten million U.S. children under age 12 have vision problems that make it hard to cope at home and school. School screenings can be misleading, because they do not test for these types of vision problems. Basic eye exams are intended to test for eye diseases and a need for eyeglasses. They may not detect vision-related learning problems.

Dr. Bradley E. Habermehl, local optometrist, offers specialized testing to diagnose vision problems that can be related to learning problems, including symptoms of A.D.D. "Children may see clearly, but not without discomfort or strain. They may even be seeing double at times, and it has simply been overlooked," states Habermehl.

An undiagnosed vision problem may be the missing piece for your child. Parents and students share the difference it made for them: "Katie began having problems with reading and math four years ago, especially tests and endless hours of homework! After being tested and going through the program, Katie enjoys reading. She gets all her homework done in school, and needs minimal to no help from mom with homework," one parent shares. "Her last report card was an A+ in Math, an A+ in English, and a B+ in Social Studies. Hooray!"

Another parent adds, "I can't say thank you enough. Matt improved in his reading. He is able to do homework in a short amount of time, and without complaining of headaches. His grades have improved consistently, and his self-esteem has improved too. His teachers are excited over the improvements he has made in his schoolwork and willingness to participate in class. Thank you for convincing him that he could when he thought he couldn't."

Symptoms of a vision-related learning problem:

- Avoids reading or other near work. Cannot sit still and finish a task.
- Loses place while reading. Skips words or has to use his/her finger to follow along.
- Tilts the head or leans while working up close. May cover one eye.
- Complains of headaches.
- Poor spelling - may pass the test but forgets the words soon after.
- Short attention span

Research more on this topic at: www.visiontherapygroup.com

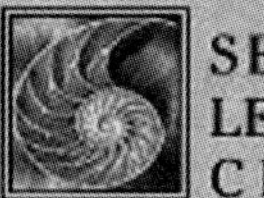

SENSORY LEARNING CENTER

Dr. Bradley Habermehl

810-736-6673

Located at 4091 Richfield Rd., Near Center Rd. in Flint

FIGURE 30-6. Newspaper advertisement is an affordable method of marketing. This example serves to educate the public on the issue to learning problems and provides effective marketing for the practice

Radio It is important to remember that radio is another excellent media source. Although it is more costly than newspaper, radio has the potential to reach thousands of new patients. A 30-second spot is commonly used and provides ample time to explain the "who" and "what" concerning the practice, and why it is important for patients to visit. Most radio stations provide help in writing and delivering the content of the infomercials as most practitioners are not accomplished writers or public speakers. In addition, radio programs may be saved and uploaded to the practice Web site or Facebook page. Many doctors choose to save their recordings for use at a later date. For example, the same "back to school special" presentations can be used for several years in a row.

Another way to advertise on radio is to connect with a local call-in radio show. It is common for local radio stations to have call-in shows on a variety of topics, including health care. Gaining a periodic spot on such a show not only educates potential patients but gets the practitioner's expertise front and center.

Television Television is one of the most costly media to use, but the results are probably the most immediate. A 30-second spot is usually the minimum amount of time you need to have your message heard. With television, the market audience can be selected in order to maximize the impact. For example, a spot aired during a news special highlighting the struggles of working with a child on the autistic spectrum would have a greater impact than one aired during a horror movie.

The practice Web site address and telephone number should be displayed the entire time the spot is playing. These videos can also be embedded on the home page of your Web site. Be sure to check with the local cable companies as they are an affordable option rather than using an actual television station.

Screenings Vision screenings are an effective marketing option that is relatively inexpensive. Local libraries are usually willing to partner with an office if the screening is free and promotes the library as a place to go to receive the vision screening. This becomes a win–win situation for all involved as it helps the children, library, and practice. It allows the office to have direct contact with the potential patient and the family and to make a necessary referral for further care if an abnormality is uncovered. Bookmarks, balloons, pencils, and other novelties may be used before the screening to promote the event. Always check with the Board of Optometry to ascertain if this is permitted because some states do not allow optometrists to do screenings. Remember that if the vision screening is perceived as only being a way to direct patients to the office, an invitation to return may not be forthcoming. It may be advisable to have a listing of doctors who provide outstanding care to give to those who need referral. Of course, this should be printed on the office's stationery.

In-service Programs When considering possible referral sources, do not forget fellow optometrists, as well as other professionals. Our colleagues in the health care field often need reminders of the services offered. Consider contacting these offices directly and offering a list of services provided as well as ways these services can be used to treat the eye and vision problems associated with conditions such as traumatic brain injury, stroke, sensory processing disorder, autism spectrum disorder, and attention deficit hyperactivity disorder.

In-service programs should be offered free of charge and built into any marketing program. Plan to spend one afternoon or morning presenting the in-service program, giving a tour of the office, and answering any questions that arise. Do not hesitate to break the in-service attendees into groups in order to demonstrate what services are provided. Make a point to have each and every attendee experience at least one diagnostic test or therapy procedure.

It is also important to follow up with all referral sources since they have entrusted the office with the care of their patients. A phone call or letter explaining the treatment and progression of therapy is always recommended. Be certain to check back with the referral sources a few times each year to ask if they may need additional information about the office, and if they do, send previously prepared packets, pamphlets or research articles.

Parent Advocates The best and least expensive marketing tool is word of mouth from a patient or parent advocate. A parent advocate is usually someone whose child or grandchild has completed your program successfully. They often add a tremendous amount of credibility to marketing because it is not you who brings the message.

Local parenting support groups are always looking for speakers who are able to bring topics of interest to their members. Support groups on a variety of topics and conditions can easily be found on the Internet. Taking along a parent advocate is always suggested so that they too can speak to the support group about their experiences. Many parents love to share their success story and are often the best marketers for a practice. There is nothing better than a passionate parent who wants to share his or her success with other parents in the community.

The secret to a good marketing program is consistency. Establish a monthly budget that adequately tells all about the patient-friendly services and materials offered. Research has shown that a message must be seen multiple times before it is acted upon. Repetition not only makes sure that potential patients hear the message but reminds them of all that can be done for those served.

CONCLUSION

Whatever the practitioner's goal, regardless of profession, the topics covered in this chapter are essential.

Mastering and implementing each of the discussed topics will not only enhance the look and feel of the practice but also improve the financial picture. A thriving practice is one that spends significant time focusing on business development. This makes it possible to focus on successfully treating patients, allowing them to reach their potential.

REFERENCES

1. Convergence Insufficiency Treatment Trial Investigator Group. Randomized clinical trial of treatments for symptomatic convergence insufficiency in children. Arch Ophthalmol. 2008;126:1336–49.
2. Vision Therapy Supplies and Sources, Optometric Extension Program Foundation. Available from: http://www.oepf.org/CCVTList.php. Last Accessed February 25, 2011.
3. Optometric Extension Program Foundation. Available from: www.oepf.org. Last Accessed February 25, 2011.
4. College of Optometrists in Vision Development. Available from: www.covd.org. Last Accessed February 25, 2011.
5. Neuro Optometric Vision Rehabilitation Association. Available from: www.nora.cc. Last Accessed February 25, 2011.
6. American Optometric Association. Available from: www.aoa.org. Last Accessed February 25, 2011.
7. American Academy of Optometry. Available from: www.aaopt.org. Last Accessed February 25, 2011.
8. Medicare Benefit Policy Manual, Covered Medical and Other Health Services. Available from: https://www.cms.gov/manuals/Downloads/bp102c15.pdf. Last Accessed February 25, 2011.

CHAPTER 31

Leonard J. Press, OD, FAAO, FCOVD
Nancy Torgerson, OD, FCOVD

The Process of Communication

INTRODUCTION

There is a saying, attributed to an old African proverb, that *It Takes a Village to Raise a Child.* The phrase is appropriate in conveying that the entire office is involved in the effort to establish and maintain effective communication with the special needs patient and his or her family. Although the patient with special needs need not be a child, the preponderance of our practices are devoted to children with special needs. When we refer to the "family" of the patient, it may involve a parent, grandparent, spouse, guardian, acquaintance, or caretaker. Communications is a broad area that permeates all chapters in this text, but in this chapter we focus specifically on intake and history forms, examination data recording forms, and samples of reports to the multidisciplinary team typically involved in the care of the patient with special needs.

SECTION 1: INTERNAL COMMUNICATION

History Forms/Questionnaires For the family of a patient with special needs, time is a precious commodity. Anything that can be done to streamline the completion of forms prior to coming to the office makes the office visit more efficient. It enables the focus to be on the patient from the time of entry.

History forms should have information related to the patient's medical, ocular, visual, nutritional, developmental, and academic histories, as well as a symptom checklist. This enables the parent to recognize pertinent items without having to worry about spelling. It is helpful to know if the child already has a diagnosis or, in the case of multiple handicaps, multiple diagnoses such as being on the autism spectrum, or having cerebral palsy, Down syndrome and any visual impairment.

If the child has had prior interventions or therapies, what has been the outcome to date? A significant number of children with special needs have had early intervention services consisting of occupational, physical, and speech therapy. Most therapies that these children receive persist for years. Services may be provided by the state in the patient's home- or school-based environment and in many instances continue in a private practice group environment such as a children's therapy center.

Children on the autistic spectrum may have often had targeted interventions such as Applied Behavioral Analysis (ABA), Floor Time Therapy (DIR), or some form of auditory processing therapies or listening programs such as Tomatis or Samonas. (Chapter 8, Autism) If so, were the therapies completed? If not, how much additional time is projected? Reading prior reports, factored together with information supplied by the parents or caregivers, will provide key information to elaborate the history. Activities and behaviors in the home may be quite different than the way the child functions in an office, institutional, academic, or therapeutic environment. If background information is used to initially probe history, ask open-ended questions that give the adult the opportunity to offer their perspective, for example:

1. "Why do you feel your child needs a visual evaluation?"
2. "Briefly describe your child as a person."

This information enables you to prioritize the sequence of the evaluation. You want to allocate your time wisely since there is often a limited window of opportunity during which the child will be a willing participant. The history can illustrate how the family dynamics and stressors are involved, and which factors need to be considered in the recommendations and treatment plan.

You should inquire about any special tutoring, therapy, or remedial assistance, as well as the source, duration, and results of these interventions. Probe the child's attitude and experiences toward reading, school, teachers, and peers. For some questions, such as a history of epilepsy or seizures, a parent may be unsure of the relevance of the answer to visual care. For other questions, such as the use of glasses, the understanding and intent will be more apparent. The answers to all these questions may take up much more space than what is provided on the history form. These forms are an inventory that serves as the basis for further discussion and documentation.

There will be instances when a parent has a different perspective than what is indicated in a prior report. It will be important to compare what is written with what a parent notes. Parent conference sessions can be useful and should take place at a time distinct from the evaluations to gain agreement on any differences. For example, a child may have difficulty with eye contact or socialization, but the parent does not feel that a diagnosis of autism is warranted. Conversely, a parent may indicate that a child has a specific diagnosis from another professional, such as attention deficit hyperactivity disorder (ADHD), primarily because that is the best descriptor that enables the child to qualify for certain interventions, services, or accommodations (Appendix A).

Acquired brain injury (ABI) presents a unique set of circumstances, requiring targeted questions overlaid on a more generalized history form. The questions address a description of the injury or accident, its source or origin, posttraumatic consciousness state, associated visual signs and symptoms, and subsequent care. The names of other professionals who have examined the patient along with results of their evaluations and recommendations must be considered. In contrast with developmental disabilities, ABI presents more of an opportunity for comparison of changes in function and performance compared to a known state prior to specific events that caused the ABI. As a general rule, parents of a special needs child may know the child better and have more insights than the professionals who have performed the evaluation. When a patient has an ABI, functions and behaviors may be puzzling to family members but more recognizable to a professional. Other associated ABI injuries may involve sports concussions, and determining the timeline of these brain injuries is an important component of the history. The case history will need to be extensive and comprehensive for patients with special needs (Appendix B).

Symptom checklists are useful supplements to history questionnaires. The most common checklists in practice and for research purposes are either the College of Vision Development-Quality of Life (COVD-QOL) symptom checklist (1) or the Convergence Insufficiency Symptom Survey (2). For special needs populations, the COVD-QOL is more pertinent, though by no means exhaustive. (The COVD-QOL is discussed in greater detail in Chapter 16, Comprehensive Examination Procedures.) Similar checklists can be adapted for your own purposes. As adapted for ABI, a symptoms checklist can be further differentiated into phases. As an example:

Sign/Symptom	**New Problem**	**Present Before But Worse Since Brain Injury**
Poor visual memory	X	
Double vision		X
Difficulties reading	X	

One important aspect in assessing symptoms in patients with special needs is that they in fact may be asymptomatic. In an study of 202 subjects with either mental illness or a dual diagnosis of mental illness and intellectual disability who were taking oral medications, Donati et al. showed that the most common complaint was "no complaint" (46.16% MI and 46.84% DD). Blurred vision (17.74% MI and 17.72% DD) and the need for new glasses (11.29% MI and 17.72% DD) were common complaints. Given that the medications that this group as a whole were taking, the amount of complaints were expected to be higher. Clinicians should not be surprised if objective and subjective findings are not well correlated (3).

Examination Forms Examination forms serve as a bridge between internal and external communication. Some practitioners have an individual in the room who can serve as a scribe to improve efficiency during the exam. In addition, proper examination forms, whether electronic or paper, can streamline documentation of the encounter. With parental consent, the evaluation may be audio/video recorded allowing for transfer of information to the patient's record at a subsequent time. Efficient documentation enables the focus to be on the patient from the time of entry and helps get the information needed to make the proper diagnosis, management, and treatment plan. Specialized forms should be created for different types of examinations: children versus adults, new patients versus former patients, strabismic or amblyopic evaluations and visual rehabilitation evaluation related to ABI, stroke, or motor vehicle accident.

The basic form can be used to make documentation of the visual evaluation as straightforward as possible. Places to circle answers or check answers or behaviors allow the doctor more time to interact with the child. Having open space for recording observations or thoughts on a supplemental form is crucial as there is great variability when working with those with special needs. Consider, for example, visual field testing. Standard preliminary testing may be a checklist item, but this may need to be performed differently for poorly responding patients. Because of motor challenges, cognitive or processing delays, or lack of attention, the patient with special needs may not be able to perform automated perimetry. The test may need to be simplified such as performing confrontation fields with large objects and assessing peripheral awareness of the target from nonseeing to seeing field of view. These results would be best recorded on a supplemental form (Appendix C). The top of each page of the examination form should have vital information such as the patient's name, date of birth, and date of evaluation. Documentation of the time of day may be useful in determining the patient's future progress.

For patients with special needs, behavioral responses and qualitative observations will be important to record. For example, observations about ocular motility will be enhanced by either digital or video recording, or illustration of the patient's responses, including head posture, body posture, and emotional responses or signs of sensory overload versus calming effects of various stimuli. The illustration of the use of digital images for communication purposes is described in the sample reports discussed later in the chapter.

Particularly when first working with patients with special needs, the examination form can help guide the clinician on the flow of visual evaluation, as well as in communicating this information to others. When a test does not fit the ability of the child or when there are outbursts during the examination, the clinician needs to improvise. A quick glance at a well-designed examination form will aid the clinician to stay on task. Appendix D illustrates a form that is useful for recording observations and effects of yoked prisms during the eye examination and in therapy.

SECTION 2: EXTERNAL COMMUNICATION

Patient Reports Writing a report that summarizes examination or treatment information is an essential component of the care process for patients with special needs. Coordination of care is becoming increasingly important as it has become commonplace for a single child to be concurrently enrolled in multiple therapies (4,5). Despite the importance of communication in patient care, it is not pervasive among practitioners. In a study of 963 patients referred to specialists from primary care physicians, only about half of pediatricians reported communication either before or after the consultation (6). In a second study of 412 primary care and specialty pediatricians, only 28% reported receiving information frequently (more than 60% of the time) from the referring primary care physician although 70% reported frequent communication back from the specialist. Reported barriers included inefficiencies in phone contact, transcription delay, and failure to keep all providers informed when more than one specialist is involved (7). Communication between doctors and other providers was a particular area of weakness in a survey of parents of children with special needs. Only 37% of parents reported communication as very good to excellent (8).

It is a good idea to wait to write the report until after the conference, as sometimes issues arise that tempers the recommendations. Increasingly, technology is used to convey findings, including flip video recordings, external digital images, and biomicroscopic images. The three sample reports with images found below show the variety of information and detail needed to facilitate communication among parents, physicians, as well as other professionals who are taking part in patient care.

CASE 1: HISTORY OF CEREBELLAR HYPOPLASIA

To Whom It May Concern

XX was evaluated in my office on December 14, 2009. She has a reported history of cerebellar hypoplasia. Her mother reported that she has been exhibiting tic/blinking behavior and has hearing aids in both ears. I originally evaluated XX in 2006 upon referral from _____, her physical therapist. XX has been evaluated by Dr. _____, a pediatric neurologist, and her pediatrician is Dr. _____.

Mrs. _____ noted that XX seems to scan quickly and that her eyes are often well ahead of her motor response capabilities. XX uses a DynaVox assistive communication device at a distance of approximately 20 inches. She reportedly is not responsive to this or other material presented below eye level. During my examination, XX exhibited some behaviors that were not present during my last evaluation of her on April 15, 2008. She used some "stimming behaviors" with her hands, as visually impaired children tend to do. Although I was not able to obtain preferential looking responses to Snellen-equivalent stimuli, I was able to obtain good optokinetic nystagmus responses.

From a functional standpoint, XX was able to see relatively small targets of interest, so her useful functional vision remains high. She did however show an aversion to convergence, or looking at a target within 20 inches. When I interposed lenses during nearpoint retinoscopy, XX showed an aversion to looking through the lenses. I conducted confrontation visual fields, and XX was responsive to three of the four primary visual quadrants—upward, leftward, and rightward, but as reported by her mother she was unresponsive to looking at targets below eye level. This was the case even though the targets were of interest to her in the other positions of gaze.

I therefore decided to put on a trial pair of base-down yoked prisms. The theory behind the use of these lenses is that they shift space in the direction opposite to the base of the prism. In this instance, the base-down prism moves targets below eye level upward and more into the patient's field of visual capture. XX's visual responses were photodocumented as follows:

The first photo shows XX unable to converge, or move her eyes inward to follow an approaching target. This was also her response when visual stimuli were presented below eye level.

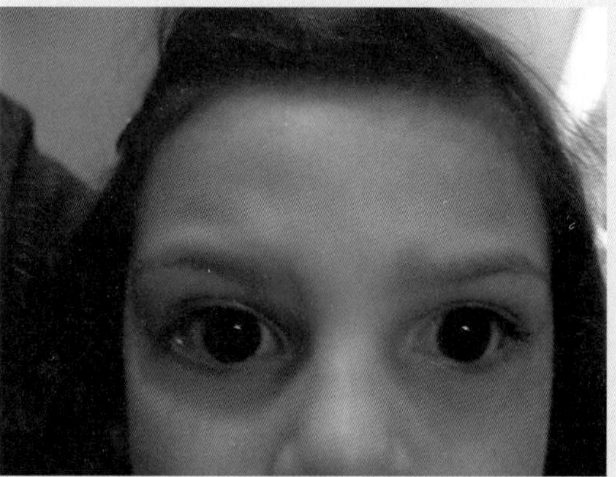

The second figure shows XX converging to the approaching "Big Bird" finger puppet target with the yoked prism lenses in place.

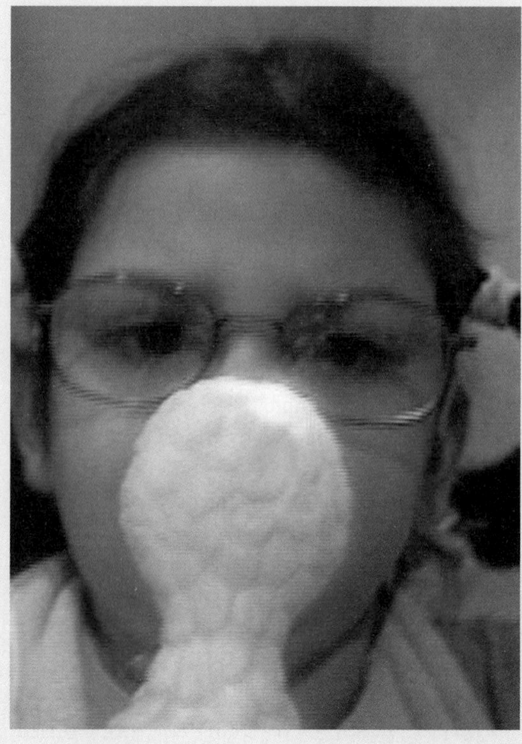

The third photo shows XX looking at a central target at eye level with yoked prism lenses in place.

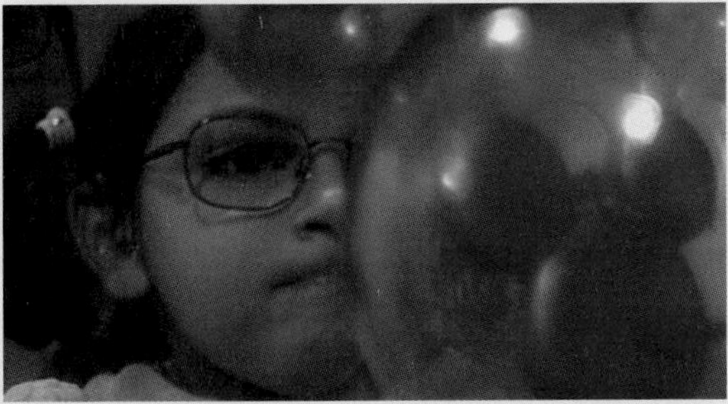

The fourth photo shows XX looking at a target below eye level with yoked prisms in place.

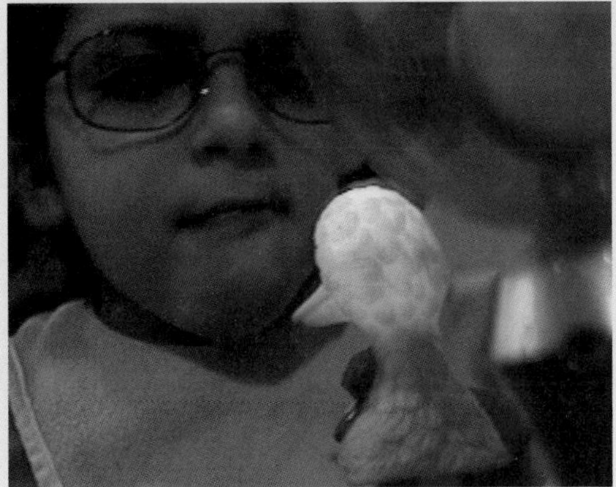

XX's responses were encouraging, so we dispensed the loaner pair of glasses that contained +0.50 power in both lenses (slight magnification) with three prism diopters yoked bases down. I saw XX in follow-up on January 14, 2010, and her mother reported excellent responses to wearing the lenses in school. In addition to being able to converge and attend to material below her eye level, important due to motor control and postural issues, XX's blinking or tic movements have reportedly stopped.

Given the positive responses, we made XX her own lenses and advised Mrs. ____ to have XX wear them as much as possible. To further expand XX's near function, I suggested that her therapists continue to use visual targets of interest. XX was very responsive to tracking targets across her midline. I indicated that convergence and field awareness can be worked on therapeutically in a manner similar to the testing arrangement photodocumented above. Targets should slowly be moved inward and outward along the midline, as well as from the outward position inward, coming from one side and then from the opposite side.

CASE 2: AUTISTIC SPECTRUM PROFILE

This is a report written to the referring Occupational Therapist:

Dear _____,

I had the pleasure of evaluating YY in my office on November 11, 2009, pursuant to concerns you raised that may be related to visual issues. The concerns included tripping, stumbling, clumsiness, inattentiveness, eye–hand coordination difficulties, visual motor difficulties, and the appearance of her eyes turning in at times (not being in midline).

She is neurologically impaired and in a full-day ABA program at _____. Her mother notes that YY does not seem to be able to scan reading materials from a normal reading distance, and that she tilts her head in one direction when watching television. Both parents accompanied her to the evaluation, the results of which are as follows.

YY adopts a habitual head posture with her face rotated toward the right, favoring gaze toward her left side. In general, it is more difficult for her to track to her left. (See Photos A and B).

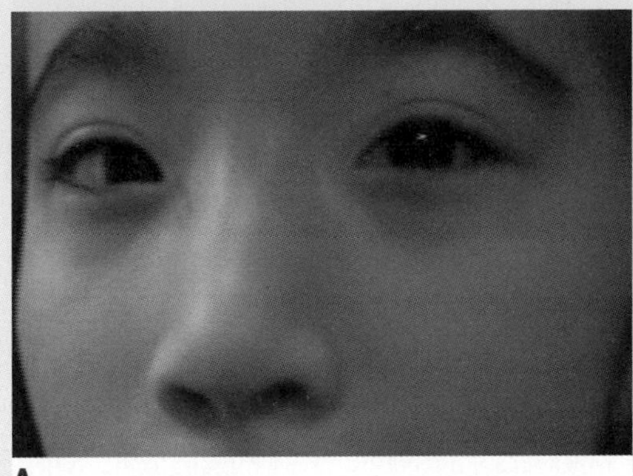

A

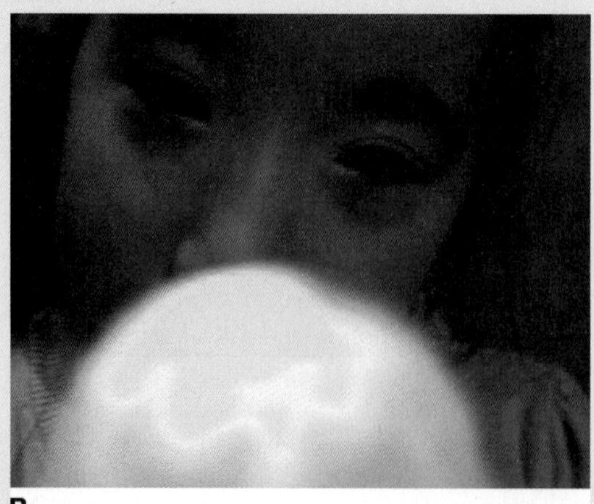

B

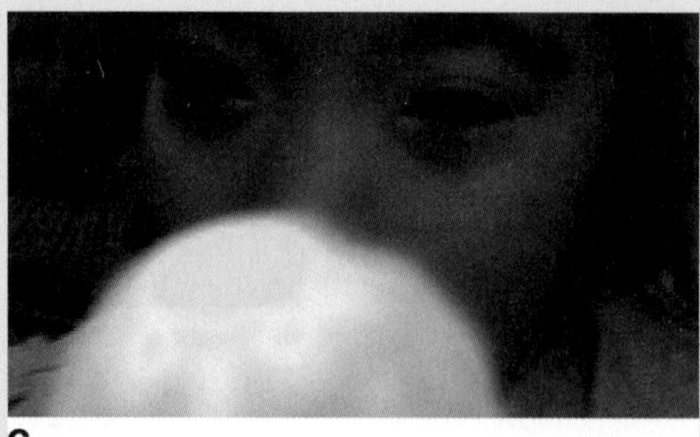

C

YY was able to attend to puppet face targets on the midline at near, but again rotated her head to the right and tilted her head to the left as noted above. (See Photo C).

When a child has a habitual head turn of this nature, it is sometimes related to an inability to abduct, or move the opposite eye outward. We ruled out a compensatory head turn by lightly restraining YY's head turn while she followed a target of interest to the right. She was able to abduct, or move the right eye outward, fully as noted below. (See Photo C).

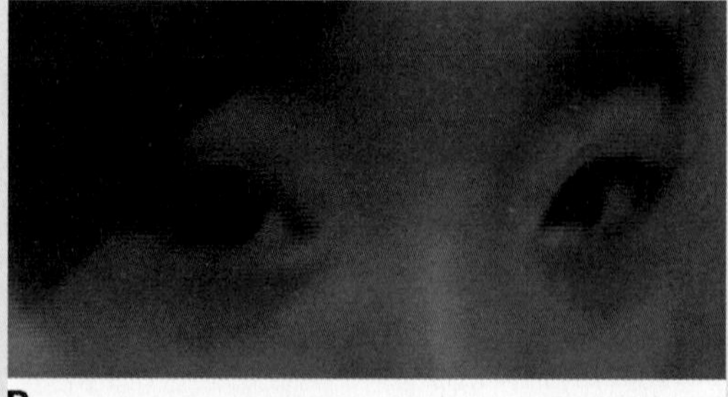

D

YY demonstrated normal reflex eye movement patterns with the pediatric optokinetic nystagmus drum targets consisting of caricatured animals and vertical line gratings, in both the naso-temporal and tempero-nasal directions. The symmetry in her reflex motor responses supports the absence of strabismus (misalignment of the eyes) as well as the ability to scan in all directions equally. YY is able to converge her eyes accurately and is able to maintain binocular eye contact on the midline when she attends to targets of interest, as evidenced below. Hirschberg corneal light reflexes indicated alignment, and Bruckner reflexes were normal. She does, however, lose interest in visual fixation quickly, necessitating frequent changes in target selection. YY was able to cross the midline effectively, with mild head restraint, when tracking a "Mickey Mouse" target. To sustain interest, we alternated between the target being illuminated and nonilluminated. When illuminated, the target has internal spinning lights. She did not exhibit any seizure-like activity in response to the flicker.
YY exhibited normal preferential looking responses to large grating patterns, and retinoscopy yielded no significant nearsightedness, farsightedness, or astigmatism in either eye. Red reflexes and internal eye structures were healthy and normal in appearance. Lastly, we were able to obtain normal confrontation visual field responses when having YY fixate a central target, while a peripheral target was illuminated.

In conclusion, YY has normal eye health, and her eyesight is adequate for all visual tasks. She is not in need of spectacle lenses at this time. She did not display any change in performance through yoked prism probes, as do some children having developmental and/or neurologic delays. We therefore conclude that the issues you're observing are not due to primary visual or ocular motor problems, but secondary to primary postural skews and global attention issues. YY will benefit from continued visual stimulation, particularly with regard to tracking visual targets of interest toward her right side. This may have to be done with mild head restraint to reduce her skew in rotating her head toward the right rather than her eyes. Ultimately her visual abilities will be gated by her overall ability to attend rather than any primary visual or eye limitations.

I will be having a conference with her parents this afternoon to review these findings, and recommendations for ongoing Occupational Therapy and Physical Therapy. Optometric vision therapy may be of benefit with lenses, prisms, and/or filters, but would be very challenging at this time. I would like to reassess her progress in 6 months. Thank you, _____, for your excellent observations, and for suggesting that YY's parents have her undergo a developmental optometric examination.

CASE 3: ACQUIRED BRAIN INJURY

This is a letter written to the patient's case manager:

Dear _____,

I had the pleasure of evaluating ZZ in my office on April 7, 2010 and subsequently on April 19. Her history is well known to you. Automated visual field testing confirmed that ZZ has a right homonymous hemianopsia, requiring her to scan toward her right visual field to maintain awareness of objects in that field. She has a constant large angle left exotropia, which is a drift of the left eye outward of approximately 40 prism diopters. (See Photo A) The acuity of that eye is reduced to between 20/50 and 20/60. This is in contrast to her right eye, which has acuity between 20/25 and 20/30.

ZZ has a variable ptosis or drooping of the eyelid of the left eye. This may be occurring subconsciously so that her brain can ignore what would otherwise be a double image coming from the left eye. She can exhibit brief voluntary convergence to try and align the eye. (See Photo B)

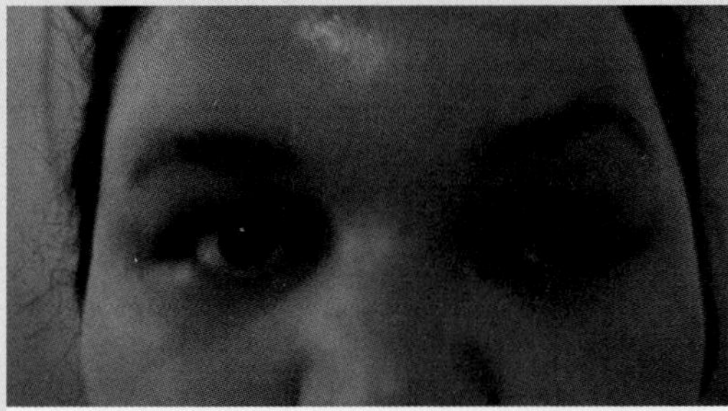
A

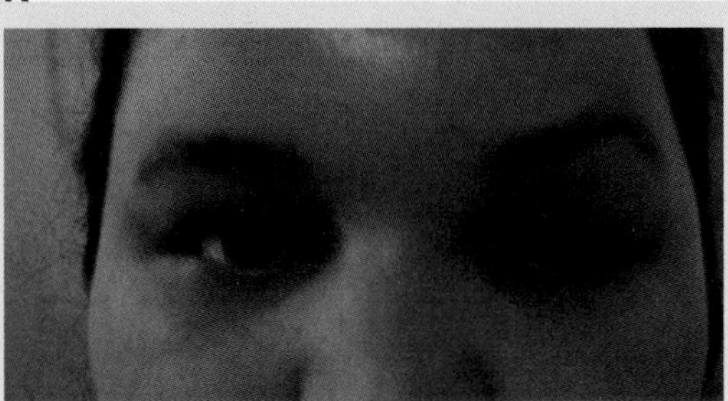
B

I spoke with ZZ's neurologist, Dr. _____, who was concerned about ruling out papilledema, or swelling of the optic nerves. I reassured him that while the optic nerves have some pale tone, there is no edema around the disk, and sent him photographs that document this (See Photos C and D).

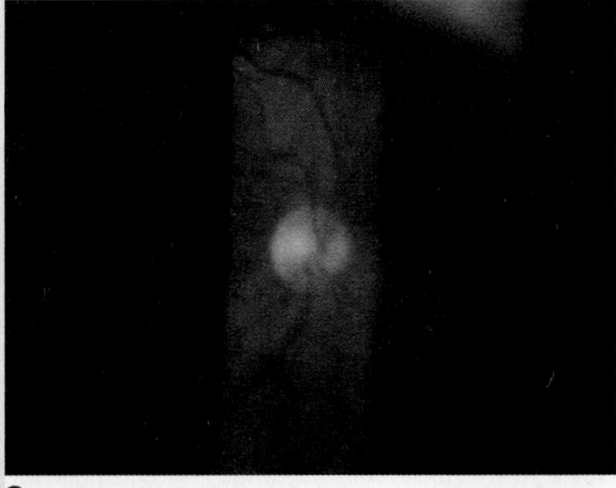
C

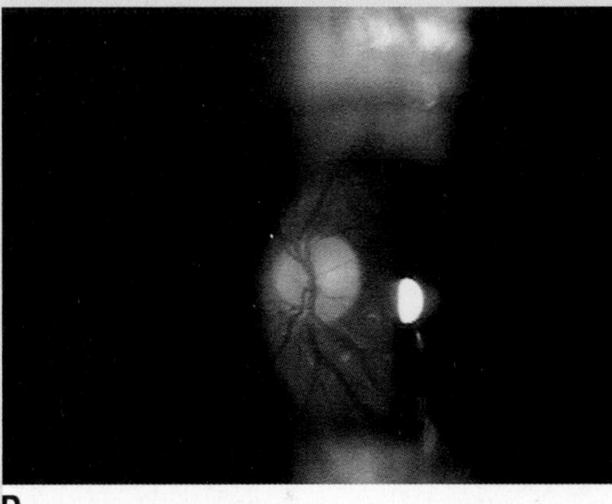
D

On all fusion tests, ZZ exhibited diplopia (double vision) when both eyes were open. Predictably, she has no measurable binocular depth perception. We recorded her eye movements with the Visagraph, and she was able to comprehend a passage with her left eye shut, though the scan path with her right eye showed erratic movements. With both eyes open, she saw double and was unable to read.

Acquired exophoria or tropia, the outward drift of ZZ's left eye, is common after ABI as occurred during her motor vehicle accident, as are various forms of visual field loss. I have prescribed a program of optometric vision therapy that will improve ZZ's fusion, the ability to use both eyes together simultaneously, and also work toward expanding her visual field awareness. Although we did not obtain a positive response initially to the use of prisms, we will continue to probe their application as related to field awareness and facilitating fusion.

CONCLUSION

Developing one's ability to communicate more efficiently also provides the opportunity to educate more effectively. As we have demonstrated, there are three principal areas or patient constituencies that communications serve:

1. **The Patient**—Having forms that are well organized helps streamline observations if you are recording while attempting to examine. If you have a chairside assistant recording your observations and findings, you may be less reliant on preprinted forms, but with the approaching ubiquity of EHR (Electronic Health Records), at some level your examination findings will be organized with uniformity. That will assist you as well as staff members in your office in communicating with the patient on subsequent visits.
2. **The Parent, Spouse, or Caretaker**—History checklists and surveys provide the opportunity to educate the family or other caregivers on areas of mutual concerns. There are numerous aspects of the developing or recovering visual system that may not have been associated with ocular or ophthalmic implications by the patient's support network. Seeing the items listed often opens the door to further discussion, specialized testing, or other considerations for management.
3. **Other Professionals**—Care of the patient with special needs involves a multitude of professionals. Much as the developmental/rehabilitative optometrist is enlightened and informed by reports from others, the written report generated will serve to inform and educate others about optometric care.

Communication regarding patients with special needs will progressively reflect the sophistication in emerging technologies. We envision that this will involve telemedicine consultation involving digitally embedded visuals, streaming audiovisual communication, and other forms of media on the horizon. For the foreseeable future, however, nothing substitutes for the human touch, and that must be evident in your communications.

APPENDIX A

CHILDREN'S VISION QUESTIONNAIRE

Appointment: Day ______________ Date ________________ Time _____________

Patient's Name:____

Patient's Nickname:____

GENERAL INFORMATION

Were you referred to our office? Yes ☐ No ☐

If yes, whom may we thank for this referral? ____________ Phone: ______________

Address: ________________________________Profession:_______________

Child's Full Legal Name: ______________________________Male _____ Female ____

Birth Date: __________________________ Age: _________years ________months

Home Address: ____

City: ____________________State:_____ Zip:_____Home Phone: ______________

Name and address of school: ____________________________________

Grade: ______________ Teacher:_______________________________________

Child's dominant hand (circle): right / left / undetermined?

Please list the names and birth dates of your family:

Father/Caretaker ____________________________Birth Date ________________

Mother/Caretaker ____________________________Birth Date ________________

Sibling ____________________________________Birth Date ________________

Sibling ____________________________________Birth Date ________________

Sibling ____________________________________Birth Date ________________

Sibling ____________________________________Birth Date ________________

ACCOUNT RESPONSIBLE INFORMATION

Person Responsible for Account: ______________________ Relationship to Patient: ______________

Account Responsible Address: ____

Account Responsible SSN: ___________________________ Home Phone: _______________

Father/Caretaker's Occupation: _______________________ Work Phone: _______________

E-mail: ____ Cell Phone: _______________

Mother/Caretaker's Occupation: ______________________ Work Phone: _______________

E-mail: ____ Cell Phone: _______________

In Case of Emergency Contact: _______________________ Phone: ____________________

Do you have Vision Insurance? Yes ☐ No ☐ If so, who is the carrier? ___________________

Insurance Address: _________________________________ Insurance Phone: ______________

Subscriber Name: ________________________ DOB: ______________ SSN: _______________

Subscriber ID# (incl. letter prefix): _____________________ Group #: ___________________

Do you have Medical Insurance? Yes ☐ No☐ If so, who is the carrier? ___________________

Insurance Address: _________________________________ Insurance Phone: ______________

Subscriber Name: ________________________ DOB: ______________ SSN: _______________

Subscriber ID# (incl. letter prefix): _____________________ Group #: ___________________

PLEASE REMEMBER TO BRING YOUR INSURANCE CARD(S) WITH YOU TO YOUR APPOINTMENT.

MEDICAL HISTORY

Pediatrician's Name: ____

Child's current state of health: ____

Medications currently using, including vitamins and supplements: ______________________________

____

For what condition(s)? ____

____

Any allergies to medications?______________________________

List illnesses, bad falls, high fevers, etc.:

Age	Severe	Mild	Complications

Is your child generally healthy? Yes ☐ No ☐

If no, explain: ______________________________

Are there any chronic problems like ear infections, asthma, hay fever, allergies? Yes ☐ No ☐

If yes, please list: ______________________________

Has your child been diagnosed on the autism spectrum? Yes ☐ No ☐

Does your child have a seizure disorder? Yes ☐ No ☐

Does your child have a sleep disorder? Yes ☐ No ☐

Has a neurological evaluation been performed? Yes ☐ No ☐

By whom? ____________________ Results and recommendations: ____________

____

Has a psychological evaluation been performed? Yes ☐ No ☐

By whom? ____________________ Results and recommendations: ____________

____

Has an occupational / speech / physical therapy evaluation been performed? Yes ☐ No ☐

By whom? ____________________ Results and recommendations: ____________

____

Has your child or a family member been treated for any condition related to:

	Patient	**Family**	**Whom**		**Patient**	**Family**	**Whom**
Eyes	☐	☐	____	Neurological	☐	☐	____
Ears, Nose, Throat	☐	☐	____	Endocrine Disorder	☐	☐	____
Cardiovascular health	☐	☐	____	Genitourinary	☐	☐	____
Respiratory	☐	☐	____	Skin	☐	☐	____

Gastrointestinal health	☐	☐	______	Musculoskeletal	☐	☐	______
Psychiatric	☐	☐	______	Hematological/lymphatic	☐	☐	______
Allergic/immunologic	☐	☐	______	Other	☐	☐	______

Specifically is there any history of the following? (Please check if there is a history)

	Patient	**Family**	**Whom**		**Patient**	**Family**	**Whom**
Diabetes	☐	☐	______	High Blood Pressure	☐	☐	______
"Cross"/"Wall" eye	☐	☐	______	Learning Disability	☐	☐	______
Chromosomal Imbalance	☐	☐	______	Amblyopia (lazy eye)	☐	☐	______
Thyroid Condition	☐	☐	______	Epilepsy or Seizures	☐	☐	______
Glaucoma	☐	☐	______	Multiple Sclerosis	☐	☐	______
Macular Degeneration	☐	☐	______	AutismSpectrum Disorder	☐	☐	______

If other, please explain: ______________________________

NUTRITIONAL INFORMATION

Current Diet: Excellent ☐ Good ☐ Fair ☐ Poor ☐

Does your child: Like sweets ☐ or crave sweets ☐

If yes, what types? ______________________________

Is your child active? Yes ☐ No ☐

moderately? Yes ☐ No ☐

extremely? Yes ☐ No ☐

Are there periods of: very high energy? Yes ☐ No ☐ very low energy? Yes ☐ No ☐

Explain: ______________________________

DEVELOPMENTAL HISTORY

Full-term pregnancy? Yes ☐ No ☐

Did the mother experience any health problems during the pregnancy? Yes ☐ No ☐

If yes, explain: ______________________________

Normal birth? Yes ☐ No ☐

Any complications before, during or immediately following delivery? Yes ☐ No ☐

If yes, explain: ______________________________

Birth weight: ______ Apgar scores at birth: ____ After 10 minutes: ______

Were forceps used? Yes ☐ No ☐

Was there ever a reason for concern over your child's general growth or development?

Yes ☐ No ☐

If yes, why? ______________________________

Did your child crawl (stomach on floor)? Yes ☐ No ☐ At what age? ____________

Did your child creep (on all fours)? Yes ☐ No ☐ At what age? ____________

If not, describe: ______________________________

At what age did your child walk? ______________________________

Was your child active? Yes ☐ No ☐

Speech: First words: ______________________________ At what age: ____

Was early speech clear to others? Yes ☐ No ☐

Is speech clear now? Yes ☐ No ☐

VISUAL HISTORY

Has your child's vision been previously evaluated? Yes ☐ No ☐

If so, Doctor's Name: ____________________ Date of last evaluation: _______

Reason for examination: ______________________________

Results and recommendations: ______________________________

Were glasses, contact lenses, or other optical devices recommended? Yes ☐ No ☐

If yes, what? ______________________________

Are they used? Yes ☐ No ☐ If yes, when? ______________________________

If not used, why not? ______________________________

Members of the family who have had visual attention and the reason:

Name	Age	Visual Situation
____________________	___	______________________
____________________	___	______________________
____________________	___	______________________

PRESENT SITUATION

Why do you feel your child needs a visual evaluation? ______________________________

How long has this problem/difficulty been observed? ______________________________

Is there any evidence from the school, psychological, or other tests that indicates some visual malfunction may be present? Yes ☐ No ☐

If yes, what? ______________________________

____

DOES YOUR CHILD REPORT ANY OF THE FOLLOWING:

	Yes	**If yes, when?**
Headaches	☐	________
Blurred vision	☐	________
Double vision	☐	________
Eyes hurt	☐	________
Eyes tired	☐	________
Words move around on the page	☐	________
Motion sickness / car sickness	☐	________
Dizziness	☐	________
Frequent sties	☐	________

List any other complaints your child makes concerning his/her vision: ________________

____

HAVE YOU OR ANYONE ELSE EVER NOTICED THE FOLLOWING:

	Yes	**If yes, when?**
Moves head when reading	☐	________
Skips, re-reads or omits words	☐	________
Loses place while reading	☐	________
Reads slowly	☐	________
Uses finger as a marker	☐	________

Eyes frequently reddened	☐	________
Frequent eye rubbing	☐	________
Frowning	☐	________
Bothered by light	☐	________
Frequent blinking	☐	________
Closing or covering one eye	☐	________
Head close to paper when reading or writing	☐	________
Focus goes in and out	☐	________
Avoids reading	☐	________
Prefers being read to	☐	________
Tilts head when reading	☐	________
Tilts head when writing	☐	________
Confuses letter or words	☐	________
Reverses letter or words	☐	________
Difficulty copying from chalkboard	☐	________
Vocalizes when reading silently	☐	________
Confuses right and left	☐	________
Poor reading comprehension	☐	________
Comprehension decreases over time	☐	________
Tires easily	☐	________
Difficulty recognizing same word on different page	☐	________
Poor word attack skills	☐	________
Difficulty with memory	☐	________

Remembers better what hears than sees	☐	____________
Responds better orally than by writing	☐	____________
Seems to know material, but does poorly on tests	☐	____________
Dislikes / avoids near tasks	☐	____________
Short attention span / loses interest	☐	____________
Poor large motor coordination	☐	____________
Poor fine motor coordination	☐	____________
Difficulty with scissors / small hand tools	☐	____________
Dislikes / avoids sports	☐	____________
Difficulty catching / hitting a ball	☐	____________
Writes or prints poorly	☐	____________
Writes neatly but slowly	☐	____________
Does not support paper when writing	☐	____________
Awkward or immature pencil grip	☐	____________
Frequent erases	☐	____________

TELEVISION VIEWING/LEISURE TIME ACTIVITIES

Does child watch TV? Yes ☐ No ☐

If yes, how much? ____________ How often? ____________ Viewing distance? ________

Does your child spend time using computer/video games? Yes ☐ No ☐

If yes, how much? ____________ How often? ____________ Viewing distance? ________

What other activities occupy your child's leisure time? ________________________

Are there any activities your child would like to participate in, but doesn't?

Please explain: ____

____

SCHOOL

Age at time of entrance to: Pre-school _____ Kindergarten _____ First Grade __________

Does your child like school? Yes ☐ No ☐

Specifically describe any school difficulties: ____

____

Has your child changed schools often? Yes ☐ No ☐

If yes, when? ____

Has a grade been repeated? Yes ☐ No ☐

If yes, which and why? ____

Does your child seem to be under tension or pressure when doing school work?

Yes ☐ No ☐

Has your child had any special tutoring, therapy, and/or remedial assistance?

Yes ☐ No ☐

If yes, when? ____

Where and from whom? ____

How long? ____

Results: ____

Does your child like to read? Yes ☐ No ☐

Voluntarily? Yes ☐ No ☐

Does your child read for pleasure? Yes ☐ No ☐

What? ____

What is your child's attitude toward reading, school, his/her teachers, other youngsters?

____

Overall schoolwork is: above average ☐ average ☐ below average ☐

WHICH SUBJECTS ARE:

Above average: ____________________

Average: ____________________

Below average: ____________________

Does your child need to spend a lot of time/effort to maintain this level of performance?

Yes ☐ No ☐

How much time on average does your child spend each day on homework assignments?
____

To what extent do you assist your child with homework? ____________________

Do you feel your child is achieving up to potential? Yes ☐ No ☐

Does the teacher feel your child is achieving up to potential? Yes ☐ No ☐

GENERAL BEHAVIOR

Are there any behavior problems at school? Yes ☐ No ☐

If yes, what? ____________________

Are there any behavior problems at home? Yes ☐ No ☐

If yes, what? ____________________

What causes these problems? ____________________

Child's reaction to fatigue? sags ☐ irritable ☐ other ☐

Child's reaction to tension? avoidance ☐ irritable ☐ other ☐ ____________________

Does your child say and/or do things impulsively? Yes ☐ No ☐

Is your child in constant motion? Yes ☐ No ☐

Can your child sit still for long periods? Yes ☐ No ☐

FAMILY AND HOME

Please indicate which adult(s) he/she lives with? ☐Mother ☐Father ☐Stepmother

☐Stepfather ☐Foster Parents ☐Adoptive Parents ☐Grandmother ☐Grandfather

☐Aunt ☐Uncle ☐Other Caretaker (please specify): ______________________________

Does your child spend time with any other person, not in the home? Yes ☐ No ☐

Please explain: ____

Has your child ever been through a traumatic family situation (such as divorce, parental loss, separation, severe parental illness)? Yes ☐ No ☐ If yes, at what age: ____________

Does your child seem to have adjusted? Yes ☐ No ☐

Was counseling /therapy undertaken? Yes ☐ No ☐

If yes, is it on-going? Yes ☐ No ☐

Is family life stable at this time? Yes ☐ No ☐

If no, please explain: ____

How does your child get along with:

Parents/other caretakers? ______________________________________

Siblings? ____

Classmates in school? ______________________________________

Playmates at home? ______________________________________

Did father or anyone in father's family have a learning problem? Yes ☐ No ☐

If yes, who? ____

Did mother or anyone in mother's family have a learning problem? Yes ☐ No ☐

If yes, who? ____

Do any, or did any, of the other children in the family have learning problems?

Yes ☐ No ☐

If yes, who? ____

To what extent? ____

____

GIVE A BRIEF DESCRIPTION OF YOUR CHILD AS A PERSON: ______________________

____

____

____

____

____

APPENDIX B

VISION REHABILITATION QUESTIONNAIRE

Date: _________

Patient's Name:___________________________________ **DOB:** _____________________

Date of injury/accident: ____

TYPE OF INJURY OR ACCIDENT:

- ☐ Motor vehicle ☐ Medication-related ☐ Cord around neck ☐ Stroke
- ☐ Fall ☐ Drug abuse ☐ Industrial Accident ☐ Aneurysm
- ☐ Blow to head ☐ Poison/toxic substance ☐ Carbon dioxide ☐ Hemorrhage
- ☐ Other: ____

WHAT PART OF YOUR HEAD WAS AFFECTED? (check all that apply):

Forehead ☐ Right side ☐ Left side ☐ Back of head ☐ Top of head ☐ Face ☐

Was the injury OPEN HEAD (bleeding) or CLOSED HEAD (non-bleeding)? ____________________

Did you lose consciousness? Yes ☐ No ☐ If yes, for how long? _________________________

Were you in a coma? Yes ☐ No ☐ If yes, how long? __________________________________

SYMPTOMS IMMEDIATELY FOLLOWING ACCIDENT/INJURY: (check all that apply)

- ☐ Double vision ☐ Vomiting ☐ Flashes of light ☐ Neck pain/whiplash
- ☐ Headache ☐ Restricted motion ☐ Disorientation ☐ Loss of memory
- ☐ Blurred vision ☐ Pain in/around eyes ☐ Loss of balance ☐ Restricted field of view
- ☐ Dizziness ☐ Other: ____

INITIAL TREATMENT

When did you first see a doctor regarding your accident/injury? ____________________________

Name of Doctor: ____________________________________ Specialty: ___________________

Where were you seen? ____

Were you hospitalized? Yes ☐ No ☐ How long? ______________________________________

What were you and your family told? ______________________________

What did the initial treatments consist of? ______________________________

What prognosis/recommendations were you given? ______________________________

Were you given medications? Yes ☐ No ☐ Medication: ______________________________

For what condition(s)? ______________________________

List any medications, including vitamins and supplements used at the current time: ______________

____

Do you have any allergies to medications? ______________________________

SUBSEQUENT/OTHER PROFESSIONAL CARE

WHAT TYPES OF PROFESSIONAL CARE HAVE YOU RECEIVED OR ARE YOU CURRENTLY RECEIVING? (check all that apply and describe):

☐ Physicians Name: ______________________________ Date: ____________

Results and recommendations: ______________________________

☐ Physiatrist Name: ______________________________ Date: ____________

Results and recommendations: ______________________________

☐ Neurologist Name: ______________________________ Date: ____________

Results and recommendations: ______________________________

☐ Neuropsychologist Name: ______________________________ Date: ____________

Results and recommendations: ______________________________

☐ Osteopathic Physician's Name: ______________________________ Date: ____________

Results and recommendations: ______________________________

☐ Physical Therapist Name: ______________________________ Date: ____________

Results and recommendations: ______________________________

☐ Occupational Therapist Name: ______________________________ Date: ____________

Results and recommendations: ______________________________

☐ Speech / Language Therapist Name: ______________________________ Date: ____________

Results and recommendations: ______________________________

☐ Psychologist / Psychiatrist Name: ______________________________ Date: __________

Results and recommendations: ____

☐ Other / Name: ____ Date: __________

Results and recommendations: ____

Has a neurological evaluation been performed? Yes ☐ No ☐

If yes, by whom? ____________________________________ Date: ________________

Results: ____

Has a psychological evaluation been performed? Yes ☐ No ☐

If yes, by whom? ____________________________________ Date: ________________

Results: ____

Has a speech and language evaluation been performed? Yes ☐ No ☐

If yes, by whom? ____________________________________ Date: ________________

Results: ____

Has a visual evaluation been performed following the injury? Yes ☐ No ☐

If yes, by whom? ____________________________________ Date: ________________

Were any additional tests, treatments, or therapies recommended concerning your vision?

Yes ☐ No ☐

If yes, what? ____

Did you undergo these treatments? Yes ☐ No ☐ Explain: ____________________________

Results and recommendations: ____

IN ADDITION DO YOU CURRENTLY EXPERIENCE ANY OF THE FOLLOWING:

Yes	Prior to Injury	
☐	☐	Difficulty with dressing
☐	☐	Difficulty with peripheral vision
☐	☐	Difficulty with bathing / personal hygiene
☐	☐	Difficulty following a series of directions
☐	☐	Difficulty using both sides of the body together
☐	☐	Dislike heights
☐	☐	Awkward, poor balance
☐	☐	Confusion / disorientation
☐	☐	Get lost often
☐	☐	Bothered by noises
☐	☐	Bothered by touch
☐	☐	Difficulty remembering things heard
☐	☐	Difficulty remembering things seen
☐	☐	Difficulty remembering name of objects
☐	☐	Difficulty remembering people's names
☐	☐	Difficulty recalling information known in the past
☐	☐	Difficulty remembering formerly familiar people / objects
☐	☐	Difficulty performing tasks formerly easy / routine
☐	☐	Difficulty with time management
☐	☐	Difficulty with numbers
☐	☐	Difficulty counting money

LIFESTYLE

Do you feel your vision interferes with activities of daily living? Yes ☐ No ☐

Is this new since the accident/injury? Yes ☐ No ☐

If yes, please explain (please include effects involving home, work, hobbies, social and personal relationships): ______________________________

____

____

What activities comprise the majority of your daily life since your accident/injury? ______________

____

____

____

What activities can you no longer engage in due to your visual or other difficulties? ______________

____

____

____

What other changes/limitations in your daily life do you attribute to your accident/injury? __________

____

____

What do you hope a Visual Rehabilitation Program can do for you? ______________________

____

____

____

What goals have you set up that you would like us to help you meet? What are your short term and long term goals?______________________________

____

____

EMPLOYMENT/EDUCATION INFORMATION (IF APPLICABLE)

What is current employment position? ____________________

If a student, what is the major course of study? ____________________

How many hours daily are spent at a desk? ____________________

How many hours daily are spent working at near/distance? ____________________

How many hours daily are spent reading/studying? ____________________

How many hours daily are spent with a computer? ____________________

APPENDIX C

Name: ______________________ Date of Birth: __________ Age: ______ Sex: M F

Date: ________________ Time: ______am/pm

Dr.Torgerson Dr.Jensen Exam / Consult ______ Dr **In** ______ Dr **Out**

Current Rx: Date of Rx:

	Sph	Cy1	Axis	Prism	Base	Add
OD						
OS						

NCT / Digital / Goldman
OD _____ mmHg
OS _____ mmHg
@ ______am/pm

Biopter: **Tech:**

Vertical Phoria	R.Hyper / L.Hyper
Lateral Phoria	Over 1 2 3 4 5 6 7 CONVERGENCE 8 Under 15 14 13 12 11 10 9
Central Fusion	
Color	8 15 5 35 All Correct
Lateral Phoria	Over 1 2 3 4 5 6 7 CONVERGENCE 8 Under 15 14 13 12 11 10 9
Central Fusion	

Visual Field: CF Humphrey Vision Disk
OD
OS

Visual Acuity: **Unaided VA** **Aided VA** Spec CL

DX OD 20/ OS 20/ OU 20/ OD 20/ OS 20/ OU 20/

NR OD 20/ OS 20/ OU 20/ OD 20/ OS 20/ OU 20/

Letters Symbols #'s E Cardiff Letters Symbols #'s E Cardiff

Single Line Full-chart Single Line Full-chart

Motilities:
Full range Smooth Hyperdys Hypodys Impaired Head Mvmt + / **- 2.00** tropia / double / blur

Cover Test: Far w w/o Near w w/o Bruckner Reflex:

PT Exo Eso O Hyper Hypo Alt Int PT Exo Eso O Hyper Hypo Alt Int

NPC: ___/___ **Worth 4 Dot:**

Randot Stereo:
Circles _______ Animals ________ Forms _______

Pupils: **Mid-line shift:**
P E R R L +/-A P D

Keratometry	
OD	
OS	

Retinoscopy/Autorefractor	
OD	
OS	

Subjective Refraction	
OD	20/
OS	20/
	Add: Near 20/ OU

Wet Refraction Cyclogel Tropicamide	
OD	
OS	

SLE: (7)	Normals	OD	OS	Abnormal Findings
Lids	Clear	☐	☐	
Lashes	clear	☐	☐	
Bulbar Conj	white	☐	☐	
Palp Conj	clear	☐	☐	
Orbit/Adnex	normal	☐	☐	
Cornea	clear	☐	☐	
Tear Film	clear	☐	☐	
Iris	clear	☐	☐	
AC	D & Q	☐	☐	
Lens	clear	☐	☐	

Angles: OD 1 2 3 4 OS 1 2 3 4

Binocular Testing:	Dsubj/spec Distance	Dsubj/Xy1/Nsubj Near
Lateral Phoria		
Vertical Phoria		
Base Out Range		
Base In Range		
	Cross Cylinder	
	PRA gross/net	
	NRA gross/net	

Last DFE: ☐ Discussed Dilation Warning

DPAs: 0.5%1.0% Trop/Cyclo/Proparacaine/Paremyd/Pheny12.5
gtts @ am pm

DFE: (2) ☐defers DFE ☐prefers Optomap ☐R/S DFE

78D/90D/B10	Normals	OD	OS	Abnormal Findings
Cup/Disc H/V		/	/	
Rim	Pink & distinct	☐	☐	
☐essels	Clear	☐	☐	
Ratio	2/3	☐	☐	
Macula	Clear	☐	☐	
Foveal Reflex	(+)	☐	☐	
Vitreous	clear	☐	☐	
Periphery	No holes, tears, or RD	☐	☐	

New Rx:

	Sph	Cyl	Axis	Prism	Base	Add
OD						
OS						

CC:(HPI:location, quality, severity, duration, timing, context, modifying factors, associated S&S)
Brief (1-3) Extended (4-8)

PMH: Problem pertinent (1) Extended (2-9)
ROS ☐All other ROS are negative

Neurologic
☐A+O to TPP
☐Mood good

Med:

Allergies: + / - env + / - med

PFSH: Pertinent (1) Complete: Est Ptn (1 from 2 of 3 areas) New Ptn (1 from 3 areas)
Past: illness/operation/injuries ☐ none noted

FHx: DM/HTN/GLAUC/ARMD ☐ none noted

SHx: Smoke/Drink/Rec Drugs

Accompained by:

Assessment:
__ Cataract Cong./NS/CS/PSC
__ Dry Eye Syndrome
__ Glaucoma Suspect
__ ARMD
__ Diabetes c̄ / s̄ Retinopathy

__ Strabismus exo/eso/hyper/accom/alt/int
__ Amblyopia (ref) or (acquired)
__ Diplopia
__ Nystagmus
__ Oculomotor Dys (s) or (p)
__ Convergence Insuff
__ Binocular Dys
__ Accommodative Dys

__ Myopia
__ Hyperopia
__ Astigmatism
__ Presbyopia
__ Anisometropia

__ Ocular Health Normal

Plan: Recommend
☐ Rx Dist/Near FT/PT Polycarb/Trivex Bifocal/PAL
☐ CL (discussed to see referring Dr.)
☐ Optomap / R/S DFE
☐ Score DEM
☐ Visual Hygiene
☐ Workshop
☐ Websites
☐ VT Recommended (give info. packet)
☐ Schedule VT
☐ Loan Struggles bk
☐ Insurance Predet / Self Call
☐ Report:____________________
☐ Thank You:____________________
☐ Referral to:____________________
☐ F1 Chase(M/B) / Thumb Pursuits(M/B) / Marsden Ball(M/B
☐ Focus Flex
☐ Pencil Pushups / Eccentric O's / 3 Dot Card
☐ Schedule VIP Testing / WACHS Battery
☐
☐
☐

Next Visit:
RTC:1 2 3 4 6 8 10 12 dy wk mo yr

OV15 OV30 DFE CY5/15 CEE

W/ Dr. T J

Signatures:

1. ____________________ O.D. Date:________

2. ____________________ O.D. Date:________

APPENDIX D

Yoked Prisms Behavioral Effects

Activity:____________________	Prism Power : √ + –				
	Δ	Up	Down	Left	Right
Ability to perform task					
Posture					
Visual awareness					
Spatial localization					
Increase or decrease in sensory seeking behaviors					
Gait					
Organization					
Eye contact people or objects					
Mood, facial expression					
Gross motot skills					
Fine motor skills					

REFERENCES

1. Maples W. Test-retest reliability of the College of Optometrists in Vision Development Quality of Life Outcomes Assessment. Optometry. 2000;71:579–85.
2. Borsting EJ, Rouse MW, Mitchell GL, et al. Validity and reliability of the revised convergence insufficiency symptom survey in children aged 9 to 18 years. Optom Vis Sci. 2003;80:832–8.
3. Donati RJ, Maino DM, Bartell H, Kieffer M. Polypharmacy and the lack of oculo-visual complaints from those with mental illness and dual diagnosis. Optometry. 2009;80:249–54.
4. Stille CJ, Antonelli RC. Coordination of care for children with special health care needs. Curr Opin Pediatr. 2004;16:700–5.
5. Stille CJ. Communication, comanagement, and collaborative care for children and youth with special healthcare needs. Pediatr Ann 2009;38(9):498–504.
6. Forrest CB, Glade GB, Baker AE, et al. Coordination of specialty referrals and physician satisfaction with referral care. Arch Pediatr Adolesc Med. 2000;154(5):499–506.
7. Stille CJ, Primack WA, Savageau JA. Generalist-subspecialist communication for children with chronic conditions: a regional physician survey. Pediatrics. 2003;112:1314–20.
8. Stricklan B, McPherson M, Weissman G, et al. Access to the medical home: results of the national survey of children with special health care needs. Pediatrics. 2004;113:1485–92.

INDEX

Page numbers in *italics* indicate figures; page numbers followed by t indicate tables.